# FUNDAMENTALS OF OBSTETRICS AND GYNAECOLOGY

## Volume I: **OBSTETRICS**

*By the same author:*

FUNDAMENTALS OF OBSTETRICS AND GYNAECOLOGY
    Vol. II GYNAECOLOGY

EVERYWOMAN

BREAST FEEDING: HOW TO SUCCEED

HERPES, AIDS AND OTHER SEXUALLY TRANSMITTED DISEASES

# FUNDAMENTALS OF OBSTETRICS AND GYNAECOLOGY

## Volume I

# OBSTETRICS

**Derek Llewellyn-Jones** OBE, MD, MAO, FRCOG, FRACOG

*Associate Professor of Obstetrics and Gynaecology,*
  *University of Sydney, New South Wales, Australia*
*Visiting Obstetrician and Gynaecologist,*
  *St Margaret's Hospital, Sydney*

## FIFTH EDITION

*Illustrations by Audrey Besterman*

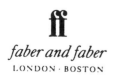

*faber and faber*
LONDON · BOSTON

First published in 1969
by Faber and Faber Limited
3 Queen Square London WC1N 3AU

Reprinted 1971 with revisions
Second edition 1977
Reprinted 1979
Third edition 1982
Fourth edition 1986
Fifth edition 1990
Printed and bound in Great Britain
by Richard Clay Ltd, Bungay, Suffolk
All rights reserved

*British Library Cataloguing in Publication Data*

Llewellyn-Jones, Derek
    Fundamentals of obstetrics and gynaecology.—
    5th ed.
    Vol.1: Obstetrics
    1. Gynaecology        2. Obstetrics
    I. Title
    618      RG101

ISBN 0–571–14227–3 (v.1) Pbk

# Contents

31   Infectious Disease in Pregnancy   248

32   Iso-immunization in Pregnancy   255

33   Tumours of the Genital Tract Complicating Pregnancy   261

34   Abnormalities of the Placenta and Membranes   265

35   Variations in the Duration of Pregnancy: Fetal Maturity   269

36   The At-risk Fetus in Pregnancy and Labour   277

37   Occipito-posterior Position   288

38   Breech Presentation   293

39   Other Malpositions and Malpresentations   308

40   Multiple Pregnancy   315

41   Prolapse of the Cord   319

**Part 4: ABNORMALITIES OF LABOUR AND THE PUERPERIUM**

42   Dystocia: Faults in the Passenger   323

43   Dystocia: Faults in the Passages   327

44   Dystocia: Faults in the Powers   339

45   Prolonged Labour and Obstructed Labour   347

46   Postpartum Haemorrhage   351

47   Damage to the Genital Tract   358

48   The Complicated Puerperium   369

**Part 5: OBSTETRIC OPERATIONS**

49   Termination of Pregnancy and Induction of Labour   381

50   Forceps   391

51   Caesarean Section   404

52   Other Obstetric Operations   410

53   Oxytocics   415

**Part 6: EPIDEMIOLOGY OF OBSTETRICS**

54   The Epidemiology of Obstetrics   421

**Part 7: THE INFANT**

55   Neonatal Physiology and Care of the Newborn   433

56   Examination of the Newborn: Congenital Defects   440

57   Hypoxia in the Newborn   450

58   Birth Injuries   456

59   Neonatal Infections   460

60   The Low Birth-weight Baby   462

     Bibliography   471

     Glossary   476

     Index   479

# Preface to the Fifth Edition

Changes in obstetric practice and the impact of technological innovations have made it necessary to revise *Fundamentals of Obstetrics and Gynaecology* once again. The revisions have been extensive and reflect to some extent my concern that, in the wish to use the new technologies, assessment of clinical policies is being neglected. In 1972, A. C. Cochrane in his Rock-Carling Lecture rated obstetrics as the least scientifically based specialty within medical practice. My experience in reviewing the literature confirms that Cochrane's opinion largely is valid.

The remedies are in the hands, and minds, of medical students, family doctors and obstetricians. New innovations, for example the routine screening of all pregnant women using ultrasound; the use of beta-agonists to suppress preterm labour; the management of hypertension in pregnancy need to be evaluated rigorously.

These two paragraphs were written in the preface to the Fourth Edition. The comments I made then are still relevant.

In the past four years developments in the scientific basis of obstetrics and gynaecology have continued to be made. The purpose of antenatal care and the procedures used have come under critical scrutiny: many of the procedures currently practised could be eliminated, providing more time for the patient and the doctor to talk with each other.

Other advances which are discussed in this edition include: chorionic villus sampling, herpes simplex virus infection in pregnancy, the management of 'high risk' pregnancy, psychiatric problems in pregnancy and the puerperium, prolonged pregnancy, deep venous thrombosis and cerebral palsy.

Once again many changes (amounting to over 20 000 words) have been made so that the book is as up to date as possible. Some of the older ultrasound pictures have been replaced and I am grateful, once again, to Dr John Anderson for his help. My secretary, Barbara Laing, and my librarian, Janet Heywood, have helped in many ways and I am grateful to them.

The work of reviewing the literature, evaluating its content and rewriting *Fundamentals* has continued to be enjoyable and rewarding.

It is in the hope that readers will continue to find *Fundamentals of Obstetrics and Gynaecology* useful that I once again dedicate the book to students of obstetrics, past and present.

DEREK LLEWELLYN-JONES
*Sydney 1990*

*Part One*

# THE PHYSIOLOGY OF PREGNANCY AND LABOUR

*The object of maternity care is to ensure that every expectant and nursing mother maintains good health, learns the art of child care, has a normal delivery, and bears healthy children. Maternity care in the narrower sense consists of the care of the pregnant woman, her safe delivery, her postnatal care and examination, the care of her newly born infant, and the maintenance of lactation. In the wider sense it begins much earlier in measures aimed to promote the health and well-being of the young people who are potential parents, and to help them to develop the right approach to family life and to the place of the family in the community. It should also include guidance in parentcraft and in problems associated with infertility and family planning.*

World Health Organisation Technical Report Series, 1952, 51, 3

# Chapter 1

# Elements of Reproduction

During each menstrual cycle, under the influence of follicle stimulating hormone (FSH) released by the pituitary gland, several Graafian follicles develop in the ovary. One, occasionally more, of these outstrips the others in growth and it is from this follicle that an ovum will be released. The stimulated follicles synthesize and secrete oestradiol 17 beta, the serum concentration of which rises. This leads to a 'positive feedback' to the hypothalamus-pituitary, and results in a sudden surge and release of the second gonadotrophic hormone, luteinizing hormone (LH). The LH surge further stimulates the growth of the largest, most mature follicle, which by this time has pushed through the ovarian stroma and is protruding through its capsule (Fig. **1/1**). This event occurs between 9 and 16 days before the next menstrual period.

## OVULATION

On the same or the next day, between 10 and 24 hours after the LH peak, the distended follicle ruptures, releasing the ovum surrounded by a mantle of granulosa cells. The follicle which contained the ovum collapses and its cells are altered, under the continuing influence of LH, to synthesize oestradiol 17 beta and progesterone. The cells become luteinized (and yellow) and the collapsed follicle is called a corpus luteum (or yellow body).

The freed ovum is swept up by micro-filaments projecting from the cells of the fimbrial end of the Fallopian tube, and is slowly moved by them and by gentle, rhythmic muscular contractions of the tube into its lumen (Fig. **1/1**).

At this time, 1 to 2 days after ovulation, the ovum is about $100 \mu m$ in diameter. In the centre is the small nucleus, which has reached metaphase of the second maturation division and is surrounded by a yellowish cytoplasm, the vitellus, which contains much carbohydrate and amino-acids. The ovum has already undergone the first meiotic division which has reduced its chromosome complement to 23, and led to the appearance of the first polar body (Fig. **1/2**(2)). A second meiotic division will occur after the sperm penetrates the egg with the production of a second polar body (Fig. **1/2**(4)).

Surrounding the ovum is a condensation of an opaque substance 5 to $10 \mu m$ in thickness, the zona pellucida, and this is partially separated from the ovum by a space, the perivitelline space, into which the polar bodies are extruded. The zona pellucida is penetrated by tiny channels through which substances can pass from the cells of the corona radiata. Spermatozoa also penetrate the corona radiata but, except for one, are unable to penetrate the zona. External to the zona pellucida is a mantle of granulosa cells, the corona radiata (Fig. **1/2**(1)). This mantle is shed within the first 48 hours after ovulation, by the action of tubal secretions, and sperm penetration of the ovum is made more easy.

The ovum at this time is ready for fertilization, and should this not occur within 36 hours it will degenerate. The effective life cycle of the ovum is therefore very short, and as the spermatozoon has a life cycle of only 48 hours, fertilization can only take place within 2 days of ovulation.

## SPERM TRANSPORT

Millions of spermatozoa are ejaculated in the semen and temporarily bathe the cervix and upper vagina. At the time of ovulation the cervical mucus is abundant, has low viscosity and contains a high proportion of sodium chloride, and, under the influence of oestrogen, rearranges its macromolecular structure. The molecular rearrangement creates small channels,

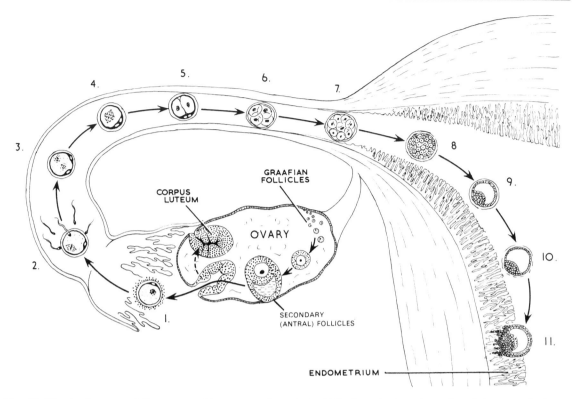

**Fig. 1/1** The development of the ovum and its passage through the Fallopian tube into the cavity of the uterus is shown diagrammatically: (1) unsegmented oocyte; (2) fertilization; (3) pronuclei formed; (4) first spindle division; (5) two cell stage; (6) four cell stage; (7) eight cell stage; (8) morula; (9) and (10) blastocyst formation; (11) zona pellucida lost, implantation occurs

or passages, in the cervical mucus. It is through these channels that the sperms penetrate, moved by the flagellation of their tails. Of the millions reaching the cervix, only hundreds of thousands survive to reach the uterine cavity, and only thousands pass into the tubes. Less than one hundred reach the outer portion of the tube where the ovum lies waiting; only a few succeed in penetrating the corona radiata (if any of its cells remain) and the zona pellucida; and only one enters the ovum proper, traversing the vitellus, and fusing with the female pronucleus.

## FERTILIZATION

The spermatozoon is only able to penetrate the zona pellucida after its structure has been altered. This ability (capacitation) is thought to have two parts: an increase in the DNA concentration in the nucleus; and an increase in the permeability of the lipoprotein

coat of the plasma membrane of the sperm head allowing the release of hyaluronidase. The capacitated spermatozoon first has to 'bind' with the zona pellucida. This ability appears to reside in a protein on the head (the acrosome) of the sperm and a specific receptor (a glycoprotein) on the surface of the zona pellucida. The binding is usually species specific.

Although several hundred spermatozoa may 'bind' on the zona pellucida, only one sperm is able to penetrate it. This may be because penetration by a single sperm alters the electrical potential of the zona pellucida. This helps to inhibit any further penetration. The penetration by the spermatozoon also induces the cytoplasm of the ovum to release enzymes in the perivitelline space and through the 'canals' in the zona pellucida. These enzymes also inhibit further sperm penetration, perhaps by altering the receptor protein or by altering the penetrability of the zona pellucida. Once inside the ovum cytoplasm, the nuclear membrane of the sperm disappears leaving a naked male pronucleus. The entry of

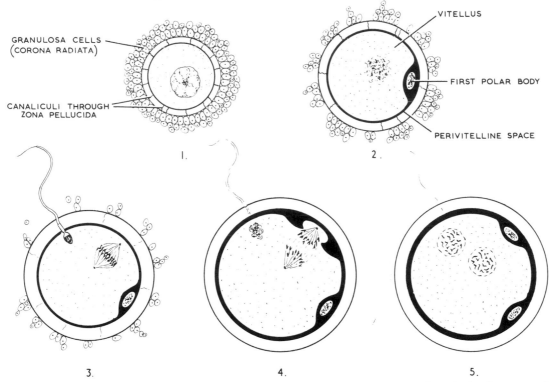

GRANULOSA CELLS
(CORONA RADIATA)

CANALICULI THROUGH
ZONA PELLUCIDA

VITELLUS

FIRST POLAR BODY

PERIVITELLINE SPACE

1.

2.

3.

4.

5.

**Fig. 1/2** Formation of the ootid and fertilization: (1) primary oocyte; (2) secondary oocyte formed after first maturation division, first polar body pinched off. Both oocyte and polar body have undergone reduction division and now each has a haploid number of chromosomes (23); (3) second maturation division stimulated by sperm penetrating into vitellus; (4) second polar body forming. The first polar body may also undergo a reduction division; (5) male and female pronuclei formed

the spermatozoon into the ovum has another effect: it stimulates the resumption of the second meiotic division of the female nucleus which had been arrested at metaphase. Anaphase, followed by telophase, occurs and the ovum divides, the second polar body being pushed to one side (Fig. **1/2**(4)). The ovum and the polar bodies have a haploid complement of 23 chromosomes. The spermatozoon pronucleus already has a haploid number of chromosomes.

## FORMATION OF THE ZYGOTE

Both male and female pronuclear material form nuclear membranes and within the membrane there is synthesis and condensation of DNA (Fig. **1/2**(5)). The two pronuclei approach and fuse, the nuclear membrane once again disappearing. Chromosomes appear in the condensed DNA, and those from each pronucleus move together to unite and form the

zygote of maternal and paternal genetic material. The new individual has begun its march through life to death.

After an interval of variable duration, but probably short because of the rich supply of amino-acids and enzymes within the cytoplasm of the ovum, a metaphase plate forms and the first cleavage division of the zygote occurs, within a few hours of fertilization.

## CLEAVAGE AND TRANSPORT OF THE EGG

Once division of the egg starts it proceeds rapidly, so that within 3 days a solid mass of uniform cells has formed. This is the *morula* stage (Fig. **1/1**(8)). The energy required for this division, and the materials required to synthesize the DNA prior to each division are obtained from the vitellus and consequently its volume is greatly reduced, which balances the increase in the size of the morula so that the zona pellucida remains intact. During the process of morula formation, the egg is gently propelled along the tube into the uterine cavity by the movement of the cilia of the endosalpinx. In the journey the zona pellucida acquires a thin coating of mucus and albumin, probably from the cells of the endosalpinx. The muscular activity of the uterus is relatively low, owing to progesterone, and the egg comes to lie in one of the folds of the velvet-like secretory endometrium, usually on the anterior or posterior wall in the fundal area, 3 to 4 days after ovulation (Fig. **1/1**(11)). During two-thirds of this time, the ovum remains in the ampulla of the oviduct, which is where fertilization occurs. The transit of the fertilized egg through the isthmus and interstitial portions of the oviduct is rapid, probably taking only a few hours.

Once the ovum embeds in the decidua, fluid from the decidual cells passes through the canaliculi of the zona pellucida and separates the cells of the morula, so that a central cavity is formed, and the egg is now termed a *blastula* or *blastocyst*. With blastula formation, the zona pellucida becomes distended, thinned and disappears in patches leaving the blastula cells in contact with the decidua. Deprived of the zona pellucida, the cells develop an adhesiveness and alter in appearance to form primitive trophoblastic cells. Eventually all the surface cells of the blastula have differentiated into trophoblast. At the same time, some deep cells at one pole of the blastocyst aggregate to form the *inner cell mass* from which the embryo will develop, and the blastocyst collapses (Fig. **1/3**).

## IMPLANTATION OF THE BLASTOCYST

The adhesion of the surface cells to the maternal endometrial epithelium is followed rapidly by invasion. Invasion of maternal tissues is a late evolutionary development, and is found only in mammals. How invasion by trophoblast occurs remains speculative, but some facts are known. In the rabbit, by the time the blastocyst has formed, most of the cytoplasm has been used up and the cell has to find new energy sources to continue mitotic division. This energy is obtained from anaerobic glycolysis with the production in the surface cells of lactic acid, which is buffered and accumulated as bicarbonate.

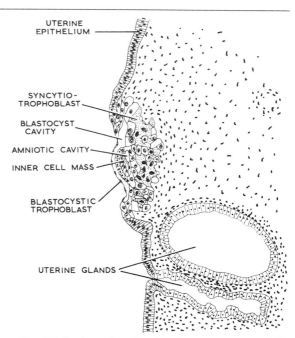

**Fig. 1/3** Section of a $7\frac{1}{2}$ day human ovum partially implanted in secretory endometrium ($\times 100$). The embryo is represented by the inner cell mass; the blastocyst has collapsed (by courtesy of Drs Rock and Hertig)

At the same time the endometrium is accumulating carbonic anhydrase. With adhesion between trophoblast and endometrium a reaction between the bicarbonate and carbonic anhydrase occurs with release of carbon dioxide which is discharged through the trophoblastic plasma membrane, across the endometrial cells and stroma to reach the capillary circulation of the endometrium. The alteration in pH towards alkalinity leads to a disintegration of the epithelial cells and permits penetration of the trophoblast. The penetration supplies the trophoblast with glycogen from the disintegrated endometrial cells and the invasion continues until a maternal capillary is reached when the trophoblast can obtain its energy supplies and nutrients from glucose and amino-acids in the maternal blood by aerobic metabolic pathways. Further invasion by the trophoblast then ceases.

The alternative view is that the trophoblast is actively invasive, and the invasion is restrained by maternal immunological factors once a certain penetration has occurred. The evidence for this view is that in the macaque monkey the columnar epithelial cells of the endometrium show degenerative changes soon after contact with the trophoblast, and an ever-widening area of cells is lost so that the tropho-blast increasingly comes into contact with the stroma. The stromal cells also show congestion, and altered structure, perhaps due to the liberation of some substance from the trophoblastic cells. The damaged cells supply nutritive material to the tropho-blast which undergoes rapid proliferation, and forms two layers: an inner cellular layer, and an outer syncytium in which all cell barriers have gone. The invasion is controlled probably by 'blocking an-tibodies' produced by the mother. A 'fibrinoid layer' forms a few millimetres below the endometrial sur-face which is normally not penetrated by tropho-blastic cells. A reduction in maternal resistance (or overactivity of trophoblast) would permit deeper tro-phoblastic penetration with the possible subsequent formation of a partial or complete hydatidiform mole.

By the 8th day after ovulation, the human ovum has become partially implanted in the secretory endometrium, the two layers of trophoblast have formed, as has the inner cell mass, and the blastocyst has largely collapsed. The trophoblast has prolifer-ated greatly and has begun to surround endometrial capillaries and small spaces have appeared within the syncytium (Fig. **1/4**).

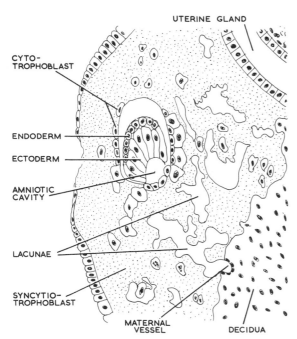

Fig. **1/4** A section through the middle of the Hertig–Rock 9 day embryo (redrawn from Hertig, A. J. and Rock, J. *Contrib. Embry. Carnegie Inst.* 1941, **29**, 127)

Three or four days later the implantation is com-plete, the blastula having penetrated so far that it is completely embedded in the stroma, and uterine epithelium is growing over the entrance. The tropho-blast has proliferated and penetrated more deeply. The spaces have increased in size and since a capil-lary or a larger vessel has been reached, are by now filled with blood. The spaces, or lacunae, become confluent to form the primitive intervillous spaces. The stromal cells of the endometrium have also reacted to the invasion by becoming polyhedral in shape and filled with glycogen and lipid, which supply the nutritive needs of the trophoblast. This change transforms the stroma into a *decidua*, and is due to the persisting activity of oestrogen and pro-gesterone (Fig. **1/4**).

As a result of the formation of the lacunae, the trophoblast is now composed of irregular strands, some of which reach to fix onto the stroma, others being free in the lacunae. The development of the trophoblast is not uniform. It is least marked to-wards the uterine lumen, and most marked towards the decidual base, where it will eventually form the placenta (see Chapter 2).

Trophoblast cells also penetrate the lumina of the intradecidual part of the spiral arteries and invade the vessel's wall. The effect of this is to convert relatively thick-walled spiral arteries into thin-walled funnel-shaped vessels. This permits a much greater maternal blood flow to the uteroplacental area.

## DEVELOPMENT OF THE EMBRYO

Concurrent with the development of the trophoblast, changes are occurring within the egg. The inner cell mass becomes two-layered by the 7th day after ovula-tion, the outer layer being formed of polyhedral ectodermal cells, and the inner of smaller cuboidal endodermal cells. A day later, the ectodermal cells are separated from the implanting trophoblast by a cleft, which later enlarges to form the amniotic cavity. The nutrition of the developing cells has by now much improved as maternal blood fills the lacu-nae in the syncytium, and consequently nutrients pass into the blastocyst which once again distends. By the 10th day the ovum consists of a bilaminar inner cell mass and two cavities: one, the amniotic cavity which is lined by epithelial cells, and the other, the re-formed blastocyst cavity in which the endodermal cells of the inner cell mass lie. A day later active proliferation of material (mesoblast)

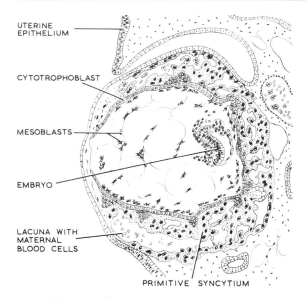

UTERINE EPITHELIUM

CYTOTROPHOBLAST

MESOBLASTS

EMBRYO

LACUNA WITH MATERNAL BLOOD CELLS

PRIMITIVE SYNCYTIUM

**Fig. 1/5** Section of an $11\frac{1}{2}$ day human embryo (Barnes embryo). The blastocystic trophoblast has differentiated into primitive syncytium and cytotrophoblast. Mesoblast has differentiated from the inner surface of the latter and almost fills the original blastocyst cavity. Lacunae have appeared in the actively growing syncytium, and maternal blood cells have seeped into several of them. Buds are appearing at intervals on the syncytium, these are the forerunners of chorionic villi (redrawn from Hamilton, Boyd and Mossman. *Human Embryology*. Heffer, Cambridge, 1962)

from the inner surface of the cellular layer of trophoblast leads to the differentiation of the third embryonic layer – the mesoderm. By the 12th day the cavity is filled with mesoblastic stellate cells which line the trophoblast and the outer surface of the amniotic cells, and cover the embryonic endoderm (Fig. **1/5**). Very rapidly, however, a space in the mesoderm appears below the endoderm which is lined by mesoblast and is continuous with the endoderm. Endodermal cells soon migrate to cover the mesoblastic lining of the cavity and form the yolk sac (Fig. **1/6**). With the formation of the yolk sac on the 13th day, the remaining mesoblast forms the extra-embryonic mesoblast. This becomes condensed and small spaces appear within it which become confluent, forming two layers of mesoblast. One lines the trophoblast, the other the embryo and yolk sac (Fig. **1/6(C)**). The space between the two increases in size and forms the extra-embryonic coelom. This separates the embryo and yolk sac from the trophoblast, except at one point, where a tube of mesoderm connects the two, and forms the body stalk or umbilical cord. This has occurred by the 16th day and mesoderm from the body stalk area has by now penetrated between the two layers of ectoderm and endoderm, to form the trilaminar embryo. The further development of the embryo is from these three layers. At the same time primitive

| Period of gestation (in weeks from the first day of the last menstrual period) | Period of gestation (in weeks from fertilization) | Length of fetus (crown to rump in centimetres) | Characteristics |
|---|---|---|---|
| 8 | 6 | 2.3 | Nose, external ears, fingers and toes are identifiable but featureless, head is flexed on the thorax |
| 12 | 10 | 6.0 | External ears show main features, eyelids fused, neck has formed, external genitals formed but undifferentiated |
| 16 | 14 | 12.0 | External genitals can be differentiated, skin transparent red |
| 20 | 18 | 15.0 | Skin becoming opaque, fine hair (lanugo) covers the body |
| 24 | 22 | 21.0 | Eyelids separated, eyebrows, eyelashes and fingernails present, skin wrinkled due to lack of subcutaneous fat |
| 28 | 26 | 25.0 | Eyes open, scalp hair growing |

**Table 1/1** Characteristics indicating maturity of the fetus

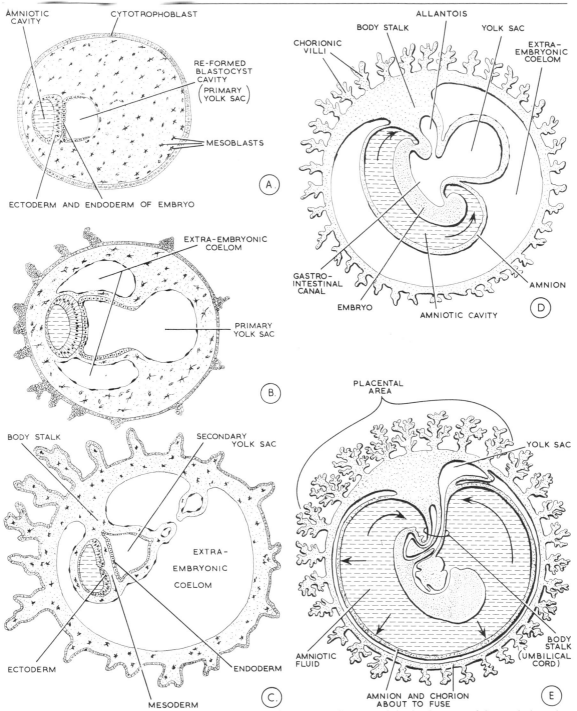

**Fig. 1/6** Formation of the amniotic cavity. (A) Formation of the inner cell mass, and the development of the amniotic cavity and the primary yolk sac. (B) Spaces appear in the mesoblast to form the extra-embryonic coelom. (C) The primary yolk sac diminishes in size as the extra-embryonic coelom enlarges. (D) The amniotic sac develops and begins to occupy the extra-embryonic coelom. (E) By the 45th day, the amniotic sac has surrounded the embryo which is suspended in the protective liquor amnii

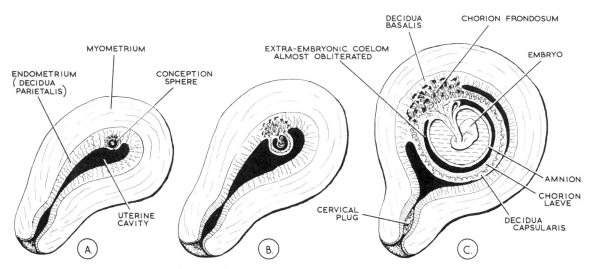

**Fig. 1/7** Diagram to show the relationship of the chorionic sac, amnion and developing embryo to the endometrium and uterine cavity at successive stages in early pregnancy. A: three weeks, B: five weeks and C: ten weeks after the last menstrual period

blood vessels are forming in the mesoblast wall of the yolk sac and in the mesoblastic lining of the blastocyst, by delamination from the cells of the wall. Mesoblast also appears by differentiation in the core of the trophoblastic villi, and here too angiogenesis begins.

**The amniotic sac**

It has been noted that a cleft appears between the ectodermal cells of the embryonic plate and the inner layer of trophoblast on the 7th day, and this enlarges to form the amniotic cavity which soon fills with fluid. The activity of the cells lining the amniotic cavity is high for it increases in size rapidly and by the 15th day it is equal in size to the yolk sac, thereafter continuing to grow whilst the yolk sac

diminishes in size (Fig. **1/6**D and E). By the 50th day after ovulation (8th to 10th week after the menstrual period) the amniotic cavity has surrounded the embryo completely and has fused with the chorion laterally and covered the cord joining with the fetal ectoderm medially. The embryo therefore floats freely and in a weightless condition in the amniotic fluid (Fig. **1/7**).

**Growth of the embryo**

The development of the embryo is dealt with at length in textbooks of human embryology but in Table **1/1** salient points are noted. Quite often following an abortion it is important to know the duration of the gestation period and some indication can be obtained from the table.

# Chapter 2
# The Placenta

The word 'placenta' connotes a functional union between fetal and maternal structures, and in the human this union has developed to a remarkable degree, as a consequence of the evolutionary development which has followed internal fertilization of a single ovum and the retention of the embryo within the mother for a relatively long time.

## PLACENTATION

Just before implantation the trophoblast differentiates into two layers, an inner cellular one, the cytotrophoblast and an outer layer, the syncytiotrophoblast, which lacks cell membranes. Proliferation of the inner layer pushes the knobs of trophoblast deeply into the decidua and by the 10th day after fertilization there is much intermingling of trophoblast and maternal tissues. Within the projecting knobs of trophoblast, a third layer of primitive connective tissue, the mesoblast, is differentiated from the inner surface of the cytotrophoblast. The mesoblast proliferates rapidly and not only forms the core of the projecting knobs of trophoblast but also lines the cavity of the blastocyst which is now termed a chorionic sac. With further proliferation the trophoblastic knobs assume a finger-like shape and are termed chorionic villi (Fig. **2/1**). Spaces appear between the closely packed trophoblastic projections, so that they are split into separate villi, and by coalescence the spaces (lacunae) increase in size. By this time the tips of the villi have reached the endometrial capillaries and have surrounded and eroded their walls so that maternal blood provides nutriment for the trophoblastic cells and seeps into the lacunae. However, the trophoblastic invasion is not uniform and ridges of maternal decidua persist amongst the trophoblast which form the placental septa seen on the maternal surface of the delivered placenta and which divide the placenta into lobes and lobules. Within a day or two, further trophoblastic growth surrounds and erodes into the endometrial spiral arterioles, and blood under pressure fills and expands the lacunae which coalesce further, creating large blood-filled spaces separated by chorionic villi. In this richly nutritive atmosphere, syncytial sprouts appear on the sides of the main villi, and these develop, subdivide and branch complexly forming free villi within the blood lake. Some of the original villi retain their attachment to the maternal endometrium and are termed anchoring villi.

By the 19th day the entire ovum is covered with growing chorionic villi, some attached to the endometrium, or as it is now termed, the decidua, but most floating freely within the blood lakes, which are surrounded by trophoblast. The trophoblast on the decidual side of the blood-filled spaces is less active than that forming the free villi and further penetration of the decidua is prevented, once the spiral arterioles have been surrounded, by chemical or immunological mechanisms. In this way a zone appears between normal trophoblast and normal decidua in which both types of cell are replaced by collagen – the fibrinous layer of Nitabusch, through which pass the undamaged spiral arteries and veins draining the decidua. Cleavage in this zone at delivery leads to separation of the placenta and the decidua.

Since the maternal blood supply is greatest on the deep surface of the ovum the trophoblast grows most profusely here, whilst that covering other zones of the conception sphere begins to degenerate by the 50th day. The actively proliferating trophoblast covering the deeper zone forms a many-branched villous system, which is termed the *chorion frondosum*, or the shaggy chorion, whilst the chorion over the remainder of the sphere degenerates to form the smooth chorion, or *chorion laeve*.

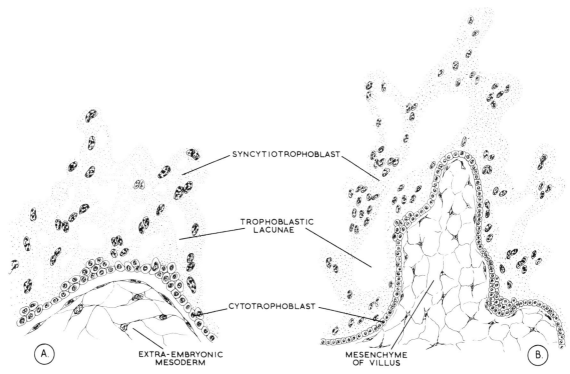

**Fig. 2/1** Early stage in development of chorionic villi. (A) The trophoblast projection has occurred with the development of lacunae, and much intermingling with maternal tissue, which for clarity is not shown. No mesoblastic core has yet entered the villus. (B) The mesoblastic core is now developing within the villus (redrawn from Patten. *Tend. Act. Gynecol. et Obstet.* 1959, Beauchemin, Montreal)

The chorion frondosum forms the definitive placenta and by the 70th day its formation is complete. The placenta is composed of about 200 trunks of trophoblastic cells, which project into the lacunae and divide and subdivide into limbs, branches and twigs, rather like a tree. Each of the main trunks and its subdivisions forms a *fetal cotyledon*, and these vary in size, 10 being large, 40 of medium size and the remainder small and of little functional significance (Fig. **2/2**). By the 70th day, the complement of fetal cotyledons is complete, and no new ones develop, although the 50 functional cotyledons increase in size to term as daughter villi are budded off the smaller branches.

**Primitive blood vessels**

By the 18th to 20th day after fertilization primitive blood vessels and blood cells have formed in the mesoblastic core of the main and secondary villous trunks. By the 23rd day the vessels have joined up with blood vessels forming, at the same time, in the mesoderm of the inner cell mass and the mesoblast of the yolk sac. Once established the primitive fetal circulation forms an increasingly complex mesh of anastomotic capillaries within the villi, which renders the terminal villi erectile and able to float more freely, and exchange nutrients and waste products more readily, in the blood-filled spaces of the placenta.

**The intervillous space**

As the blood lakes coalesce, a large space is formed which is filled with blood and occupied by chorionic villi, most of which are floating but some are attached to the decidua. The roof of the space is formed from chorion (the chorionic plate) and the floor from trophoblast and decidua (the decidual plate). On the maternal side the space is partly divided by septa of varying heights and shapes haphazardly distributed (Fig. **2/3**), but on the fetal side

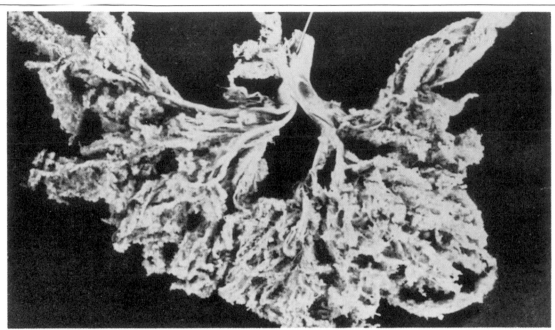

**Fig. 2/2** A fetal cotyledon dissected out to show its branching, tree-like form (from Crawford. *J. Obstet. Gynaecol. Brit. Emp.* 1956, **63**, 542)

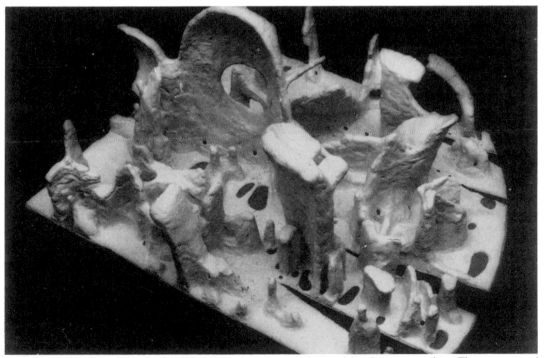

**Fig. 2/3** Maternal surface of the placenta. Model showing septa and the arterial and venous openings. The venous openings are large and are not related to the bases of the septa, whilst the majority of the arterial openings are at this site. Note the great irregularity in the height and shape of the maternal septa (from Brosens, I. and Dixon, H. G. *J. Obstet Gynaecol. Brit. Cwlth.* 1966, **73**, 357)

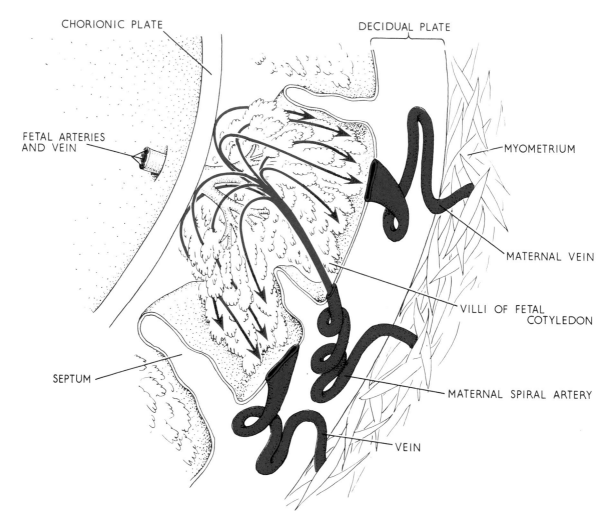

CHORIONIC PLATE

DECIDUAL PLATE

FETAL ARTERIES
AND VEIN

MYOMETRIUM

MATERNAL VEIN

VILLI OF FETAL
COTYLEDON

SEPTUM

MATERNAL SPIRAL ARTERY

VEIN

Fig. 2/4 Diagram of an intervillous space. A fetal cotyledon can be seen, in which the 'fountain' effect of the maternal arterial blood is demonstrated. The blood cascades over the tree-like villi to escape through the maternal veins

a very free intercommunication exists. Thus the appearance from the maternal side is of a complex series of intercommunicating spaces, whilst on the fetal side a single space is found. The spiral arteries enter each intervillous space at the base of the maternal septa and between 100 and 120 separate arteries have been counted, each supplying one fetal cotyledon. Drainage from the spaces occurs through veins which tend to form venous lakes in the decidua. During systole the arterial blood spurts into the intervillous space like a fountain, at a pressure of 80mmHg and pushing the villi aside to reach the

chorionic plate, flows laterally and cascades down, bathing the branched villi, to escape slowly through the decidual veins. Thus even during diastole the pressure in the space is maintained, and it is this 'pulsatile flow' of blood which keeps the intervillous space distended (Fig. 2/4).

The pulsatile flow of maternal blood is increased in the second quarter of pregnancy when trophoblast cells invade the lumina of the spiral arteries, this time in their myometrial sections. The trophoblast cells infiltrate the artery's wall, destroy the fibro-muscular tissue of the wall and induce deposition of

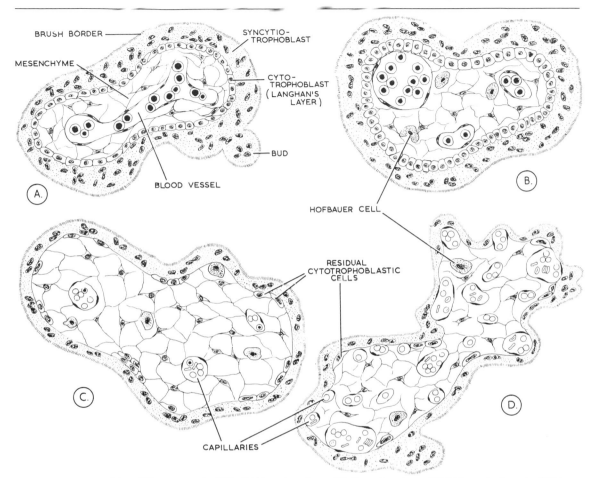

**Fig. 2/5** Chorionic villi at different ages ( × 350). (A) 4 week embryo; (B) 6½ week embryo; (C) 14th week placenta; (D) term placenta (redrawn from Patten, 1959)

fibrinoid material. This process converts the relatively rigid artery into a thin-walled flaccid vessel, permitting a greater flow of maternal blood. Failure of this process to occur is a factor in fetal growth retardation and in so-called placental dysfunction (see p. 277).

The maternal blood flow through the entire placenta has been estimated to rise from 300ml per minute at 20 weeks to 600ml per minute at 40 weeks. The total volume of the entire intervillous space (excluding villi) has been estimated at 150 to 250ml, and since there are about 60 functional fetal cotyledons, the blood flow over each is about 3 to 9ml per minute. The surface area of the villi has been calculated to be at least 11m² so that opportunity for exchange of nutrients is considerable.

## CHANGES IN THE CHARACTER OF THE VILLI AS PREGNANCY ADVANCES

With increasing placental age the structure of the villus changes. In early pregnancy (10th to 20th week) the villus is covered with syncytiotrophoblast which is sometimes condensed at its tip. Beneath this is a layer of cellular cytotrophoblast, which is initially two cells thick, and a relatively acellular mesoblastic core containing the fetal vessels which are quite small. The cytoplasm of the syncytium contains numerous round foamy vesicles, which are believed to be areas of protein synthesis but these decrease in number as pregnancy progresses, and as the fetal liver takes over protein synthesis.

By the 25th week of pregnancy, the syncytium has not changed, but only isolated collections of cytotrophoblastic cells remain, the stroma is more cel-lular and compact containing phagocytic cells and the vessels larger and closer to the trophoblastic covering. By the 36th week the cytotrophoblastic cells have largely disappeared, the syncytium has become attenuate and aggregations of nuclei (syncy-tial clumps) appear within it, but trophoblastic tissue always intervenes between the maternal and fetal circulations. With ageing, deposition of calcium occurs within the vasculature of the villi, and foci of intervillous fibrin are deposited on the surface of many of the villi, both occurrences having the effect of reducing exchanges of substances, but this is coun-tered by the smaller distance between the fetal vessels and the thinned syncytium cover the villi, both fac-tors enhancing the exchange of nutrients (Fig. **2/5**).

### 'INFARCTS'

*Fibrin deposition* on the surface of the villi appears to be progressive from implantation to term; so much so that its appearance is normal in the term placenta. The cause is unknown but may be due to the release of coagulation material by syncytiotropho-blast in response to the mechanical forces of the blood spurts striking its surface. The degree of fibrin deposition varies from microscopic deposits on in-dividual villi, to much larger deposits below the chorionic roof of the intervillous space. These pre-sumably occur by coalescence of small deposits, and if large may interfere with intervillous circulation, although this is uncommon. Any villus within the area of the fibrin loses contact with maternal blood and dies, thus forming a true infarct.

However, perivillous fibrin deposition has no del-eterious effect on the baby. In some cases, par-ticularly diabetes and Rhesus iso-immunization, fi-brinoid material appears within the syncytium of the villus and extends inwards but does not invade the stroma, the trophoblastic basement membrane re-maining intact, 'fibrinoid necrosis' eventually occur-ring. In 'uncomplicated' pregnancies the placenta shows fewer than 3 per cent of the abnormal villi. In 'complicated' pregnancies the incidence ranges from 18 to 40 per cent. The earlier the termination, the higher the incidence which may be considered evi-dence of a feto-maternal immunological reaction. For example, it has been shown that fluorescein-labelled antiserum tends to localize in the villi show-ing 'fibrinoid necrosis'.

In some placentae, one or more of the spiral arteries supplying the intervillous space may undergo spasm with reduction of the blood flow, and subse-quent coagulation. In these cases, the entire basal portion of the villi which lie between the placental septae, may become 'infarcted' or more correctly this space is occupied by *intervillous fibrin deposition*, which is usually found adjacent to the floor of the intervillous space.

Alternatively a number of vessels may become occluded beneath the decidual plate with extravasation of blood and partial separation of that area of the placenta. All the villi in the spaces supplied by the occluded vessels will of course die, and a large infarct will be seen in the placenta if it is examined after delivery. This mechanism occurs in *abruptio placentae*.

### FETAL VASCULAR PATTERN

The pattern of the fetal blood vessels is best under-stood if they are traced from the umbilicus where they join with the fetal vessels formed in the embry-onic mesoderm, to the tips of the chorionic villi, and back to the umbilicus.

The umbilical cord is a mesoblastic structure covered by an amniotic sheath and measures between 15 and 120cm (mean 50cm) in length. It is filled with mesoderm which becomes increasingly jelly-like as pregnancy advances. Within the substance of the jelly, one vein and two arteries are formed by diffe-rentiation from the mesodermal cells. The vein is thin-walled and joins the ductus venosus within the fetus. The arteries are thick-walled and in places the

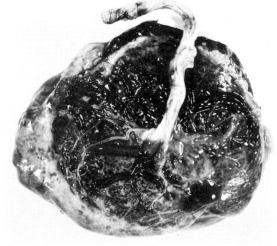

**Fig. 2/6** The fetal surface of the placenta showing the radial distribution of the vessels

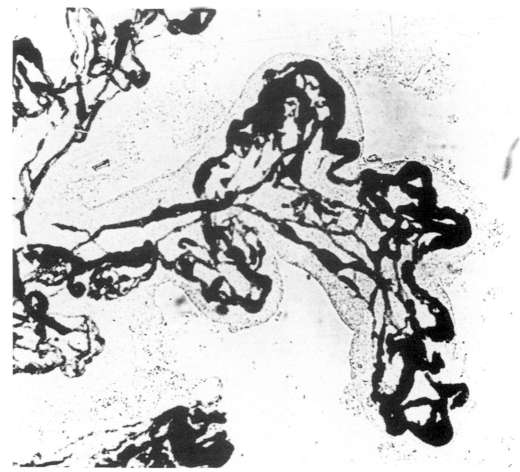

**Fig. 2/7** Injected vessels in the growing end of a villus which is 'budding off' daughter villi. The complex anastomosis of the vessels can be seen (Crawford, J. M. *J. Obstet. Gynaecol. Brit. Emp.* 1959, **66**, 885)

muscular layer is condensed to form crescentic rings (Hoboken's valves). Within the fetus the two arteries join the fetal internal iliac arteries, and peripherally they coalesce with the arteries formed within the chorionic villi. Just before entering the placenta, the two arteries form an anastomosis which has the effect of balancing the arterial blood flow to each side of the placenta.

## VASCULAR SYSTEM OF THE CHORIONIC VILLI

Within the placenta, just below the fetal surface, the vessels are enclosed in chorion and divide into branches, rather like the spokes of a wheel (Fig. **2/6**). At each division a proportion of the arteries perforate the placenta to supply a main villous trunk.

In addition perforating branches arise from the under surface of the arteries as they pass over the placenta to supply other villous trunks. Within the villi further branching occurs to supply each daughter villus as it is budded off (Fig. **2/7**). In the terminal villi, the arteries end as a capillary plexus which lies in close contact with the maternal blood, separated only by the trophoblastic cells which form the chorionic villi, and the placenta is referred to as a *haemochorial placenta* (Fig. **2/8**). The capillary structure of the placental villus is not dissimilar in structure from that in the renal glomerulus when examined under the electron microscope.

The pressure gradient in the fetal vessels of the lamb is shown in Fig. **2/9**, and there is every reason to suppose that similar conditions apply in man. It can be seen that most of the vascular resistance

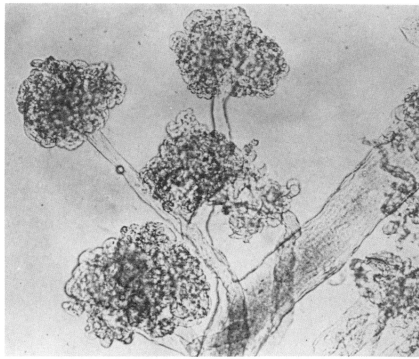

**Fig. 2/8** Terminal vascular divisions and capillary tufts in chorionic villi. These tufts present a large area of fetal blood to the maternal blood with only a thin placental barrier in between (Crawford, J. M. *J. Obstet. Gynaecol. Brit. Emp.* 1959, **66**, 885)

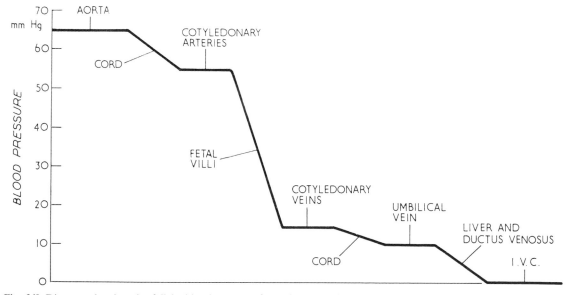

**Fig. 2/9** Diagram showing the fall in blood pressure from the aorta through the umbilical circulation and liver to the inferior vena cava in the mature fetal lamb (re-drawn from Dawes, G. S. *Amer. J. Obstet. Gynecol.* 1962, **84**, 1643)

occurs in the capillary tufts of the villi, and that the fetal arterial blood pressure is most important in maintaining the villous circulation. On the afferent side of the capillary tuft, the direction of exchange of substances is from fetus to mother, on the efferent side it is the reverse. However, the blood pressure on the efferent side never falls below 15mmHg probably because of a sphincter-like action in the ductus venosus, so that in systole and in diastole the villi are erectile and better able to function. The drainage from the villi is by venules and veins, and these follow the course of the arteries but only one vein enters the umbilicus.

### Abnormalities of vascularity

The human placenta functions as an extracorporeal fetal circulation, in many ways similarly to the 'artificial kidney' but more efficient. It also serves the function of an 'artificial lung', again with remarkable efficiency, and these two functions depend predominantly on a normal vascular system. The paramount importance of this can be deduced from the fact that when only one artery is present (this occurs in 1 per cent of singleton births) the incidence of fetal abnormalities is 25 per cent and they are incompatible with life in half of the cases.

# CLINICAL ASPECTS OF THE PLACENTA

## THE NORMAL PLACENTA

Examined after delivery the normal placenta is discoid in shape and weighs about one-seventh the weight of the baby. The fetal surface is covered with amnion and chorion and the fetal vessels can be seen coursing across it. The maternal surface is covered with greyish remnants of decidua and is divided into between 15 and 30 lobes or 'maternal cotyledons' by the placental septae which may reach almost to the chorionic plate.

## GROSS ABNORMALITIES IN PLACENTATION

By the 70th day the definitive placenta has been formed and the remaining chorionic villi have disappeared leaving a fairly smooth chorion and thin decidual layer covering the remainder of the conception sac. With further growth of the embryo this layer, the decidua capsularis, becomes apposed and fixed to the decidua vera. The definitive placenta has a fixed number of fetal and maternal cotyledons which do not increase to term, although the size and weight of each fetal villus does increase throughout pregnancy.

The shape of the placenta is therefore determined at the time of placentation, and variations from the typical round or disc-shaped placenta are found (Fig. **2/10**). The majority of these have no significance and are due to implantation on unfavourable sites. For example, a placenta attached to the side of the uterus may spread out onto the anterior and posterior wall and hence have a bi-lobed appearance. The shape of the placenta is altered by the place of union with the umbilical cord. Generally the cord enters the placenta at its midpoint, but sometimes the junction is at a placental edge, the *marginal insertion* of the cord (battledore placenta), or the umbilical vessels may run for some distance through the membranes before entering the placenta (vasa praevia). This is referred to as the *velamentous insertion* of the cord, and if the vessels lie across the cervix they may be compressed by the fetal head leading to fetal distress.

Certain grosser abnormalities have clinical significance and are mentioned in decreasing order of frequency.

### 1. Placenta extrachorialis

In normal placentation the size of the chorionic plate is approximately equal to that of the decidual plate, and trophoblastic invasion is at right angles to the surface of the decidua. However, in certain circumstances, which are not yet clear, the area of the chorionic plate is reduced and the trophoblast, having invaded deeply, is stimulated (or inhibition is removed) and further invasion takes place in a lateral direction. This invasion is irregular and most marked in the deeper decidua, the superficial decidua being largely spared, although some trophoblastic villi may invade this area. The capillary supply in the superficial decidua is not good, and the capillary walls are

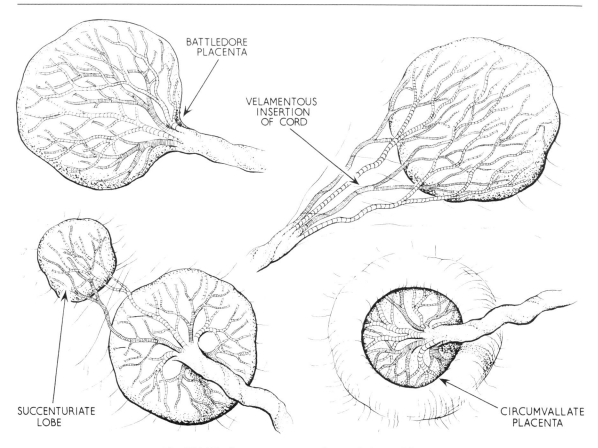

**Fig. 2/10** The four most common abnormal placental forms

friable so that small haemorrhages are common. Unable to obtain oxygen, the villi die and proper intervillous spaces are not formed. Thus in the superficial layers, decidual cells, dead villi and old clot or fibrin are found. In the deeper layers normal placentation with trophoblastic villi filling the intervillous spaces occurs. In this way the area of the chorionic plate is less than that of the decidual plate and some of the placenta is outside the chorionic plate – the *placenta extrachorialis*. Since the superficial decidua is largely spared it appears as a ring or band on the surface of the placenta (*placenta marginata*) or the membranes may be folded to enclose decidua (*placenta circumvallata*). Both types may be found on the fetal surface of the placenta and may partially or completely encircle the placenta. The condition occurs in about 18 per cent of all pregnancies.

The clinical significance of the condition is not great and the only finding is a higher incidence of antepartum haemorrhage indistinguishable from that of mild accidental haemorrhage or lateral placenta praevia. The haemorrhage is due to rupture of the maternal capillaries in the superficial decidual zone. Usually the haemorrhage is small and the blood rapidly clots, the clots being replaced by fibrin, but in about 10 per cent of cases the degree of haemorrhage is greater and blood tracks between the membrane and decidua to reach the vagina. Since the placenta is in no way damaged there is no fetal risk.

## 2. Placenta membranacea

In these placentae, implantation takes place deeper into the decidua, and the trophoblast over most, or all, of the sphere develops into, and is maintained as a placenta. The entire fetal membranes are covered with a thin but functioning placenta and the thickness of the placenta is in inverse proportion to its area.

### 3. Placenta succenturiata

In this variety the main placenta is connected to an accessory and small placenta by an artery and a vein which pass through membranes. Its origin is supposed to be due to the development of some of the villi of the chorion laeve, but this is uncertain. The clinical significance of placenta succenturiata is that the accessory lobe may be overlooked at delivery and left in utero, and give rise to haemorrhage, infection and the clinical finding of a 'placental polyp'. A second rare complication is that the vessels connecting the two placentae may be ruptured during childbirth leading to fetal exsanguination.

### 4. Placenta accreta, increta and percreta

In a few instances the trophoblastic villi penetrate deeply into the decidua, or even through the layer and into the muscle without disturbing the gestation. The condition is due either to excessive aggressiveness of the trophoblast or to thinness and lack of vascularity or resistance in the decidua. It can only be diagnosed by examining the removed uterus. In such studies portions of the decidua basalis are seen to be absent and the chorionic villi attach directly onto myometrial cells (*placenta accreta*), penetrate the cells to some degree (*placenta increta*), or even penetrate through to the serosal surface of the uterus (*placenta percreta*).

### 5. Haemangiomata of the placenta

These tumours are relatively common, being found in approximately 1 per cent of all placentae. Most tumours are small and without clinical significance but a few are large and are associated with hydramnios, antepartum haemorrhage and premature labour.

## Chapter 3

# The Feto-placental Unit

In order to grow, the fetus must be able to obtain oxygen, amino-acids, minerals and vitamins from the mother and must discharge carbon dioxide and waste products into the maternal circulation. This exchange is effected through the placenta, which in addition has certain other functions, some of which it shares with the fetus. The functional interdependence of the fetus and the placenta has led to the concept of a feto-placental unit.

The placenta is (1) the organ of respiration and excretion of the fetus, (2) the organ of nutrient transfer to the fetus, (3) by forming an immunological 'barrier', it protects the fetus (which contains paternal as well as maternal genes) from undergoing immunological rejection by the mother, and (4) in collaboration with the fetus, it synthesizes certain hormones which affect the maternal economy more than the fetal, and consequently are considered in Chapter 4 as well as here.

## TRANSPORT MECHANISMS THROUGH THE PLACENTA

The trophoblast through which the transfer occurs has been studied using the electron microscope. The syncytium consists of a sheet of cytoplasm, which is elevated into minute fingers (microvilli) on the free maternal side, and contains many irregularly dispersed nuclei (Fig. **3/1**). The cytoplasm is liberally supplied with lysosomes and mitochondria. On the fetal side the plasma membrane abuts onto the cells of the cytotrophoblast, and where these have disappeared, onto the collagen fibres and phagocytes of the mesoblast, which is relatively thin and contains the fetal capillaries. At all periods of pregnancy, a cellular membrane separates the maternal and fetal circulations, and all of the placental functions are mediated in, or act through this 'barrier'. These functions require a great expenditure

of energy, and the rate of metabolism of the placenta is comparable to that of the adult kidney or liver.

Transport of substances through the placenta takes place by:

1. Passive transport    a. simple diffusion
                                    b. facilitated diffusion
2. Active transport     a. enzymatic reaction
                                    b. pinocytosis.

### Passive transport

The majority of substances pass through the placenta by *simple diffusion*, moving from a high to a low

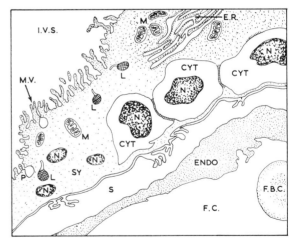

**Fig. 3/1** Part of a chorionic villus seen under the electron microscope. The thinner 'alpha' zone on the left is thought to be concerned with transport of substances, the thicker 'beta' zone on the right with synthesis of protein. (IVS, intervillous space; MV, microvilli; M, mitochondria; P, pinosome; L, lysosome; ER, endoplasmic reticulum; SY, syncytiotrophoblast; CYT, cytotrophoblast; N, nucleus; BM, basement membrane; S, connective stroma (mesoblast); ENDO, endothelium; FC, fetal capillary; FBC, fetal blood cell)

concentration area. A few substances pass through more rapidly than might be expected, their passage being *facilitated* by the shape and structure of the molecule.

**Active transport**

Special transport systems involving temporary combinations with enzyme systems are required for most inorganic ions and some substrates. The transport of more complex molecules is mediated by *pinocytosis* when the microvilli enlarge to engulf molecules; or by the development of phagolysosomes, in which the phagocytosed substance is joined by a wandering lysosome, and *enzymatic* reactions take place within the organelle. Transfer from trophoblast to fetal capillary through the stroma may be aided by the specialized phagocytes of the villi (Hofbauer's cells).

## RESPIRATORY FUNCTIONS OF THE FETO-PLACENTAL UNIT

The very large area of the fetal vasculature of the villi, and the relatively slow diffusion of maternal blood through the intervillous space permits a good exchange of oxygen and carbon dioxide. The gaseous exchange takes place by simple diffusion across the semipermeable trophoblastic cell membrane (Fig. 3/2).

Oxygen is carried to the intervillous space by the erythrocytes in the form of oxyhaemoglobin. The blood entering the intervillous space is 90 to 100% saturated, has a $pO_2$ of 90 to 100mmHg, and supplies about 17ml of oxygen per 100ml blood. The oxygen needs of the placenta and fetus are met by this blood, and since the placenta has a high metabolic rate, about one-third of the available oxygen is utilized by it. The remainder diffuses across the placenta and is taken up by the haemoglobin of the fetal erythrocytes, the umbilical vein blood being 70% staturated and having a $pO_2$ of 30 to 40mmHg, a partial pressure which is quite adequate for all fetal needs. The fetal blood which enters the umbilical arteries is equal to half the total output of the heart, and the pressure of this blood drops to low levels during its passage through the fetal villi, so that a pool of slowly moving blood in the capillary mesh of the villi is able to absorb a relatively high proportion of oxygen and discharge much of the contained $CO_2$. Fetal blood, moreover, is better able to take up oxygen than is adult blood. Not only is

the haemoglobin concentration higher, but at a given pH it has a greater affinity for oxygen than maternal blood.

Carbon dioxide ($CO_2$), like oxygen, diffuses rapidly across the placenta, and any change in maternal $pCO_2$ leads to a rapid rise of erythrocyte carbon dioxide content, where the gas is converted into

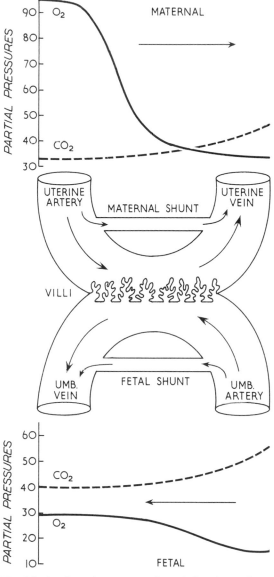

**Fig. 3/2** A schematic representation of the placental gas exchange. It can be seen that fetal blood has a much lower partial pressure of oxygen than the adult, and the fetus in utero has been described as living in conditions of oxygenation resembling those of the top of Mount Everest

bicarbonate and returned to the plasma to be converted into carbonic acid. Because of this, hydrogen ion concentration of the blood rises to produce a 'respiratory acidosis'. The fetus is hardly affected by these changes because, although carbon dioxide diffuses so rapidly across the placenta, rendering the fetal blood temporarily more alkaline, this simultaneously increases its oxygen capacity, whilst the increased acidity of the maternal blood enhances oxygen release. The fetus therefore obtains more oxygen, and the increased carbon dioxide is buffered in the fetal blood.

The placenta also transfers hydrogen ions, bicarbonate and lactic acid between mother and fetus, so that the acid-base status of the mother and her fetus are closely related. However, this transfer tends to occur fairly slowly. In a normal labour a mild degree of maternal acidosis is usual, but the fetus is not affected as it is able to buffer the additional acidity from its own reserves. But if maternal acidosis is aggravated by dehydration or acido-ketosis, the fetal buffering system may be unable to cope with a resulting fetal metabolic acidosis.

The efficiency of the system depends on adequate perfusion of the placental bed with maternal blood, an adequately functioning placenta (in so far as gas and ionic exchange are concerned), and a well-functioning fetal circulation through the umbilical vessels. Should maternal blood perfusion be reduced due to disease, such as pregnancy-induced hypertension or chronic renal disease; or should placental function decrease, due to ageing as in prolonged pregnancy, or to insufficient time for exchange, as in uterine over-activity; or should the feto-placental circulation be deranged, as when cord compression occurs, oxygen supplies may be reduced and fetal acidosis will occur independently of maternal acidosis. This may be hazardous to the fetus, and is most likely to occur in the late first stage and the second stage of labour.

## NUTRIENT TRANSFER THROUGH THE PLACENTA

The rate at which substances can be transferred across the placental trophoblastic membrane depends to some extent on their concentration on either side. The rapid diffusion rate of water confirms that the trophoblastic membrane is similar to all other animal membranes in allowing the free passage of water. Halogens (bromine, fluorine, iodine) pass less readily because of the presence of calcium salts within the placenta, but still diffuse relatively quickly. Of the alkalis, sodium and potassium diffuse easily and rapidly. The diffusion of sodium increases as pregnancy advances and the trophoblastic layers of the villi are reduced. Certain simple substances, such as amines, urea and uric acid as well as the gases are transferred by diffusion, moving from an area of higher concentration to that of a lower. Thus urea and uric acid in excess in the fetus are easily transferred to the maternal circulation.

Other substances which are in higher concentration in the maternal plasma are *actively* transported by complex enzyme systems. Most are first broken down into relatively simple compounds in the maternal circulation and are resynthesized in the placenta. For example, carbohydrates are broken down into glucose, and the simpler compound is actively transported into the syncytium, where the more complex substance is reconstituted, before being discharged into the fetal villous capillary network. Little or no fructose or glycogen crosses the placenta. Most proteins are broken down into amino-acids before transfer, but a few proteins are transferred intact, the transfer taking place slowly, probably by pinocytosis. Examples are immunoglobulin G and probably albumin. Minerals conjugate with enzymes to be transferred, those with low atomic weights being more readily transferred than those with high atomic weights. Vitamins are reduced to simpler forms and reconstituted within the trophoblast, the fat-soluble vitamins passing through more slowly than the water-soluble ones. In most investigations using isotope-tagged substances, transfer and reconstitution occur rapidly, often within 30 to 60 minutes (Table 3/1). Oddly, lipids do not appear to be transferred across the placenta. The evidence is that the placenta bars lipid transfer, although it absorbs a small quantity of lipids from the maternal circulation, probably as free fatty acids. Within the syncytiotrophoblast the limited supplies of free fatty acids are resynthesized into phospholipids and other lipids, which are stored and released into the fetal circulation for transport to fat storage areas in adipose tissue as pregnancy advances. This means that most maternal lipids are retained by the mother for her energy needs, thus sparing carbohydrate for transfer to the fetus. Until the last ten weeks of pregnancy all the fetal phospholipids are derived from the placental stores, as the fetal liver is not capable of lipid synthesis.

The quantity of nutrients transferred depends on the adequacy of the maternal uterine blood flow. In

| Maternal blood | Intervillous space | Placental transfer methods | | |
| --- | --- | --- | --- | --- |
| | | Passive | Active | Pinocytosis |
| $H_2O$, $O_2$, $CO_2$, urea, Na, K | ⟶ | + | | |
| Glucose | Facilitated by carrier molecule | | + | |
| Polysaccharides ⟶ | Mono- and di-saccharides | | + | |
| Protein ⟶ | Amino-acids | | + | |
| Fat ⟶ | Free fatty acids | | + | |
| Vitamin A ⟶ | Carotene | + | | |
| Vitamin B complex, Vitamin C | ⟶ | | + | |
| Iron, phosphorus | ⟶ | | + | |
| Antibodies | Only IgG | + | | |
| | ⟶ | ± | | + |
| Erythrocytes | ⟶ | | | ?+ |

**Table 3/1** Transfer of substances through the placenta

certain diseases there is a reduction in the maternal blood flow through the uterine vessels and reduced perfusion of the placental villi. In some of these cases, the result is an inadequate transfer of nutrients to the fetus, with consequent retarded fetal growth in utero due to malnutrition. In some cases the supplies of nutrients and oxygen may be so reduced that the fetus dies. In other cases the supply of nutrients is sufficient to maintain fetal growth, but ageing of the placenta, which occurs in prolonged pregnancy, may reduce placental function and lead to fetal death either before or during labour.

**Fetal energy metabolism**

The fetus has been called a glucose-dependent parasite. This is because over 90 per cent of its energy requirements are obtained from glucose, (and about 10 per cent from amino-acids) transferred from the mother. The fetus rapidly utilizes the transferred glucose, and fetal blood glucose levels are about two-thirds those of the mother, which facilitates glucose transfer.

The quantity of glucose transferred increases after the 30th week of pregnancy. Towards the end of pregnancy about 10g of glucose per kilogram body-weight is retained daily and the excess over immediate metabolic requirements is converted into glycogen and fat by the placenta and fetal tissues. The glycogen is stored in the liver, the skeletal muscles and the heart, whilst fat is deposited around the heart and behind the scapulae. It has been calculated that in the last 10 weeks of pregnancy a daily synthesis of 2g of fat occurs, so that by 40 weeks, 15 per cent of the fetal weight is made up of fat, constituting an energy reserve of about 21 000kJ (5000kcal). These reserves of fat and glycogen are needed immediately after birth as a source of energy for metabolic functions and especially for the regulation of body temperature.

As has been noted, if the placenta receives inadequate supplies of glucose and other nutrients, the growth of the fetus will be retarded, fat deposition will be impaired and a 'dysmature' (small for dates) infant will be born.

**Drug transfer**

Since drugs are chemical substances, their transplacental transfer is no different from that of nutrients, and all pass to some degree. The rate is governed to some extent by the fat solubility of the ionized molecule (the higher the solubility, the more rapid the transfer), and by the thickness of the trophoblastic barrier. As pregnancy progresses the thickness diminishes, whilst the placental area increases and the more rapid passage of drugs is favoured.

Table **3/2** shows the rapidity of the passage of drugs commonly used in pregnancy.

| Drug | Route of administration | Percentage fetal serum concentration | | |
|------|------|------|------|------|
| | | Less than 30 min | 30 to 59 min | 60 to 120 min |
| *Antibiotics* | | | | |
| Penicillin | Intramuscular | | | 50 to 75 |
| Streptomycin | Intramuscular | | | 50 |
| Tetracycline | Oral | | | 50 |
| Erythromycin | Oral | | | 25 |
| Sulphonamide | Oral | | | 75 |
| *Sedatives* | | | | |
| Barbiturates | | | | |
| (quick-acting) | Intravenous | 100 | | |
| (medium-acting) | Oral | | 75 to 100 | |
| *Tranquillizers* | | | | |
| Phenothiazines | Intravenous | 100 | | |
| *Narcotics* | | | | |
| Morphine | Intramuscular | | 75 | |
| Pethidine | Intramuscular | | 75 | |

**Table 3/2** Transplacental passage of drugs

## STEROID METABOLISM IN THE FETO-PLACENTAL UNIT

The placenta has a wide spectrum of synthesizing and catabolic functions, especially steroidogenesis. In this activity the syncytiotrophoblast is the active synthetic layer, containing many enzymes (including acid phosphatase). However, several important enzymes are missing in the placenta (at least from mid-pregnancy onwards), whilst others are absent in the fetus.

In this respect the placenta and the fetus act as an integrated unit for the synthesis and metabolism of steroid hormones, particularly oestrogens. The placenta is able to produce human chorionic gonadotrophin, human placental lactogen, human chorionic thyrotrophin, progesterone and androgen from precursors supplied by the mother, but requires the participation of the fetus for the production of oestrogens.

The synthesis of oestrogen is the main example of the close relationship of the placenta and fetus in steroidogenesis. Acetate and cholesterol are supplied to the placenta from maternal sources, together with a small quantity of dehydroepiandrosterone synthesized in the maternal adrenals. Within the placenta, the cholesterol is converted into pregnenolone and then to progesterone, which is transferred into the maternal and fetal circulations (mainly the former). That portion transferred into the maternal

circulation acts at cellular level and is then rapidly converted in the target cells and in the liver into pregnanediol in which form it is excreted in the urine.

The synthesis of oestrogens is much more complex, as the placenta lacks certain enzymes necessary to complete the synthetic pathways. These are C 17, 20-desmolase and 16-hydroxylase. Current belief is that pregnenolone is synthesized in the placenta from maternally supplied acetate and cholesterol, and is transferred to the fetal adrenals where together with fetally synthesized pregnenolone it is hydroxylated and sulphurylated. It is then converted into dehydroepiandrosterone sulphate (DHAS). The DHAS is then transferred to the fetal liver where it is 16-hydroxylated, and returned to the placenta for aromatization and conversion into oestriol (Fig. **3/3**).

Further discussion of the various hormones produced by the feto-placental unit is continued in Chapter 4 'The Physiology of Pregnancy', as they affect the entire range of physiological alterations which occur in pregnancy.

## IMMUNOLOGY OF TROPHOBLAST

The placenta is of fetal origin and thus formed of maternal and paternal elements. It can, therefore, be considered an allograft, yet it is not rejected by the mother. The explanation of this phenomenon is by no means clear. It is known that transplantation

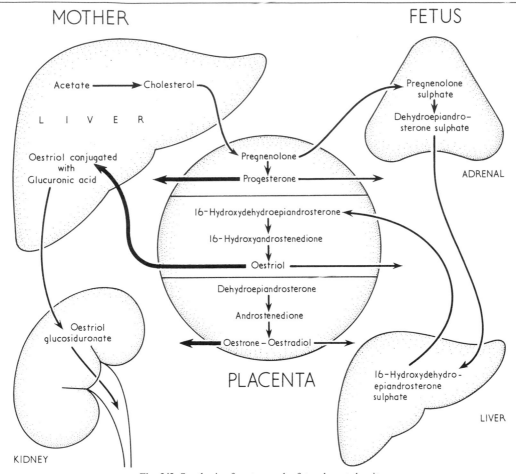

**Fig. 3/3** Synthesis of oestrogen by feto-placental unit

antigen sites are present on the plasma membranes of the cytotrophoblast, and may be present on the syncytiotrophoblast.

One hypothesis is that the antigen induces maternal production of a blocking immunoglobulin G antibody which binds on to antigen sites on trophoblast and on maternal leucocytes. Bound to the sites it induces the production of fetal immunosuppressor cells. By 'masking' the antigen sites and by stimulating fetal suppressor cells, the 'foreign' fetus is not rejected and pregnancy continues. If both parents share several histocompatibility antigens (HLA), there may be an inadequate stimulus by the fetus to the production of blocking IgG, making fetal rejection (abortion) more likely (see p. 188) and possibly increasing the chance that pregnancy-induced hypertension will occur if the pregnancy continues.

A second hypothesis is that allogenic (foreign) trophoblast is not attacked by maternal immuno-competent cells because it synthesizes increasing quantities of the hormone, human chorionic gonado-trophin (HCG). In experiments HCG has been shown to block the destructive action of immuno-competent lymphocytes. These hypotheses seek to explain why the placenta and fetus are not rejected by the mother, but they are only hypotheses.

The other cells forming the placenta and the fetus are antigenic and will provoke an immune reaction if injected into the mother, but the fetus itself has only a poor capacity to produce antibodies in response to invasion by maternal antigens or by bacteria. From the 20th week of pregnancy, or earlier, the fetus is able to synthesize immunoglobins in response to a challenge. These are produced by B cells, and initially IgM is synthesized, later IgD, then IgG and IgA are produced. Cellular immunity (a function of T immunocytes) develops about the same time.

The fetal immune response is supplemented by the passage of certain maternal antibody molecules, provided they are not too large, into the fetus, which gives it passive protection. The antibodies are all of the 7S variety of immunoglobulins, and if the mother is infected during pregnancy with measles or hepatitis, or receives variola, poliomyelitis or diphtheria vaccine, antibodies pass to the fetus throughout pregnancy and give it passive protection against these diseases for about 4 months after birth. During this period the passive antibodies may interfere with the early active immunization in the infant.

## FETAL PHYSIOLOGY AND GROWTH

Nearly weightless in its heat-controlled uterine capsule, the fetus is dependent upon the placenta for its respiratory and excretory functions, shares with the placenta the latter's hormonal synthesis function, and relies upon the placenta for its nutritional requirements. Its growth during the 40 intra-uterine weeks is determined by many factors, both genetic and environmental. Of the latter, adequate placental perfusion by maternal blood and adequate function of the placenta appear crucial. Maternal nutrition is consequently not a limiting factor to fetal growth, except in prolonged famine conditions, although deficiencies in maternal food intake may lead to curtailment of pregnancy and an increased perinatal mortality rate.

The primacy of efficient placental perfusion and function is exemplified in dysmature babies and in multiple pregnancies. The dysmature, or growth-retarded, baby is often found in patients who have pregnancy-induced hypertension or chronic renal disease. In these cases the blood flow to the uterus is reduced; and degenerative changes occur in the placenta. In multiple pregnancy the size of the placenta is larger but it probably receives a reduced blood flow per unit area of villus surface. It may well be that a limiting factor on fetal growth is the villus surface area. The growth of the fetus accelerates after the 20th week of pregnancy, and efficient placental function is vital after this time.

To sustain its growth, the fetus must obtain amino-acids, minerals and vitamins from the mother, and energy supplies to convert them into the more complex substances required for cell division and

organ growth. The energy requirements are obtained almost entirely from carbohydrate which is the principal metabolic fuel. Lipids, as free fatty acids, only cross in small amounts until the last 15 weeks of pregnancy.

The fetus, as mentioned earlier, is carbohydrate-dependent and fetal insulin appears crucial in regulating its growth. Because of the good insulation provided by the amniotic fluid, and because of its relative weightlessness, the fetus makes minimal energy demands for temperature control and muscle function, so that most of the energy is used for growth. Any excess carbohydrate is converted into glycogen or lipids, in the fetal liver. However, prior to the 30th gestational week the liver is poorly able to convert the excess carbohydrate, so that glycogen storage and lipid deposition are low before that time.

From the 30th week the liver becomes increasingly efficient (Fig. **3/4**), and conversion into glycogen is effected rapidly so that the fetal blood glucose concentration is kept low, usually lying between 20 and 30mg/dl. The actual level fluctuates and depends on the amount of glucose transferred across the placenta, the rate of peripheral utilization of glucose and the rate of storage and release of fetal glycogen. Glycogen is also stored in the fetal heart muscle, the skeletal muscles and the placenta. Should hypoxia occur for any reason, the fetus is able to mobilize the liver and

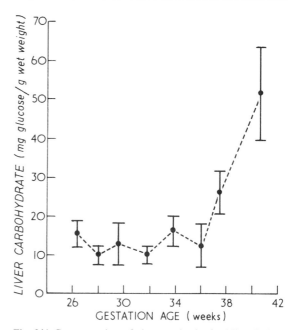

**Fig. 3/4** Concentration of glycogen in the fetal liver in late pregnancy

heart glycogen (but not the skeletal muscle stores) for anaerobic glycolysis (see Chapter 36).

A proportion of the carbohydrate is converted into lipids, and this proportion increases as term approaches. Before the 30th gestational week the fetal liver is largely unable to synthesize lipids, and until that time the greater proportion of fetal lipids are synthesized by the trophoblast from free fatty acids absorbed from the maternal circulation. Liver function increases rapidly after the 30th week, and increasing amounts of carbohydrate are converted into fat, which is stored in fetal adipose tissue.

The fetus has two kinds of adipose tissue. Brown fat cells have multiple small fat vacuoles and consequently a greater contact between mitochondria and the lipid vacuoles. White fat cells have a single large vacuole. White adipose tissue covers the body of the infant at term, and acts mainly as a lipid store and as an insulator. Brown adipose tissue plays a significant part in non-shivering heat production once the fetus has been born. The brown fat is deposited mainly around the neck, between the shoulder blades, behind the sternum and around the kidneys. The initial deposition of fat occurs when the fetus weighs about 800g, and at this stage (24 to 26 weeks' gestation) 1 per cent of its body-weight is fat. From this time the fat deposition increases, so that by term 15 per cent of the fetus' body-weight is fat, and the increments are greatest after the 35th week. This is the reason why premature infants have smaller stores of fat and are less well able to survive exposure to cold. It has been found that the brown adipose tissue is almost totally depleted of fat in extremely premature infants who have been exposed to cold and subsequently died.

The amino-acids required for protein synthesis are obtained from the maternal blood by active transfer methods, and the concentration of amino-acids is higher in the fetal blood than in the maternal blood. Protein synthesis exceeds protein breakdown, and when the latter occurs the fetus reuses the resulting amino-acids for synthesis of new proteins. Indeed such studies as have been made indicate that the rate of synthesis of protein in various fetal organs is greater than in adult organs. It appears that the fetus synthesizes its own nucleic acids and does not rely upon any transfer of maternal nucleic acids.

The fetus also produces a specific protein, alpha fetoprotein (AFP) in its liver. The concentration of AFP rises to a peak between the 12th and 16th week of pregnancy and then slowly decreases to term. AFP is secreted by the fetus in its urine and the amniotic fluid level parallels that of the fetal plasma. Normally, amniotic AFP is swallowed by the fetus and degraded in its gut. Raised levels are found in multiple pregnancy, or if the fetus is unable to swallow, or if extra AFP leaks into the amniotic fluid from fetuses with open neural tube defects. From the second quarter of pregnancy onwards, AFP appears in the maternal blood plasma, presumably from the amniotic fluid or the fetal plasma by some indirect mechanism.

## CARDIOVASCULAR SYSTEM

The circulatory pattern of the fetus is described on page 433 and it should be noted that over 56 per cent of the cardiac output passes through the umbilical arteries, to perfuse the placenta. The cardiac output increases as term approaches, and in the last weeks about 200ml/kg/minute is usual. To obtain this output, the heart rate varies between 110 and 150 beats per minute, and the two ventricles work in parallel, the right ventricle pumping out more blood than the left. The blood flow through the umbilical arteries is, therefore, about 140ml/kg/ minute, and the pressure in excess of 50mmHg. The pressure falls considerably in the placenta as has been discussed (p. 23), but even in the umbilical vein, it is maintained at a level in excess of 15mmHg, perhaps by the sphincter-like action of the ductus venosus, thus keeping the villi constantly in a turgid state, and enabling placental function to continue at all times.

The fetal arterial blood pressure also increases through pregnancy, and in the last 4 weeks has a mean value of 75mmHg systolic and 55mmHg diastolic.

There is a progressive increase in the red cell count, the haemoglobin level and the packed cell volume as term approaches. At 14 weeks' gestation the mean haemoglobin concentration of fetal blood is 10g/dl, and all the erythrocytes contain fetal haemoglobin (HbF). By term, the haemoglobin concentration is 18g/dl, and the proportion of cells containing HbF has fallen to 70 per cent, the remaining 30 per cent of erythrocytes containing adult haemoglobin (HbA); but there are wide variations between individuals. The life-span of fetal erythrocytes is probably the same (about 120 days) as in the adult. Erythrocytes containing HbF are qualitatively different from those containing HbA: they are more resistant to haemolysis but less resistant to trauma, which suggests that the cell membrane is altered. More important, as far as oxygen transport is concerned, the altered cell function permits fetal haemoglobin to become more saturated with oxygen at a given partial oxygen pressure.

## ENDOCRINE ACTIVITY

From about the 14th week of gestation, fetal TSH is secreted, which leads to the release of $T_3$ and $T_4$ into the fetal circulation. The quantity of $T_3$ is low, but a relatively large amount of biologically inactive 'reverse $T_3$' is produced.

Immediately after birth, a sudden surge of TSH occurs, mainly because of the neonate's exposure to the extra-uterine environment. This causes a surge release of $T_3$ and $T_4$, and, at the same time, the amount of 'reverse $T_3$' falls.

## THE RENAL SYSTEM

The fetal kidney develops from the metanephros, and new glomeruli continue to be formed up to the 36th week of gestation. Renal function starts in fetal life, urine being secreted by the 16th week and probably earlier. The rate of urine flow is not known in the human fetus, although in monkeys a flow rate of 5ml/kg/hour is found in the last weeks of gestation. The urine is voided into the amniotic fluid. The functional efficiency of the kidney increases as pregnancy advances, at least as measured by secretion of bilirubin.

## THE LUNGS

The lungs in the early embryo are made up of epithelial tubes surrounded by mesoderm. With further development the epithelium becomes folded and glandular in appearance and primitive alveoli are formed. By the 24th to 26th week an adjacent capillary supply has been developed and the lung is capable of gas exchange should the infant be born. By full gestation three or four further generations of alveoli have developed. The epithelium, which has a cuboidal appearance, becomes flattened with the first breath.

The fetal lung secretes fluid which partly distends its passages. At about 20 to 24 weeks' gestation, it also begins to produce a surface-active lipoprotein which facilitates expansion of the lung at birth, and subsequently has a role of great importance in allowing the air-containing lung to maintain its normal volume.

Real-time ultrasound scanning has shown that the fetus has periods of respiratory movements ('breathing') and of body movements. In early pregnancy the movements are sporadic and inco-ordinate, but after mid-pregnancy they become regular, and increase in frequency as the pregnancy advances. A diurnal variation occurs with both respiratory and body movements: a normal fetus having periods of respiratory movement, of body movement and of inactivity. Body movements occur most often in the early morning and late evening, whilst respiratory movements are more frequent during the day-time. Fetal 'hiccups' also occur but have no relationship to the time of the day or the stage of the pregnancy.

Fetal respiratory activity results in the inspiration of amniotic fluid into the large bronchi and bronchioles, as beyond this the fluid secreted by the alveoli is under considerable pressure. However, episodes of hypoxia late in pregnancy or during delivery stimulate gasping efforts of respiratory muscles, and inhalation deep into the pulmonary tree of liquor contaminated with meconium.

## THE GASTRO-INTESTINAL TRACT

Since the fetus is supplied with energy in the form of carbohydrate transferred from the mother, its intestinal tract is relatively quiescent. It is true that the fetus swallows liquor amnii, and the cellular material contained in this enters the gut, where it is acted upon by the various enzymes and converted into meconium. This remains in the gut unless an episode of severe hypoxia leads to 'defaecation' of meconium into the amniotic sac. Pancreatic enzymes such as lipase are found from the 16th week of gestation, trypsin activity occurs at about 26 weeks when the fetus weighs 1000g, and increases slowly to term, whilst amylase activity is absent. Liver function is generally depressed in utero, as the placenta performs many of its homeostatic functions. However, glycolytic and glycogen synthetic functions are developed and increase in efficiency towards term. Its ability to conjugate with glucuronides is defective and only reaches an adequate capacity after birth. Because the placenta clears the fetal blood of bilirubin and other metabolites requiring a transferase activity, the fetal and neonatal liver is deficient in certain transferases. Until these deficiencies are corrected, in the neonatal period, bilirubin may accumulate in the infant's blood, a matter which is of some consequence in haemolytic disease of the newborn.

## Chapter 4

# The Physiology of Pregnancy

During the weeks of pregnancy great changes occur in the physiology of the female designed to give to the fetus the nutrients required for growth, and the mother the additional energy she may require for labour and subsequent lactation. Most of the changes occur before the fetal need arises. This is because the trophoblast of the placenta is the key regulator in the process. The trophoblast is a highly active tissue, removing substances from the maternal blood, converting some and elaborating others, returning some, such as oestrogen and progesterone, into the mother's blood, and passing others such as protein and vitamins to the fetus. All the chemicals necessary for this activity are derived from the maternal blood, and to enable adequate quantities to reach the placental bed, a quiescence of metabolism occurs, with delay in the exchange between maternal blood and tissues. The quiescence also enables the mother to conserve energy and the placid, plethoric appearance of the pregnant woman is well known.

Discussion of the physiological alterations of pregnancy should start at the placenta, for here complex hormones are elaborated which affect the economy of the whole body.

## HORMONAL SECRETION IN PREGNANCY

### PLACENTAL HORMONE PRODUCTION

Within days of implantation of the conceptus into the uterine decidua, the trophoblast is elaborating hormones, the main ones being chorionic gonadotrophin (HCG) and human placental lactogen (HPL) which are hormones unique to pregnancy, and the sex steroids, the oestrogens and progesterone (Fig. **4/1**).

#### Human chorionic gonadotrophin

HCG is formed by trophoblast from its earliest days and can be detected in the serum by radioimmunoassay (for the beta sub-unit of HCG) within 10 days of conception; but as only about 10 per cent is excreted in the urine, it is rarely detectable in urine until about 30 days after conception. Production, and consequently excretion, of HCG rises rapidly to a peak between the 60th and 80th days of pregnancy, and this is followed by a fall to a level which is maintained for the rest of pregnancy. During the peak between 500 000 and 1 000 000IU of HCG are secreted each day; the quantity falling to about 80 000 to 120 000IU each day in the last quarter of pregnancy (Fig. **4/2**). The peak persists for longer in multiple pregnancy and in abnormal conditions such as trophoblastic tumours. After delivery, detectable HCG disappears from the urine and serum in 7 to 10 days but persists for longer in the blood. The high circulating levels of HCG in early pregnancy suggest that its function is mainly to maintain a local environment favourable for implantation and growth of the embryo.

Initially its action is to maintain the corpus luteum's secretion of oestrogen and progesterone,

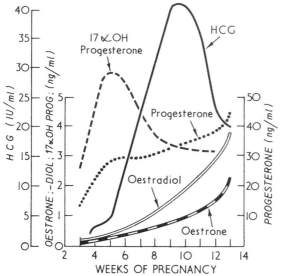

Fig. 4/1 Hormone secretion in early pregnancy

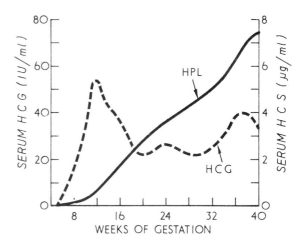

Fig. 4/2 Concentration of chorionic gonadotrophin in the serum at varying times during pregnancy. The urinary gonadotrophin excretion parallels that of the serum (Hytten and Leitch. *The Physiology of Human Pregnancy*. Blackwell, Oxford, 1964)

until the placenta has developed sufficiently to take over all steroid production, after which time the level of HCG falls. But it is probable that it has additional functions which persist unaltered throughout pregnancy. These are to regulate oestrogen production by the placenta, and to suppress maternal immunological reactions against the fetus.

**Protein hormones**

The syncytiotrophoblast secretes a number of pregnancy-specific hormones. These include human placental lactogen (HPL) and pregnancy-specific betaglycoprotein (SP-1). The physiological functions of these proteins are not fully known. The secretion of HPL appears to complement that of HCG. As the level of HCG falls from its peak, that of HPL begins to rise, continuing to do so until late pregnancy (Fig. **4/3**). HPL does not appear to enter the fetal circulation, so that all its effects are on the mother's physiology. The principal effect of HPL is to alter the maternal metabolism so that the fetus thrives in utero, and to initiate the changes which enable lactation to begin after the fetus is born. At cellular level HPL encourages protein synthesis on the ribosomes. It is partly responsible for mammary growth in pregnancy and it may be involved in the production of colostrum. Its involvement in the synthesis of milk is uncertain and its role, if any, small compared with that of human prolactin.

The most important pregnancy preserving functions of HPL are its metabolic actions. It exerts a glucose-saving effect on the mother so that glucose is diverted to the fetus, which, as has been mentioned, is largely a glucose-dependent parasite. HPL does this by mobilizing free fatty acids from maternal body stores, and this lipolytic effect reduces maternal glucose utilization by offering her a ready source of energy supply. The raised blood glucose levels enable the fetus to obtain glucose more readily for its needs.

Fig. 4/3 HCG and HPL secretion in pregnancy

HPL stimulates insulin secretion centrally, but inhibits its effect at peripheral sites. This may be a major reason for the known diabetogenic effect of pregnancy. HPL may cause nitrogen retention, but this effect has not been clearly established.

HPL also enhances the transfer of amino-acids to the fetus, and prevents the reduction of progesterone to its less biologically active metabolite, 20α dehydroprogesterone, thus maintaining higher concentrations of progesterone.

SP-1 is secreted entirely into the maternal circulation, and its concentration rises, paralleling that of HPL. Its function is unknown and clinically its measurement seems to offer little in the management of the 'at risk fetus', as there is no correlation between the concentration of the protein and placental function. As well, its half-life of 24 hours (compared with HPL's half-life of 20 minutes) makes it an inappropriate hormone to evaluate placental function.

Measurement of SP-1 may help in determining the outcome of threatened abortion: in several studies low SP-1 levels have correlated with subsequent abortion, whilst normal levels indicated a continuing pregnancy. However, the usefulness of measurements of the placental proteins compared unfavourably with that of ultrasound in evaluating the outcome of complications in early pregnancy.

### Prolactin

Recent research has found that the oestrogen-primed, progesterone-stimulated endometrial decidua synthesizes prolactin. In pregnancy the prolactin is secreted into the amniotic fluid. The functions of endometrial prolactin in pregnancy probably include: (1) Regulation of amniotic fluid osmolarity. In women who present with chronic polyhydramnios, a defect in amniotic prolactin receptors has been found. (2) Involvement in the modulation of prostaglandin synthesis by the chorio-amnion, and thus an influence in the onset of labour. (3) Stimulation by fetal lung alveolar pneumocytes to produce surfactant (see p. 436).

### Human chorionic thyrotrophin

Recent work suggests that the placenta synthesizes human chorionic thyrotrophin which on radioimmunoassay is similar to, but not identical with, thyrotrophin. HCT does not enter the fetal compartment but is responsible for the raised levels of thyrotrophin in the mother's plasma. These are two or three times the non-pregnant levels.

### Oestrogens

In pregnancy the main source of oestrogen production is the placenta. As described in Chapter 3, the synthesis of oestrogens is a complex process involving the fetus, as the placenta lacks certain essential enzymes necessary to complete the synthesis. More than 20 oestrogen have been identified but only three appear to have clinical significance. These are oestrone, oestradiol and oestriol. Oestriol is the relatively inactive form and most organs produce only oestrone and oestradiol, which are then rapidly converted into the inactive oestriol in the liver. The placenta is capable of producing oestriol in addition, and retaining it selectively. This is shown by the fact that the ratio of oestriol:oestradiol:oestrone in the non-pregnant woman is 3:2:1, but in pregnancy rises to 30:2:1 so that oestriol accounts for 90 per cent of the oestrogens secreted.

The actions of oestrogens are important and complex. At the cellular level oestradiol, which is the most active form, acts upon enzyme systems (the main one of which is cyclic AMP) and through this mechanism, or directly, enhances RNA and protein synthesis by the cell. In addition oestradiol alters the polymerization of acid mucopolysaccharides. This has the effect of increasing the hygroscopic qualities and reducing the adhesion of the collagen fibres in connective tissue. This effect is most marked in the cervix, which becomes swollen and soft in pregnancy. Oestradiol aids the growth of uterine muscle, either by enzymatic action or by increasing uterine blood flow. In the breast, oestradiol increases the size and mobility of the nipple, and causes duct and alveolar development. There is also evidence that it plays a part in causing the water retention found in pregnancy (Fig. **4/4**).

### Progesterone

Progesterone is secreted initially by the corpus luteum and the trophoblast, but by the 35th day after fertilization, the placental syncytiotrophoblast takes over all significant synthesis from maternally supplied precursors, mainly cholesterol. At this stage of pregnancy the plasma progesterone is about 50ng/ml. A small fall may occur in the next three weeks, but from then on a linear rise begins, to reach a level of 150ng/ml at term (see Fig. **4/1**).

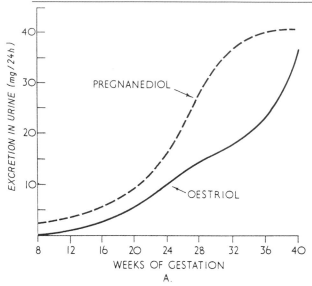

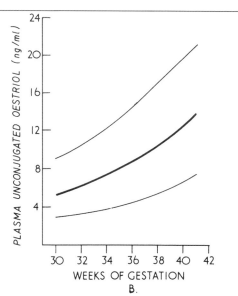

**Fig. 4/4a** Excretion of oestriol and pregnanediol in normal pregnancy

**Fig. 4/4b** Plasma unconjugated oestriol in the last ten weeks of pregnancy

Progesterone is removed from the blood rapidly and is converted in a wide variety of tissues into pregnanediol, in which form it is excreted in the urine. However, only between 6 and 27 per cent of progesterone is excreted in this form so that urine pregnanediol assays give no accurate estimate of progesterone production.

In most tissues the concentration of progesterone is low, but in the myometrium relatively large amounts of the steroid are maintained, because of a specific binding protein which has a special affinity for progesterone.

The main effect of progesterone in pregnancy is to reduce smooth muscle excitability, and, because of the high myometrial concentration, this effect is maximal in the pregnant uterus. It is believed that the smooth muscle relaxing effect operates also on the ureters, the stomach and the gut. This would account for the ureteric dilatation, and the reduced intestinal peristaltic activity which occurs in pregnancy.

Progesterone also regulates the storage of body fat to some extent, and is hyperthermic, leading to the temperature rise of 0.5 to 1°C found in pregnancy. By its action on the brain cells it may be responsible for the 'placidity' commonly found in pregnant women. It is implicated in the hyperventilation of pregnant women. A small amount of placental progesterone enters the fetal circulation,

where it is carried to the adrenal glands to act as a precursor for fetal corticosteroids.

**Pituitary gland**

There is evidence that ACTH, prolactin, thyrotrophin and melanocyte hormone activity increases as pregnancy advances, as does the production of the posterior pituitary hormones. It is also possible that a hormone, placentotrophin, is produced which enhances HCG production by the placenta, although the evidence for this is still equivocal.

Prolactin levels in blood plasma rise progressively during pregnancy (especially up to the 30th week), and may be a factor in producing the depression of pituitary gonadotrophic function which occurs. FSH and LH levels in plasma become very low by the 8th week of pregnancy and from then on, little synthesis of FSH or LH occurs. The reason may be the negative feedback of oestrogen and the supressing effect of prolactin on the gonadotrophic cells in the pituitary.

**Adrenal gland**

Total corticosteroids increase progressively during pregnancy, which could account for the pregnant woman's tendency to develop abdominal striae, glycosuria and hypertension, and also for the heavier features so commonly seen in pregnant women.

## Thyroid gland

The thyroid may enlarge in pregnancy, occasionally to twice its normal size, but there is no evidence of increased thyroid activity, and the enlargement is mainly due to colloid deposition. This in turn is in response to a reduced level of plasma iodine, due to the increased ability of the kidneys to excrete iodine in pregnancy. A rise in the circulating levels of thyroxine ($T_4$) and tri-iodothyronine ($T_3$) also occurs. This is not due to increased thyroid activity but to an oestrogen-stimulated secretion of thyroxine-binding globulin by the liver. The raised levels do not indicate hyperthyroidism, as TSH levels are unaltered and the *free* thyroxine levels are within the normal range. However, tests for thyroid function are altered in pregnancy and the diagnosis of hyperthyroidism made difficult (Table **4/1**).

|  | Normal non-pregnant | Normal pregnant |
|---|---|---|
| Total $T_4$ | $119 \pm 33$nmol/litre | $136 \pm 34$nmol/litre |
| Total $T_3$ | $2.4 \pm 1$nmol/litre | $3 \pm 0.8$nmol/litre |
| $T_3$ resin | $98\% \pm 16\%$ | $78\% \pm 18\%$ |

**Table 4/1** Alterations in tests for thyroid activity in pregnancy

## GENITAL TRACT

### Uterus and vagina

The effect of the hormonal stimulation is most marked upon the tissues of the genital tract, and the uterine muscle fibres grow to 15 times their pre-pregnant length during pregnancy, whilst uterine weight increases from 50g before pregnancy to 950g at term (Fig. **4/5**). In the early weeks of pregnancy the growth is by hyperplasia and more particularly by hypertrophy of the muscle fibres so that the uterus becomes a thick-walled spherical organ. From the 20th week, growth almost ceases and the uterus expands by distension, the stretching of the muscle fibres being due to the mechanical effect of the growing fetus. With distension the wall of the uterus becomes thinner and the shape cylindrical (Fig. **4/6**). The uterine blood vessels also undergo hypertrophy and become increasingly coiled in the first half of pregnancy, but no further growth occurs after this, and the additional length required to match the

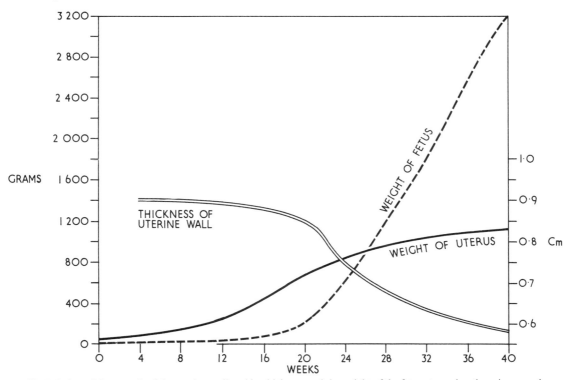

**Fig. 4/5** Relation of the growth of the uterine wall and its thickness and the weight of the fetus at varying times in normal pregnancy

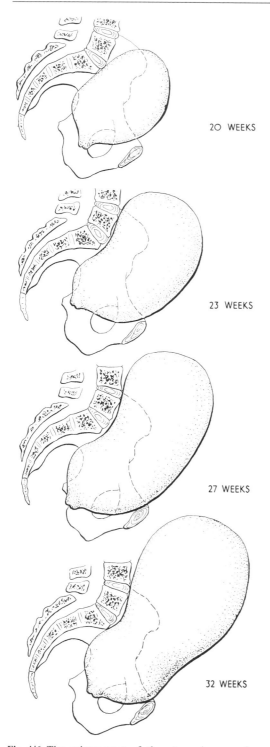

**Fig. 4/6** The enlargement of the uterus in normal pregnancy, drawn from radiographs

continuing uterine distension is obtained by uncoiling the vessels.

The uterus is derived from the two Mullerian ducts and the myometrium is made up of a thin external, largely longitudinal, layer; a thin inner, largely circular, layer and a thick intricately interlaced middle layer, which comprises two spiral systems of interdigitating muscles derived from the two Mullerian ducts. The proportion of muscle to connective tissue is greatest in the fundal area and diminishes as the lower segment of the uterus and cervix is approached, the lower half of the cervix having no more than 10 per cent of muscle tissue.

The effect of the uterine distension is to stretch both interdigitating spiral systems, and the angle of crossing of the fibres is greatest in the thick fundal area, and least in the thinner lower segment area where the fibres cross at an angle of about 160° and are less stretched. Incision of the myometrium in this zone is anatomically more suitable, and experience of lower segment caesarean section confirms that healing is better (Fig. **4/7**).

The lower uterine segment is that part of the lower uterus and upper cervix lying between the line of attachment of the peritoneum of the uterovesical pouch superiorly and the histological internal os inferiorly. It is that part of the uterus where the proportion of muscle diminishes, being replaced increasingly by connective tissue (mainly collagen fibres) which forms 90 per cent of the cervical tissues (Fig. **4/8**). Because of this it becomes stretched in

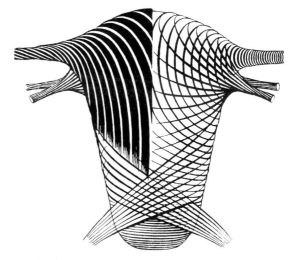

**Fig. 4/7** Representation of the obliquity of decussation and interweaving of myometrial fibres. The obtuse angle of decussation in the lower segment can be seen (from Bumm)

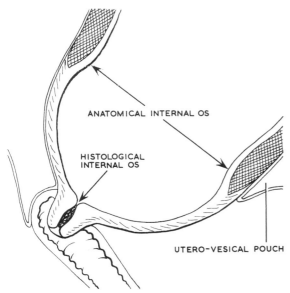

**Fig. 4/8** The lower uterine segment in late pregnancy (*see also* Fig. 7/8)

late pregnancy as the thickly muscled fundus draws it up from the relatively fixed cervix.

## Cervix

The cervix becomes softer and swollen in pregnancy so that the columnar epithelium lining the cervical canal becomes exposed to the vaginal secretions. This change in the cervix is due to oestradiol which increases the hygroscopic qualities of the cervical connective tissue and loosens the acid mucopolysaccharides (glycosaminoglycans) of the collagen-binding ground substance.

In addition, prostaglandins act on the collagen fibres especially in the last weeks of pregnancy. The cervix becomes softer and more easily dilatable, the so-called 'ripening' of the cervix. In this way the cervix is more easily able to dilate in labour.

## Vagina

The vaginal mucosa becomes thicker, the vaginal muscle hypertrophies and there is an alteration in the composition of the surrounding connective tissue, with the result that the vagina dilates more easily to accommodate the fetus in parturition. The changes, initiated by oestrogen, occur early in pregnancy and there is an increased desquamation of the superficial vaginal mucosal cells with increased vaginal discharge in pregnancy. Should pathogens, whether bacterial, fungal (such as candida) or parasitic (such as trichomonads) enter the vagina they can more easily establish themselves, and vaginitis is consequently more frequent.

## THE CARDIOVASCULAR SYSTEM

The *blood volume* increases in pregnancy apparently to fill the additional intravascular space caused by the development of the placenta and the blood vessels. The *plasma volume* increases from the tenth week of pregnancy reaching a maximum of 3800ml by the 32nd to 34th week when the increase is about 1200 to 1500ml, 50 per cent above the non-pregnant plasma volume. It then increases slightly to term. The *red cell mass* increases in a linear fashion to term from 1400ml in the non-pregnant to 1700ml in the last quarter of pregnancy. This is a 30 per cent increase (Fig. **4/9**). The red cell mass and red cell production, which is more rapid in pregnancy, are adjusted closely to, and regulated by, the increased demand for oxygen transport in pregnancy. Because the total increase in the red cell volume is proportionately less than the total increase in plasma volume, the concentration of the red cells in the blood falls, with a reduction in the haemoglobin concentration. This has been called the physiological anaemia of pregnancy, but it is a misleading term for although the *haemoglobin concentration* falls to about 12g at the 32nd week, the pregnant woman has a larger total haemoglobin than when non-pregnant (Table **4/2**).

During pregnancy iron is removed from the iron stores held in the bone marrow, the liver and the spleen, for use by the mother and are transferred to the fetus. The decrease in the quantity of stored iron is reflected by a fall in serum ferritin levels. A decrease in blood viscosity occurs, which provides a haemodynamic benefit.

As well as a rise in red cells, there is an increase in *white cells*, to about 10 500 per ml and an increase in *blood platelets*. The serum protein pattern alters, total protein, albumin and gamma globulin falling in the first quarter and then rising slowly towards term, whilst the beta globulin and the fibrinogen fractions rise. Because of the latter the erythrocyte sedimentation rate increases fourfold and cannot be used as a diagnostic measure in pregnancy. Serum lipids, particularly cholesterol, which is the precursor of oestrogen and progesterone, also increase in pregnancy.

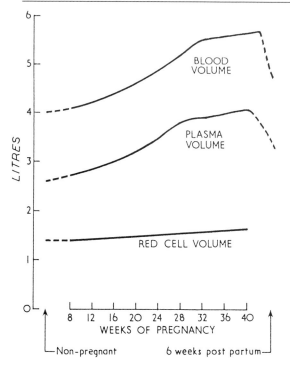

**Fig. 4/9** Blood changes in pregnancy (information obtained from Hytten and Leitch)

|  | Non-pregnant | Weeks of pregnancy | | |
|---|---|---|---|---|
|  |  | 20 | 30 | 40 |
| Plasma volume (ml) | 2600 | 3150 | 3750 | 3850 |
| Red cell mass (ml) | 1400 | 1450 | 1550 | 1650 |
| Total blood volume (ml) | 4000 | 4600 | 5300 | 5500 |
| Body hematocrit (%) | 35.0 | 32.0 | 29.0 | 30.0 |
| Venous hematocrit (%) | 39.8 | 36.4 | 33.0 | 34.1 |

**Table 4/2** Plasma volume, red cell volume, total blood volume and hematocrit in pregnancy

### Cardiovascular dynamics

To deal with the increased blood volume and additional requirements for oxygen, the cardiac output increases by 30 to 50 per cent in pregnancy, a rise from 5 litres per minute at the 10th week of pregnancy to 6.5 litres at about the 25th week. The raised level is then maintained to term (Fig. **4/10**). Most of the increased cardiac output is due to an increase in the stroke volume of the heart, due to the high circulating levels of oestrogen, but the heart rate also increases by about 15 per cent (Fig. **4/11**).

The increased cardiac output is balanced by a reduction in the peripheral resistance of the blood

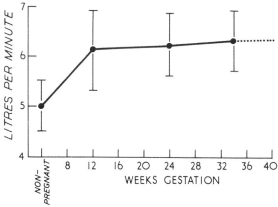

**Fig. 4/10** Cardiac output in pregnancy

vessels, owing to the effect of oestrogen and progesterone. For this reason the blood pressure is altered only minimally. In non-hypertensive women the diastolic blood pressure does not fall between the 15th and 25th week of pregnancy, as was once thought, but there is a tendency for it to rise after the 30th week.

In common with other vessels, the veins of the legs become more distensible, and with the obstruction offered to the venous return by the higher pressure of blood returning from the uterine veins, and the mechanical pressure of the uterus, the venous pressure rises and varicosities appear in those women

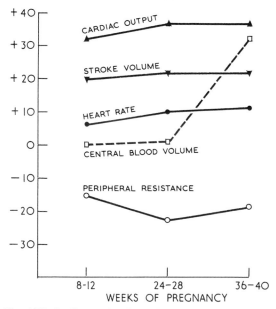

**Fig. 4/11** Cardiovascular dynamics: percentage alterations over non-pregnant levels occurring in pregnancy

with poor valves in their leg veins. The venous dilatation also occurs in the pulmonary vascular bed, and this explains the increased vascularity and enlarged pulmonary vessels seen on radiography in pregnancy.

### Regional distribution of blood flow

The uterus receives the greatest proportion of the increased blood flow, and recent evidence suggests that the flow increases from 75ml per minute at the 10th week of pregnancy to about 500ml in the 35th to 40th week. This increased uterine blood flow is vital to the fetus. In uterine systole, blood is forced under pressure into the chorio-decidual space from the endometrial arteries, and spurts through the intervillous lake to reach the chorionic plate. The stream loses velocity, surrounds and cascades over frond-like villi, allowing an exchange of nutrients and waste products to take place before it drains away through the endometrial veins in uterine diastole, to be replaced by a further spurt with the next systole.

In the kidneys, renal blood and plasma flow increase to 400ml per minute above non-pregnant levels by the 16th week, the flow remaining at this level to term. The blood flow through the skin and mucous membranes also increases, reaching a maximum of 500ml per minute (an increase of 70 per cent over non-pregnant flow) by the 36th week. The increased flow is associated with peripheral vasodilatation and this accounts for the clinical observation that pregnant women 'feel the heat', sweat easily and frequently complain of nasal congestion (Fig. 4/12).

## OTHER SYSTEMS

### The respiratory system

Breathing remains diaphragmatic in pregnancy, but because of the reduced movement of the diaphragm, pregnant women breathe more deeply and so increase the tidal volume, allowing for a better mixing of gases and an increased oxygen consumption which rises by 20 per cent. This is due to an increase in the ventilation rate from 7 litres per minute to 10 litres per minute (an increase of 40 per cent). This in effect causes 'overbreathing' and a lower arterial $pCO_2$. It is probably an effect of circulating

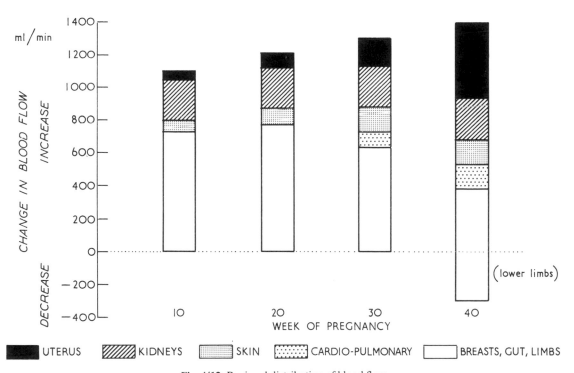

**Fig. 4/12** Regional distribution of blood flow

progesterone, and may contribute to the common complaint of dyspnoea. With advancing pregnancy the lower ribs flare out to accommodate the enlarging uterus, and do not always return to their normal position, to the annoyance of some of the more figure-conscious mothers.

### The alimentary system

Although there is no evidence of increased dental decay in pregnancy, the gums may become 'spongy', probably due to hormonal influences which lead to intracellular fluid retention. The entire musculature of the intestinal tract is relaxed and this is the cause of many minor discomforts in pregnancy. Oesophageal reflux due to relaxation of the cardiac sphincter may cause heartburn. Gastric secretion is reduced, and the food remains longer in the stomach. Delayed stomach emptying is particularly marked during labour, when food can remain in the stomach for up to 48 hours. The relaxed intestinal muscle also leads to lowered motility, and although this permits more complete absorption of foodstuffs, it leads to constipation which often occurs in pregnancy.

### The renal system

The smooth muscle of the renal pelvis, the ureters and the bladder undergo relaxation in pregnancy leading to dilatation of the renal pelvis and ureters (Fig. **4/13**). The dilatation begins about the 10th week of pregnancy and is mainly of the abdominal portion of the ureter which has relatively less muscle and is loosely supported by connective tissue. The loose support can also lead to kinking in the middle portion. The effect of dilatation is to increase the capacity of the renal pelvis and ureters from 12 to 75ml, and to increase the risk of urinary stasis. Relaxation of the muscle of the bladder also encourages urinary stasis, and the risk of infection of the urine in the bladder and ascending infection to the renal pelvis is greatly increased.

In early pregnancy water excretion by the kidney is increased, and causes frequency of micturition which may be misdiagnosed as due to infection. The increased ability to excrete water diminishes as pregnancy advances, and the frequency of micturition in late pregnancy is due to the pressure of the fetus and uterus upon the bladder.

The renal blood flow increases until the 16th week of pregnancy when it levels off, remaining at the

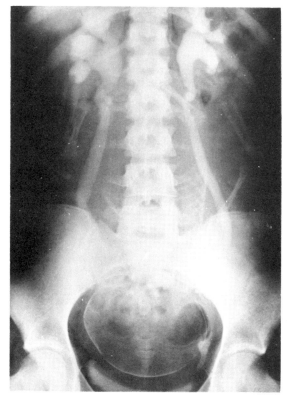

**Fig. 4/13** Dilatation of the renal pelvis and ureters in pregnancy, as shown by radiology

higher level until delivery. More important, the glomerular filtration rate rises by 60 per cent in early pregnancy, and remains at this high level until the last 3 or 4 weeks of pregnancy when it falls significantly. As tubular reabsorption is unaltered, the clearance of many solutes is increased and urea, uric acid, glucose, amino-acids and folic acid are more readily excreted. The increased glomerular filtration rates, augmented by the natriuretic effect of progesterone, would also lead to the excess loss of sodium, were it not for a compensatory mechanism. To conserve sodium, the renin–angiotensin–aldosterone system is stimulated. Renin produced in the kidney acts on its substrate to produce angiotensin. This in turn acts on the adrenal cortex inducing aldosterone secretion, which in turn enhances the resorption of sodium from the renal tubules, so that maternal electrolyte homeostasis is preserved.

Because of the increased secretion of renal renin the level of plasma renin rises, but there is a parallel decline in responsiveness to angiotensin II.

### Immune system

Serum levels of IgG, IgA and IgM decrease significantly from about the 10th week, reaching their lowest level at the 30th week and then levelling off. This reduction is probably due to the effect of haemodilution and of immune suppression; it may account for the increased risk of infection which occurs during pregnancy.

## THE EFFECT OF THE PHYSIOLOGICAL ALTERATIONS

Many of the changes outlined are the result of the increased production of oestrogen and progesterone by the trophoblast, and most are anticipatory of fetal needs, since they occur when fetal demands are insignificant. Later when fetal metabolism increases, additional oxygen and nutrients have to be brought to the placenta for elaboration and transfer to the fetus, and fetal waste products have to be removed and returned to the maternal circulation. The key organ in all these complex chemical reactions is the placenta.

So that the transfer of nutrients between maternal blood and trophoblast may be readily effected, there is a quiescence of maternal metabolism, and exchange between the mother's blood and her own tissues is reduced allowing a higher concentration of nutrients to reach the placenta. This quiescence leads to a reduction in insulin sensitivity, so that glucose remains in the blood longer, and a reduction in thyroid activity, which further slows metabolism and permits increased fat deposition. Further energy is conserved by the reduction of muscle tone. The conservation of energy continues throughout pregnancy and is thought to be an evolutionary safeguard so that the mother can feed her baby should she herself be unable to obtain extra food after delivery.

An effect of the higher blood concentration of nutrients and delayed exchange between maternal blood and tissues, is that a higher concentration reaches the kidneys. Since glomerular filtration is increased but tubular reabsorption unaltered, there is a greater loss of nutrients, which is part of the price paid for the quiescent metabolism. The blood volume increases to fill the additional intravascular space created by the placenta, and the heart rate and stroke volume rise to cope with the increase. Owing to the greater proportionate increase in the plasma volume, the constituents of the blood alter, the haemoglobin concentration falling and the serum protein pattern altering considerably. However, there is more total haemoglobin available and this adjusts precisely to the increased oxygen required by the fetus. The oxygen is obtained by a better exchange of gases in the lungs. The entire female organism adapts to preserve and nourish the fetus growing within the uterus, and with the anabolic metabolism comes a mental tranquillity and somnolent beauty.

# WEIGHT GAIN IN PREGNANCY

A healthy normotensive primigravida may expect to gain 12.5kg (28lb) in pregnancy, of which 9kg (20lb) is gained in the last 20 weeks. This 'ideal' weight gain is only a guide and individual variations must be allowed: an undernourished woman should be encouraged to gain more weight.

An obese woman should be encouraged to lose weight before becoming pregnant as obesity is associated with an increased risk that pregnancy-induced hypertension will occur, and the woman is more likely to have a large baby, which may cause a difficult childbirth. During pregnancy an obese woman should eat a prudent, but not a restricted diet, as dietary restriction has not been shown to confer any advantage either to mother or her baby. A woman who is underweight (Body Mass Index less than 19) should avoid becoming pregnant until she has gained weight, as she has a 20 per cent chance of giving birth to a growth-retarded infant, particularly if ovulation has been induced in the menstrual cycle in which she conceived. Apart from these dangers, women who gain weight excessively in pregnancy find it difficult to return to their pre-pregnant weight, and permanent obesity may persist. Since most women are concerned about keeping their figure, the doctor may stress that a weight gain of more than 15kg (33lb) in pregnancy is usually followed by a permanent increase in weight, and women should be advised to gain no more than 0.5kg (1.1lb) per week in the last 20 weeks of pregnancy.

The weight gain in pregnancy is made up of several components:

1. The products of conception
   a. The fetus, the placenta and the liquor amnii.
2. The maternal components
   a. The uterus and breasts
   b. The increased blood volume
   c. Fat and protein storage
   d. Water storage.

**The fetus**

The average birth-weight increases with higher socio-economic groups, and babies born to women in Australia, Britain and the USA are heavier than those born to women in Asia and Africa. The average birth-weight of a British or an Australian child is 3300g (7.5lb) whilst that of an Indian child is 2900g (6.5lb) but the latter is no less vital and able to survive. Birth-weight is not affected by maternal age, but increases with birth order, later babies being heavier, and is reduced by cigarette smoking.

In the uterus, the fetus initially gains weight only slowly, but after the 20th week a steady increase occurs. The weight of the placenta follows a reverse pattern, the most rapid gain occurring in the first 15 weeks, with a steady increase to 20 weeks and then a slow increase to term. Before the 15th week the placenta weighs more than the fetus, but after this time forms a progressively smaller proportion of the products of conception and by term its weight is about 20 per cent short of that of the baby (Fig. **4/14**)

**The liquor amnii**

The liquor amnii increases rapidly from the 10th week of pregnancy reaching a total of 300ml at 20 weeks, 600ml at 30 weeks and 1000ml at 35 weeks, after which a slow decline occurs to 600ml at term, and rapid drop after this so that by the 43rd week only 250ml of liquor remains. The liquor maintains the fetus at a constant temperature and protects it from injury. Almost weightless in the liquor, the fetus is able to move with minimal energy loss. As well as this, recent research shows that the liquor possesses antibacterial activity against both Gram-positive and Gram-negative organisms.

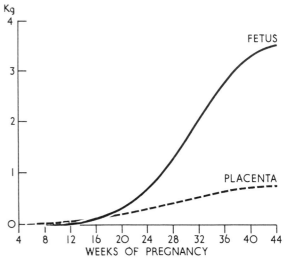

**Fig. 4/14** Fetal and placental weight curves compared at various gestation periods

**The maternal components**

The weight of the *uterus* increases through pregnancy, more rapidly in the first 20 weeks, when hyperplasia is maximal, and then slowly to 40 weeks. At term the organ weighs about 900g more than its non-pregnant weight. The *breast weight* increases throughout pregnancy, as does the *blood volume. Fat deposition* in healthy pregnant women who live in the developed nations is variable, depending on the woman's intake of fat and carbohydrate. A gain of between 2.5 and 3.0kg of fat is usual, of which 90 per cent is deposited before the 30th week of pregnancy. This stored fat can liberate between 90 and 105MJ (21 000 and 25 000 kcal) of energy after childbirth for various activities, including breast-feeding. *Protein deposition* occurs throughout pregnancy but the extra amount retained is small.

In normal pregnancy the total body fluid increases by 6 to 8 litres, of which between 2 and 4 litres are extracellular. Sodium is retained with the water and about 900mmol is retained by the end of pregnancy. Most of the fluid is retained after the 30th week of pregnancy, and this accounts for much of the weight gain during this period. A normal woman, without any evidence of oedema, retains between 2 and 3 litres of extracellular fluid, mainly in the last 10 weeks of the pregnancy.

Excessive fluid retention may be detected by regular weighing before the appearance of clinical oedema, and an increase of more than 1kg (2.2lb) in any one week of pregnancy after the 30th week

| | |
|---|---|
| Fetus | 3300g |
| Placenta | 600g |
| Uterus | 900g |
| Breasts (glandular tissue) | 400g |
| Blood | 1200g |
| Fat deposited | 2500g |
| Fluid (extracellular) | 2600g |
| | 11 500g |

**Table 4/3** The components of the weight gain in pregnancy

should be viewed with suspicion, as excessive weight gain may be an early sign of impending pregnancy-induced hypertension.

In instructing pregnant women to avoid excessive weight gain common sense must be used, and compli-cated regimens avoided. Variability from the norm is usual and pregnancy should be treated as a pleasant physiological event, and not made into a pathological nightmare by officious, malinstructed physicians.

**The energy costs of pregnancy**

The extra energy required for the growth of the fetus and the placenta, the increase in the size of the maternal organs, the extra fat, and the increased metabolic rate, is about 250MJ (60 000kcal) over the entire pregnancy. This works out at about 0.9MJ (230kcal) a day – an amount provided by two slices of bread and 100ml of milk!

## Chapter 5

# The Diagnosis of Pregnancy

Most patients first believe that they are pregnant and visit their physician to confirm this belief. A few deliberately falsify their symptoms, knowing that they are pregnant, in an attempt to procure termination of the unwanted pregnancy. A few have many of the symptoms and signs of pregnancy without any fetus in the uterus. The diagnosis of pregnancy is of importance to all these groups. It is more informative to divide the pregnancy into four periods of 10 weeks, rather than three periods, or trimesters, which is the conventional method.

### FIRST QUARTER

*Amenorrhoea* in a woman who has previously menstruated regularly must be considered due to pregnancy, until disproved. Of course, pregnancy is not the only cause of amenorrhoea, which may occur because of emotional stress, hormonal imbalance or local uterine conditions, but it is the commonest cause. Some women become pregnant during a period of amenorrhoea, either during a period of emotional stress, during lactation or at the time of the menopause. In a few women pregnancy may be present despite menstrual-like bleeding, occurring at the correct cyclical time. Bleeding in these episodes is usually scanty, and has been referred to as the 'placental sign' which is the rule in monkeys. With these provisos, any woman who becomes amenorrhoeic after regular menstruation should be considered pregnant until disproved.

*Nausea and vomiting.* Nausea occurs in over 50 per cent of pregnant women, usually between the 4th and 9th week after the last menstrual period.

*Bladder irritability.* Frequency of micturition, due to physiological changes, is common in the first trimester.

## SIGNS

### Breasts

Abnormal heaviness and enlargement of the breasts, with associated symptoms of tension, are usual in early pregnancy, particularly in women who develop breast tension in the premenstruum. With pregnancy, the nipple and areola increase in size and become darker in colour, and the area around the areola often becomes discoloured, with distended veins. In the primary areola, Montgomery's tubercles become prominent. The breast changes may be the earliest indication of pregnancy, particularly in the primigravida.

### Vagina

Owing to the increased vascularity occasioned by the increased oestrogen secretion, a dusky bluish discoloration may be seen in the vulva, extending up the anterior vaginal wall. The vagina and cervix become softer and more distensible. These symptoms are apparent from the 4th week, but since they are due to vascular congestion, may be brought about by other conditions such as uterine myomata and other pelvic tumours.

### Uterus

The uterus enlarges and softens in preparation for the growing fetus, and the uterine development anticipates the growth of the ovum. Between the 6th and 10th week, the embryo only occupies the upper part of the uterus, the lower part being empty. On bimanual examination, the softened lower part can be easily compressed between the fingers, in contradistinction to the firmer cervix below and the globular fundal area containing the fetus above. This

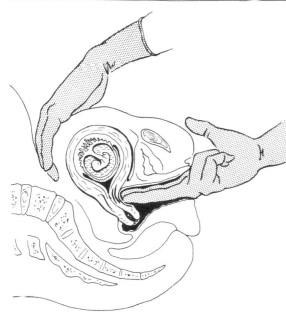

**Fig. 5/1** Hegar's sign

is Hegar's sign (Fig. **5/1**). Once the entire uterine cavity is occupied by the growing embryo, the sign disappears. This occurs at the end of the 10th week.

### Immunological tests for pregnancy

With the development of trophoblast, the syncytium synthesizes and releases into the circulation large amounts of human chorionic gonadotrophin (HCG),

especially of the beta sub-unit of HCG, which can be measured by a sensitive monoclonal anti-HCG antibody test. The test can detect small amounts of beta HCG ( > 0.8IU) in plasma or urine. These quantities are found at the time of the missed period. The test can be made in a laboratory, or the woman can purchase a home-testing kit.

The measurement of beta HCG: (1) enables pregnancy to be detected very early, (2) ectopic gestation to be excluded by two negative tests on successive days, and (3) trophoblastic disease follow-up to be performed.

### Ultrasound

Ultrasound can be used to visualize the fetus as early as 6 weeks, and in cases of doubt may be helpful (Fig. **5/2**).

## THE REMAINING THREE QUARTERS OF PREGNANCY

The symptoms of nausea, vomiting and bladder irritability usually cease by the 14th week, whilst the amenorrhoea continues. At about the 18th to 20th week in primigravidae, and 2 weeks earlier in multigravidae, the first faint fluttering movements of fetal activity ('quickening') will be felt. The movements increase in strength as pregnancy proceeds.

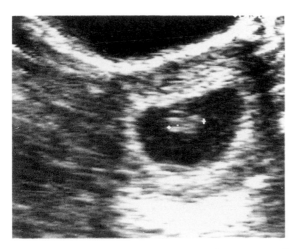

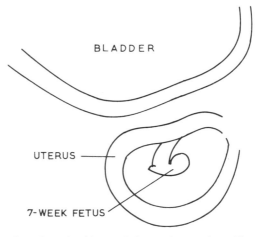

**Fig. 5/2** Ultrasound scan showing normal fetus at 7 weeks. The patient showed evidence of threatening to abort. The pregnancy continued to term. Line drawing shows identification of landmarks

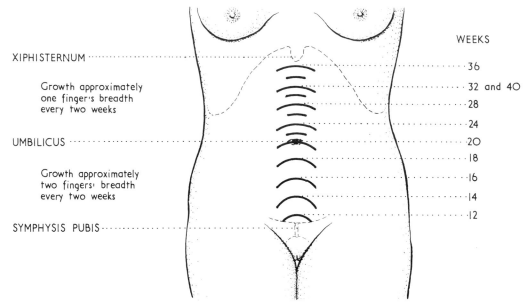

XIPHISTERNUM

Growth approximately
one finger's breadth
every two weeks

UMBILICUS

Growth approximately
two fingers' breadth
every two weeks

SYMPHYSIS PUBIS

WEEKS

36

32 and 40

28

24

20

18

16

14

12

**Fig. 5/3** The abdominal markings of uterine growth related to the number of weeks after the last menstrual period

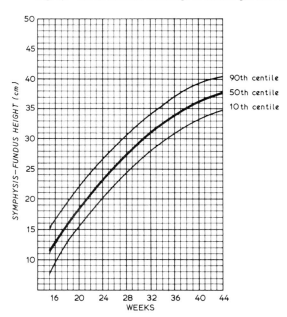

90th centile

50th centile

10th centile

**Fig. 5/4** Gestational age estimated from symphysis-fundal height

## SIGNS

### Uterus

In the second quarter, the uterus becomes palpable

on abdominal examination, and some estimation of the duration of the pregnancy can be obtained by determining the height of the fundus (Fig. **5/3**). The accuracy of this estimation is variable, and depends on the tenseness of the abdominal muscles and the obesity of the abdominal wall. A more accurate method is to measure the symphysis-fundus height. The patient lies on her back, with her legs straight and her bladder empty. The height of the fundus is determined with gentle pressure of the ulnar border of the hand and is marked. The distance from the upper border of the symphysis to the fundal mark is measured and compared with the expected height by referring to a chart (Fig. **5/4**). This technique is also useful in determining if the fetus is small-for-dates in the second half of pregnancy (Chapter 36).

On vaginal examination the enlarged uterus will be detected, and it may be felt to contract. Enlargement of the uterus due to myomata, or to the presence of an ovarian cyst (Fig. **5/5**), may lead to confusion, but if the uterus is pushed forward by the fingers in the anterior fornix, the fetus may be felt to leave and then return to the finger. This is called internal ballottement.

### Fetal heart sounds

The fetal heart can be observed beating from the 6th week of pregnancy by real-time ultrasound, and can

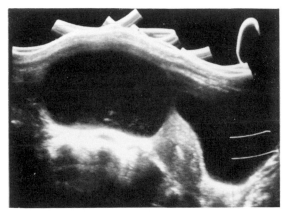
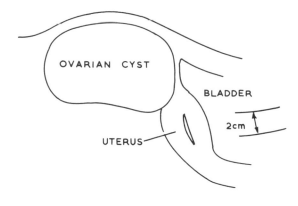

OVARIAN CYST

BLADDER

2cm

UTERUS

**Fig. 5/5** Sagittal scan showing an ovarian cyst. Line drawing shows the identification of relevant points

be heard using an ultrasonic detector from the 10th week of pregnancy. At this stage the machine's accuracy is 40 per cent, by the 15th week it increases to 95 per cent.

Clinical examination of the mother's abdomen, using a stethoscope (or a fetal heart detector) detects the fetal heart from about the 20th week of pregnancy. The sounds are best heard over the fetal back and the rate varies between 120 and 160 beats per minute.

**Palpation of fetal parts**

The fetus can be directly palpated after the 25th week of pregnancy, and its position and presentation can be defined. These may vary from examination to examination.

**Medical imaging of the fetus**

Ultrasound has largely replaced radiology in the detection of fetal abnormal conditions. Some obstetricians routinely examine all patients between the 12 and 20th week (see also p. 58). The examination (1) confirms the gestation period, (2) establishes the presence or absence of a multiple pregnancy, (3) identifies some fetal malformations. In cases of suspected fetal growth retardation a further ultrasound examination at about the 34th week may provide an additional diagnostic help. In cases of suspected intra-uterine fetal death, real-time ultrasound establishes the diagnosis by failing to detect fetal heart pulsations.

**Uterine contractions**

Although these occur at long intervals from early pregnancy, they become increasingly frequent and stronger after the 30th week (i.e. in the last quarter of pregnancy) when they are palpable and may even cause discomfort. At this time they are known as Braxton Hicks contractions (see Chapter 9).

**PSEUDOCYESIS**

Emotional disturbance such as the intense desire for pregnancy, fear of losing a husband or lover, or desire to achieve parity with other women, can cause stimulation of the hypothalamus and the release of gonadotrophic hormones. The patients complain of all the symptoms of pregnancy, but often in a bizarre order. All have amenorrhoea. The breasts become heavy, with secretion of cloudy fluid from the nipples, the abdomen enlarged because of fat or flatus. Indeed, on physical examination the patient appears to be pregnant, with the exception that the uterus is not enlarged (Fig. 5/6).

Once the absence of pregnancy has been determined, the patient should be given sympathetic psychiatric attention.

**DIAGNOSIS OF PREVIOUS PREGNANCY**

The breasts show pigmentation of the areolae, the

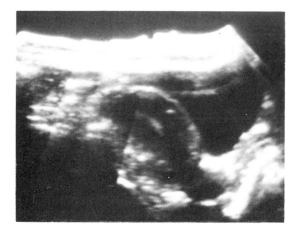 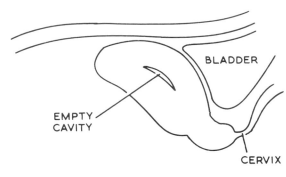

**Fig. 5/6** An ultrasound picture showing an empty normal uterus in a woman who had pseudocyesis (longitudinal scan). Line drawing shows the identification of relevant points

abdominal wall may show striae, and the abdominal muscles may be stretched. On vaginal examination, the hymen is replaced by small tags (carunculae myrtiformes) and evidence of a repaired perineal tear or a gaping introitus may be present. On specu-lum examination, the external cervical os is slit-like, and not round.

The diagnosis can be difficult, as the abdominal signs are produced by other conditions, and a firm opinion can seldom be given.

# Chapter 6

# Antenatal Care

It is only in the past 50 years that as much attention has been paid to the 40 weeks of pregnancy as is paid to the 14 hours of labour. During this time there has been a marked, and progressive, reduction in both maternal and fetal mortality and morbidity, and the availability of adequate antenatal care is largely responsible for this.

The aims of adequate antenatal care are to ensure:

(1) that the mother reaches the end of pregnancy as healthy as, or even healthier than, she was at the outset
(2) that any physical or psychological problems are detected and treated
(3) that any complication of pregnancy is either prevented or detected early and managed adequately
(4) that the mother is delivered of a healthy baby
(5) that the mother has the opportunity to discuss her anxieties and fears about the pregnancy, and the right to be informed about proposed procedures
(6) that the couple are prepared for childbirth and child rearing (including receiving information about diet, child care and family planning).

These objectives may be met in several ways depending on local conditions, facilities, personnel and custom, but several assumptions can be made. First, antenatal care may (and should) be provided by family doctors as well as obstetric specialists. Second, trained nurse–midwives can play a major role in community-based and hospital outpatient obstetric care. Third, in many instances obstetric units or hospitals are not the most appropriate place for the provision of routine antenatal care. Fourth, highly trained specialist obstetricians, neonatologists and their hospital-based teams have the major role in managing complicated pregnancies, particularly when the newer technologies are involved.

Antenatal care is largely an exercise in preventive medicine, and during the antenatal period, in addition to detecting any abnormality which may arise, instruction should be given in general hygiene and in the care of the baby.

So that doctors and other members of the obstetric team may best fulfil their roles as advisers or confidantes of the expectant mother, it is essential that they have knowledge of the psychological and nutritional requirements of the pregnant woman, and are able to communicate easily and clearly with her. For these reasons, before the organization of antenatal care is discussed, the psychological preparation for motherhood and elements of nutrition will be considered.

## THE PSYCHOLOGICAL PREPARATION FOR MOTHERHOOD

The idea that a mother is a passive, ignorant receptacle for a growing fetus, who is best kept uninformed about the changes occurring within her, has been a long time dying. All too often, whether in hospital, or midwife-controlled antenatal clinics, or in the consulting rooms of doctors, the patient is shunted on a sort of conveyor belt system to be processed, but never has the reason for the procedures explained to her. Added to this are the cultural misconceptions regarding pregnancy and labour which are handed down by word of mouth from mother to daughter in all communities. The attitudes derived from this ancestral information are frequently disadvantageous and often dangerous to the health of the mother and her baby.

Since one of the purposes of antenatal care is to prepare the mother for labour, and for the care of her newborn baby, the attendants of the pregnant woman have a unique opportunity to inform, instruct and educate women in elements of hygiene, in baby care and to demolish the accumulated racial myths related to parturition.

Naturally the approach will differ in different communities, but in all, an informed patient is the more co-operative in accepting the need for antenatal care, and labour is to her a much less frightening and traumatic episode. In Christian societies, the idea that 'in sorrow shall you bring forth your child', and that this is a retribution for the influence Eve had in inducing Adam to taste the forbidden fruit, is in the racial consciousness, although it is accepted that it is both unchristian and mythical.

The idea that pregnancy and labour are normal physiological functions of viviparous mammals must be suggested to the patient as often as possible.

It is well established that most primigravidae, and a large number of multigravidae, experience an increase in anxiety during pregnancy and have doubts or fears about childbirth. There is some evidence that the greater the anxiety, the greater is the chance that labour will be more difficult. The most usual anxieties are that the baby will die in utero, will not be born normally and will not be healthy. The second most common concerns are that childbirth will be traumatic and that pain relief will not be provided. Other anxieties relate to contraception after the birth, that drugs taken in pregnancy may cause birth defects, and that the birth of the child will alter the relationship between the woman and her husband.

Opportunity must be given for pregnant women to talk about their anxieties to empathetic, informed, communicative medical attendants. If everyone has the appearance of being rushed, the patient will feel that she cannot ask questions as the 'doctor is too busy'. The doctor and the nurse-midwife should talk to the patient during the antenatal examinations. They should seek to allay her fears, and obtain her co-operation by describing the changes which are occurring in her body and explaining the purpose of each investigation they make. No question which the patient asks, no matter how stupid it seems, should ever be ridiculed, but should be answered directly. The patient is naturally interested in the welfare of her baby, and its size and position should be told her after abdominal palpation.

Another hidden anxiety is a fear of the pain of childbirth. All too often the young mother is told of the gruesome imagined experience of older women, or else has a cultural myth which she has heard from childhood. These fears and anxieties should be dispelled by simple explanations of the nature and course of labour. Books are available (for example, my book *Everywoman, A Gynaecological Guide for Life*). In many hospitals instructional classes are held, but every attendant can reduce the anxiety of the mother by sympathetic explanation.

# ELEMENTS OF NUTRITION

To live and grow, man requires food. He needs food to supply energy for his essential functions, he needs food to maintain the structure of the tissues of the body. The cells of the body are not static structures; there is a constant turnover, many cells being broken down whilst others are being formed. It is true that many of the breakdown products can be used again, but inevitably additional substances are required to replace those lost in metabolism, in the faeces and in the urine. In pregnancy, the development of the fetus within the uterus places an additional demand for nutrients upon the mother.

The chemical components of the diet are termed the nutrients, and these include carbohydrates, fats, proteins, alcohol, water, minerals and vitamins.

### Carbohydrates

The main dietary carbohydrate is starch, which is present in all cereal grains, in potatoes, and in other tubers. In the body, starch is broken down into sugar, and of course the average diet has sugar added in the form of sucrose obtained from sugar-cane or sugar beet. Starch and sucrose supply about

50 to 80 per cent of the total calories in the diet. The proportion provided by carbohydrates is higher in the developing countries and amongst the poorer section of the community in the developed countries. This is because carbohydrates, usually in the form of rice, maize or wheat, are a relatively cheap source of energy. Carbohydrates break down in the body to carbon dioxide and water, and in the breakdown release about 16.8kJ (4kcal) per gram of carbohydrate ingested. A normal diet contains 300 to 500g of carbohydrate, which provides 5028–8380kJ (1200 to 2000kcal).

## Fat

The second main source of energy is fat, which in the richer countries of the world provides a man with 40 per cent of the energy he needs. The 'average' man or woman in the developed countries eats about 140g of fat a day, mainly as butter, or in the fat present in cakes, puddings and sauces. One gram of fat releases 38kJ (9kcal), so that about 5279kJ (1260kcal) are added to the energy supply each day. In the poorer countries of the world, the average person has a smaller intake of fat, as foods rich in fat are expensive. In India, for example, an average of 10 to 20g of fat is eaten daily. Fats (or more correctly lipids) are mainly triglycerides, which are saturated fatty acids. In addition to them, the diet needs to supply certain essential unsaturated fatty acids, which the human is unable to synthesize. However, the requirement is very low, and is provided by even the poorest diet.

Most of the ingested fats are oxidized in the body via aceto-acetic acid to carbon. In cases when carbohydrate intake is greatly reduced, as in persistent vomiting, or when its metabolism is disturbed as in diabetes, energy is obtained by breaking down stored fats. These release quantities of aceto-acetic acid, which circulates in excessive amounts and is excreted in the urine. The condition is known as acido-ketosis.

## Protein

An adequate intake of protein is essential in order to replace the continuous breakdown of body proteins which make up the bulk of the muscles of the body. Each day between 200 and 400g of protein, which represents 3 per cent of the total body protein, is broken down into its constituent amino-acids, and is re-synthesized. Most of the amino-acids are used again, but some are lost and must be provided in the diet, or disease will result. Protein breakdown also provides energy, 1g releasing 16.8kJ (4kcal). The average diet of a woman in the Western developed countries provides between 70 and 100g of protein, which is more than is necessary to maintain tissue repair. There are two forms of protein. First-class proteins are mainly animal proteins, i.e. those found in meat, eggs and milk. These proteins contain all the essential amino-acids. The second group are second-class proteins, which lack certain amino-acids, and are mainly vegetable proteins. Fortunately these vegetable proteins have different amino-acid constituents, and a mixture of them will provide all the essential amino-acids needed. In the developing countries, where first-class proteins are too expensive for the average family, protein deficiency can be avoided if the family eats a mixture of vegetable proteins. Unfortunately protein deficiency is all too common in these countries, particularly in children. This leads to much ill-health and a higher mortality rate in childhood.

It is considered that ideally an individual should eat 0.5g/kg protein per day, and that preferably this should contain a mixture of first-class and second-class protein.

Proteins break down in the body to amino-acids, which are the building blocks of new proteins. During this process, energy and nitrogen are released. The nitrogen combines with body substance, to form, particularly, urea, and 90 per cent is excreted in the urine.

In pregnancy, particularly after the 20th week, there is an increased requirement for protein, which is needed for the growth of the fetus. It is for this reason that it is recommended that a pregnant woman obtain about 1g protein/kg per day.

## Minerals

Minerals are essential for normal metabolic processes. The principal minerals required are sodium (Na), potassium (K), calcium (Ca), magnesium (Mg), phosphorus (P) and iron (Fe). With the exception of iron, the diet of most pregnant women contains adequate amounts of minerals. Iron deficiency is fairly common, however, and is considered in Chapter 28. In addition to these minerals, trace elements are needed. These include cobalt, copper, fluorine, iodine, manganese and zinc. Deficiency of these trace elements, except in gross starvation, is rare.

## Vitamins

Vitamins are compounds which are essential for the proper functioning of enzyme systems in the body. Enzyme systems implement most cellular activity. Unfortunately the human is unable to synthesize most vitamins, and these must be supplied in the diet. Vitamin deficiency is much less common today, but vitamin deficiency diseases continue to occur in the developing countries. They include beri-beri, pellagra, keratomalacia, scurvy and rickets.

The term vitamin was suggested because the substances were thought to be 'vital amines'. Originally they were given capital letters as each new one was discovered. Today the chemical compositions of the vitamins are known, and it would be better to use the chemical names. Vitamins can be divided into two main classes – the fat-soluble vitamins and the water-soluble vitamins. Since the body has stores of fat in which vitamins may be deposited, vitamin deficiency due to lack of water-soluble vitamins tends to occur earlier and to be more severe. Fat-soluble vitamins pose a further problem: if too much of the vitamin is ingested in the mistaken belief that if a little is good for you, a lot must be better, the vitamin may be stored in excess in the liver and lead to toxic side-effects. Water-soluble vitamins are excreted readily in the urine, so that this problem does not arise with them.

## Fat-soluble vitamins

### RETINOL, OR VITAMIN A

Retinol is present in dairy foods, liver, and particularly in fish-liver oils. The vitamin can also be formed in the body from carotene, which is a pigment widely found in fruits and vegetables. In the average European diet, about half the supply of retinol comes from carotene, and half from dairy products. In the developing countries of Asia, Africa and South America, vitamin A deficiency is not uncommon, as dairy products are too expensive and the diet may contain inadequate supplies of fruit and vegetables.

The first sign of vitamin A deficiency is night blindness, but in more severe deprivation epithelial surfaces are unable to shed the superficial cells and these pile up as a thickened (keratinized) layer. This particularly affects the cornea of the eye, which becomes opaque and softened (keratomalacia). Quite

quickly the cornea collapses and infection enters leading to permanent blindness. Because breast milk of the poorer mothers may be deficient in retinol, and because of nutritional deficiencies after weaning, keratomalacia and blindness is still far too common in the poorer countries of the world.

The recommended requirement of vitamin A for a pregnant or lactating woman is 6000IU per day. In Western countries this is provided in the normal diet, and supplements are only required exceptionally.

### CALCIFEROL, OR VITAMIN D

Calciferol is involved in the metabolism of calcium. It promotes the absorption of calcium from the gut, and encourages its deposition in bone. Vitamin D is obtained from dairy products, cheese, milk, butter, and from eggs and liver. Fish-liver oil is a particularly rich source of the vitamin. As in the case of retinol, calciferol can be synthesized in the body from precursors in the skin by the action of ultraviolet light. It is not yet known how much of the needs are provided in the diet, and how much by sunlight acting on dehydrocholesterol in the skin.

Deficiency of vitamin D, operating during childhood when the bones of the legs and pelvis are soft and malleable, produces rickets. The word is appropriate, for it comes from the old Anglo-Saxon word, *wrikken* – to twist. If the deficiency occurs later in life and is associated with a calcium lack, the shape of the pelvis is markedly distorted, the condition being called osteomalacia.

The Industrial Revolution of the late eighteenth century brought thousands of countrymen into the newer industrial cities of Western Europe. Here they huddled in poor, overcrowded housing, received minimal wages, whilst overhead a pall of smoke blocked out the sun. The children were deprived of adequate supplies of dairy foods, and lacked sunshine, so that vitamin D deficiency occurred and rickets was very common. In Britain, rickets disappeared after World War II, when sensible dietary measures ensured that no pregnant woman or her child was deficient in vitamin D. This single measure changed the practice of obstetrics considerably, and contracted pelvis due to rickets is now most unusual. Cases of rickets, however, still occur in the Asian immigrant population.

Evidence has been presented recently that pregnant Asian women in Britain have reduced 25-hydroxy vitamin D levels, and a number of their babies develop symptomatic hypocalcaemia in the neonatal period. The cause of the vitamin deficiency is uncertain. It may be due to an inadequate intake in the diet (particularly if the woman is a vegetarian) or to lack of exposure to sunshine. It seems that most Asian pregnant women in Britain should receive a daily supplement of calciferol 1000IU.

Although the people of the developing countries do not eat many dairy products, the abundant sunshine reduces the likelihood of rickets, with one main exception. Muslim women in North India are still often kept in purdah, and because of the lack of exposure to sunshine, vitamin D deficiency may occur with resulting osteomalacia.

It is recommended that a pregnant woman takes 400IU of calciferol a day. The diet of most women in the developed countries of the world easily supplies their need.

## TOCOPHEROL, OR VITAMIN E

It has been claimed that lack of tocopherol is responsible for abortion, infertility and muscular ailments. These claims have not been supported by any controlled scientific study and vitamin E has no place in the treatment of abortion or any other disorder in adults.

## VITAMIN K

Except in newborn babies, vitamin K deficiency is unknown in man. This is because it is synthesized in the intestine by the action of the intestinal bacteria.

## Water-soluble vitamins

## ASCORBIC ACID, OR VITAMIN C

Deficiency of ascorbic acid leads to swollen and bleeding gums, to bruising and to haemorrhages in various internal organs – a disease entity called scurvy. The vitamin, which is a sugar, is obtained from fruit and vegetables, and these are the only sources. Of the vegetables, green leafy vegetables such as cabbage have the highest concentration, but potatoes provide an adequate amount. Unfortunately, ascorbic acid is easily destroyed by moderate temperatures, and consequently the peculiarly Anglo-Saxon habit of cooking vegetables in large quantities of boiling water is to be condemned.

The requirement of a pregnant woman is about 50mg per day. This is easily provided in a normal diet, as an orange supplies 30mg, a slice of papaya (or pawpaw) 30mg, an ordinary helping of green leafy vegetables 20mg, and a good helping of potatoes (say 100g, or 3oz) about 10mg. Only in instances where fresh fruit and leafy vegetables are not eaten is a dietary supplement necessary.

## THIAMINE, OR VITAMIN B$_1$

Thiamine is found in all living cells, and the main source in foodstuffs is in the aleuron of the cereal grain. Machine milling of wheat and rice removes the husk, and consequently reduces the thiamine intake. Wholemeal bread and unpolished rice provide ample thiamine, as do peas, beans and other pulses. In Western countries, thiamine deficiency is unusual, but in Asia it is not uncommon. The disease produced is called beri-beri. Pregnant and lactating women require about 1 to 1.5mg of thiamine a day.

## RIBOFLAVINE, OR VITAMIN B$_2$

Deficiency of this vitamin leads to fissuring of the skin, particularly at the angles of the mouth. It is most unusual in the developed countries, as the vitamin is found in many foods, milk, beer, cereals and pulses being excellent sources, supplying more than the required 1.5mg of riboflavine a day.

## NICOTINIC ACID

Nicotinic acid, which cannot be obtained from the nicotine absorbed by smokers, is required for enzymatic processes in epithelial layers. Its deficiency leads to pellagra – an eczematous skin condition which is frequently associated with diarrhoea and mental disturbances. Nicotinic acid is found in meat, particularly offal, and fish, in milk, and in yeast and yeast extracts. It is also present in whole wheat grain in abundance, and when white flour is preferred many countries insist that nicotinic acid be added to the flour before it is used for bread-making. Nicotinic acid deficiency is exceptional in developed countries. The daily requirement of 15mg is exceeded in a normal diet.

## FOLIC ACID

Folic acid, which is the generic name for a group of acids, is an essential enzyme for the synthesis of nucleic acids. If folate deficiency occurs, rapidly dividing cells, which require to build up a supply of nucleic acids before division, are unable to do so. Folic acid deficiency particularly affects blood cells, and if folate deficiency occurs, megaloblastic anaemia may result. The need for folic acid is about 300 to 600µg per day in pregnancy, and this is generally provided in green vegetables and butcher's offal. In certain conditions, such as multiple pregnancy, it is probably wise to give folic acid supplements, but these do not need to exceed 1mg a day.

# DIET IN PREGNANCY

More nonsense has been published about diet in pregnancy in recent years than on any other medical subject. In the years before World War II, it was considered that diet taken during pregnancy affected fetal growth and survival. Post-war studies cast doubt on this, and present opinion is that, within the normal range of diets available, the influence of diet on birth-weight is small, and on difficult labour it is negligible. As far as obstetrical efficiency is concerned, nutrition during infancy and childhood has as much influence as nutrition during pregnancy. For this reason, instruction of the pregnant woman regarding her diet in pregnancy and proper feeding of her child is important, but fanciful, confusing, vague diets are of little value, and possibly damaging.

What then should a pregnant woman eat? To a large extent this will depend on her cultural habits and on the income available for food. The lower the income, the greater is the reliance upon filling carbohydrate foodstuffs, and the less the intake of high-class animal protein. In affluent societies the advice should be buy all you can afford from the butcher, the greengrocer and the dairy, and spend only little at the confectioner, the grocer and the chemist. A woman can understand this, but the mass media keep up a constant stream of propaganda telling her to eat this concentrate, that frozen foodstuff, the other vitamin preparation, so that dispassionate appraisal is difficult, and inaccurate information about protein, mineral and vitamin needs is widespread.

At present we have insufficient physiological information about the needs of women in pregnancy, and any recommendation can only be a guide and must not be considered absolute. This is especially so as women have different physiques, live in different climates, and follow different occupations; their only common factor being that they are pregnant. With this proviso, the daily allowances shown in Table **6/1** should adequately provide for all needs.

| Calories | 2200–2500 (kj) |
|---|---|
| Protein | 65g |
| Calcium | 1000mg |
| Iron | 15mg |
| Vitamin A | 6000u (750µg) |
| Vitamin D | 400u (10µg) |
| Thiamine | 1mg |
| Riboflavine | 1.5mg |
| Nicotinic acid | 15mg |
| Ascorbic acid | 50mg |
| Folic acid | 1mg |

**Table 6/1** Daily allowances of nutrients suggested for pregnant women (from 20th week)

If this is translated into the foodstuffs the woman buys, she should try each day to drink a pint of milk (either raw, or made up in milk drinks and puddings, or as cheese); eat 120g (4oz) of fish or meat, and one egg daily; eat an orange, an apple or a slice of papaya daily; and have green leafy vegetables at least three times a week. Apart from this, she can eat what she likes, so long as she pays attention to her weight gain.

Astute advertising has convinced many doctors and most patients that vitamin and mineral supplements are essential for the well-being of mother and unborn child, and that the woman who does not take them is depriving her child of a good start to life. Whilst in a few instances this is true, the majority of women do not require most of the vitamins, minerals and trace elements so beautifully packaged by pharmaceutical houses. In an affluent society, provided that the patient eats the diet outlined, and that her haemoglobin concentration exceeds 10.5g/dl it is probable that iron supplementation in pregnancy is unnecessary, certainly before the 28th gestation week. Over 95 per cent of pregnant women in the developed nations do not need iron, although a single tablet of an iron salt (which provides about 85mg of elemental iron) may be taken daily without harm. Iron supplements should be reserved for those women who have genuine iron deficiency as demonstrated by examining the appearance of the erythrocytes in a stained blood slide. Most of these women are in the lower socio-economic groups and many are under the age of 20. These women and most pregnant women in the developing nations do require iron and vitamin supplements in pregnancy. Iron tablets should be given to provide at least 200mg of available iron (of which 10 to 30 per cent will be absorbed). This dose is provided by ferrous sulphate 200mg thrice daily, ferrous gluconate 400mg thrice daily, or ferrous fumarate 200mg thrice daily. The tablets should be taken at 8-hourly intervals, not related to meals, as these hinder iron absorption. In addition, a vitamin tablet containing ascorbic acid 50mg, folic acid 1mg, thiamine 2 mg, riboflavine 2mg, and nicotinic acid 15mg should be taken daily.

# ANTENATAL SCREENING

Much of antenatal care is concerned with screening, that is, seeking an abnormality in an apparently healthy individual. Screening is meant to enable a health professional to select a sub-group of a larger population with a higher risk of developing a pathology, which could then be confirmed or denied by further testing. Screening is not a diagnosis and, by definition, some women who are selected by the screening process will not have any pathology. This implies that the use of screening processes should be cheap, preferably non-invasive and relatively effective in identifying patients with the condition (i.e. have a high sensitivity in detecting true positives). The terms sensitivity and specificity have special meanings in this regard (Table **6/2**).

Screening may be simple. The age, parity and past or family history may identify some women who are at a greater risk of having an abnormal pregnancy. The routine measurement of blood pressure will identify women who have, or who develop,

|  | People having the condition | People who do not have the condition |
|---|---|---|
| *Positive:* people who appear to have the condition | True positives (a) | False positives (b) |
| *Negative:* people who do not appear to have the condition | False negatives (c) | True negatives (d) |

$$\text{Sensitivity} = \frac{a}{a + c} = \text{the probability that the test will be positive when the condition is present}$$

$$\text{Specificity} = \frac{d}{b + d} = \text{the probability that the test will be negative when the condition is absent}$$

$$\text{Positive predictive value} = \frac{a}{a + b} = \text{the probability that the condition is present when the test is positive}$$

$$\text{Negative predictive value} = \frac{d}{c + d} = \text{the probability that the condition is not present when the test is negative}$$

**Table 6/2** Screening test results

hypertensive disease in pregnancy and whose fetus is at greater risk of dying. Vaginal bleeding in pregnancy is another example. In recent years, with advances in medical technology, conditions which previously were undiagnosable before birth can now be identified in pregnancy. Some of these matters are considered before the technique of antenatal care is described.

## THE MEASUREMENT OF BLOOD PRESSURE IN PREGNANCY

A significant rise in blood pressure in pregnancy is an early warning that the patient may develop pregnancy-induced hypertension. Because of this a pregnant woman's blood pressure is measured at each antenatal visit. In order to detect a 'significant' rise of blood pressure it is helpful for the examiner to know what the woman's blood pressure was before she became pregnant, and to take her blood pressure during the first 10 weeks of pregnancy, to provide a baseline. It must be remembered that blood pressure is a quality, not a quantity above which it is 'bad' and below which it is 'good'. Although the mean blood pressure rises with age, this is of little consequence in the reproductive years. During pregnancy, in normal women, the blood pressure tends to remain constant until the last quarter, when a rise of less than 10 points in the diastolic pressure may occur.

By convention (since most 'normal' pregnant women have a blood pressure below this level) a systolic reading of 140 or more and a diastolic reading of 90 or more is the 'threshold' for diagnosing hypertension in pregnancy. However, as blood pressure is a quality, it is as useful to use a change from the baseline as well as an absolute level. One such change indicating possible pathology is an increase in the systolic pressure of 30mmHg or more and in the diastolic pressure of 15mmHg or more. Unfortunately, the measurement of blood pressure (by indirect readings) may be inaccurate for a variety of reasons: posture, the size of the cuff, the time of the day, the environment and the emotional state of the patient. In an attempt to reduce the variables, the blood pressure of a pregnant woman should be taken after she has rested for 10 minutes, and is sitting, or lying on her left side; if an elevation is found, the procedure is repeated after an interval. Her arm should be horizontal at heart level. The systolic pressure is recorded easily, but in pregnancy

the diastolic pressure to be recorded is that associated with the change in sounds from a hard to a muffled thumping (Korotkoff IV). If the disappearance of sound is widely divergent from Korotkoff IV, this should also be recorded. The use of Korotkoff IV to determine the diastolic pressure in *pregnancy*, is based on meticulous studies comparing intra-arterial and indirect blood pressure readings.

## SCREENING FOR PRENATAL DEFECTS

Prenatal screening is currently available to detect Down's syndrome, open neural tube defects (spina bifida and anencephaly) and single autosomal defects when a previous child has had such a defect (Table 6/3).

Prenatal screening for Down's syndrome and other genetic abnormalities may be made by chorion villus sampling (CVS) or by amniocentesis and cell culture. Screening for open neural tube defects is made by the measurement of alphafetoprotein in the maternal serum and the amniotic fluid.

### Chorionic villus sampling

This technique is now well established. Between the 9th and 11th gestational week a sample of about 20mg of chorionic tissue is removed from the placental edge of the chorion frondosum, by sucking it through a narrow cannula. Under ultrasonic guidance the cannula is introduced through the cervix until its tip is just within the chorion (Fig. 6/1). The

- Pregnancies in women over 35 years of age
- Pregnancies at increased risk for fetal neural tube defects (i.e. previously affected child)
- History of Down's syndrome or other chromosomal abnormality in the family
- Previous pregnancy resulting in the birth of a chromosomally abnormal child, or one with multiple malformations
- Known chromosomal abnormality in either parent
- History of sex-linked disease (e.g. thalassaemia, haemophilia, Duchenne muscular dystrophy)
- Couples at risk for detectable inborn errors of metabolism

Table 6/3 Possible indications for diagnostic tests in first half of pregnancy

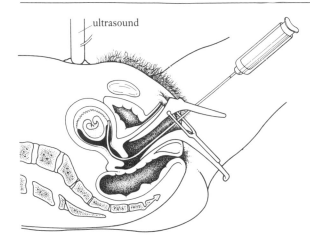
ultrasound

**Fig. 6/1** Chorionic villus sampling

karyotype of the sample can be determined within 24 hours and single gene defects can be detected using DNA probes.

Chorionic villus sampling (CVS) is used to detect chromosomal abnormalities, cystic fibrosis, thalassaemia, haemophilia, polycystic kidney disease, Huntington's disease and some muscular dystrophies. CVS is attended by a fetal loss of 3 per cent, which is 1 per cent more than would be expected for the spontaneous abortion of normal (not blighted) fetuses at the same period of gestation.

### Amniocentesis

This procedure is performed at about the 15th week of pregnancy. A needle is thrust through the abdominal wall into the amniotic sac, guided by ultrasound to avoid the placenta and fetus, and amniotic fluid is removed. This is centrifuged and the fetal cells obtained are placed in a culture medium. About three weeks later the cells are harvested and a karyotype is made. Following amniocentesis, about 1 per cent of fetuses are aborted. This is twice the rate expected in the late second quarter of pregnancy.

### Screening for open neural tube defects

Routine screening all pregnant women for open neural tube defects remains controversial. Open neural tube defects (anencephaly and open spina bifida) occur in between 2 and 5 pregnancies per 1000. The cost to the parents of a defective baby in emotional unhappiness and in money for its care, is believed to outweigh the costs and dangers associated with prenatal diagnosis and termination of the pregnancy. The Clinical Genetics Society in Britain has recommended that all pregnant women should be offered prenatal 'screening' by measuring the level of serum alphafetoprotein (AFP) at about week 16. In cases of open neural tube defects (NTD) the serum AFP is usually raised, while a low serum AFP may help in diagnosing Down's syndrome (p. 443).

The routine recommended is as follows:

If a raised serum AFP (above the 97th percentile or more than $2\frac{1}{2}$ times the median of the week of pregnancy) is found and confirmed by repeating the test a week later, the woman may have a baby with a neural tube defect (NTD).

Raised serum AFP levels also occur in other circumstances, notably error in gestation dates, threatened or missed abortion and multiple pregnancy.

The next step is to exclude these by an ultrasound examination which (1) confirms the accuracy of the gestation date, and (2) excludes a multiple pregnancy or a missed abortion. Having established that the woman has a single fetus of at least 16 weeks gestation, an amniocentesis is made to obtain a sample of amniotic fluid, so that the amniotic-AFP level can be determined (Table **6/4**). If the amniotic-AFP level is raised (5 standard deviations above the mean, or 3 times the median value for the gestational week) the chance that the woman has an affected baby is over 95 per cent and termination of pregnancy can be offered, by using prostaglandins.

Several problems remain before the policy can be fully recommended. First, serum AFP levels are not raised in every case of NTD, particularly if it is a closed lesion. Second, in about half of cases in which amniocentesis is thought appropriate, the amniotic AFP level is not raised and the fetus is normal. Third, about 1.5 per cent (range 0.25–10) of these normal fetuses are aborted spontaneously within 4 weeks of the procedure; and the incidence of later complications in pregnancy, abruptio placentae, premature rupture of the membranes, hyaline membrane disease and orthopaedic postural abnormalities are increased.

Because of these problems, controversy continues over *routine* screening for NTD affected fetuses by measuring the mother's serum AFP, although most authorities agree that when a woman has previously had an affected baby the service should be offered.

If the service is offered each woman is entitled to

Offer the service to all mothers, allowing any mother to withdraw from the programme at any stage.

**Table 6/4** A scheme of routine screening for NTD. The service may be offered to all mothers, but any woman participating must be allowed to withdraw from the programme at any stage.

the explanation (1) that serum AFP does not detect every open NTD affected fetus (about 10 per cent are missed), (2) that, even when the AFP level is raised in both maternal serum and amniotic fluid, about 5 per 1000 babies will not have an NTD – in other words the test carries a false positive rate of 0.5 per cent, and (3) that amniocentesis carries the risk that a normal fetus will subsequently be aborted spontaneously or that the continuing pregnancy may be complicated by antepartum haemorrhage. The risk of one of these events occurring is about 0.5 per cent.

A recently developed biochemical test may prove more specific and may add to the precision of alpha-fetoprotein tests. This is to measure acetylcholin-esterase (AChE) in amniotic fluid using a qualitative gel electrophoretic test. AChE is released by imma-ture nerve terminals into the cerebrospinal fluid and, in cases of neural tube defect, into the amniotic fluid. The diagnostic value of AChE measurements is currently under study.

A suggestion has been made that the incidence of neural tube defects will be reduced if the mother-to-be takes a large vitamin (and mineral) supplement from the time of conception. This suggestion is cur-rently under investigation in Britain, but should not be adopted until the results of the trial are known because no information is available about the safety of the supplement in early pregnancy.

## ROUTINE BIOPHYSICAL AND BIOMEDICAL SCREENING

In spite of considerable enthusiasm by some obste-tricians the place of routine screening by biophysical or biochemical methods has not been evaluated in well-designed trials, with the exception of the simple expedient of asking a pregnant woman to note (and in some cases record) the frequency of her baby's movements. At each antenatal visit after the 24th week of gestation, the woman should be asked about the frequency of fetal movements (kicks), and in certain cases she should be asked to complete a fetal movement chart (see p. 279).

## 'ROUTINE ULTRASOUND' EXAMINATIONS

A number of obstetricians believe that every preg-nant woman's uterus should be screened by ul-trasound either between the 10th and 13th week (Fig. 6/2) or between the 16th and 20th week (Fig. 6/3). A further screening at about the 34th week may also be advised.

Ultrasound screening between the 5th and 7th gestational week will usually detect an intra-uterine fetus and can estimate the size of the amniotic sac. This is helpful in cases of threatened abortion. Ultra-sound is helpful in diagnosing some cases of ectopic gestation, particularly if a vaginal probe is used.

Screening between the 10th and 13th week is useful in determining the period of gestation of a woman who is uncertain when she became pregnant. At this time the measurement of the fetal crown–rump length gives the gestational age with an accuracy of + or − 4 days in 95 per cent of patients. Screening at this time will exclude or confirm a suspected tropho-blastic tumour.

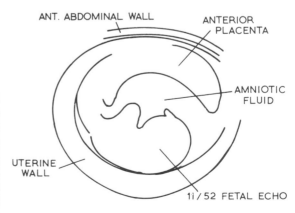

ANT. ABDOMINAL WALL

ANTERIOR PLACENTA

AMNIOTIC FLUID

UTERINE WALL

1i/52 FETAL ECHO

**Fig. 6/2** Transverse scan showing normal fetus at 11 weeks' gestation. Line drawing shows the relevant identifying points

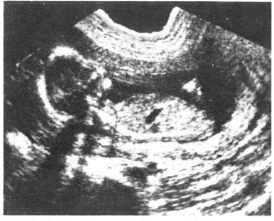 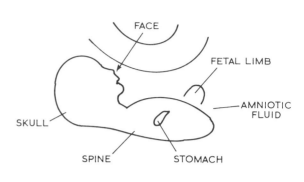

**Fig. 6/3** Ultrasound scan showing normal fetus at 18 weeks' gestation. Line drawing shows the relevant identifying points

Apart from the above cases, screening at about 18 weeks' gestation provides the most useful compromise between accuracy of gestational age and the best visualization of fetal anatomy. If the fetus is found to have short femurs and a nuchal skin fold thickness 6mm or more, an amniocentesis should be made to exclude Down's syndrome. Neural tube defects can be detected at this time and, if desired, termination of pregnancy can be offered. Multiple pregnancy can be detected readily at this period of gestation, and it avoids the problem of the 'disappearing twin' (p. 315). The position of the placenta can be determined, although a low-lying placenta found before the 30th week does not necessarily indicate placenta praevia.

The value of ultrasound examinations in selected cases is undoubted (for example when the date of the last menstrual period is unknown or no clinical examination has been made in the first 10 weeks; or if twins are suspected) but the cost benefits of *routine* ultrasound examinations have not been established.

## BIOCHEMICAL TESTS

In the past some centres routinely measured urinary oestriol and serum HPL at intervals from the 30th week of pregnancy. This routine screening has been shown to have no real value; and most centres have abandoned biochemical tests.

# THE TECHNIQUE OF ANTENATAL CARE

### THE FIRST ANTENATAL VISIT

The importance of establishing a good relationship between the patient and her medical advisers – doctor and nurse-midwife – cannot be overemphasized. If the patient is treated as an intelligent woman, interested in her pregnancy at this stage, her full co-operation in her prenatal care will be obtained. It is the duty of doctor and nurse-midwife to obtain this co-operation, and their attitude to the patient is of great importance.

Ideally, each pregnant woman should be seen first before the 10th week of pregnancy. The advantages of this early visit are that a baseline can be obtained against which the physiological changes occurring in pregnancy can be assessed, and any abnormalities can be noted and treated before they have a detrimental effect. Unfortunately at present some women do not seek antenatal care until after the 20th week. If the doctor, and his medical associates, working in the community, could induce all pregnant women, whether single or married, to visit a doctor, or a clinic, in the first quarter of pregnancy, many subsequent potential problems would be avoided. Community action in this regard, using the media, is urgently required.

At the first visit several matters are considered and the findings carefully recorded.

## The history of present pregnancy

The date of the first day of the last menstrual period is recorded, and the patient is questioned about her menstrual cycle. If the menstrual cycle is of normal duration (25 to 34 days), it is easy to calculate the estimated date of the childbirth. This calculation relies on the fact that the average duration of pregnancy is 266 days from conception, and 280 days from the date of the first day of the last menstrual period in a woman whose menstrual cycles are normal. The calculation is made by adding one year and 10 days to the date of the first day of the last menstrual period, and subtracting 3 months from the total.

Thus, if the first day of the last menstrual period was 12 June 1990, the baby will be due on 22 March 1991. Of course, if the menstrual cycle is of longer duration than normal, or is irregular, this must be allowed for in the calculation. One of the reasons for requesting the patient to attend for examination before the 10th week of pregnancy is to be sure that the patient recalls accurately the date of the last menstrual period, and to enable the doctor to check the calculated period of gestation against the size of the enlarging uterus.

Recently a complication in calculating the date of the delivery has arisen with women who have used oral contraceptives for a while and then decided to have another baby. Normally ovulation occurs about midcycle, but is often delayed for from 2 to 4 weeks in the first cycle after stopping the Pill. These women may have conceived 2 to 4 weeks later than they would normally, and the estimated date of delivery is consequently 2 to 4 weeks later than that shown by the normal calculation. Expectant mothers should be asked if they have used oral contraceptives, and whether they conceived in the first cycle after ceasing to take the Pill.

Once the calculation has been made, as accurately as possible, the patient should be told when her baby is expected.

If the woman is uncertain about the date of her last menstrual period or has infrequent menstruation, and if the clinical examination is inconclusive, an ultrasound examination should be made. This may be made between the 12th and 24th week, when the expected date of childbirth can be determined with an accuracy of 7 days. Ultrasound can also detect some congenital defects and can diagnose multiple pregnancy. Some obstetricians advise routine ultrasound screening of all antenatal patients, but, as mentioned, the cost-benefit of this procedure has not been established.

Enquiries are made about the progress of the pregnancy so far, and abnormal happenings are recorded so that the doctor may investigate them further.

## The history of previous pregnancies

A great deal of information about the obstetric performance of a patient can be obtained by enquiring about previous pregnancies. Special attention is paid to noting abnormalities which occurred in a previous pregnancy. For example, a patient may have had hypertension previously, or may have had an urinary tract infection. The outcome of the pregnancy is recorded, and if any of the pregnancies ended in an abortion, the duration of the pregnancy when this occurred is noted. The duration of the previous labours and the sex and weights of previous babies are recorded. Once again, this is most informative. For example, if a patient delivered a 4000g baby after a labour of 8 hours, it is highly improbable that she has a contracted pelvis! Abnormal occurrences in the puerperium of previous confinements are noted, with particular reference to postpartum haemorrhage, venous thrombosis, and whether the babies were breast-fed or not.

## The history of past illnesses or operations

Inquiries are made about any previous illnesses or operations which the patient may have had, and information is sought about the presence of diabetes or hypertension in either of the expectant mother's parents or in any of her siblings. This is of importance, as certain familial diseases, such as diabetes, may become manifest in pregnancy.

## The physical examination

Once the history has been obtained – and in many clinics this is done by the nurse-midwife – the patient is ready for the physical examination, and for the necessary laboratory tests. The order in which these are made differs in different clinics.

The initial physical examination must be made by a doctor. He will check and record the patient's height and weight, and will then do a systematic examination of her cardiovascular system (including her blood pressure), her respiratory system, and her gastrointestinal system. He will examine her breasts, paying particular attention to the nipples and to her desire to breast-feed. If the patient wishes to breast-feed and the nipples are retracted, he will advise remedial treatment, which is usually supervised by the nurse-midwife.

Next he will make a vaginal examination. It is important to take a cervical smear for exfoliative cytology to exclude cancer, although the 'pick-up' is very low. However, the patient is shown that the procedure is painless, and a further smear, made at the postnatal visit, enables the doctor to assert with confidence that no cervical epithelial abnormality is present. If these two smears are negative, further cytology need only be made at 3-year intervals. Following the cervical smear, the doctor does a bimanual examination to determine the size, position and shape of the uterus, and to exclude tumours of the uterus, ovaries or of the bony pelvis.

If a cervical smear has been made in the previous twelve months, and a routine pelvic ultrasound examination is intended to be made at about the 10th to 12th week, the vaginal examination may be omitted.

### Laboratory tests

These are made in the clinic, or the patient is referred to the pathological laboratory. The following tests must be performed at the first visit, and some at each visit.

1. *Blood*
   Haemoglobin concentration (normal 10.5–15g)
   Haematocrit (PVC) (normal $> 35$)
   MCV and MCH (if patient southern European, African or Asian)
   ABO and Rhesus group
   If Rhesus negative, Rhesus antibodies
   All patients: irregular antibodies
   VDRL or similar (to exclude syphilis)
   Hepatitis B surface antigen (HBsAG)
   Anti-rubella antibodies

2. *Urine*
   Urinalysis (specific gravity, protein, sugar)
   Culture for bacteriuria (see p. 222)

3. *Further tests in pregnancy*
   a. All women: repeat irregular antibody test at 36 weeks

b. Rhesus negative women: rhesus antibodies at 20, 24, 28, 32, 36 weeks
   c. Haemoglobin re-estimate between 30 and 36 weeks and/or serum territin
   d. Random blood sugar when 'booking' and at about 28 weeks (see p. 241)

### Summing up

The results of all the questions, the examination and the laboratory tests are carefully recorded, and the doctor, or the nurse-midwife, should now make time available to talk with the patient and to answer any questions she may have. Every opportunity should be taken to explain what is being done and why, and the full co-operation of the patient should be sought.

For antenatal care effectively to meet the objectives stated on page 49, the patient should visit a doctor (or midwife) at regular intervals. At each visit sufficient time should be set aside to discuss the patient's feelings, expectations and any perceived fears in addition to performing the screening procedures. The usual recommendation (dating from 1929) is that a 'normal' pregnant woman should be seen every 4 weeks to the 28th week of pregnancy, every 2 weeks to the 36th week and weekly from then until the baby is delivered. Patients who are identified as being at 'higher risk' of losing the baby (for example, women with cardiac disease, essential hypertension, diabetes or blood disorders) require to be seen more often. Recently much discussion has taken place in Britain about whether the schedule suggested over 50 years ago is appropriate today for 'normal' pregnant women. One suggestion is that whilst normal primigravidae should be seen according to the schedule, normal multigravid women need only be seen in the first 10 weeks of pregnancy, about the 22nd week and again at the 30th week before entering the schedule of visits.

## VISITS UP TO WEEK 28

Time should be given so that the patient may ask questions about matters which worry her, and should be answered clearly.

The examination consists of a general and an obstetrical assessment.

Although it is customary to weigh the patient at each antenatal visit, it is of minimal value and can be abandoned. If the obstetrician chooses to continue to weigh the patient, a weight gain of up to 4kg may be expected before the 20th week of pregnancy. After that a gain of not more than 0.5kg a week is 'ideal', and if the weight gain is greater than this, reasons should be sought, and advice given. No weight gain, or weight loss, may indicate fetal problems and should be investigated.

The woman's blood pressure is measured at each visit and her urine examined for the presence of protein and glucose (using dipsticks). Her ankles are examined for the presence of oedema. A rise in blood pressure which persists after rest may be a sign that pregnancy-induced hypertension is likely to occur. Unfortunately, it presupposes that the examiner knows what the blood pressure was in early pregnancy. It has been pointed out that blood pressure is a quality, not a quantity above which it is 'bad' and below which it is 'good'. It is also known that average blood pressure increases with age, but of course in the reproductive years this is not a matter of much concern. So that the most information can be obtained, it is of great help to know the expectant mother's pre-pregnant blood pressure, or if that cannot be obtained, to know her blood pressure in the first quarter of pregnancy. The mean blood pressure does not alter in pregnancy, except in women who have pre-existing hypertension, when a fall between the 15th and 25th week may be observed, and in women who develop pregnancy-induced hypertension. For this reason a rise of 15 points of the diastolic, or 30 points of the systolic pressure, persisting after rest for 20 minutes, must be regarded with concern, the patient being seen again after 3 to 7 days. For convenience (and since most 'normal' women have a blood pressure below this level), a systolic reading above 140 or a diastolic reading above 90 are considered abnormal. There is evidence that a rise above this level is more significant than a relative rise of diastolic blood pressure if it is below this arbitrary limit. My experience is that if an absolute level must be made, the patient whose blood pressure is less than 140/90 is in no danger.

Until recently, the diastolic pressure was taken when all sounds disappeared on listening over the brachial artery with a stethoscope. The recent studies show that in pregnancy the change in sound *from a hard thumping to a soft beat* records the diastolic pressure more accurately. However, if this reading and the disappearance of all sounds are widely separated, both should be recorded.

**The obstetrical examination**

The obstetrical part of the examination at each visit consists of measuring the height of the fundus of the uterus above the pubis, and determining its relationship to the estimated duration of the pregnancy. Marked discrepancies require investigation. For example, an excessively large uterus is suggestive of multiple pregnancy, or the development of hydramnios; whilst failure of the uterus to grow between visits is suggestive of poor fetal growth or even fetal death.

The time of 'quickening' is noted but, as this varies between the 16th and 24th week of pregnancy, it is of limited value except to the patient, who now knows that she has a living child within her womb. After the 24th week the doctor should enquire about fetal movements at each visit.

The position of the fetus within the uterus is of interest to the mother and to the medical attendant but, as the fetus is so mobile, this is usually not sought until the 28th week. At each visit after this time, the lie, presentation, and position of the baby are determined, and the mother is told where the baby lies in her uterus.

## THE BABY IN PREGNANCY

Since the baby is growing in an enclosed water-filled sac, it is relatively weightless and able to move about freely. For this reason its lie, position, presentation and attitude may vary from visit to visit. The *lie* is the relationship of the long axis of the fetus to the long axis of the mother; the *presentation* refers to that part of the fetus nearest the pelvic brim; the *position* indicates the relation of the presenting part to a particular part of the pelvic wall; and the *attitude* refers to the relationship of the various parts of the fetus one to the other.

In late pregnancy, the baby normally *lies* longitudinally in the uterus, *presenting* by the head, which is close to the mother's pelvic brim, the *position* of the occiput is lateral, and the fetus is in a flexed *attitude*, the chin being flexed on the chest and the upper and lower limbs being folded across the fetal trunk. Occasionally, particularly before the 32nd week of pregnancy, the fetus may present as a breech, and rarely it may lie transversely. In about 1 in 80 pregnancies, two babies (or more) are present.

All this information can be obtained by gentle abdominal palpation and, when the information has been obtained, it should be given in simple language to the mother as well as being carefully recorded.

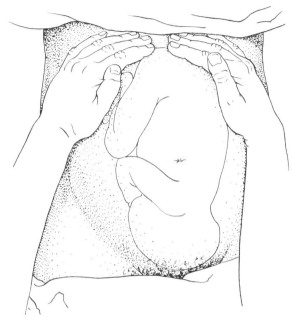

**Fig. 6/4** Abdominal palpation. Step 1 – fundal palpation

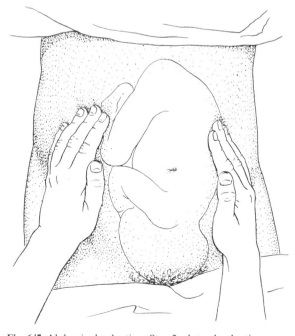

**Fig. 6/5** Abdominal palpation. Step 2 – lateral palpation

## The method of abdominal palpation

The patient lies on her back with her head and shoulders slightly raised, having previously emptied her bladder. The medical attendant usually stands on the patient's right side, and examines the abdomen gently and to a routine. In a way the procedure can be considered a piece of detection by educated fingers, in which the finding of the fetal head is the main clue. To do this, four manoeuvres are practised.

### FIRST MANOEUVRE, FUNDAL PALPATION (Fig. **6/4**)

The height of the fundus above the symphysis is determined with the ulnar border of the left hand, and then the fundal area is gently pressed between the two hands in an attempt to determine which pole of the fetus (the breech or the head) is occupying the fundal area.

### SECOND MANOEUVRE, LATERAL PALPATION (Fig. **6/5**)

The hands are now gently slipped along the side of the uterus, and quick, gentle palpations are made of the corresponding sides of the uterus. By this means, the back is identified as an elongated firm mass on one side of the midline, and the limbs as small irregular shapes in an area which is relatively empty when compared with the other side of the uterus. Often the examiner will feel the fetus move under his hands.

### THIRD MANOEUVRE, PELVIC PALPATION (Fig. **6/6**)

The medical attendant now turns and faces the patient's feet and places his hands on the lower part of the uterus, well to the sides. With the fingers extended, he gently presses downwards, and from side to side, attempting to recognize the presenting part. Usually it is the head, which is firm, large and rounded, and unless fixed in the pelvis, can be balloted from side to side between the fingers. If the presenting part cannot be readily identified because it is fixed in the pelvis, the fingers are slipped further downwards and inwards until they dip into the pelvic brim. If the hand which is on the same side as the fetal back slips more deeply than the other into the pelvis, it can be assumed that the head is well fixed. If the patient cannot relax her muscles, she should

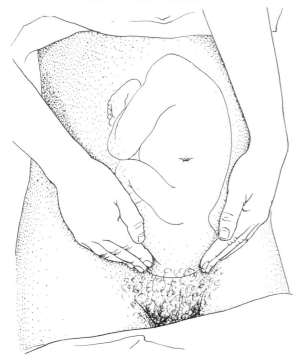

**Fig. 6/6** Abdominal palpation. Step 3 – pelvic palpation

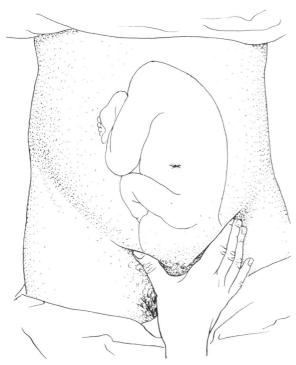

**Fig. 6/7** The Pawlik manoeuvre

flex her legs slightly and the fingers should be slipped in more deeply each time the patient forcibly breathes out.

### THE PAWLIK MANOEUVRE (Fig. 6/7)

This fourth manoeuvre is not always necessary and, unless performed gently, may be painful. Facing the patient's head, the right hand is spread widely and is pressed into the suprapubic area above the inguinal ligament. When the fingers and thumbs are approximated, the presenting part can be felt between them and its mobility above the pelvic brim determined.

Although palpation is usually easy, occasionally the patient may be tense and the uterus contracted. In such cases it is better to wait for a while rather than to persist in palpating, and above all to be gentle!

If there is doubt about the presentation of the fetus, *auscultation* of the fetal heart may resolve the matter. In vertex presentations, the fetal heart sounds are best heard below the umbilicus.

## VISITS FROM THE 28TH WEEK

The patient attends every 2 weeks if normal, or more often if any abnormality is detected, from the 28th to the 36th week; and then every week until delivery. At each of these visits, enquiries are made about her health, and her questions are answered in a clear way. She should be encouraged to talk about her attitude to pregnancy and to labour, and the opportunity should be taken to correct any misconceptions. At each visit, the blood pressure is estimated, the urine examined for protein, and the position of the baby in the uterus is checked. During this period, two examinations of considerable importance are made. The first is to estimate once again the haemoglobin level, or haematocrit, at about the 36th week of pregnancy; the second is for the obstetrician to perform a vaginal examination and pelvic assessment. This is essential in all primigravidae, and in some multigravidae, where the capacity of the pelvis is in doubt. In a primigravida, the fetal head may be expected to fix (become engaged) in the pelvis by the 37th week, and this event gives a useful guide of the presence or absence of disproportion between the fetal head and the bony pelvis. The pelvic assessment is therefore best made by the obstetrician at about the 37th week of pregnancy.

### The pelvic assessment

Before the examination, the patient should have emptied her bladder and bowels. The patient is most easily examined in the dorsal position, with the legs flexed at the thighs and knees. The vulva is inspected and the presence of varicosities noted. The right hand is gloved, the vulva swabbed with chlorhexidine solution (1 in 1000) and the labia minora separated with the left hand. The index finger and middle finger are lubricated with chlorhexidine obstetric

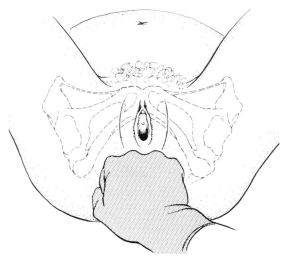

**Fig. 6/8** Estimating the size of the pelvic outlet with the clenched fist

cream, and are introduced into the vagina, the sensitive clitoral area being avoided. The condition of the vaginal walls, the texture and degree of shortening (effacement) and dilatation of the cervix are noted. The degree of engagement of the head is determined or, if it is not engaged, it is pushed into the pelvis by downward and backward pressure of the left hand. The examining fingers now press deeply and diagonally upwards across the pelvis to determine if the sacral promontory can be reached. The curve of the sacrum is next palpated, and the prominence of the ischial spines noted. The sacrospinous ligament is palpated, and should accommodate the two examining fingers. Finally the lateral pelvic walls are palpated and the fingers withdrawn. The distance between the ischial tuberosities is measured with the closed fist, which should be accepted between them, and the shape of the pubic arch is determined (Fig. 6/8).

### Engagement of the fetal head

With better nutrition during childhood in the developed nations, cephalopelvic disproportion has ceased to be a major problem. However, it is important to ascertain that the fetal head 'fits' into the maternal pelvis. In other words if the head is 'engaged'. Some obstetricians express the degree of engagement of the fetal head in fifths (Fig. 6/9), others believe that it is impossible to be so accurate and use the terms unengaged, engaging, engaged.

| COMPLETELY ABOVE | SINCIPUT +++ OCCIPUT ++ | SINCIPUT ++ OCCIPUT + | SINCIPUT + OCCIPUT JUST FELT | SINCIPUT + OCCIPUT NOT FELT | NONE OF HEAD PALPABLE |
|---|---|---|---|---|---|
| 5/5 | 4/5 | 3/5 | 2/5 | 1/5 | 0/5 |
| | | | | | |
| 'FLOATING' ABOVE THE BRIM | 'FIXING' | NOT ENGAGED | JUST ENGAGED | ENGAGED | DEEPLY ENGAGED |

Level of pelvic brim

**Fig. 6/9** Descent of the fetal head

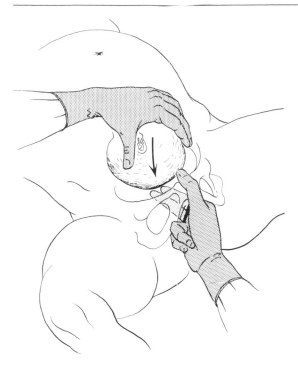

**Fig. 6/10** Estimating the relative size of the fetal head and the maternal pelvis by Muller-Kerr 'head fitting' test

In the majority of primigravidae, the fetal head will have become engaged in the maternal pelvis by the 37th week of pregnancy, but in multiparae, engagement is frequently delayed until false labour, or true labour, supervenes. The fact that the fetal head has engaged in the pelvis does not necessarily imply that labour is imminent. The converse (in primigravidae), that the head is unengaged by the 37th week, requires investigation.

The <u>causes of lack of engagement of the fetal</u> <u>head are:</u>

1. Lack of adequate formation of the lower uterine segment
2. Malposition of the fetal head
3. Cephalopelvic disproportion or contracted pelvis
4. Tumours in the pelvis obstructing the entry of the fetal head
5. Placenta praevia
6. Incorrect estimation of the period of gestation.

The cause can only be determined by a clinical assessment of the pelvis by digital examination, supplemented in cases of doubt by radiological pelvimetry. As has been pointed out, the pelvic assessment should be made routinely at about the 37th week, and should form part of the normal obstetrical examination. Abdominal palpation will give some indication of the size of the fetus and of the position of the fetal head. Pelvic examination will detect any tumour occupying the pelvis, and will enable the obstetrician to assess the size of the bony pelvis. The presence of disproportion can be further assessed by the Muller-Kerr method (Fig. 6/10). In Kerr's words 'the external hand pushes the head downwards and backwards into the pelvis while the fingers of the other hand estimate the relative size of pelvis and head . . . The patient is placed in the dorsal position and the obstetrician stands at her side facing her. Two fingers of the right hand are passed into the vagina. These determine the consistency and manner of engagement of the fetal head. Further information is obtained by utilizing the thumb externally, which is passed along the brim and estimates the degree of overlapping.'

If the test is positive at the 37th week, and the head enters the pelvis, cephalopelvic disproportion is not the cause of the lack of engagement. It may then be due to an under-developed lower uterine segment, or a malposition of the fetal head, and both may alter in the succeeding weeks.

## THE ONSET OF LABOUR

A particular worry is that labour will start and that the patient will not know and will deliver before she can be helped. At one of the visits in the last month of pregnancy, the signs of the onset of labour should be described simply to the patient. She should be told that generally labour coincides with the regular onset of uterine contractions. Initially the contractions are at 30-minute intervals, but become stronger and more frequent over the next few hours. When they cause discomfort and are at about 10-minute intervals, the patient should come to hospital or send for the midwife if she is to deliver at home. The character of the contractions is that the abdomen becomes hard, and discomfort, or pain, is felt in the lower abdomen and back. Less often a 'show' of blood or mucus precedes the contractions, and it should be explained that the 'show' is due to the separation of the plug of mucus which blocks the cervix. If the 'show' is heavy, and largely bloody, soiling at least one pad, the patient should be told not to be alarmed but to come at once to hospital. Occasionally the first sign may be rupture of the membranes (the 'bag of waters') which to the patient may be a frightening event. She should be told that if this occurs, she should come into hospital without awaiting the onset of uterine contractions.

An explanation of the first stage of labour should also be given, and her co-operation ensured. In hospitals where psychoprophylaxis is practised, the course of labour is explained at lectures, but the doctor and nurse-midwife should reinforce these with explanation at the antenatal visits. The patient often feels that no progress is being made

in the first stage of labour, and the physiology of cervical dilatation should be described.

The woman often will ask if she will be given drugs to 'kill the pain'. She should be reassured that analgesics are readily available when, and if, she requires them, but that if she enters labour healthy, confident and with knowledge of what occurs during labour, she is unlikely to need much analgesia. A great fear is that she will be left alone in labour, and that during this time the birth will take place. A woman must never be left alone in labour, and if she and her husband desire it, he should be permitted to stay with her throughout this time.

# PSYCHOPROPHYLAXIS IN PREGNANCY AND LABOUR

In many cultures, sex and childbirth are considered shameful matters to be hidden from view and not discussed. A consequence is that many women are ignorant of the process of parturition, and because of racial myths and overheard whispers, have acquired a 'conditioned reflex' in which childbirth is associated with pain and danger of death. Psychoprophylaxis seeks to eliminate this 'conditioned reflex' and to replace it by a new one in which the cortical perception of labour pain is suppressed by altering the brain's threshold to sensation. The method, which originated in Russia and has been adapted in France, depends on the Pavlovian theory that conditioned reflexes can be acquired and altered by training, and that the perception of pain is particularly responsive. In an explanation of the physiology of this theory, Vellay suggests that the brain has a threshold below which pain is not perceived. Normal vegetative stimuli are not felt as they do not reach the threshold of perception, but the threshold can be reduced by conditions such as fear, emotional upset, shock, hunger and cold. In these conditions stimuli, normally non-painful, cross the lowered threshold and are translated as pain. In labour the cultural ignorance about childbirth, and the fear of pain and death, reduce the threshold so that pain is felt; psychoprophylaxis raises the threshold by explanation and 'neuromuscular' training, so that active participation of the patient in labour may take place. The purpose of the latter, according to Vellay, is to convert cerebral activity 'into motor activity' with the resulting raising of the pain thresh-

old. Over 90 per cent of women in Russia and 70 per cent of French women are taught the method with reportedly great success. Psychoprophylactic preparation follows two lines. (1) Fear of labour is reduced or eliminated by a series of lectures and discussions over 10 weeks in which feelings and expectations about labour and birth are shared and explored. Also, information regarding the anatomy of the female genital tract, physiological changes in pregnancy, fetal development, the process of normal labour and delivery, and some of its complications, hospital routines and procedures and the effects of drugs during pregnancy and labour are given to replace fear with understanding. (2) Relaxation, massage, controlled breathing exercises and general body awareness are taught to enhance the conditioned reflex and convert 'cerebral activity into motor activity'.

Throughout Australia, the method is promoted by over 50 childbirth preparation organizations and offered by many hospital and private physiotherapists.

## CURRENT TEACHING

Current teaching reflects a change in emphasis from formal physical exercises to understanding the process of childbirth. However, the use of the conditioned reflex to raise the pain threshold and neuromuscular control to aid breathing and relaxation remains the foundations of psychoprophylaxis.

## 1. The conditioned reflex

The re-education of the woman is achieved through lectures and discussions as previously mentioned, so that during childbirth understanding, acceptance and activity replace fear and tension. Contractions are seen as signals for relaxation and controlled breathing, not for tension and pain.

## 2. Breathing exercises

Several levels of breathing are taught to raise the pain threshold and maintain relaxation as the stress of labour increases. Slow diaphragmatic, moderate chest, and rapid mouth breathing methods provide a means of controlled respiration to cope with the increasing intensity and frequency of contractions throughout the first stage. Quick, shallow breathing with breath blown out at regular intervals is taught to enable the woman to maintain control during the difficult transition phase.

The time of transition from the first to the second stage is one during which the woman requires particular support from the birthing team. The physical signs of the period, and the emotions she may expect, have been taught but need to be reinforced.

Relaxation must be maintained into second stage so that the breathing remains responsive and controlled. Prolonged breath holding and pushing are discouraged allowing the second stage to flow without great exaggeration and stress.

## 3. Neuromuscular control

The woman is taught about reciprocal muscle activity to enable her to be aware of tension in her body during labour and to learn to relax and release the tension should this occur. Massage and relaxation techniques are also taught to develop this greater body awareness so she can understand and work with her contractions, not try to become totally distracted from them.

* By achieving this awareness she can relax and control the muscles of the pelvic floor at important times such as transition, second stage and crowning.
* Reinforcement of her learning and support for her efforts during labour and delivery come from the encouragement of her partner who is usually fully aware of her breathing levels, preparation and practice.
* Practical labour rehearsals are enacted many times

during preparation to practise skills and give the partner or support person some indication of their role as a member of the birthing team.
* For successful outcome, the woman needs her partner, her doctor, the midwives and perhaps a childbirth educator or 'monitorice' encouraging her and informing her as to her progress during childbirth.

The essential difference between the psychoprophylactic method and the earlier methods of 'relaxation' of Grantly Dick-Read is that in the latter the active participation of the patient is not sought, and the need for analgesics is considered a failure on the part of the patient. Using psychoprophylaxis, about 45 per cent of patients require no analgesia, 45 per cent require one, or at the most two, injections of pethidine, and about 10 per cent are not helped.

The success of psychoprophylaxis depends on the attitude induced in the mother during pregnancy, and on the attitudes of her attendants during labour, as much as upon the specific exercise.

## 4. Patient participation 'active birth'

A further development has been to encourage the patient (and her partner) to become more involved in the process of childbirth. The proponents of this variation of psychoprophylaxis teach the woman relaxation techniques and simple breathing techniques. The breathing taught is for the woman to breathe in slowly and deeply initially, increasing the rate and reducing the depth as the pain of the uterine contraction increases. The proponents of active birth believe that labour is painful for most women, and teach the woman to accept the pain rather than anticipate a painless labour. At the end of each contraction the woman breathes out slowly and relaxes completely. In other words, she concentrates on natural breathing during the contractions and on becoming sensitive to the demands of her body. At special times, for example, during the transition stage and while the fetal head is being born, she may need to take rapid, gentle breaths, sighing out with each expiration.

As well, the woman is able to choose which position she finds most comfortable at various times during labour. She may choose to walk about between contractions or to lie on her side. During contractions she may choose to stand, to lie, to squat or to support herself on her hands and knees, or to be supported by her partner.

# ANTENATAL INFORMATION

Certain matters affecting the mother during pregnancy should be discussed at the early visits.

### Alcohol

Heavy alcohol consumption in pregnancy ($>120$g or 12 standard drinks a day) is associated with fetal growth retardation, developmental delay and neurological complications in the baby. There is some evidence that moderate alcohol consumption ($>100$ to 120g a day) may be associated with an increased risk of spontaneous abortion, and a smaller fetal head circumference. A consumption of 100g a day or less does not appear to have any damaging effects on the fetus or mother. Nevertheless, a pregnant woman should be advised to limit her consumption of alcohol during pregnancy.

### Clothing

In general, the patient should wear the clothes she prefers which enhance her attractiveness. The clothes should be comfortable and non-constricting. Unless she is accustomed to wearing a girdle or has abdominal muscles stretched by previous pregnancies, a maternity support is not needed. She may wear what shoes she likes, but should be told that as pregnancy advances and her centre of balance alters, she should avoid high heels except on special occasions.

### Dental care

An early visit to the dentist is advised, so that any dental care required can be carried out in the first half of pregnancy.

### Employment

In current economic conditions many pregnant women choose or have to work. Provided the woman does not become too tired, and that her enlarging abdomen does not interfere with the job; and provided that industrial conditions in the office, factory or store are appropriate, work during pregnancy will harm neither the mother nor the fetus. In most developed countries paid maternity leave is granted for 6 weeks before the expected date of the childbirth.

### Exercise

Exercise is to be encouraged if this is the usual habit of the patient, but need not be insisted upon if the patient is usually sedentary. She should take walks, and may play ball games if she wishes. She should neither become a fanatic for exercise nor become a vegetable. If she enjoys swimming, she may continue to swim. In general, she should not alter her regimen of exercise just because she is pregnant.

### Immunization

If about to travel overseas, antityphoid or cholera inoculations may be given. All pregnant women who have not been immunized against poliomyelitis, or whose immunity has lapsed, should be immunized in early pregnancy.

### Sexuality during pregnancy

Many doctors fail to discuss sexuality during pregnancy, and many women feel inhibited about asking. Because of this many couples are inadequately informed, and have considerable misconceptions.

Studies have shown that many women have reduced sexual desire and activity, especially in the early weeks of pregnancy and after the 30th week. The reason for this decline in libido is unclear. Some women find sexual intercourse uncomfortable, others fear that coitus and orgasm may damage the fetus or bring on premature labour. Others see themselves as unattractive. Others find the physical awkwardness of coitus in late pregnancy inhibiting.

It is appropriate to talk with the couple. There is no evidence that coitus, cunnilingus or masturbation, whether leading to orgasm or not, have any damaging effect on the fetus, or induce labour prematurely. All forms of sexual enjoyment are permissible in pregnancy, with the proviso that, during cunnilingus, the man should be warned not to blow, forcing air into the woman's vagina, as this has led to air embolism in pregnancy.

Many pregnant women want additional closeness from their partner, and he should be supportive and gentle at all times. In late pregnancy, coitus with the man on top may be uncomfortable, but other coital positions are not, and non-coital sexual satisfaction may be preferred. Coitus can continue, if the couple wish, up to term without any damage to mother or baby.

### Smoking

Pregnant women should be advised not to smoke cigarettes, or if they are unable to break the habit, to restrict smoking to one cigarette after a main meal. This advice is given because cigarette smokers (especially women who smoke more than 20 cigarettes a day) have a slightly greater chance of aborting and their baby's birth-weight, at all stages of gestation, is between 150 and 300g less than the weight of a baby of a non-smoker, and the perinatal death rate may be slightly higher. One reason for the damaging effect of smoking in pregnancy is that smokers have a reduced intervillous blood flow and higher blood levels of carbon monoxide. These findings suggest that if the adverse effects of cigarette smoking are to be minimized, cigarette smoking should be avoided from the time of conception. However, smoking behaviour is affected by many psycho-social factors, and the woman may find smoking an appropriate method for her to reduce stress, and tension, so that the success of a non-smoking campaign in pregnancy may be limited. This is important to know as fortunately there is no evidence that smoking during pregnancy has any effect in the long-term mental or motor development of the child.

### Travelling

Provided the journey can be made in a leisurely and comfortable way, there need be no restriction on travelling during pregnancy.

# Part Two

# NORMAL LABOUR

# Chapter 7

# The Passages

## THE HARD (BONY) PASSAGES

The pelvis is made up of four bones, which are united at three joints. They are the two innominate bones, the sacrum and the coccyx. Each innominate bone derives from three bones which fuse completely at about the time of puberty, to form the single innominate bone; they are the ilium, the ischium and the pubis.

The articulated pelvis is formed by the innominate bones antero-laterally and by the sacrum and coccyx posteriorly. When the individual stands erect the pelvis is inclined forwards, and the antero-superior spine of the ilium is in the same vertical plane as the pubic spine.

The bony pelvis is divided into the false pelvis and the true pelvis by the pelvic brim, which is bounded by the pubic crest, the iliopectineal line on the innominate bone and the anterior border of the ala and promontory of the sacrum. The false pelvis, formed mainly by the flaring ilia, has little obstetric significance, but the shape and structure of the true pelvis is of great importance (Fig. 7/1).

The normal true pelvis is cylindrical in shape with a bluntly curved lower end, and it is slightly curved anteriorly. Anteriorly the canal is short, being

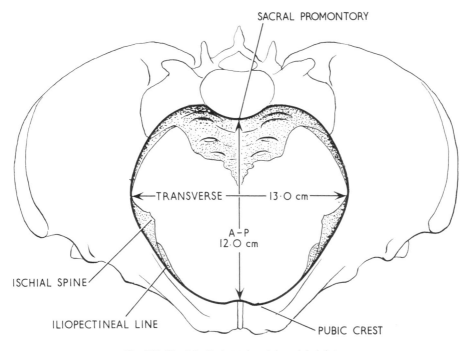

**Fig. 7/1** The 'ideal' obstetric pelvis: pelvic inlet

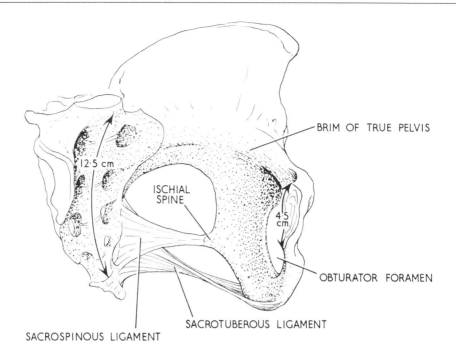

**Fig. 7/2**  The pelvic cavity. The right innominate bone has been removed in order to show the extent of the cavity

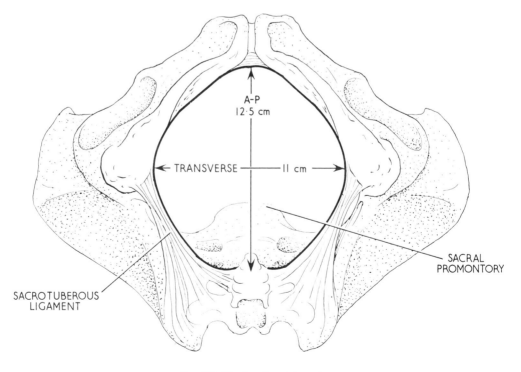

**Fig. 7/3**  The female pelvic outlet

formed by the posterior surface of the symphysis pubis, which measures 4.5cm; posteriorly it is formed by the curved sacrum and measures 12cm. Laterally its sides narrow slightly from above downwards and are formed from the pubic rami, the ischium, part of the body of the ilium and by the sacrum and coccyx (Fig. **7/2**). The obturator foramen creates a large opening in the antero-lateral wall of the cavity which is covered by the obturator internus muscle. On the postero-lateral walls the great and lesser sciatic foramina form large gaps in the bones and are filled by the piriformis muscle and tendon of obturator internus. The two sciatic foramina are separated by the sacrospinous ligament which stretches from the lateral border of the fifth sacral and first coccygeal vertebrae to the ischial spine, and is covered with the coccygeus muscle.

The outlet of the pelvis is bounded by the arcuate pubic ligament and the pubic arch anteriorly, the ischial tuberosities and the sacrotuberous ligaments laterally and by the sacrum and coccyx posteriorly (Fig. **7/3**).

## PELVIC ZONES

The contour of the birth canal varies at different levels and for descriptive purposes four zones can be defined (Fig. **7/4**).

The *zone of the pelvic inlet* is bounded by the upper border of the pubis in front, the iliopectineal line laterally and the sacral promontory posteriorly. The antero-posterior measurement, from the innermost margin of the pubis to the most anterior portion of the sacral promontory, measures 12cm amongst Europeans (Caucasians) and 0.5 to 1cm less in Asian women. The *transverse diameter of the brim* is that of the greatest transverse diameter and measures 13cm in Caucasians and 0.5 to 1cm less in Asians. The *available transverse diameter* of the brim is the width of the pelvis at the mid-point of the antero-posterior diameter, and measures 12.5cm.

The *zone of the cavity* is wedge-shaped in profile and in section almost round, the antero-posterior diameter being 13.5cm and the transverse diameter 12.5cm. It is the most roomy part of the pelvis.

The *zone of the mid-pelvis* passes through the apex of the pubic arch, the spines of the ischium, the sacrospinous ligament and the tip of the sacrum. It is the narrowest zone of the pelvis and is ovoid in shape. The most important diameter is that between the ischial spines (the ischial bispinous diameter)

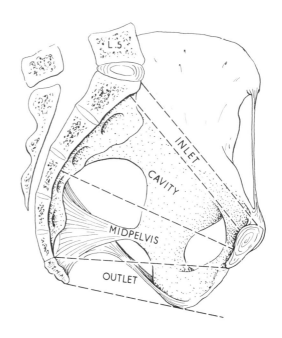

**Fig. 7/4** The 'zones' of the pelvis

which measures 10.5cm. This zone is sometimes contracted, and as the fetal head normally rotates into the antero-posterior diameter of the outlet at this level, rotation may be prevented.

The *zone of the outlet* passes through the arch of the pubis, the tuberosity of the ischium, the sacrotuberous ligament and the coccyx. This zone is pyramidal in shape, the apex being at the line joining the two tuberosities. The transverse diameter measures 11cm and the antero-posterior diameter 12.5cm when the coccyx is pushed back. The angle between the pubic rami – the subpubic angle – is of great importance, for the narrower the pubic arch the more is the fetal head displaced backwards and the less the room available for it. Normally the subpubic arch is rounded and the subpubic angle measures 85° (Fig. **7/5**).

## THE INCLINATION OF THE PELVIC BRIM

In the erect position the pelvic inlet makes an angle of about 55° with the horizontal but this varies among individuals and from race to race. Races which rarely squat have a greater angle, those which

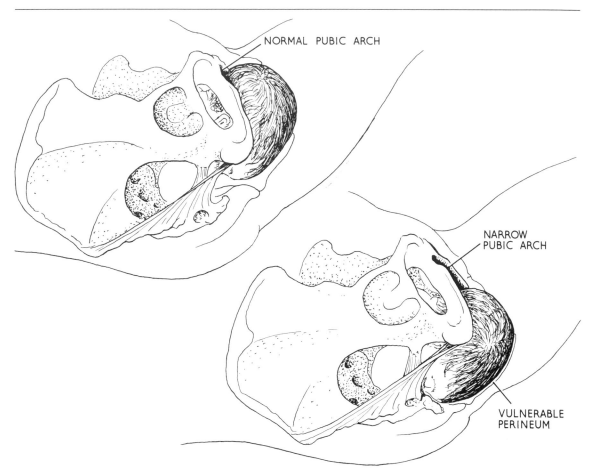

NORMAL PUBIC ARCH

NARROW
PUBIC ARCH

VULNERABLE
PERINEUM

**Fig. 7/5** The subpubic arch. When the arch is narrow the fetal head is forced backwards and tears of the perineum are common

habitually squat a lesser one. The average pelvic inclination amongst Japanese is 40° and amongst Americans 60°. In the reclining position the angle is considerably reduced to about 25° below the horizontal.

The greater the angle, the harder it is for the fetal head to engage and the greater the chances of prolonged labour (Fig. **7/6**).

## THE AXIS OF THE BIRTH CANAL

The axis corresponds to the direction the fetal head takes during its passage through the pelvic cavity. The head descends in a straight line through the zone of the brim and the zone of the pelvic cavity until it reaches the level of the ischial spines (zone of

the mid-pelvis). This area corresponds to the attachments of the pelvic floor and the course of the head is changed from downwards and backwards to downwards and forwards. The axis of the birth canal thus takes an angled turn (Fig. **7/7**).

|  | UK, USA, Australia | Malaysia, Philippines |
|---|---|---|
| Antero-posterior of brim (obstetric conjugate) | 12cm | 11cm |
| Transverse of brim | 13cm | 12cm |
| Ischial bispinous | 10.5cm | 10cm |
| Antero-posterior of outlet | 11.5cm | — |
| Transverse of outlet | 10.5cm | — |
| Subpubic angle | 85° | 85° |

**Table 7/1** Radiographic measurements of the pelvis

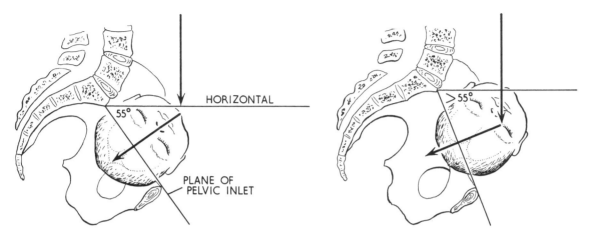

**Fig. 7/6** Diagram showing the effect of the inclination of the pelvic brim on the engagement of the fetal head

## THE IDEAL OBSTETRIC PELVIS

Correlation between pre-delivery radiological pelvimetry and the ease of delivery permits a description of the ideal obstetric pelvis.

1. The brim should be round, or oval transversely with no undue projection of the sacral promontory. The antero-posterior diameter (obstetric conjugate) should measure 12cm and the available transverse diameter 12.5cm. In the erect position the pelvic brim should be inclined at an angle of 55° to the horizontal.
2. The cavity should be shallow with straight side walls from which the ischial spines do not project unduly. The sacrum should have a smooth concave curve, from above downwards, and the sacro-sciatic notches should be large, the sacrospinous ligament being at least 3.5cm long.
3. The pubic arch should be rounded and the inter-tuberous distance at least 10cm.

## FACTORS INFLUENCING PELVIC SHAPE

Gross deformities of pelvic shape due to the effects of childhood rickets or adult osteomalacia are relatively uncommon because of rising affluence and better dietary habits in the developed countries; and because sunshine and calcium are relatively abundant in the developing countries. Minor alterations in shape, however, have been observed more fre-

quently since radiological pelvimetry became available, and epidemiological studies have been applied.

Although racial factors influence the size of the pelvis – and races of small stature are likely to have small pelves – the factors do not seem to have much effect in producing abnormal shapes. Minor abnormalities of shape are due to inadequate nutrition in infancy and childhood, particularly just before puberty when pelvic bone growth is rapid and the

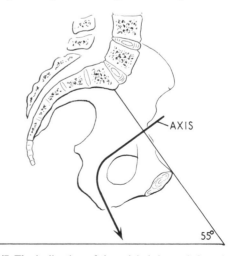

**Fig. 7/7** The inclination of the pelvic brim and the axis of the birth canal. The plane of the pelvic brim makes an angle of about 55° with the horizontal in the erect patient, and the plane of the outlet about 10° with the horizontal. The axis of the birth canal is angled, the alteration in direction occurring at the pelvic floor

bones are still malleable. Amongst Scottish women a height of less than 155cm is associated with a significantly higher incidence of minor pelvic deformity, particularly flattening of the brim. These small women are often in poor health and the combination of poor health, small body stature and minor pelvic deformities are probably due to poor living conditions, poor nutrition and poor hygiene. In Asian countries the association of small stature and pelvic deformity is not so marked and the reasons for this are less clear.

### THE PLACE OF PELVIMETRY IN THE DETECTION OF MINOR PELVIC ABNORMALITIES

The work of Thoms (1935) and Caldwell and Molloy (1940) established pelvimetry as a valuable method of detecting pelvic bony abnormalities. But, as with many discoveries, the method was overused and abused, and complex classification sought to include every possible pelvic shape. It became recommended that every primigravida should have a routine radiological pelvimetry, but despite the information obtained, no reduction in the incidence of complicated labour occurred: for, except when the pelvis is grossly contracted, the final arbiters of vaginal delivery are the quality of the uterine contractions and these cannot be assessed by radiology.

Radiological pelvimetry has now found its correct place: it is an invaluable method of confirming or denying a clinical impression of cephalopelvic disproportion. It should not be used routinely, but only when clinical assessment prior to labour indicates that the pelvis may be contracted, or during labour that cephalopelvic disproportion is present and may interfere with vaginal delivery of the baby. Radiological pelvimetry is discussed in more detail in Chapter 19.

# THE SOFT TISSUES OF THE PELVIS

### THE UTERUS

The uterus can be divided into three functionally different portions: (1) the upper segment; (2) the lower segment; and (3) the cervix, and these will be discussed separately.

#### The upper uterine segment

The muscle of this portion of the uterus undergoes the greatest degree of hyperplasia and hypertrophy during pregnancy, and is the most active contractile portion in labour. It consists of the fundus and that portion of the uterus lying above the reflection of the vesico-uterine fold of peritoneum.

#### The lower uterine segment

This area of the uterus has been subject to much controversy. It is that part of the uterus lying between the vesico-uterine fold superiorly and the fibromuscular junction of uterus and cervix inferiorly. With the effacement and dilatation in labour the cervix also becomes incorporated into the lower segment (Fig. **7/8**).

The myometrial fibres cross at an obtuse angle in this area and consequently the stretch is less than in the fundus, so that during early pregnancy the lower uterine segment is relatively poorly formed. In late pregnancy, when fundal myometrial activity increases, the lower uterine segment develops more rapidly and is stretched radially to permit the fetal head to descend (Fig. **7/9**).

In obstructed labour the full force of the contracting muscle of the fundus of the uterus impinges upon the lower segment, the fibres of which become increasingly distracted, and thinned, so that uterine rupture is a possibility.

After normal delivery and especially after an obstructed labour, the tone of the muscle fibres of the lower uterine segment is less than that of the firmly contracting fundus and on palpation the area is flabby and folded. This hypotonicity is of short duration and within 5 days the lower segment has become incorporated in and is indistinguishable from the upper segment of the uterus.

#### The cervix uteri in pregnancy and labour

The cervix uteri is that portion of the uterus which extends from the fibromuscular junction above to the external os below. The upper margin of the cervix is not a fixed point, as the myometrial fibres

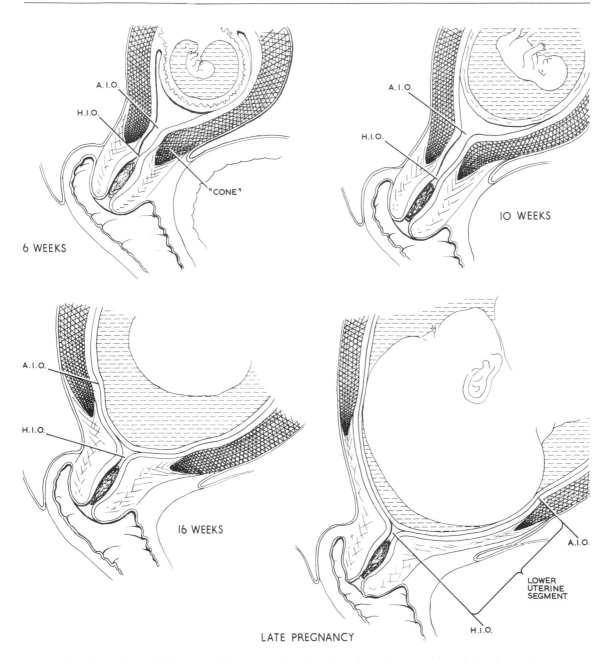

**Fig. 7/8** The formation of the lower uterine segment based on the observations of C. P. Wendell-Smith. Cone = the condensation of muscle at the junction of the body of the uterus and the cervix; A.I.O. = anatomical internal os; H.I.O. = histological internal os.

become attenuated and end as a cone of variable length, from which individual groups of fibrils project like hairs. These myofibrils are surrounded by the collagen characteristic of the parenchyma of the cervix. At the level of the utero-cervical junction the endometrium changes into the single-layer cubical cells characteristic of the endocervix. The endocervical cells invade the collagen matrix in a series

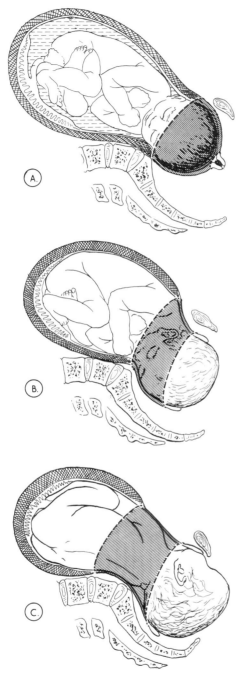

**Fig. 7/9** A. The lower uterine segment in late pregnancy. B. The lower uterine segment in late labour. It has dilated circumferentially and has thinned but is shorter. C. In obstructed labour the dilated and thinned lower uterine segment stretches and is in danger of rupture. Redrawn from Danforth, D. N. and Ivy, A. C. *Amer. J. Obstet. Gynecol.* 1949, **57**, 831

of deep clefts and tunnels, which unfold during cervical dilatation and by offering a greater surface area, prevent epithelial damage occurring during delivery. The endocervical cells are mucin-secreting, but because of the influence of progesterone, the mucus becomes thick and viscid and forms a cervical mucus plug (Fig. **7/10**).

The action of oestrogen and progesterone during pregnancy increases the hygroscopic qualities of the cervical connective tissues and loosens the acid mucopolysaccharides of the binding substance between the collagen fibres. This softens the cervix and permits its more ready dilatation in labour. It also increases the volume of the cervix, and since the endocervix is the least supported area, leads to the eversion of cuboidal endocervical cells onto the vaginal portion of the cervix. The increase in volume occurs radially, but the length of the cervix is not increased, so that in pregnancy the cervix feels soft but is not longer than in the non-pregnant woman. Oestrogen also increases the number and size of cervical blood vessels.

Further alterations occur in the cervix in late pregnancy, and are due to the greater activity of the myometrium. The changes vary from person to person and are more marked in multigravidae. In essence they consist of a variable degree of shortening of the length of the cervix (effacement) and a variable degree of dilatation of the cervical canal. In addition the texture of the cervix becomes softer, resembling the feel of the lips rather than that of the tip of the nose. These findings are collectively called cervical 'ripening' and the feel of the texture of the cervix is the most important of them. The changes may occur gradually or abruptly, and can occur at any time from the 34th week of pregnancy but usually occur nearer to term, especially in primigravidae. However, if examined at the 34th week, 20 per cent of primigravidae and 40 per cent of multigravidae will have a cervix at least 2cm dilated.

Cervical ripening is due to physical alterations in the collagen fibre of the cervix. The changes are probably initiated by prostaglandins, and probably blocked by high levels of circulating progesterone. The effects of the prostaglandins are most marked when a low progesterone:oestrogen ratio exists, which occurs in late pregnancy.

At the onset of labour, the primigravid cervix is ripe, either partly or not effaced and 1.75cm dilated (1 finger-breadth). The multigravid cervix is ripe and usually effaced and 2cm or more dilated (1 to 2 finger-breadths) (Fig. **7/11**). With each uterine con-

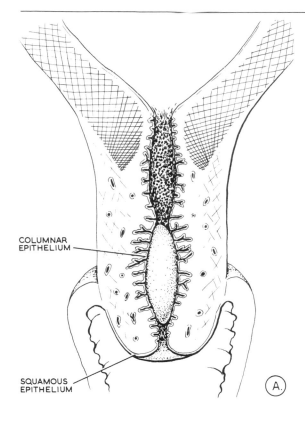

COLUMNAR
EPITHELIUM

SQUAMOUS
EPITHELIUM

(A)

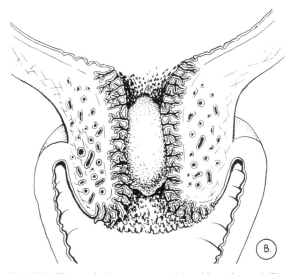

(B)

**Fig. 7/10** The cervix in pregnancy. (A) at 10 weeks; and (B) at 38 weeks. With advancing pregnancy there is an increased vascularity and softening of the cervical tissues, and a marked thickening of the endocervical mucosa, which pouts through the external os giving the appearance of an 'erosion'. Note that the cervix has shortened considerably by the 38th week

traction, there is concurrent slight retraction of the uterine muscle and this force is transmitted to the collagenous cervix. Unable to resist the force, the weak cervix is first effaced completely and then progressively dilates, opening circumferentially, and the presenting part is pushed down onto it. The process is repeated until the entire cervix is incorporated into the body of the uterus and the utero-vaginal canal forms a single tube (Fig. **7/12**).

Following the birth of the baby, the utero-vaginal tube collapses, the uterus contracts and retracts maximally, but the distension of the elastic muscle fibres has gone, and consequently the tension on the cervix is reduced so that it hangs down like a curtain, has little tone and readily admits 3 fingers. It dilates again, this time by pressure, to allow the placenta to pass, but for the first 48 hours of the puerperium is a congested toneless organ of stretched collagen fibrils covered with hyperplastic epithelium.

During the next 14 puerperal days, as oestrogen is withdrawn, there is a rapid reduction of cervical size, its texture becomes increasingly firm, and the ectopic cuboidal epithelium is drawn into the cervical canal, leaving a greater or lesser area which during pregnancy has been transformed by metaplasia into stratified epithelium (the transformation zone).

## THE PELVIC FLOOR

Apart from the uterus and vagina, which will be considered separately, the bony pelvis contains a variety of muscles, the rectum and the bladder. Of most obstetrical interest are the muscles which make up the pelvic floor, for the direction of the rotation of the presenting part, be it head or breech, is profoundly influenced by them.

The main element in the pelvic floor is the group of muscles collectively known as the levator ani, which arise from the lateral pelvic wall and decussate in the midline between the urethra, the vagina and rectum. The levator ani rises from the pelvic aspect of the pubis, from the condensed fascia, known as the white line, which covers the obturator internus muscle, and from the pelvic aspect of the ischial spine (Fig. **7/13**). From this broad origin the fibres sweep downwards, backwards and medially to be inserted into the upper vagina, the perineal body, the anal canal, the anococcygeal body, the lateral border of the coccyx and the lower part of the sacrum (Fig. **7/14**). The sides of the muscle slope downwards and forwards forming a gutter, or sling,

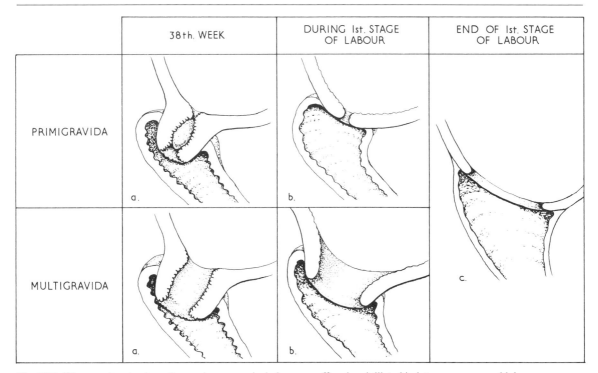

| | 38th. WEEK | DURING 1st. STAGE OF LABOUR | END OF 1st. STAGE OF LABOUR |
|---|---|---|---|
| PRIMIGRAVIDA | a. | b. | c. |
| MULTIGRAVIDA | a. | b. | |

**Fig. 7/11**  Diagram showing how the cervix progressively becomes effaced and dilated in late pregnancy and labour
  1. Primigravida. (a) 38th week of pregnancy. Little or no effacement or dilatation has occurred. (b) First stage of labour. Effacement has occurred but dilatation is not yet marked. (c) End of the first stage of labour. The cervix is fully effaced and dilated.
  2. Multigravida. (a) 38th week of pregnancy. Dilatation has begun but no effacement has yet occurred. (b) First stage of labour. Effacement and dilatation are occurring simultaneously

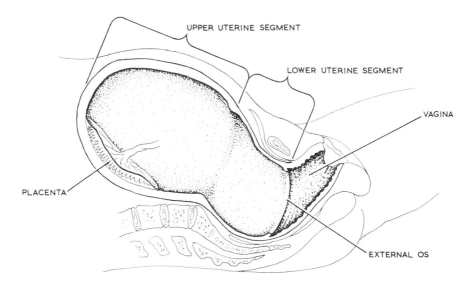

**Fig. 7/12**  The birth canal of a patient in the second stage of labour

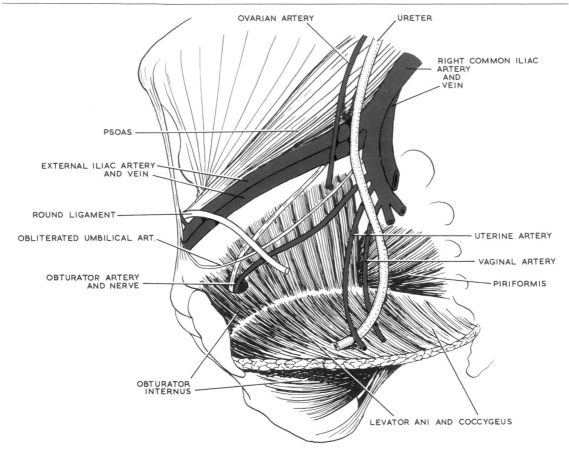

**Fig. 7/13** The lateral pelvic wall

through which the urethra, vagina and rectum pass. To some extent the vagina is supported by this sling, but to a much greater extent the rectum lies suspended by the sling of the levator ani. When the leading part of the fetal head impinges on the gutter formed by the two levator ani muscles it tends to rotate in an anterior direction (Fig. **7/15**).

Above the levator ani muscles are the vessels supplying the uterus and cervix, the ureters and the condensations of areolar tissue which form after stress and by fusing with the fascia which ensheathes the bladder, rectum and cervix uteri and is called the 'cardinal ligament' (Fig. **7/16**). In fact it is not a ligament, but a composite mass of tissue formed from the areolar tissue, collagen and the muscle walls of the venous plexuses which surround the cervix. With full dilatation of the cervix, this tissue is drawn out of the way, but should the patient attempt to push the fetus through an undilated cervix, permanent lengthening of the cardinal ligament is likely.

Anteriorly to the cervix is the bladder, with the bladder base and neck (the vesico-urethral junction) resting on a condensation of fascia, the interdigitating fibres of the levator ani and the muscular wall of the vagina. Should the anterior vaginal wall be damaged during delivery, prolapse of the bladder is likely. This is known as a cystocele.

As the fetal head descends into the pelvis the bladder base is lifted upwards and forwards appearing to rotate about the vesico-urethral junction. The amount of movement depends upon the size of the fetal head; the tighter the fit, the greater the movement. At the same time the vesico-urethral junction and urethra are pushed closer to the posterior surface of the symphysis pubis (Fig. **7/17**). In cases of obstructed labour or traumatic forceps delivery, these two areas, the lower part of the bladder base and vesico-urethral angle, are subject to pressure or damage, which may eventuate in a vesico-vaginal fistula.

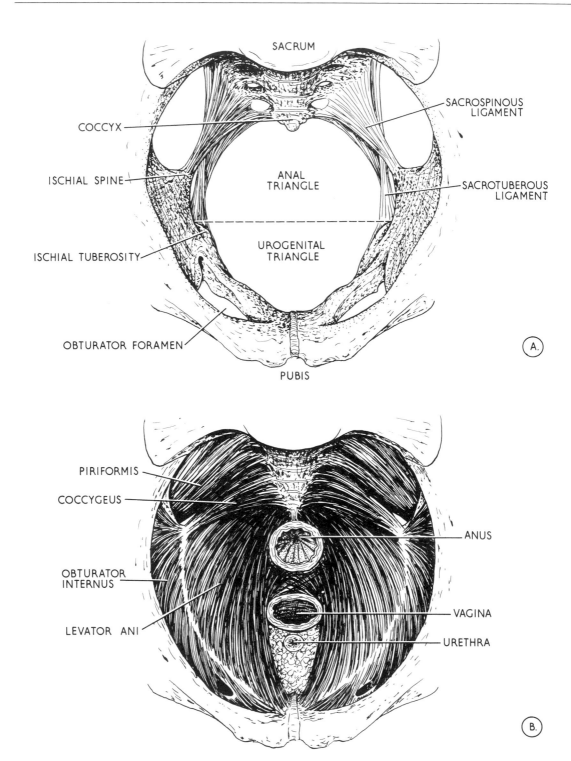

**Fig. 7/14** The muscles which form the pelvic floor viewed from above

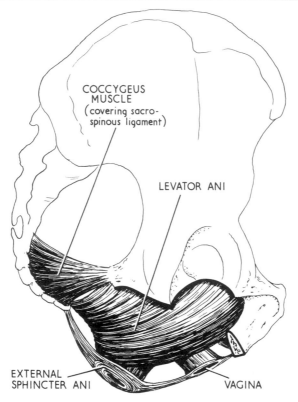

**Fig. 7/15** The pelvic diaphragm: lateral view

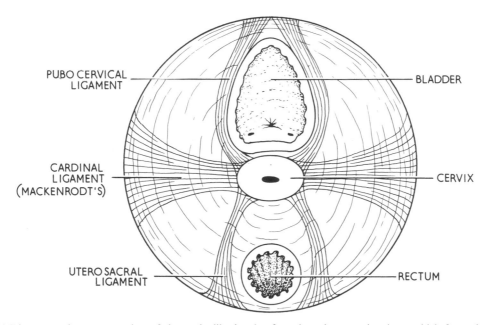

**Fig. 7/16** Diagrammatic representation of the spoke-like bands of condensed connective tissue which form the cardinal 'ligament'

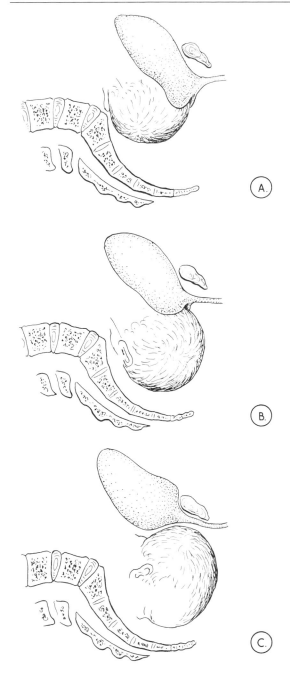

Fig. 7/17 The bladder in labour. Primigravida. (A) One hour in labour. Cervix 3.5cm dilated, bladder base beginning to lift; (B) Fifteen hours in labour. Cervix 7cm dilated; (C) Nineteen hours in labour. Cervix fully dilated, head on perineum. Bladder neck drawn up, urethra elongated (redrawn from radiological studies by Malpas, P., Jeffcoate, T. N. A. and Lister, U. *J. Obstet. Gynaecol. Brit. Emp.* 1949, **56**, 949)

The descending head also presses on the rectum but it is rarely damaged since it is well protected by fat, and has the hollow of the sacrum into which to retreat. Lying behind the rectum and emerging from the sacral foramina are the nerves which form the sciatic plexus. These nerves may be subjected to pressure by the fetal head, or may be damaged by the application of forceps, but permanent injury is uncommon.

In summary the structures related to the upper concave surface of the pelvic floor are:

1. The bladder anteriorly, resting on the pubococcygeus portion of the levator ani
2. The uterus and vagina behind the bladder, the vagina passing through the gap between the levator muscles (hiatus urogenitalis)
3. The broad ligaments and pelvic connective tissue, containing the uterine venous plexuses
4. The ureters, which lie on the pelvic floor beneath the broad ligaments, and pass forwards to the bladder. They are in close relationship to the lateral vaginal fornices and cervix
5. The uterine arteries above the ureters, and the vaginal arteries below the ureters
6. The rectum lying behind the uterus and vagina and passing through the gap between the levator muscles (the hiatus rectalis)
7. Between the levator muscles, and penetrated by the urethra and the vagina, is the superior layer of condensed tissue known as the urogenital diaphragm.

## THE PERINEUM

Below the pelvic floor is the perineum. Above it is bounded by the convex surface of the levatores ani, below by the skin between the buttocks and thighs. Laterally it is bounded by the bones and ligaments of the pelvic outlet – the lower pubic rami, the ischial tuberosities, the sacrotuberous ligaments and the coccyx. In this way it forms two triangular areas, the urogenital triangle anteriorly and the anal triangle posteriorly (Fig. **7/18**).

The urogenital triangle is filled with several muscles which meet at the mid-point of the perineum between vagina and rectum and are bounded above and below by layers of superficial fascia. This area is particularly vulnerable to injury by the birth of the fetus and perineal tears commonly occur during delivery unless a preventive incision, known as an episiotomy, is performed.

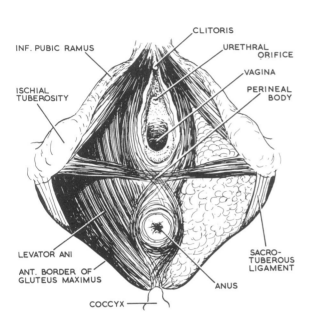

INF. PUBIC RAMUS

ISCHIAL
TUBEROSITY

LEVATOR ANI

ANT. BORDER OF
GLUTEUS MAXIMUS

COCCYX

CLITORIS

URETHRAL
ORIFICE

VAGINA

PERINEAL
BODY

SACRO-
TUBEROUS
LIGAMENT

ANUS

**Fig. 7/18** The muscles of the female perineum. In the left half of the diagram the fat pad which fills the space has been removed to show the lower surface of the levator ani which forms the roof of the space

## THE FORMATION OF THE BIRTH CANAL

When myometrial contraction and retraction has led to full dilatation of the cervix the head descends into the vagina which expands to encompass it. Normally an apparent space, the vaginal muscle has hypertrophied and the epithelium become folded during pregnancy so that it can accommodate the fetus without damage. As the fetal head descends it encounters the pelvic floor and the leading point is directed forward by the gutter formed by the levatores ani. The fetus must now pass through the urogenital diaphragm. The levator muscles stretch and are displaced downwards and backwards so that the anus receives the full force of the descending head and, dilating, gapes widely to expose the anterior rectal wall. Pressure is also exerted on the lower part of the vagina, and the central portion of the perineum, and as the head is born the tissues may tear.

The descent of the fetus from the uterus to the world is straight to the level of the ischial spines, then it moves in an anterior curve around the lower border of the symphysis pubis. If the pubic arch is wide, the head will stem close behind the symphysis, and the perineum will not be so stretched. If the angle is narrow, the head is forced back, the direction of the curve is more obtuse and perineal damage likely.

## Chapter 8

# The Passenger

The fetus may influence the course of labour by its size and position. A large baby, with a large hard head, may cause difficulty as it is propelled through the birth canal. Of all the parts of the fetus, the head is the most important as it is the least compressible and pliable part, and the one liable to suffer the most damage.

The face of the newborn baby is small relative to the cranium which makes up most of the head. The cranium is made up of five bones held together by a membrane which permits their movement during birth and in early childhood. They eventually fuse to form the firm rigid skull of adult life. The bones are the two frontal, the two parietal bones and the occipital bone, and the areas where they impinge upon each other are called *sutures*. Some of the bones have rounded corners so that wide spaces are left, covered by membrane. These are termed *fontanelles* (Fig. **8/1**).

The frontal bone is separated from the two parietal bones by the coronal suture, and is itself divided by the frontal suture. The two parietal bones are separated by the sagittal suture, and are separated from the occipital bone by the lambdoid suture. Each parietal bone posteriorly is protuberant and this region is known as the parietal eminence.

At the junction of the sagittal, frontal and coronal sutures is a diamond-shaped space, the anterior fontanelle. Between the two parietal bones and the occipital bone is a triangular space, which becomes obliterated in labour as the occipital bone slips under the parietal bones. However, the edges of the parietal bones remain palpable, and with the posterior part of the sagittal suture have the shape of a Y, the leg of the Y being the sagittal suture. This is the posterior fontanelle.

The regions of the skull are distinguished by special names which aid in the description of the presenting part palpated per vaginam during labour (Fig. **8/2**).

The *occiput* is the area lying behind the posterior fontanelle.

The *vertex* is the area of the skull lying between the anterior and posterior fontanelles and two parietal eminences.

The *bregma* is the area of the anterior fontanelle.

The *sinciput* is the area lying in front of the anterior fontanelle. The sinciput can be further subdivided into:

The *brow* which is the area between the anterior fontanelle and the root of the nose.

The *face* which is the area below the root of the nose and the orbital ridges.

## THE DIAMETERS OF THE FETAL SKULL

The region of the skull which presents in labour depends on the degree of flexion of the head, and the area involved may be related to the diameter of that region. In the occipital presentation the diameter at right angles to the occiput is the suboccipito-bregmatic diameter which measures 9.5cm. In the vertical position the diameter is the occipito-frontal which measures 11.5cm. If the brow presents, the relevant diameter is the mento-vertical measuring 13cm and the head in this presentation is unlikely to negotiate the pelvis. If the face presents, the short submento-bregmatic diameter presents (Fig. **8/3**). Two other diameters of the fetal skull are also important, the biparietal which measures 9.5cm and the bitemporal of 8cm. In summary it can be seen that the fetal skull is an irregular ovoid, narrow in front, broad behind, mainly because of the two parietal eminences.

If the fetal head can pass through the pelvis, the rest of the body can usually follow without difficulty. Occasionally there is difficulty with the shoulders

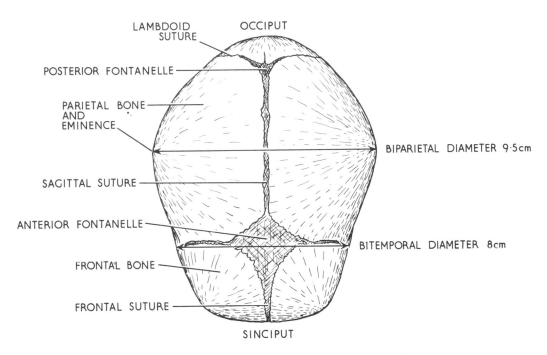

LAMBDOID SUTURE
OCCIPUT
POSTERIOR FONTANELLE
PARIETAL BONE AND EMINENCE
BIPARIETAL DIAMETER 9·5cm
SAGITTAL SUTURE
ANTERIOR FONTANELLE
BITEMPORAL DIAMETER 8cm
FRONTAL BONE
FRONTAL SUTURE
SINCIPUT

**Fig. 8/1** The fetal skull from above showing important obstetrical diameters

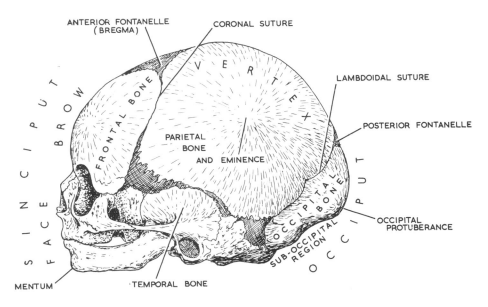

ANTERIOR FONTANELLE (BREGMA)
CORONAL SUTURE
LAMBDOIDAL SUTURE
POSTERIOR FONTANELLE
VERTEX
SINCIPUT
BROW
FRONTAL BONE
PARIETAL BONE AND EMINENCE
OCCIPITAL BONE
OCCIPUT
SUB-OCCIPITAL REGION
OCCIPITAL PROTUBERANCE
FACE
MENTUM
TEMPORAL BONE

**Fig. 8/2** The fetal skull from the side, showing landmarks

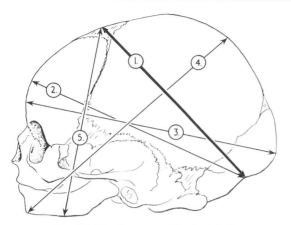

**Fig. 8/3** The diameters of the fetal skull

|   | Diameter | Length | Presentation |
|---|----------|--------|--------------|
| 1. | Suboccipito-bregmatic | 9.5cm | Flexed vertex |
| 2. | Suboccipito-frontal | 10.5cm | Partially deflexed vertex |
| 3. | Occipito-frontal | 11.5cm | Deflexed vertex |
| 4. | Mento-vertical | 13.0cm | Brow |
| 5. | Submento-bregmatic | 9.5cm | Face |

and the width of these is taken between the two acromial processes. This diameter, known as the *bis-acromial*, measures 11.5cm.

If the buttocks present, the measurement of the presenting part is taken as the distance between the trochanters of the two femora. This diameter, which is called the *bi-trochanteric* diameter, measures 9cm.

## MOULDING OF THE SKULL

As the fetal head passes through the pelvis it is subjected to considerable pressure. Owing to the mobility of the bones within their membranous cover-ing, its shape may be modified without damage to enable it to mould into the pelvis. During moulding the parietal bones slip under each other and the occipital bone and the frontal bones slip under the parietal bones (Fig. **8/4**). If the amniotic sac has ruptured the ring of the cervix presses firmly against the scalp, and venous return and lymphatic drainage is diminished from the encompassed area of the scalp, producing a swelling called the *caput suc-cedaneum*. The size of the caput, which is soft and boggy to touch, varies with the degree of pelvic contraction, but disappears within a few days of birth (Fig. **8/5**).

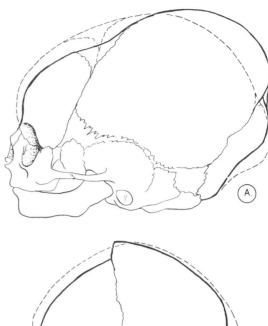

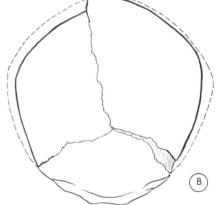

**Fig. 8/4** Moulding of the fetal skull. (A) lateral view; (B) posterior view. The dotted line shows the shape before moulding

## THE DISPOSITION OF THE FETUS IN THE UTERUS

Although the fetus in labour is compressed to some extent into a cylinder and little able to move, for convenience of description certain terms are used.

The *lie* refers to the relationship of the long axis of the fetus to the mother. The fetus may be in a longitudinal (vertex or breech), or an oblique, or a transverse lie. Ninety-nine per cent of babies enter labour in a longitudinal lie, either presenting cephal-ically (in 95 per cent) or as a breech (in 4 per cent) (Fig. **8/6**).

The *attitude* of the fetus is defined as the relation of the various fetal parts to each other. Normally in labour the fetus is flexed at all joints.

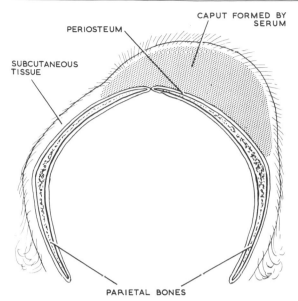

**Fig. 8/5** The caput succedaneum

The *presentation* relates to that part of the child which occupies the lower segment of the uterus. When the head occupies this zone, the presentation is cephalic; if the buttocks occupy the zone, it is a breech presentation, whilst if the child lies obliquely, the shoulder generally occupies the lower segment and it is a shoulder presentation.

The *presenting part* is that portion of the fetus which is bounded by the cervix during the first stage of labour, or the vagina in the second stage and which is touched by the fingers on a vaginal examination. If the presentation is cephalic, the presenting part is usually the vertex, but may be the brow or the face depending on the degree of deflexion of the head on the spine. Similarly the child's legs in a breech presentation may be flexed, extended or a foot may present.

The *position* of the fetus refers to the relationship of the presenting part to the periphery of the pelvis. If the vertex presents the occiput is the point of

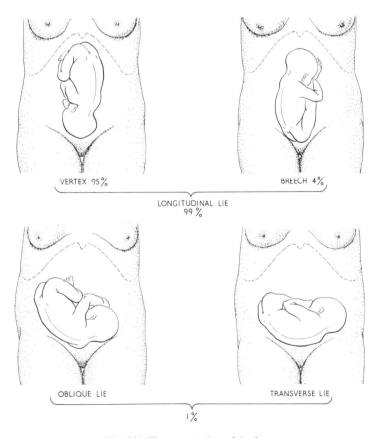

**Fig. 8/6** The presentation of the fetus

reference, if the breech presents the sacrum is the point of reference, if the face presents, the chin, or mentum, is the point of reference; if the shoulder presents the scapula is the point of reference. It is referred to the maternal pelvis, imagining the mother to be in the erect position, and dividing the pelvis into segments of 45°. Thus right refers to the right side of the mother, and left to her left side; anterior refers to her front, and posterior to her back. In the vertex presentation the eight positions occur with unequal frequency.

For ready reference the positions and frequency in the case of vertex presentations are given in Fig. **8/7**. It can be seen that in 75 per cent of cases the vertex engages in a lateral position. The reference point of the breech is the sacrum, and the eight positions are SA, RSA, RSL, RSP, SP, LSP, LSL and LSA.

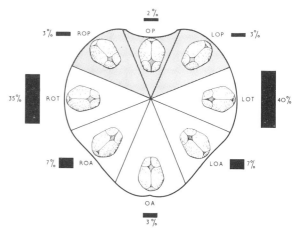

**Fig. 8/7** The positions of the vertex at the onset of labour, and their relative frequency; the shaded positions are the pessimal ones

## GROWTH OF THE FETUS

The development of ultrasound has permitted an accurate determination of fetal weight for a given gestational age. In Malmo, Sweden, the method has been used for all pregnancies since 1973. The results are shown in Fig. **8/8**. It will be observed that the fetus reaches a weight of 2500g at the end of the 35th week and that there is no slowing down of weight increase around 40 weeks.

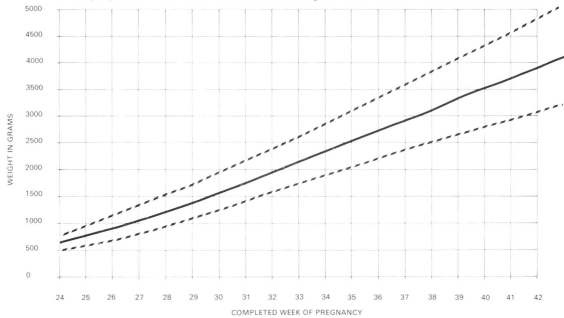

**Fig. 8/8** Fetal weight at various weeks of gestation (from 24 weeks)

*Chapter 9*

# The Powers

## THE PHYSIOLOGY OF UTERINE ACTIVITY

The myometrium is composed of interdigitating spiral fibres derived from the two Mullerian ducts which have joined at their antimesenteric borders and, by the disappearance of the central septum, formed a single muscular hollow organ. The outer longitudinal and inner circular layers are poorly developed and unimportant, and these extend the entire length of the Mullerian tract. The middle spiral, interdigitating layer is only marked in the uterine portion, and the muscle content decreases toward the cervix so that muscle forms no more than 10 per cent of the cervical tissue compared with over 90 per cent of fundal tissue.

Each muscle fibre is composed of bundles of fibrils which, in turn, are composed of spindle-shaped cells, averaging 200mm in length and 7mm in diameter. Electron microscopy has shown that these cells are themselves made up of smaller elements, and it is these which are the contractile elements of the uterus. The contractile fibril is made up of interdigitating protein chains of actin and myosin, surrounded by a membrane which alters in permeability (Fig. **9/1**).

### MUSCLE FIBRE CONTRACTION

In the presence of oestrogen and probably generated by prostaglandins, an impulse alters the electric potential of the cell membrane and permits the entry into the contractile fibril of sodium and calcium ions

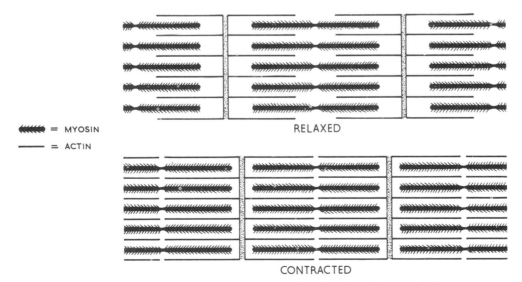

**Fig. 9/1** Diagram showing the arrangement of myosin and actin in a muscle fibre

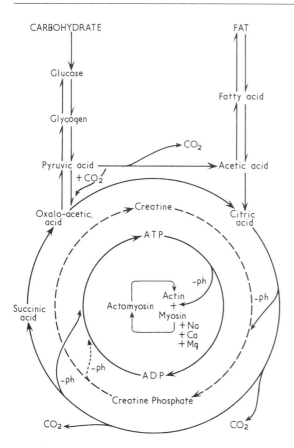

**Fig. 9/2** Biochemistry of muscle activity ATP = adenosine-triphosphate: ADP = adenosinediphosphate

## CHARACTERISTICS OF MYOMETRIAL CONTRACTIONS

Although the uterus is composed of many fibres and fibrils, in practice it functions as a single hollow muscular organ, and myometrial contractions can be measured by placing a thin polyethylene catheter into the amniotic cavity and attaching this to a recording apparatus to determine the amniotic pressure. Since this is proportional to the tension in the myometrium, it measures myometrial activity with accuracy.

Uterine muscle is never completely relaxed and in between contractions a resting *tone*, ranging between 6 and 12mmHg, is found. The contraction causes a rise in intra-uterine pressure and this rise is called the intensity, or *amplitude*, of the contraction. It has two elements, a fairly rapid rise to its peak and a slower decline to the basal tone. The *frequency* of contractions is expressed as the number per unit of time. Much of the research on uterine activity has been done in Montevideo, and the product of intensity times frequency over a 10-minute period gives a measure of uterine activity. This is expressed in Montevideo Units (Fig. **9/3**).

Recently, studies of uterine activity have been made using a cardiotocograph linked to a computer. The computer measures the area under the contraction, above the base line. This is expressed in kilopascals per 15 minutes in the print-out. In active labour, the mean contraction area is $1100 \pm 350$kPa/

which start the energy-releasing cycle, leading to a momentary electrostatic discharge being created. This pulls the actin fibrils into the spaces between the myosin fibrils (Fig. **9/2**). As the excitation wave discharge ceases, the protein chains separate again.

Prostaglandin either directly, or by potentiating oxytocin, a hypothalamic hormone, also lowers the threshold of the adjacent cell membranes to impulses and permits the excitation wave to pass from fibril to fibril, and so a contraction of the entire muscle fibre, and then of adjacent fibres occurs. The contractile wave is opposed by placental progesterone which 'blocks' the passage of the impulse from fibril to fibril. In late pregnancy the 'blocking' effect of progesterone is reduced and the stimulating effects of prostaglandin and oxytocin are increased. This has the effect of increasing the contractility of the uterus as pregnancy advances.

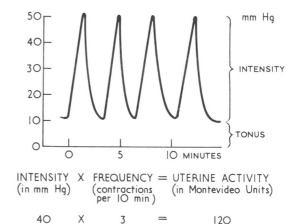

| INTENSITY (in mm Hg) | X | FREQUENCY (contractions per 10 min) | = | UTERINE ACTIVITY (in Montevideo Units) |
|---|---|---|---|---|
| 40 | X | 3 | = | 120 |

**Fig. 9/3** Quantitative measurements of tracings of uterine contractions (redrawn from Caldeyro-Barcia, R. and Poseiro, J. J. in Greenhill's *Obstetrics*, 13th edition. Saunders, 1965)

15 min. Studies have shown that kPa/15 min correlate well with Montevideo Units per 15 min, but with the appropriate equipment the former can be automatically computed.

## SPREAD OF CONTRACTIONS

The method of determining myometrial activity by measuring amniotic pressure has the disadvantage that it only records total activity and gives no information about what is happening in the various parts of the uterus. Since the descent into the pelvis of the fetus, and its later expulsion into the world,

depends largely upon the activity of the fundal muscle in dilating the cervix, it is clear that there must be a gradient of activity, stronger in the fundus and weaker in the lower pole of the uterus, or the cervix would not dilate. By placing external recorders on various parts of the abdomen over the uterus, or by inserting microballoons into the myometrium, it has been possible to record myometrial activity simultaneously in various parts of the uterus.

At the junction of the Fallopian tube and uterus on each side there is a 'pacemaker'. In each woman one or other pacemaker is dominant and it is from here that all contractile waves originate. The wave passes inwards and downwards from the pacemaker,

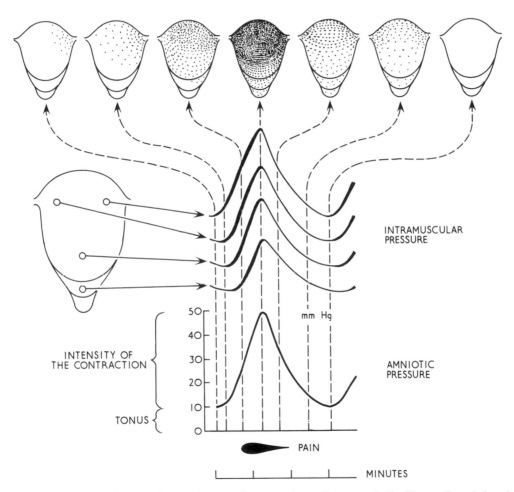

**Fig. 9/4** The normal wave of contraction passing over the uterus shown diagrammatically. The small uteri show how the wave starts and spreads, finally fading. The large uterus shows the four points at which the intermyometrial pressure was recorded with microballoons. The phase of contraction is shown by the thick ascending line. Note how the peak of contraction occurs in all parts of the uterus simultaneously (redrawn from Caldeyro-Barcia, R. *Trans. Cong. Int. Gynecol. et Obstet. 1958.* Librairie Beauchemin, Montreal, 1959)

at a rate of 2cm per second, to involve the entire organ in a contraction. In normal uterine action, the intensity and incremental stage of the contraction is greater in the upper segment as the muscle is thicker and there is a higher proportion of actomyosin to contract. In this way the contraction is co-ordinated, the maximal amount of contraction occurring in the fundal part of the uterus, and the peak of the contraction occurring in all parts simultaneously (the triple descending gradient) (Fig. **9/4**). The position of the mother during labour influences uterine activity. Uterine action is greatest in women who walk about during labour, and least amongst women who labour lying prone on a delivery bed. With each contraction there is a slight permanent shortening of the muscle fibres (retraction) and since the cervix is deficient in muscle it is progressively dilated. The dilatation of the cervix is further aided by the pressure of the fetal presenting part against it, which leads to the reflex release of additional oxytocin.

# MYOMETRIAL ACTIVITY

### Pregnancy

Up to the 30th week of pregnancy uterine activity is slight, small localized contractions of no more than 5mmHg occurring at intervals of 1 minute. Every 30 to 60 minutes a contraction of higher amplitude (10 to 15mmHg) arises which spreads to a wider area of the uterus and may be palpated (Fig. **9/5a**). These palpable contractions occur with increasing frequency and intensity after the 30th week and are referred to as Braxton Hicks contractions (Fig. **9/5b**). After the 36th week of pregnancy, uterine activity increases progressively until at a point in time labour starts (Fig. **9/5c**).

### The onset of labour

This is difficult to determine with accuracy, and consequently difficult to define. At the most it can be said to be the time after which uterine contractions cause the progressive dilatation of the cervix beyond 2cm, and painful contractions usually occur at least every 10 minutes (Fig. **9/5d**).

### Labour

In true normal labour the intensity and frequency of the contractions increase, but there is no rise in the resting tone. The *intensity* increases in late labour to 60mmHg and the *frequency* to 2 to 4 contractions every 10 minutes, or 150 to 200 Montevideo Units. The *duration* of the contraction also increases from about 20 seconds in early labour to 40 to 90 seconds at the end of the first stage, and in the second stage (Fig. **9/5e**). Contractions are most effective when they are co-ordinate, with fundal dominance, have a maximum intensity of 40 to 60mmHg, last 60 to 90 seconds and recur with a 2- to 4-minute interval between the peaks of consecutive contractions, and the uterus has a resting tone of less than 12mmHg. More frequent contractions of higher intensity diminish the oxygen exchange in the placental bed and may lead to fetal hypoxia and clinical signs of fetal distress. The efficiency of contractions is greater when the mother walks about or lies on her side during the first stage of labour, and this position also improves the placental blood supply.

The co-ordinated contractions of labour cause a permanent shortening of the muscle fibres and since this is maximal in the upper part of the uterus a distending tension is placed upon the less muscular lower part, and more particularly upon the scantily muscled cervix. The cervix therefore dilates circumferentially with each contraction, closing in at the end of the contraction; but because of the retraction of the muscle in the upper uterus, a permanent but slight dilatation occurs with each contraction.

In the second stage of labour voluntary contraction of the diaphragm and abdominal muscles, added to the uterine contraction, propels the baby downwards through the dilated vagina and overcomes the resistance of perineal muscles to its advance (Fig. **9/5f**). At the height of each bearing-down effort the total force exerted on the fetus is approximately 8000g and this is resolved into two components: one a force propelling the head downwards, and the other a dilating force, which stretches the birth canal against the resistance of the pelvic and perineal muscles. (If the membranes are intact the resultant

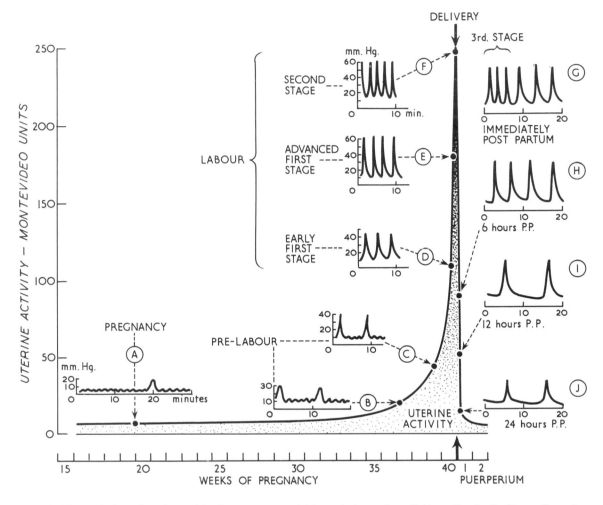

**Fig. 9/5** The evolution of uterine activity in pregnancy and labour (redrawn from Caldeyro-Barcia, R. *Trans. Cong. Int. Gynecol. et Obstet. 1958*. Librairie Beauchemin, Montreal, 1959)

propelling force is less, as the amniotic fluid balances part of it.) Since the pelvic floor muscles form an inclined groove, and since the head is ovoid, the additional pressure leads to the rotation of the occiput through 90° to lie anteriorly.

Uterine activity continues unaltered after expulsion of the fetus and leads to the expulsion of the placenta from the upper uterine segment, in between 2 and 6 minutes after the birth of the baby. Once the placenta has left the upper uterine segment, uterine activity diminishes, but contractions of an intensity of about 60 to 80mmHg still occur regularly for 48 hours after delivery, the frequency decreasing as time passes (Figs **9/5g** to **9/5j**). these contractions

and those of the third stage are usually painless, but painful contractions disturb some patients. Further painful contractions may occur with suckling, due to a reflex release of oxytocin.

## INNERVATION OF THE UTERUS

The uterus is well supplied with sensory nerve fibres, and these, together with sensory fibres from the upper vagina, pass through the felted plexus of nerve ganglia which lies adjacent to the lateral aspect of the cervix, on each side. This nerve plexus is known as the juxtacervical plexus, or Frankenhauser's

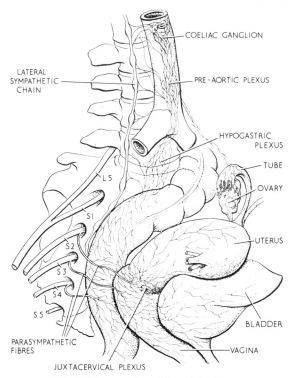

Fig. 9/6 Innervation of the pelvic viscera

plexus (Fig. 9/6). The fibres pass on to the hypogastric plexuses, the inferior of which forms the presacral nerve, and then through the lumbar and lower thoracic chains to reach the spinal cord at T11, T12 and L1. A few sympathetic fibres derive from the lumbar sympathetic chain. Parasympathetic fibres reach the plexus from the parasympathetic components of S2, S3 and S4 nerve roots, but whether these nerves pass through the plexus to reach the uterus has not been determined.

The motor nerve fibres to the uterus leave the spinal cord at the level of T7 and T8. They then pass through the hypogastric plexuses and the juxtacervical plexus to reach and spread through the uterus.

The higher level of the emergence of the motor nerves compared with that of the sensory nerves, permits the latter to be blocked by epidural anaesthesia, without the block affecting uterine activity.

**Intrinsic nerves of the uterus**

Small ganglia are found in a net of nerves lying in contact with the outer surface of the muscular layer

of vagina and cervix, but no ganglia have been detected above the level of the internal os, nor has any co-ordinating nerve plexus been found in the myometrium. It appears, therefore, that the intrinsic nerves of the uterus are all postganglionic and are distributed to both the myo- and endometrium. A few of the fibres end in nerve cells but the majority supply the arterioles. Most of these are non-myelinated (i.e. motor) and stimulation produces vasoconstriction. Myelinated (i.e. sensory) fibres are found in situations similar to those of the motor fibres.

**Functional aspects**

At the moment the functional action of the nerve supply is little understood. If the sympathetic supply has any activity other than that regulating vasodilatation it would appear to be inhibitory rather than motor, but not all impulses passing along the sympathetic fibres have the same effect, some impulses causing excitation, some inhibition. This may depend on the stimulation of one of two kinds of receptors in the vessel walls. In pregnancy the $\beta$-receptors, which are inhibitory, seem to be more responsive to stimuli, and this may be due to the hormonal ratio at the time.

Whatever the distribution of the sympathetic supply, it has little importance in uterine activity, which can continue uninterruptedly in the absence of any nervous connection. Indeed, if anything, the uterus acts more efficiently when the nerve connections are severed, suggesting that the sympathetic supply is regulatory rather than actively motor.

## THE PAINS OF UTERINE CONTRACTIONS

The cause of pain during the contractions of labour is not clearly understood, as it is known that the contractions of the puerperium, although of equal intensity, are usually painless. The confusion is increased as pain is subjective, and different pain thresholds are found in different people, and in the same person under different circumstances. The well-adjusted woman, who knows what will happen in labour and who has no hidden fears, will feel less pain than the excitable, fearful woman (Fig. 9/7).

In part, uterine pain may be due to ischaemia developing in a myometrial fibre during active contraction. Since the fibres occupying the upper uterine segment are the most active, pain from these should

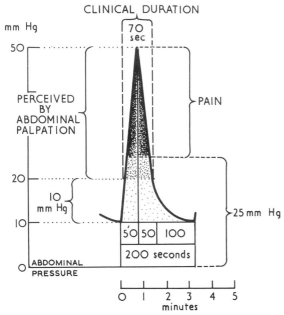

**Fig. 9/7** Pain in labour. The initial part of the contraction is painless and not perceived by abdominal palpation. The duration of the contraction observed clinically (70 s) is shorter than the duration of myometrial activity (200 s)

be felt most during a contraction. This accords with clinical experience as the pain of uterine contraction in labour is felt in the abdomen in the approximate distribution of the cutaneous nerves of T12 and L1.

The backache which occurs during cervical dilatation, and when the lower uterine segment muscle contracts more strongly than normally, is due to stimulation of sensory fibres which pass along the sympathetic nerves to the sacral central connection. From this it is clear that the more efficient the labour, i.e. the more dominant the fundus and relaxed the lower uterine segment and cervix, the less the backache and lower abdominal pain. In the second stage of labour the pain is due to stretching of the vagina and pelvic and perineal tissues. It will therefore be felt in the back, in the pelvis and may radiate down the inner surface of the thighs.

The pain of labour can be reduced or eliminated by (1) damping down the cerebral perception of pain; (2) anaesthetizing the nerves as they enter the spinal cord by the use of epidural anaesthesia which extends as far up as T12; or (3) by blocking the nerves of the juxtacervical plexus. The pain of the second stage can be reduced, or eliminated, in a like manner, or by blocking the pelvic and perineal

nerves at the ischial spines, or by a block of the perineal nerves. Pain relief in labour is discussed in Chapter 18.

## THE INITIATION OF LABOUR

The cause of the onset of labour in humans is still unknown, although in recent years more facts have been discovered, and the process is better understood in laboratory animals. The statement Reynolds made in 1965 that parturition probably began 'as a result of the gradual accelerating convergence of a number of factors, structural, humoral, nervous, nutritional and circulatory which, at a specific time in each species, and adapted to the morphologic conditions present in each, are so associated that they lead to the evacuation of the uterus of its contents' still represents most of our knowledge.

Any explanation of the mechanism which controls labour has to take into account the fact that the uterus, unlike other hollow muscular organs, is able to become distended without reflexly initiating muscular contractions in an attempt to expel the distending object. From this it seems that for labour to start, two events have to occur. The first is that the cervix 'ripens', in other words the collagen tissue alters in texture so that the progressive dilatation of the cervix is more readily effected. The second event is that the myometrial contractions become co-ordinated and the triple descending gradient of uterine activity becomes established.

During pregnancy these events are inhibited by the action of several hormones, which interact with each other in ways which remain obscure. Current evidence suggests that cervical ripening is effected by an increasing local concentration of prostaglandins and is inhibited by the action of progesterone.

The control of uterine activity, at least in so far as co-ordinated progressive activity is concerned also appears to depend on a precise interplay of several hormones.

One hypothesis is that uterine quiescence is maintained during pregnancy by progesterone, secreted by the syncytiotrophoblast. It is believed that in the human, a 'progesterone block' of uterine activity is opposed by oestrogen. Oestrogen, which causes myometrial hyperplasia and hypertrophy in the first half of pregnancy, is also thought to initiate the synthesis and release of prostaglandins by decidual cells. The released prostaglandins act *locally* on adjacent myometrial fibres which are stimulated to contract. The role of posterior pituitary oxytocin is uncertain, but there is evidence that its main function is to sensitize the myometrial fibres so that a contraction wave may pass from a muscle fibre to an adjacent muscle fibre, and so spread through the myometrium. Recently additional facts bearing on this hypothesis have been discovered. In the last 3 or 4 weeks of pregnancy a change in the ratio between free (unbound) oestriol and progesterone (measured in saliva) occurs. Oestriol levels continue to rise, whilst progesterone levels either plateau or fall slightly. This leads to a raised oestrogen/progesterone ratio. Rising oestrogen levels are known to enhance the synthesis of prostaglandins in uterine tissue. At cellular level, it has been demonstrated that progesterone is less well able to bind to receptors in myometrial cells in the last weeks of pregnancy. These findings, if confirmed, support the belief that the 'progesterone block' is less efficient as term approaches.

During the same period of time, amniotic (and presumably decidual) levels of prostaglandins rise, and the myometrium becomes increasingly sensitive until, at a particular point in time, regular progressively strong, actively propagated, co-ordinated uterine contractions begin, mediated either directly by prostaglandin, or indirectly, after the myometrium has been sensitized by endogenous, perhaps fetal, oxytocin.

Recent research suggests that in late pregnancy oxytocin receptors appear in the decidua. Oxytocin binds to the receptors and induces the release of prostaglandins (PGF2$\alpha$) from the decidua. It also appears that endometrial prolactin modulates the synthesis of prostaglandins. Prostaglandins then potentiate oxytocin-induced uterine contractions, leading to cervical effacement and the establishment of uterine activity. There is evidence that decidual prostaglandin levels have to increase for labour to progress from the quiet to the active phase (see p. 111). If this research is confirmed it appears that both oxytocin and prostaglandins are required to *initiate* labour, but to maintain progressive labour, prostaglandins alone are effective.

In some animal species, the fetus is involved in its own birth process by producing hormones, but it has not been established if the human fetus has a similar role in initiating its own birth. Up to term, the fetal pituitary only produces fragments of the ACTH molecule, but at term it produces formed ACTH. Also in late pregnancy the fetal pituitary produces increasing amounts of oxytocin. These two hormones may be involved in the co-ordinated rhythmic uterine contractions which characterize labour.

From the fragmentary evidence it would seem that labour starts not only because of a reduction in inhibiting influences but also because of an increase in stimulating influences. The balance between these influences varies between individuals and between pregnancies in an individual. The only constant fact is that the time of onset of labour is quite inconstant.

## Chapter 10

# Physiological Alterations in Labour

## MATERNAL

The effect of labour on the mother depends upon its duration, the attitude of the mother and of her attendants to labour, and her physical condition at the onset of labour. Since the aim of antenatal care is to ensure that a woman enters labour at the peak of her physical and psychological condition and is attended during labour by trained, empathetic attendants, the main factor is the length of the labour.

### Energy expenditure in labour

Labour is aptly named, for it is a period of considerable expenditure of energy. Most of this energy expenditure is due to the muscular activity of the contracting uterus, but to some extent increased cardiac activity is involved. The metabolic processes releasing energy require glucose as an initial ingredient, but carbohydrate intake in labour tends to be limited, because of the current policy of starving a woman during childbirth. This may lead to the oxidization of accumulated body fat to provide energy for skeletal and smooth muscle contractions. The metabolic process causes a rise in the level of ketones in the blood, predominantly D-3 hydroxybutyric acid and, to a lesser extent, lactic and pyruvic acids, and a consequent mild metabolic acidosis. This is most marked in the second stage of labour when uterine activity is greatest, and a fall of about 0.05 units in the maternal blood pH is usual, although the pH remains in the normal range of 7.3 to 7.4.

The mild metabolic acidosis which occurs in late labour is compensated to some extent by a mild respiratory alkalosis. This results from hyperventilation which tends to occur at this time, perhaps in response to progesterone levels and to anxiety. In the second stage of labour the respiratory alkalosis diminishes as breath-holding is usual during uterine contractions, and the metabolic acidosis tends to increase because of the stronger uterine contractions. Some degree of mild acidoketosis seems common in labour, and ketonuria often occurs (as judged by the use of Ketostix which is probably too sensitive a test as it indicates > 1mmol/litre of aceto-acetic acid). If the woman enters labour in good condition and labour lasts less than 12 hours, the mild acidoketosis can be ignored, and intravenous infusions are not necessary.

In longer labours and in difficult labours an intravenous infusion should be started. The amount should be limited to 1 500ml over a 12-hour period. Larger quantities should be avoided as women in labour have an impaired ability to excrete water and water intoxication, or maternal or fetal hyponatraemia may result. Solutions of 5 or 10 per cent dextrose should be avoided as they may provoke maternal hyperinsulinaemia and hypoglycaemia, which inhibit liver lipolysis and ketone synthesis. This in turn leads to excessive lactate formation and a reduction in the buffering capacity of the blood. Fetal hypoglycaemia and increased plasma lactate levels also occur. Hartmann's solution is an alternative, but in excess it too increases maternal and fetal lactate levels. If hydration is required in labour, normal saline should alternate with Hartmann's solution.

### Cardiovascular changes

The increased energy required in labour is not only used for uterine muscular activity, but also for increased cardiac work. Cardiac output increases by 12 per cent over prelabour baseline readings between contractions in active labour; and by 30 per cent during contractions. The increased cardiac output is shown by an increase in stroke volume and in heart rate, so that the pulse rate rises (but rarely exceeds 100 beats per minute unless ketosis develops). At the same time the mean arterial pressure rises by about 10 per cent, and in advanced labour the rise may be even greater. These two changes increase cardiac work markedly in response to a uterine contraction. The right atrial pressure may reach 40–50mmHg in the second stage of labour, and the cardiopulmonary blood volume increases simultaneously. These changes are in part due to the increased blood volume which is expressed from the uterus during a contraction. It is for these reasons that labour may pose a hazard to the uncompensated cardiac patient, or to the patient who is severely anaemic. However, a normal woman has adequate reserves to compensate for the additional strain on her heart.

Following delivery, a further rise in cardiac output occurs. Since bradycardia is usual at this time, the rise must be due solely to an increase in the stroke volume. This effect lasts for between 4 and 9 days, so that the early puerperium is also hazardous for the uncompensated cardiac patient.

The body temperature also rises slightly, but is less than 37.8°C (100°F) unless ketosis develops, when it may exceed this. Labour is a stressful condition, and increased secretion of adrenal corticosteroids occurs, with progressive alterations in the serum electrolyte pattern. The extra energy expenditure leads to increased heat production, and sweating occurs, with loss of fluids from the body. In labour the motility of the intestinal tract is reduced and gastric emptying delayed, so that the stomach contents may remain for 48 hours without moving.

**Trauma to the tissues**

Vaginal delivery is always associated with some damage to the cervix, to the lower vagina and to the perineum. Minor lacerations occur on the cervix which heal rapidly, although the lateral margins of the os may be damaged, causing a slit-shaped os. The vaginal muscle and supports are always stretched, and the shape of the parous vagina is permanently altered. The perineum is usually damaged, tears of the fourchette or perineum being common.

Retention of urine is common after delivery, and is most likely to be due to a reflex inhibition of micturition due to damage to fibres of the levator muscle.

**Blood loss at delivery**

Following expulsion of the placenta the myometrium contracts strongly, effectively strangling the spiral arteries which supply the placental bed, and permitting thrombi to form within them. Despite this, some loss of blood from the placental bed is inevitable, and to this is added the blood contained in the placenta and that coming from lacerations in the genital tract.

Clinical estimates suggest that the average blood loss in normal labour is 300 to 500ml, but recent studies using isotope measurements cast some doubt on this. One careful investigation of 19 women showed a mean blood loss of 1100ml. Although this quantity seems great it is less than the total increase in blood volume which occurs in pregnancy, so that the cardiovascular response is undisturbed, provided the patient is not anaemic.

## FETAL

The entry of mankind into the world is not gentle. Unlike other mammals, man has developed a large head and this has to traverse a bony canal. It has been calculated that the force exerted on the fetus during a contraction is 1kg per $cm^2$, and this doubles during the second stage of labour when voluntary expulsive efforts are added. The effects of this force are mainly on the head, with moulding of the skull bones and the development of the caput succedaneum. Normally the stress of labour causes the infant no harm, but if the moulding is extreme, or the baby delivered inexpertly, particularly by the use of obstetric forceps or the vacuum extractor, intracranial oedema and tearing of intracranial ligaments may occur.

Labour and delivery are attended by a greater or lesser degree of fetal hypoxia, and the effects of this are conditioned by the physiological reserves with which the baby enters labour. These in turn are related to the health of the mother before labour and to the efficiency of the placenta. If the function of the placenta has been reduced for any reason in the last quarter of pregnancy (see p. 277), when the transfer of glucose is maximal, the fetus may enter labour with diminished glycogen reserves and may be unable to compensate for the reduction in supply of glucose and oxygen which may occur if labour is abnormal or prolonged, or if excessive analgesia is used. Maternal acidoketosis may aggravate the degree of fetal acidosis directly, but the main cause of fetal acidaemia in labour is insufficient transfer from mother to fetus of glucose (due to inadequate maternal intake of glucose) and to a lack of $O_2$

transfer, due to excessive uterine activity or excessive sedation of the mother. If these circumstances are permitted the fetal reserves of glycogen may be depleted, with increasing fetal acidosis which may result in intra-uterine fetal death or irreversible brain damage if the baby survives. However, the fetus is able to withstand hypoxia better than the infant, and can obtain its energy requirements in an anaerobic energy cycle, making use of the reserves of glycogen held in the fetal liver. The cycle is relatively inefficient, and leads to the accumulation of lactic and pyruvic acid with a resulting fetal acidaemia.

### The fetal heart rate in labour

The increasing fetal acidaemia affects the fetal heart as it attempts to compensate for the relative hypoxia. The fetal heart rate is the result of a balance between the opposing effects of sympathetic nerve stimulation, which tends to produce tachycardia, and the vagal tone which tends to produce bradycardia. Normally in the fetus the vagus is dominant and exerts a constant slowing effect on the heart, stabilizing the rate at $140 \pm 20$ beats a minute. This is the *basal* fetal heart rate, and it varies from individual to individual within the limits noted.

The moderating effect of vagal tone is opposed by the cardio-accelerator action of the sympathetic nerves, which operate through a reflex arc, and is older both phylogenetically and embryogenetically than the vagus.

When fetal hypoxia occurs, the altered composition of the blood leads to a rise in the vagal and the sympathetic tones, which are different in character from one another. The vagal response occurs when the degree of hypoxia is moderate or marked, and is rapid in onset. It lasts as long as the cause operates, and then disappears rapidly. In contrast, the sympathetic response occurs in mild hypoxia. Its onset is delayed, after which it develops progressively and lasts for longer than the cause, persisting for 10 to 30 minutes after the latter has ceased to operate.

These changes have beneficial effects during periods of fetal hypoxia, as the increased sympathetic tone redistributes the blood to the brain, the coronary vessels and to the placenta, whilst causing vasoconstriction in dispensable tissues, such as the skin. The resulting tachycardia ensures that the limited oxygen is moved more rapidly to the vital organs. The changes also prevent energy waste by the fetal heart. This is due to the combined effect of the long-sustained rise in sympathetic tone, and the transient rises in vagal tone which occur after each uterine contraction, when the degree of fetal hypoxia increases. The latter reduces the fetal heart output during and immediately after each contraction, at a time when only a poor feto-maternal oxygen exchange can occur. The former (by causing tachycardia) causes a better placental blood flow and gas exchange *between* contractions.

Alterations in the fetal heart rate during labour may give an indication of the degree of fetal acidaemia and hypoxia. The alterations are difficult to detect by auscultation, since this is normally recorded *between* contractions, and has a considerable observer error. Since the vagal element slows the fetal heart rate *during* contractions, this is the most important time to detect early 'fetal distress'. Clinically, fetal distress may be detected by counting the fetal heart rate for periods of 15 seconds, with an interval of 10 seconds between each count, starting at the time of onset of a contraction and continuing for 2 minutes after the contraction has ceased. If the fetal heart rate exceeds 160, shows slowing of 30 beats or more during or just after a contraction, or is persistently less than 100 beats a minute, fetal distress may be diagnosed.

Although auscultation is less accurate in detecting 'fetal distress' in labour than a fetal heart monitor, the use of the latter is probably unnecessary unless the fetus is at 'high risk' (see Chapter 36).

## Chapter 11

# The Mechanism of Labour

In 95 per cent of cases the fetus enters labour lying longitudinally and presenting cephalically. In the last weeks of pregnancy the lower uterine segment expands to accept the fetal head, which in the case of the primigravida is generally, and in the case of the multigravida is usually fixed within the true pelvis. The descent of the fetal head into the pelvis is termed engagement, and since the fetus is relatively pliable, the head tends to be flexed upon the neck, and the vertex becomes the presenting part.

When effective myometrial contraction and retraction occurs during labour, the fetus is pushed down into the pelvis and the fetal head accommodates itself as best it can to the birth canal. Since the shape of the canal, encroached upon by the soft tissues of the pelvis, varies at different levels, there is considerable movement of the fetal head, and of the fetus, as it passes through the birth canal. Understanding of these movements is essential and the description given here should be reinforced by the use of the model pelvis and manikin.

The movements have not been completely explained but the concept of a pliable fetus with a firm ovoid head adapting itself to a curved lower birth canal fits most of the observations made.

The movements of the fetus in the vertex presentation in labour are:

1. Descent with further flexion
2. Internal rotation, or accommodation to the lower part of the pelvis
3. Disengagement by extension
4. Restitution, or external rotation
5. Delivery of anterior shoulder by lateral flexion of the trunk posteriorly
6. Delivery of the posterior shoulder by lateral flexion of the trunk anteriorly
7. Delivery of buttocks and legs of the fetus.

Although the movements have been noted serially,

in fact the whole constitutes one continuous movement, and the time of occurrence of each step depends upon the configuration of the pelvis (Fig. **11/1**).

### 1. Descent with further flexion

The vertex is engaged in the brim of the pelvis, the sagittal suture lying in the transverse diameter of the inlet (Fig. **11/2**). This suture may lie equidistant from the symphysis and sacral promontory (synclitism) or nearer to the symphysis (asynclitism – posterior parietal presentation). In exceptional instances, the suture lies nearer to the promontory (asynclitism – anterior parietal presentation) and this generally indicates some reduction of the diameters of the pelvic inlet.

During the first stage the head descends only slightly but flexion is increased (Figs **11/3**; **11/4**).

### 2. Internal rotation

Once the cervix is fully dilated, the membranes usually rupture, and the fetus rapidly descends to the level of the ischial spines, where rotation begins, as the head meets the grooved gutter of the levator muscles which form the pelvic floor. Further flexion of the head occurs and anterior rotation of the occiput takes place through 90° in the occipito-lateral, 45° in the occipito-anterior and 135° in the occipito-posterior position of the vertex. Following this rotation, which takes a variable time, the occiput lies anteriorly behind the symphysis pubis (Fig. **11/5**). Although the rotation is usually complete before the vertex reaches the vulva, it may not be completed until the actual expulsion, the head still turning as it is born.

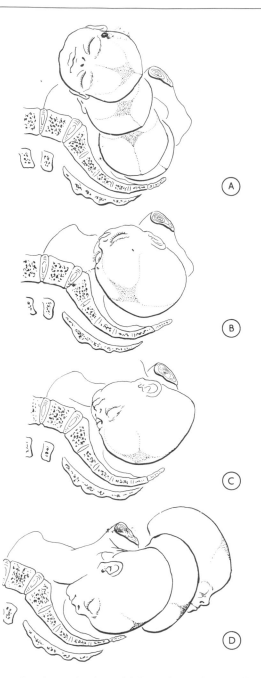

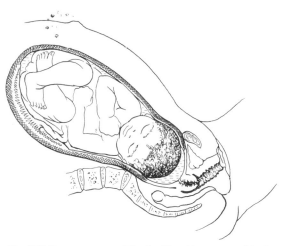

**Fig. 11/2** Late pregnancy. The fetal head has engaged in the transverse diameter of the pelvic brim, and some flexion of the head on the chest has occurred. The cervix is soft but is not yet effaced and the amniotic membranes are intact

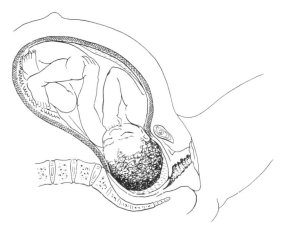

**Fig. 11/3** Early labour. There has been further flexion of the fetal head, and it has moved more deeply into the true pelvis, causing pressure on the bladder and rectum. The cervix has become effaced but has not yet begun to dilate, and the membranes are intact

**Fig. 11/1** The mechanism of labour drawn from radiographs taken in labour. Left occipito-transverse (or lateral) position of the vertex

A. Descent with further flexion
B. Internal rotation beginning
C. Internal rotation almost completed, head in the lower straight
D. Birth of the head by extension

### 3. Disengagement by extension

With further propulsive contractions, aided by the voluntary contractions of diaphragm and abdominal muscles, the head is forced further down towards the vulva, and the vertex appears, stretching the vulval orifice (Fig. **11/6**). With further contractions, extension of the head occurs and the perineum sweeps over forehead, base of nose, mouth and chin to release the head (Fig. **11/7**).

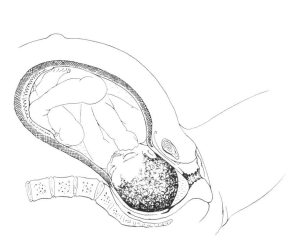

**Fig. 11/4** Late first stage of labour. The cervix is now 7cm dilated and further flexion of the fetal head has occurred. The membranes are still intact

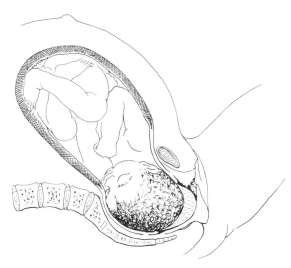

**Fig. 11/5** Early second stage. The cervix is fully dilated, and the head is beginning to rotate at the level of the ischial spines. Rotation is through 90°, so that the occiput lies in the anterior segment of the pelvis and the sagittal suture of the fetal head in the antero-posterior diameter of the pelvis. The membranes are intact and bulge in front of the head

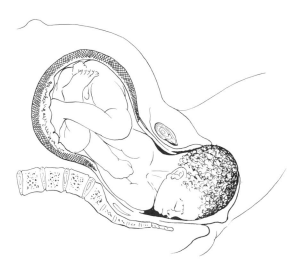

**Fig. 11/6** Late second stage. The head is broaching the vulval ring ('crowning'). The membranes have ruptured. The perineum is stretched over the head

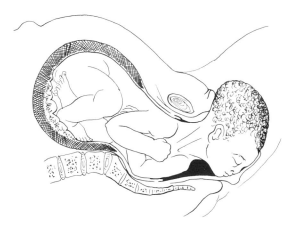

**Fig. 11/7** Birth of the head. As the fetal head is pushed through the vulval ring it extends on the neck, and the perineum is swept over the face. The direction of movement of the head is now upwards. The uterus has retracted to fit closely over the fetal body. The shoulders are still in the transverse diameter of the midpelvis

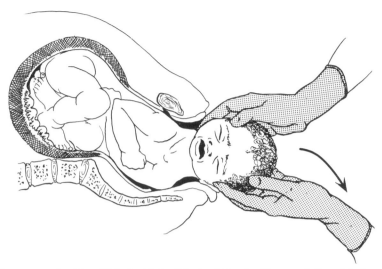

**Fig. 11/8** Birth of the anterior shoulder. With the birth of the head the shoulders reach the pelvic floor and, directed by the levator 'gutter', rotate to lie in the antero-posterior diameter of the pelvic outlet. The head therefore rotates 'externally', or undergoes 'restitution', to its position at the onset of labour. The anterior shoulder (in this case the right one) is appearing from behind the symphysis. The birth of the shoulder is aided by downward and backward traction of the head by the obstetrician

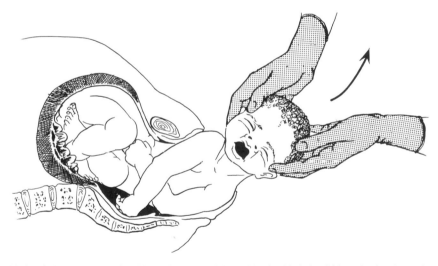

**Fig. 11/9** The birth of the posterior shoulder. The obstetrician aids the birth by lifting the head gently upwards whilst maintaining traction. This prevents damage to the perineum

#### 4. Restitution

Since the shoulders have now reached the pelvic floor, the groove of the levators induces a rotation so that the bis-achromial diameter becomes anteroposterior in relation to the pelvis. This movement is duplicated by the delivered fetal head which undergoes restitution, rotating the same number of degrees it turned previously but in the opposite direction (Fig. **11/8**).

#### 5, 6 and 7. Delivery of the shoulders and remainder of the fetus

The delivery of the shoulders takes place by lateral flexion, first posteriorly to disengage the anterior shoulder which appears from behind the symphysis and then anteriorly to disengage the posterior shoulder. With both shoulders born, the remainder of the fetus is rapidly expelled (Fig. **11/9**).

*Chapter 12*

# Clinical Course of Labour

## PRE-LABOUR

During the second half of pregnancy the activity of the uterus increases, and palpable painless uterine contractions, first noted by Braxton Hicks, may become apparent to the patient. These occur, especially at night, at 1- to 2-hourly intervals or longer. The contractions are not co-ordinated and consequently no expulsive effect is noticed.

In most primigravidae, and many multigravidae, the painless Braxton Hicks contractions merge into a *prodromal* stage which may last up to 4 weeks. During this time the lower segment expands to accept the fetal head, which enters the upper pelvis. This relieves the pressure on the upper part of the abdomen ('lightening') but increases the pressure in the pelvis. Consequently constipation and urinary frequency become apparent, and some patients complain of increased pressure in the pelvis and an increased mucoid vaginal discharge.

## 'FALSE LABOUR'

As term approaches, many women complain of painful uterine contractions, which may seem to indicate the onset of labour. However, despite the contractions, progressive dilatation of the cervix fails to occur. The condition is termed *false labour.*

In it, the triple descending gradient of uterine activity fails to become established. A reverse gradient of uterine activity is present, the lower part of the uterus contracting nearly as strongly as the upper part. Because of this, cervical dilatation fails to occur and the pain of the uterine contraction is often felt as low backache.

Clinically, the painful contractions occur more often at night, but their frequency and intensity do not increase as time passes.

A woman who complains of this pattern of uterine activity needs an explanation and, if the pains are distressing, treatment with analgesics, and perhaps a hypnotic so that she may enjoy a good night's sleep.

Often the pains of false labour recur on a number of days, and in some cases, the reverse gradient of activity changes and true labour starts.

## THE ONSET OF LABOUR

True labour may start and progress rapidly, or the start may be slow, with contractions only occurring at long intervals, the so-called 'sluggish uterus', or in a more modern idiom – prolongation of the quiet (latent) phase of labour.

If the woman is becoming distressed that labour is not progressing, a more effective pattern of uterine activity can be obtained by performing an amniotomy and by starting an intravenous infusion of oxytocin. This regimen should only be instituted if there is no cephalopelvic disproportion and the cervix is partly or wholly effaced, 2cm dilated and soft.

The onset of labour is difficult to time with any degree of accuracy, and may be heralded by several signs. (1) The false labour pains may become co-ordinate and regular, or painful contractions may alert the patient that labour has started. (2) A discharge of mucus mixed with some blood may occur. This is due to the effacement and dilatation of the cervix allowing the 'plug' which previously filled it to be released. The blood comes from minute lacerations in the cervical mucosa. The passage of the mucus and blood is known as the 'show'.

The transition into labour is gradual but labour may be said to have begun when the cervix is at least 2cm dilated and contractions become painful and regular with diminishing intervals between each contraction.

Because of the difficulty in establishing the time of onset of labour with any degree of accuracy, many obstetricians mark the onset of labour from the time the woman is admitted to hospital. This has advantages if the graphic method of recording the progress of labour (the partograph) is adopted.

# THE STAGES OF LABOUR

### First stage

During this phase the effacement of the cervix is initiated or completed, and cervical dilatation occurs. In a primigravida cervical effacement precedes dilatation, but in a multigravida both can occur simultaneously. The first stage continues until full dilatation of the cervix has occurred, and during this time there is some descent of the presenting part within the pelvis. In a normal pelvis the fetal head enters with the sagittal suture in the transverse diameter of the brim in 75 per cent of cases, obliquely (i.e. occipito-anterior or posterior) in 20 per cent, and directly anterior or posterior in 5 per cent of cases (Fig. 12/1).

The first stage of labour lasts an average of 12 hours in primigravidae, and 7½ hours in multigravidae. This period can be further divided into a relatively quiet first phase (the latent phase) during which contractions occur with increasing frequency and are of increasing duration, but are not particularly distressing to the patient, and an active second phase. In this phase the duration of the contractions increases to 60 to 90 seconds, and they recur at intervals of 3 to 5 minutes. The quiet phase lasts 8 hours on an average, the active phase 3 to 5

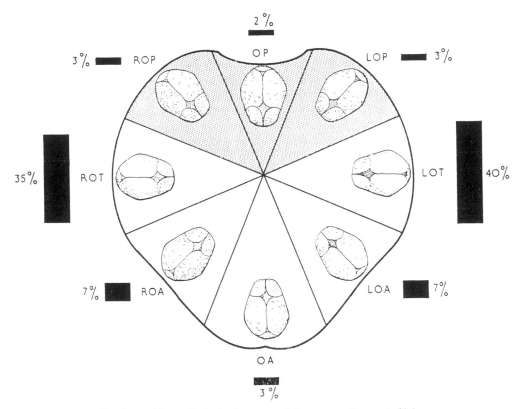

**Fig. 12/1** The position and relative frequency of the vertex at the onset of labour

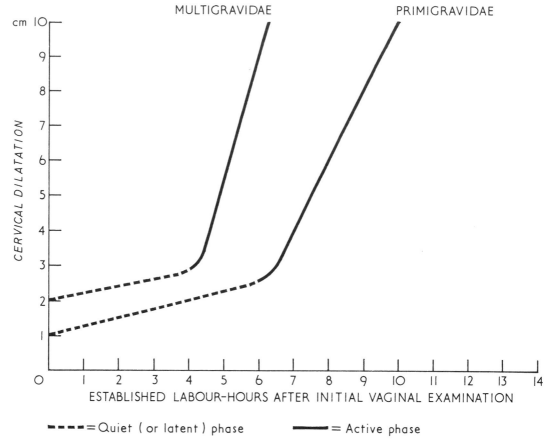

MULTIGRAVIDAE            PRIMIGRAVIDAE

**Fig. 12/2** The phases of labour

hours. The contractions are particularly distressing towards the end of the first stage when the membranes usually rupture.

Vaginal examinations at 2-hourly intervals to determine cervical dilatation and descent of the fetal head have shown that labour has two phases. The first is a quiet or latent phase, in which cervical dilatation tends to be slow. The second is an active phase which is associated with rapid cervical dilatation (Fig. **12/2**). The active phase begins when the cervix is 4 or 5cm dilated in over 90 per cent of women whose labour is normal. Studies of cervical dilatation during labour have led to the development of the *partograph* and *action lines* (p. 118). Slow cervical dilatation may occur in the latent phase (prolonged latent phase) or in the active phase (slow active phase) or cervical dilatation may cease in the active phase (arrest in the active phase).

Should labour have lasted for more than 12 hours in a primigravida, or more than 9 hours in a multigravida, investigations must be initiated to determine the cause. This matter is considered in Chapters 42 to 45. Should the investigations indicate that the mother is not dehydrated or acidoketotic, disclose an absence of cephalopelvic disproportion and find that one of the abnormal cervical dilatation patterns is present, many obstetricians recommend an aggressive, active approach, by rupturing the membranes (amniotomy) and giving an oxytocin infusion (provided the pattern of uterine activity is normal).

**Second stage**

This is the expulsive stage, during which the fetus is forced through the curved birth canal. It lasts from full dilatation of the cervix until the baby is born. The uterine contractions last from 60 to 90 seconds and recur at 2- to 5-minute intervals, and the expulsion of the baby is aided by the voluntary muscles of the abdominal wall and diaphragm. As the presenting part reaches the gutter-shaped pelvic floor, which is at the apex of the concavity of the pelvic curve, internal rotation takes place, usually anteriorly, but in 1 per cent posteriorly. The main expulsive efforts are now those of the abdominal muscles and diaphragm and the pelvic muscles reflexly relax to allow the baby to be born. During this phase the patient grunts as she pushes, and taking a breath, closes her glottis, braces her feet and by contracting her abdominal muscles and diaphragm, forces the presenting part of the fetus against her perineum. The energy required makes the patient sweat, her pulse rises during the expulsive effort, and after the contraction has passed off, she relaxes.

As the presenting part is pushed lower in the pelvis it rotates so that the occiput lies anteriorly behind the symphysis pubis. The patient may feel an intense pressure on her rectum, or complain of pains which radiate down her legs, and are due to pressure on the sacral plexus and obturator nerve. Some 15 minutes later the anus begins to open, exposing its anterior wall, and haemorrhoids, if present, become engorged. Between the labia minora the presenting part can be seen, advancing with each contraction, retreating between contractions, but making a small net advance with each. The head now presses upon the perineum. The patient complains of a 'bursting' feeling, and has a desire to push which should be restrained until a contraction occurs. Soon the head is visible at the vulva between contractions, the perineum is stretched, the skin tense and shining and the anus flattened (Fig. **12/3a**). With each contraction the head advances and a large segment of the presenting part becomes visible. If it is the head it is said to be 'crowned' by the perineum (Fig. **12/3b**). Now with an extra effort the baby is born. If the presentation is a vertex, the head is forced out, extending at the neck as it does so, so that the forehead, face, mouth and chin emerge over the perineum (Figs **12/3c**; **12/3d**). After this there is a pause of about a minute, during which time the head rotates into the transverse diameter of the outlet, so that the shoulders may enter the antero-posterior diameter of the lower pelvis (Figs **12/3e**; **12/3f**). The shoulders are then born, the anterior stemming from behind the symphysis, followed by the posterior which rolls over the perineum, and then by the trunk and legs, in one long expulsive effort. The mother relaxes, exhausted for the moment. The baby gasps convulsively once or twice and then cries vigorously. A little blood is expelled as the myometrial fibres retract to make the uterus the size it was at 20 weeks gestation. The second stage has ended.

The average duration of the second stage in a primigravida is 1 hour and in a multigravida 30 minutes. A second stage lasting more than 1½ hours in a primigravida (or more than 1 hour if she is pushing) and 1 hour in a multigravida, should be considered prolonged, and the baby delivered by obstetric manipulations.

**Third stage**

The third stage extends from the birth of the child until the complete expulsion of the placenta and membranes. Separation of the placenta takes place through the spongy layer of the decidua basalis as a result of uterine contractions being added to the retraction of the uterine muscle which occurs with the birth of the child. In this way the area of the placental bed is reduced to one quarter of its size in pregnancy, but as the placenta is unable to change in size, it buckles upwards, and the arteries and veins supplying the intervillous spaces tear, causing a retroplacental haemorrhage, and further placental separation. The process starts as the child is born and is continued by uterine contractions which persist, with no diminution of force, after the birth of the child. It is probable that placental separation is complete within 5 minutes of birth, but the placenta may be held in position by the adherent membranes which take longer to strip from their decidual juxtaposition. Traditionally no attempt is made to deliver the placenta until the signs of placental descent into the upper vagina are noted. These are: (1) a gush of blood which occurs as the retroplacental blood separates the membranes and reaches the vagina; (2) a lengthening of the cord as the placenta passes through the cervix; and (3) a rise in the height of the fundus uteri as the placenta reaches the vagina. When these signs have appeared, delivery of the placenta is effected by cord traction and suprapubic pressure to control the descent of the uterus. The delivery of the placenta is accompanied by the loss of blood which normally does not exceed 300ml. Following the birth of the placenta the uterus retracts strongly and the lattice arrangements of muscle fibres effectively strangle the blood vessels supplying the placental bed, preventing further blood loss and encouraging fibrin plug deposition in their torn ends.

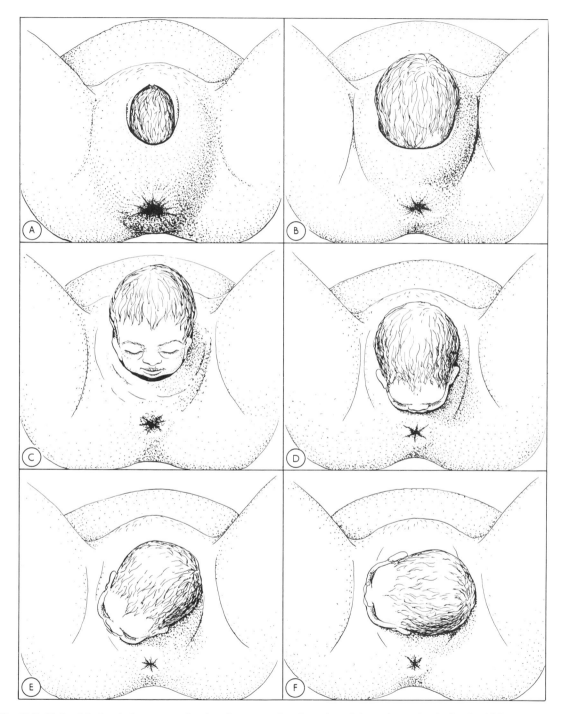

**Fig. 12/3** Birth of the head. A sequence showing the progressive distension of the perineum by the head, which extends as it is born. The perineum sweeps over the forehead, face and chin. Once the head is born it drops slightly and then restitution (external rotation) occurs

## DURATION OF LABOUR

The duration of labour is not easy to determine precisely as its onset is often indefinite and subjective. In studies of informed women, whose labour started spontaneously, there was a wide variation in the duration of labour as can be seen in Table **12/1**.

|           | *Para 0*                | *Multiparae*                      |
|-----------|-------------------------|-----------------------------------|
| 1st stage | $8\frac{1}{4}(2-12)$h   | $5\frac{1}{2}(1-9)$h              |
| 2nd stage | $1(\frac{1}{4}-1\frac{1}{2})$h | $\frac{1}{4}(0-\frac{3}{4})$h |
| 3rd stage | $\frac{1}{4}(0-1)$h     | $\frac{1}{4}(0-\frac{1}{2})$h    |
|           | $9\frac{1}{2}(2\frac{1}{4}-14)$h | $6(1-10\frac{1}{4})$h   |

**Table 12/1** The duration of labour

Labour is usually shorter when the patient knows something of the physiology of normal labour, is in good health at the onset of labour, has confidence in her attendants and is well adjusted.

Ninety per cent of nulliparous women (para 0) may be expected to deliver within 16 hours, and the same proportion of multiparous women (para 1+) will deliver within 12 hours. A labour lasting more than 18 hours should be considered prolonged (see Chapter 45).

Several factors influence the duration of labour. These include the age of the woman, her parity, her knowledge of the process of childbirth, and the size of the fetus and its position in the uterus. Labour seems to last longer amongst nulliparous women, particularly older primigravidae, and if the baby presents in the occipito-posterior position.

*Chapter 13*

# The Management of Labour

In recent years, in the developed nations, there has been an increasing tendency for pregnant women to be confined in hospital. In the USA, Canada, Australia and the Scandinavian nations, nearly all women are delivered within a hospital or a maternity unit. In Britain, the percentage of hospital confinements has risen from 75 per cent in 1965 to over 95 per cent in 1980. Even in the Netherlands where home births formed the majority of births in the 1960s, today only one woman in three gives birth at home.

By contrast, in the developing nations of the world, and particularly in the rural areas (where over 75 per cent of the population live), home confinement is the rule.

Hospital confinement has the advantage that although 85 per cent of labours are uneventful, in 15 per cent complications may arise which require urgent skilled treatment. Good prenatal care can prevent many of these, but unexpected problems may occur in labour. Against hospital confinement are the facts that the health care tends to be impersonal, 'meddlesome midwifery' is more common, and cross-infection is a risk. However, in well-organized services most of these disadvantages can be eliminated.

In nations where hospital facilities are inadequate, and home confinement is culturally accepted, the separation from the others of patients who are at a higher risk of developing complications in labour or the puerperium, can be made, and the high-risk patients can be offered hospital confinement.

The experience of a hospital in central Malaysia will serve as an example. In this institution, because of the heavy demands, priorities for hospital confinement were adopted. The following groups of women received priority:

1. Women with a history of disease or difficulty in a previous pregnancy or labour, or who develop complications during the present pregnancy

2. All primigravidae

3. All women pregnant for the fifth or subsequent time.

So that continuing obstetric care could be offered to all the women in the area, a web-network of maternity services was established. The central hospital was 'linked' to district hospitals and both types of hospital conducted antenatal clinics. These were 'linked' to a constellation of antenatal clinics in the metropolitan area, the country towns and villages. The main clinics had a doctor in attendance; the peripheral ones were conducted by midwives who had been trained at the central hospital. A patient was therefore screened, and if an abnormality arose in pregnancy or labour, could be rapidly and safely transferred to the next step in the chain. In addition, an 'obstetric flying squad' was available at the central hospital to go to the villages, bringing treatment to the patients. Patients delivering in the central hospital who were normal were discharged 24 to 48 hours after confinement and were visited in the home by trained midwives.

Since domiciliary midwifery will continue to be practised in many countries, and the aid of a doctor may be urgently required, it is essential that an 'obstetric flying squad' is organized in such areas. It is usually based upon the main hospital in the area.

The rationale of the flying squad is that in cases of emergency, particularly eclampsia and in certain cases of postpartum haemorrhage, skilled aid is better brought to the patient in the home than the patient to the hospital. The team consists of an experienced obstetrician, an anaesthetist and a trained member of the nursing staff. On receipt of a call, previously packed equipment is loaded onto an ambulance car, blood is provided in cold containers, and the team goes to the patient. Experience has shown that resuscitation by blood transfusion, and removal of a retained placenta are the most frequently required procedures. Complicated operations should be avoided. In Malaysia this service has been supplemented by the use of an 'air ambulance' for evacuation of patients from remote, inaccessible areas.

The question of who shall care for the pregnant woman is argued with passion in many developed nations. There are those who would eliminate the nurse–midwife, and those who would enhance her status; there are those who believe that all pregnant women should be confined by specialist obstetricians; there are those who would retain the family doctor to care for 'normal' pregnancies, leaving the specialist to deal only with the 'abnormal'.

The most rational approach appears to be the concept of an obstetric team, in which the nurse–midwife, the family doctor and the specialist all play well defined roles, but in which there is close harmony and good communication. Each member of the team must know his, or her, strengths and limitations and all must work in close co-operation so that better patient care and better obstetrics result.

In the past 50 years, in the developed nations, changes have occurred in the management of labour, which have resulted in childbirth becoming 'medicalized'. This concept is based on the opinion that childbirth is a pathological process. The perception of childbirth as a potentially pathological process led to the institution of many techniques which have helped to reduce the maternal mortality and perinatal mortality rates considerably since 1930. Good prenatal care by trained medical and health staff; childbirth in hospital; the availability of blood; the reduction of puerperal infections by antibiotics; technological equipment to monitor the well-being of the mother and her baby in labour and earlier intervention in prolonged labour, have made childbirth safe.

Over the same period social and demographic changes have occurred in the developed nations. Pregnant women are better nourished from infancy; and women, in general, have chosen to have smaller families (completing childbearing at an earlier age), thus reducing the risk of pregnancy and childbirth amongst older, high parity women.

These beneficial effects have a darker side. The 'medicalization' of childbirth has had a number of undesirable effects. Maternity hospitals became increasingly 'clinical' and impersonal and the expectant mother, on admission, has been subjected to procedures which 'depersonalized' her. She became the passive recipient of the skilled care of the obstetric team, who delivered her baby and cared for it, without her involvement to any significant degree.

In the past few years, many mothers, and their partners, have begun to question this approach to childbirth. They point out that childbirth is an important life-event which enhances the relationship of the couple. They point out the importance of the parents' participation in the birth of their child and the benefits of early 'bonding'. They point out that many of the routine practices in hospitals are unnecessary, and may be detrimental to the emotional and psychological well-being of women in childbirth.

From these criticisms, many justified, the concept of choice in childbirth has arisen. Women should be given the opportunity to choose the way they wish to experience childbirth, provided that medical considerations do not demand special care and intervention.

Three main choices in childbirth should be made available. These are (1) prepared, participatory childbirth; (2) conventional childbirth; (3) actively managed childbirth.

**Prepared, participatory childbirth**

In this approach to childbirth the expectant mother, and her partner, learn during pregnancy about the processes of childbirth and child care. They learn techniques of psychoprophylaxis. Childbirth is an event which is shared by the mother and father of the child, and perhaps by their other children.

Labour is supervised by trained staff but drugs are not given unless the mother requests them, and instrumental delivery is avoided unless a real medical indication arises. During labour the mother chooses how she will cope. She may walk about, sit in a chair, squat, kneel or lie in bed: it is her choice.

The birth takes place in a quiet environment and the baby is given to the mother, immediately after birth, to cuddle and so that it may suckle.

A number of women who choose prepared childbirth also believe in the teaching of Dr Leboyer. He contends that the actual birth should take place in relative silence and in soft lighting, as noise and glare are traumatic to the newborn baby. He believes that birth should be gentle. Many of his views have

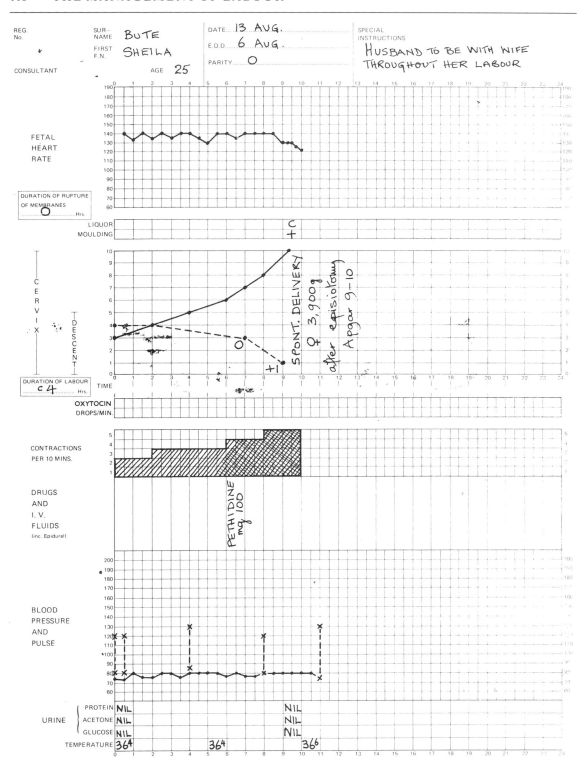

**Fig. 13/1** A partograph

a scientific basis, but some (for example, allowing the cord to cease beating before cutting it, and putting the baby in a warm bath) are of doubtful benefit.

A randomized clinical trial of the Leboyer approach and a conventional, gentle, supportive approach to childbirth failed to show any differences in maternal or infant morbidity or in infant behaviour up to 8 months of life.

However, Leboyer's concepts have reinforced the belief that a woman has a right to choose how she will experience childbirth.

Women can have a prepared, participatory childbirth in a traditional hospital environment; but the process is more satisfactory if she can give birth in a 'Birthing Centre'.

## BIRTHING CENTRES

The spread of elective induction of labour and the active management of labour, using advanced technology, has led to a reaction by some women and their partners. The reaction has been to press for a return to home births, which carries the risks of sudden unexpected fetal distress in labour, anoxia of the neonate and postpartum haemorrhage.

An alternative to this is for hospitals to offer women, whose pregnancy has been carefully screened, the facility of a Birthing Centre. A Birthing Centre is furnished like a bedroom, containing a firm double bed, chairs and curtains, with the necessary equipment for childbirth discreetly hidden. The woman and her partner, the father of the child, together with any of her children she wishes to be present, share the experience of labour and childbirth. The delivery is conducted by a nurse–midwife who is also present throughout labour, or by a doctor, depending on the woman's wishes.

As the Birthing Centre is in the hospital, close to the delivery floor, skilled medical aid and appropriate equipment are available at a moment's notice should complications arise; or the woman can be easily transferred to a traditional delivery unit.

After birth, which is conducted gently, the baby remains with its parents so that they can celebrate its birth and so that 'bonding' may take place. The mother remains in her room for between 12 and 48 hours after childbirth, when she goes home. She is visited there by 'district nurse–midwives'.

Experience of the few Birthing Centres which have been established, showed that women choosing this form of childbirth had fewer inductions of labour,

required less analgesia in labour, had more spontaneous deliveries and fewer episiotomies than women in traditional delivery units. Their babies were less hypoxic at birth. About 5 per cent of the women required medical intervention, most being transferred to the delivery floor of the maternity unit.

### 'Conventional' childbirth

In this choice, the woman is admitted to the maternity ward, in the currently conventional way, which is discussed in the next section. She is content to leave the process of childbirth in the care of the obstetric team, and to accept, without question, their management. She may or may not be told why a procedure takes place, and usually does not want her partner to support her during childbirth. She is cared for with skill but does not participate in the process of childbirth.

### Actively managed childbirth

The development of the partograph and an appreciation that most labours last less than 12 hours after

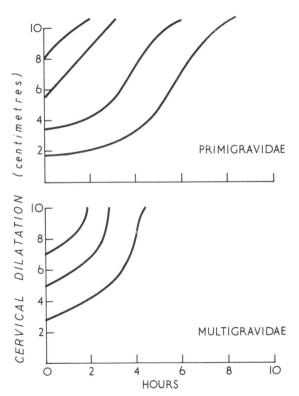

**Fig. 13/2** Action lines for the partograph

admission to hospital, has led to a new approach: actively managed childbirth.

On admission to the delivery unit, the patient's diagnosis of labour is confirmed or rejected by the medical attendants. Regular, painful contractions, the passage of bloodstained mucus (a show) or rupture of the membranes, and effacement of the cervix are used as criteria to establish that labour has started. The duration of labour is timed from this examination. A partograph is established and the progress of labour is judged by the dilatation of the cervix. Vaginal examinations are made every two hours and the cervical dilatation recorded on the partograph (Fig. **13/1**). 'Action lines' (Fig. **13/2**) printed on transparent plastic are superimposed. The slowest acceptable rate of cervical dilatation is lcm/hour. If the cervical dilatation is found to lie to the right of the 'action line' the membranes are ruptured and a dilute incremental oxytocin infusion (see p. 387) is established in nulliparous women (and a few multiparous women), provided a single fetus presents as a vertex and there are no signs of 'fetal distress'.

Progress in the second stage is judged by descent of the fetal head and its rotation. One hour is allowed for the fetal head to reach the pelvic floor (the first phase) and a further hour for delivery to occur (the second phase).

The longest acceptable duration of labour is 12 hours from admission. If the woman has not delivered by this time, a caesarean section is performed or a forceps delivery is attempted. Caesarean section is performed for delay in the first stage of labour or the first phase of the second stage. Forceps delivery is attempted for delay in the second phase of the second stage of labour.

This method has been used in the National Maternity Hospital, Dublin since 1970. Each patient is attended by one nurse and epidural analgesia is available, but is requested by less than 10 per cent of women. The incidence of prolonged labour (>12 hours) is 2.5 per cent, the caesarean section rate about 7 per cent and the forceps rate 8 per cent (nullipara 12 per cent; multipara 4 per cent).

# THE PRACTICAL MANAGEMENT OF LABOUR

The practical management of the patient in labour is the craft rather than the science of obstetrics. For this reason the written word will be greatly enhanced if the student attends patients throughout the course of labour. Unfortunately, even today, it is all too common for students to attend the delivery of the baby but to have no knowledge of the pattern of labour prior to this time, or of the woman's reaction, both mental and physical, to the process of childbirth.

The management of labour begins, in most developed nations, when the patient seeks admission to hospital. She does this when she believes, or knows, that she is in labour. For many women this is a time of considerable stress, and covert fear, although if the patient has informed herself of the process of labour, the fear will be less. The attitude of the member of the health team who admits the patient is most important, for his or her approach can reduce the patient's anxiety considerably.

On admission, it is usual to offer the patient a shower, and during the time she has it the op-

portunity is taken to obtain her antenatal records. The record is carefully scrutinized for any abnormalities in the past medical or obstetrical history, for the findings during the antenatal visits, and for the results of laboratory tests.

When the woman has had a shower, her suprapubic and pudendal hair are trimmed short, unless she has done this before coming to hospital. She should be asked if she has recently defaecated, and if not if she would like to have an enema or, preferably, a bisacodyl suppository. A mid-stream specimen of urine is obtained and examined.

During these procedures the patient is asked about the frequency and strength of the uterine contractions, how long they have been present and where they are felt most strongly. Information is also sought about the presence of a 'show' or rupture of the membranes.

The patient is next examined by the admitting doctor, the private doctor or the nurse–midwife.

A general examination is made, the temperature, pulse and blood pressure are recorded. The abdomen is palpated and the presentation and position of the baby determined. The patient is next examined vaginally. This must be performed with careful attention to asepsis. Although the vulva is usually heavily contaminated with bacteria, the upper vagina is only slightly contaminated and the cavity of the uterus is sterile. Infection must not be introduced during labour, as the placental bed after delivery is an open wound in a hot, moist atmosphere conducive to the growth of bacteria. The vaginal examination must therefore be sterile.

Until recently there was considerable argument whether the first pelvic examination, and subsequent ones to determine the progress of labour, should be vaginal or rectal. Those who supported the latter claimed that it was safer, as the introduction of bacteria into the upper vagina by the examining fingers was avoided. The matter has now been resolved and the superiority, and safety, of vaginal examinations, *carried out with a proper aseptic technique*, has been established. Not only is a rectal examination less informative and less accurate, but as the information is obtained by rubbing the posterior mid-vaginal wall over the cervix, and the fetal 'presenting part', transfer of bacteria from the relatively contaminated mid-vagina to the relatively sterile cervical area can occur.

**The vaginal examination**

The method of the vaginal examination is simple. The hands are washed in antiseptic soap or solution, for 3 minutes, and the fingernails carefully cleansed. A sterile pair of gloves is put on. The vulva is swabbed with an antiseptic solution and chlorhexidine cream 1 per cent (Hibitane obstetric cream) is poured over the vulva and into the vagina, by separating the labia minora with the fingers of the left hand. The index and middle fingers of the right hand are introduced into the vagina and the vaginal examination carried out.

The objectives of the vaginal examination are:

1. *To confirm the findings of the 37th week* vaginal examination and additionally to establish the degree of effacement (taking up) of the cervix and its dilatation. This is recorded in centimetres but is measured with the fingers. The degree of cervical dilatation measured in centimetres and in finger-breadths is shown in Fig. **13/3**.

2. *To establish the presentation and position* of the presenting part. The vertex is firm, rounded and usually the posterior fontanelle, where three sutures

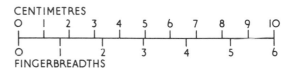

Fig. **13/3** To show the relationship between the size of the cervix measured in centimetres and in 'finger-breadths'

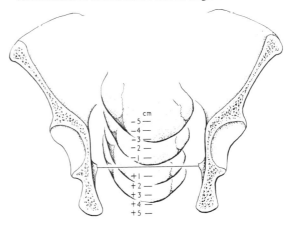

Fig. **13/4** Station of the head (redrawn from Greenhill, *Obstetrics*, 13th edition. Saunders, 1965)

meet, can be palpated in one or other lateral position. Caput formation may make the examination more difficult. A breech presentation can be detected by feeling a soft irregular mass, in place of the hard round head.

3. *To determine the station* of the presenting part. This is the level of the lowest fetal bony part in relation to an imaginary line joining the mother's ischial spines. The station of the head is measured by finger-breadths (1.6cm each) above or below the ischial spines (Fig. **13/4**).

4. If the membranes have ruptured this is noted, as is the presence of rigidity of the perineum and varicosities of the vulva.

During the course of labour, at appropriate intervals, usually 2-hourly or less, but which are determined by the individual progress, further vaginal examinations are made. On each occasion the same attention to asepsis is paid. These examinations monitor the progress of labour, by noting the following five points:

1. The degree of effacement and dilatation of the cervix
2. The station of the presenting part
3. The position of the presenting part
4. The state of the bag of membranes

5. The amount of moulding, caput formation or oedema present.

Vaginal examinations are also required (1) if the obstetrician is uncertain of the progress of labour; (2) when the membranes rupture, to exclude prolapse of the cord and to determine the degree of cervical dilatation; (3) if the patient says she feels she wants to 'bear down', which is usually a sign that the cervix is fully dilated, but it may not be so, and the point must be checked; (4) in the second stage of labour if progress is slow.

# MANAGEMENT OF THE FIRST STAGE OF LABOUR

During the first stage of labour dilatation of the cervix takes place, with slight descent of the head into the pelvis. The first stage can be divided into a quiet phase when the contractions are infrequent, short in duration and not distressing to the patient, and an active phase during which increasingly frequent and strong contractions are felt. During the first stage the patient can help most by relaxing during the contractions and not resisting them.

The end of the first stage can be a trying time. The cervix is 8 or 9cm dilated, but the patient feels an intense, often overwhelming desire to push. This period until full cervical dilatation is called the 'transition stage'. The uterine contractions are strong, pain in the back and abdomen may be intense. Considerable support is needed to help the woman avoid pushing, which will merely increase cervical oedema.

## General

Since the patient cannot help actively in this stage of labour, she must be given reassurance and encouragement from friendly unhurried attendants. In the quiet phase she should be allowed to sit or walk around, and hospitals should have first stage 'common rooms' where patients may gather and read or watch television. But if the presenting part is not engaged, the patient should stay in bed, and should not walk around. In the active phase, most patients request analgesia and many may prefer to remain in bed. But each woman should be given the choice: some women prefer to walk about, others to sit on an upright chair, others to recline in bed. Each delivery room should provide facilities for a woman to choose.

If she chooses to be in bed, she should lie on her side, or recline propped up on pillows. The reason is that in the supine position the weight of the contracting uterus reduces the placental blood flow by compressing the descending aorta and inferior vena cava, and diminishes the intensity and duration of uterine contractions.

A matter of some importance, which is often neglected, is that most women are afraid of being left alone during labour in case the baby becomes suddenly, unexpectedly at risk. If the woman wishes it, her partner should stay with her throughout labour; if she does not wish this, a nurse–midwife should be with her to reassure her and to monitor the well-being of the fetus.

## Specific

1. The frequency, duration and intensity of the uterine contractions are recorded by the nurse or doctor. The progress of descent of the presenting part can be established by abdominal palpation, but, as has been noted, not much descent occurs in the first stage of labour. The pulse, temperature and blood pressure are recorded every 2 hours in normal cases, and more frequently if there is an abnormality. A vaginal examination is made every 2 hours. The progress of labour is recorded on a partograph (see Fig. **13/1**). Because of the delayed gastric emptying time in labour, both solid food and fluids may remain in the stomach for a considerable time. Should an inhalational anaesthetic be required, the patient may then regurgitate and inhale the stomach contents. For this reason it is usual to withhold oral feeding once labour has become established, and many obstetricians routinely set up an intravenous infusion of glucose to prevent the development of ketonuria. Recently the wisdom of this approach has been questioned as glucose infusions providing more than 25g during labour may cause fetal hyperinsulinaemia and neonatal hypoglycaemia. Further, although

glucose infusion reduces maternal ketosis, it may cause maternal acidosis and fetal acidosis in some women. In other cases, infusions of fluid > 3.0 litres in 24 hours may cause neonatal hyponatraemia, leading to convulsions, respiratory and feeding problems.

It is now recommended that intravenous infusions are not generally required in the first 12 hours of labour, regardless of the presence of ketonuria. The patient's lips and mouth are kept moist and she may be given ice to suck. If intravenous fluids are thought necessary the amount should not exceed 1500ml in a 12-hour period. Normal saline 500ml should alternate with Hartmann's solution 500ml. If an oxytocin infusion is needed, the vehicle should be normal saline. The patient should be asked to empty her bladder at 4-hourly intervals when the urine is tested for the presence of albumin and acetone.

2. Vaginal examinations are performed when indicated in the way already described.

3. The fetal heart rate should be listened to every 15 minutes in the first stage of labour and every 5 minutes in the second stage. The normal variation is between 120 and 160 beats a minute. If the rate remains below 100 between contractions and particularly if meconium is passed in a cephalic presentation, 'fetal distress' may be imminent, and a full assessment of the situation must be made (see Chapter 10). In this connection the technique of auscultating the fetal heart requires consideration. Nurse–midwives are usually taught to auscultate the fetal heart for 1 minute *between* contractions. Unfortunately this method misses one early sign of fetal distress which is slowing of the fetal heart towards the end and just after a contraction. A more appropriate way to auscultate the fetal heart is to listen and count the beats for a period of 1 minute *immediately after* a contraction. If the staff are motivated, the following method is even more accurate but requires additional skill. The heart rate is counted for periods of 15 seconds, missing 5 seconds between each count, from the time the contraction is becoming strong until one minute after it ends. The individual counts are recorded and an average taken. If the heart rate has dropped by 30 or more beats from the reading between contractions fetal distress should be suspected.

4. Vaginal discharge is looked for. It may be bloody, and if slight is of no significance, but if of greater amount the cause must be investigated.

5. If the membranes have ruptured, or are ruptured artificially, the liquor should be checked for the presence of meconium. If it is present the fetal condition should be checked with a fetal monitor. The absence of meconium is a good sign: very few babies die in normal labour if meconium is absent.

The aim of the medical attendants is to make the mother as comfortable as possible during the first stage of labour; to ensure that any abnormality in the progress of labour is noted; and to give the patient adequate analgesia. This matter is discussed at greater length later, but in brief: in early labour during the quiet phase, hypnotics may be given at night to ensure that the patient sleeps. When the contractions are painful and the cervix at least 3cm dilated, pethidine 100 to 150mg (or meptazinol 100–150mg) should be given intramuscularly, and this may be repeated about 4-hourly as required. In the active stage of labour, when uterine contractions are painful, the patient can be given the choice of additional injections of pethidine, inhalations of $N_2O$ in oxygen or an epidural analgesic may be initiated (see Chapter 18).

# THE SECOND STAGE OF LABOUR

The second stage of labour begins when the dilatation of the cervix is complete. In the second stage, the contractions of the uterus, together with voluntary muscle contractions, push the baby along the birth canal to the outside world. The presenting part sinks deeply into the pelvis, and then stretches the pelvic floor and perineum to become visible between the labia minora before being expelled. In this stage the active co-operation of the mother is essential and help should be offered if she has not been delivered within 1½ hours of the onset of the second stage, or if the fetal head has been visible for 30 minutes.

The only sure way of determining the onset of the second stage is by doing a vaginal examination and noting that the cervix is fully dilated. As this is often omitted the following pointers help: (1) the final stages of dilatation of the cervix are frequently attended by very painful contractions; (2) a pause in the frequency of the contractions often occurs when dilatation is complete; (3) the membranes frequently rupture at this time; (4) the patient expresses a desire to 'bear down' with each contraction.

If there is any doubt about the matter, a vaginal examination should be made.

**Objectives**

The objectives of care in the second stage are: (1) to prevent infection of the genital tract by careful attention to asepsis and antisepsis; (2) to ensure that the child is born alive and undamaged; (3) to preserve the muscles of the perineum.

**General**

The patient either lies on her side or continues to be supported by pillows reclining at an angle of about 45° to the bed, or is supported by the father of her child. The correct position is the one she finds most comfortable. Some women prefer to squat or kneel, others prefer to stand, until the baby's head is visible at the perineum, when they return to bed for the birth.

During the second stage, the uterine contractions occur at 3- to 5-minute intervals, last 60 to 90 seconds and are strong. With each contraction the head moves towards the pelvic outlet, receding between contractions. As it descends it rotates and eventually comes into view. The fetal heart rate is recorded every 5 minutes. If marked slowing occurs, this requires investigation. Vaginal discharge, either meconium-stained or bloody, is noted and, if the latter, must be investigated. It is usually due to trauma of the cervix or vagina or to damage to vulval varicosities. Occasionally it is due to abruptio placentae.

The maternal pulse is recorded $\frac{1}{4}$-hourly, the temperature and blood pressure hourly. The bladder should be kept empty but if the patient cannot void, catheterization should be omitted until a distended bladder is noted. The patient's fluid intake is noted, sips of water or ice to suck being permitted. No parenteral analgesics are now allowed but inhalations of trichloroethylene (Trilene) or $N_2O$ and oxygen may be given when the contractions are strong; or additions are made to the epidural analgesic.

Since the co-operation of the patient in expelling her baby is of great importance, encouragement and instruction by her attendants are essential. No woman in the second stage of labour should be left unattended and the nurse, or doctor, should explain how the labour is progressing and reassure the patient that it is normal. In this stage the patient and her attendant act as a team.

# THE BIRTH OF THE BABY

As the presenting part becomes visible between the labia minora the patient must be prepared for the birth. The position of the patient for childbirth has been controversial but increasing numbers of obstetricians prefer the dorsal position to the left lateral position previously popular in Britain.

If the dorsal position is adopted the head and shoulders of the patient should be propped with two or more pillows. If the patient has not passed urine in the previous two hours she is asked to try and if she is unable to do so may require catheterization. The obstetrician scrubs up and puts on a sterile gown, mask and gloves. The patient's vulva is swabbed with cottonwool pledgets soaked in chlorhexidine (1 in 1000) solution and then covered with chlorhexidine 1 per cent cream. One sterile drape is placed beneath the patient and one covers her abdomen and sterile leggings may be used if desired. The obstetrician stands on the patient's right.

With each contraction, and as the patient pushes, the fetal head becomes more visible, retracting between contractions. Between each contraction the fetal heart is auscultated by one of the attendants.

**Delivery of the head**

Soon the area of the visible head has increased to 5cm, and the perineum is distended, the anterior rectal wall being visible. The obstetrician now increases the flexion of the head with the forefinger of his left hand, whilst a sanitary pad held in his right hand covers the anus and supports the perineum. These manoeuvres are protective and should never be used to hold back the fetal head forcibly.

In this way the birth of the head is accomplished slowly, until it has crowned (i.e. the parietal bosses have emerged through the vulva), and the frontal prominences are just visible. Once the head has crowned, the mother no longer pushes but pants during contractions so that the delivery may be performed with gentleness. To be born the head must extend, and this movement is helped by pushing the chin upwards as it lies deep to the anus, with the swab-covered right hand. The forehead, nose, mouth and chin emerge and the head is born, the perineum being pressed back beneath the chin. The eyes are swabbed with sterile water, a swab moving away from the nasal side of each eye laterally.

### Protection of the perineum

By ensuring slow delivery of the head, and by maintaining flexion, the perineal muscles are able to stretch to meet the distending force. However, they may be particularly rigid, or the skin tight, so that a jagged tear must occur before the head is born. Since a tear is likely in the delivery of most primigravidae, obstetricians are increasingly making use of a clean incision in the perineum before tearing occurs. This is an episiotomy.

### Episiotomy

When the distension of the perineum is marked, and the skin obviously stretched and glistening, 5 to 10ml of 1 per cent lignocaine is injected in a fan-like manner into the perineal tissues (unless epidural analgesia has been used, when local anaesthesia is obviously not needed). At the height of the next contraction a deliberate incision is made, either medially or in a medio-lateral direction (Fig. **13/5**). One blade of sharp 5-inch (12cm) scissors is inserted into the vagina, and the incision starts at the median raphe. The advantages of the episiotomy are: (1) a ragged tear is avoided; (2) the rectal sphincter is not damaged; (3) the head is subjected to less pressure; (4) stretching of the muscles is avoided, as this may be a factor in reducing the incidence of subsequent vaginal prolapse.

In the opinion of some doctors and many women episiotomy is performed too frequently and too little attention is paid to the morbidity of the operation.

Disabling discomfort affects over 50 per cent of women following episiotomy and lasts for a mean of 4 days (ranges 1–21 days). This requires oral or intramuscular analgesia and the use of a rubber cushion. It also hinders the establishment of lactation. More serious, perhaps, between 55 and 70 per cent of women have subsequent dyspareunia when questioned 6 weeks after childbirth, and at 12 weeks, 15 to 30 per cent of sexually active women have dyspareunia.

The way in which the episiotomy is repaired may be a major factor in the development of post-episiotomy morbidity (see p. 359).

### Delivery of the shoulders

From the moment of the birth of the head to that of the feet of the baby a full minute should elapse. Once delivered, the head will rotate through 90°, and mucus will stream from its nose and mouth. With the next contraction the head is grasped between the fingers of each hand and is gently drawn posteriorly so that the anterior shoulder is released from under the pubis. If the umbilical cord is looped around the fetal neck, the loops are disengaged by slipping them over the head of the fetus, or if they are too tightly twisted, by dividing the cord between two Spencer-Wells forceps.

The disengagement of the anterior shoulder is now completed and the posterior shoulder delivered by drawing the baby upwards in an arc towards the mother's abdomen. The mother should now have the opportunity of seeing and touching her child, after which it is laid between her legs, and the nose and fauces sucked clear of the remaining mucus, with a soft rubber catheter and bulb. By placing the baby at a level below that of the placenta, an additional 60ml of blood (equal to 55 per cent of its blood volume) is added to its circulation. One-third of this amount is added within 30 seconds and the remainder within 2 to 3 minutes of birth. In normal cases, clamping and tying the cord (and its division about 2.5cm from the umbilicus), should be delayed for 1 to 2 minutes after birth. The reason for this procedure is that babies who have received a moderate transfusion of placental blood have a lower incidence of the respiratory distress syndrome, and improved renal function.

### The newborn child

Once the child is born it moves its arms and legs and very soon the first inspiration leads to the first

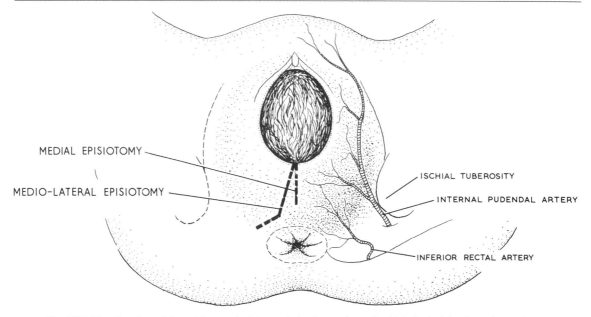

MEDIAL EPISIOTOMY

MEDIO-LATERAL EPISIOTOMY

ISCHIAL TUBEROSITY

INTERNAL PUDENDAL ARTERY

INFERIOR RECTAL ARTERY

**Fig. 13/5** The direction of the episiotomy incision and the tissues through which the incision is made are shown

cry. This may occur during the actual delivery or may be delayed until the mucus has been sucked clear. Once the baby is crying and the cord has been severed, a check is made to detect gross abnormalities (Chapter 56) and the baby is given to the mother to cuddle and to suckle. The importance of this early contact to maternal-baby 'bonding' has been stressed in recent years, and has been shown to influence their psychosocial relationship favourably.

The value of early and frequent contact between the mother and her baby in later mothering behaviour and in responsiveness in the child has been demonstrated by controlled studies in the USA and in Europe. Babies which were cuddled, usually naked, against their mother's breasts, and which were in frequent contact with the mother in the first days of life, when observed at 2 months were much more responsive and cried less than the control group. Early mother and baby bonding also favourably influenced the mother's behaviour to her child.

Unless there are medical contra-indications, the mother and father of the baby should be given the opportunity to explore and to cuddle their baby and to celebrate its birth. Most babies are alert, have good respiratory function and normal reflexes (unless the mother has been heavily sedated during labour). Most babies can be safely left in the care of their parents for a period of celebration. The medical attendant only needs to visit from time to time to

check that the mother's uterus is contracted and her baby well.

Only when this period has passed need the mother be 'tidied up', and the baby given a more complete physical examination.

During this period, the third stage of labour will have been completed.

A further more complete examination of the infant is made when the third stage is over.

Exaggerated beliefs of the value of 'bonding' should be discouraged. Whilst early parent–baby contact is to be encouraged, 'bonding' or 'attachment' between parents and baby will be as effective if it occurs later, in the first weeks (or months) of life. In certain instances, such as illness of the mother, an operative childbirth, or if the baby has had to be placed in intensive neonatal care, the parents may be anxious that the event will prevent bonding occurring. They may be reassured that if they are 'good' parents no psychological damage will occur to a baby who did not have the opportunity to be in close contact with the mother in the first days of life.

### Initiation of breathing

The great majority of infants establish respirations rapidly and require no more attention than clearing the upper air passage. A few infants are born in an hypoxic state, which may be severe or mild. These infants require resuscitation as described in Chapter 57. The degree to which the hypoxia has affected fetal vitality can be assessed by the Apgar scoring system, assessed at 1 and 5 minutes after birth (see p. 451). The management of respiratory depression is discussed on page 465. It should be noted that there is no evidence that analeptic drugs (such as lobeline or ethamivan) have any value in the initiation of respirations. They should not be used. However, if the mother has received pethidine in the previous 4 hours and the baby has an Apgar score below 6, naloxone 0.01mg/kg body-weight is given intramuscularly or intravenously.

### Prophylactic eye drops

Because of the danger of neonatal ophthalmia due to gonococci introduced during birth from the mother's vagina into the baby's conjunctival sac, it was usual until recently to place prophylactic drops into the neonate's eyes. Today, the number of cases of gonococcal neonatal ophthalmia is small, and prophylactic eye drops have been abandoned. Instead the eyes of all infants are inspected prior to discharge from hospital and mothers (particularly those at 'high risk' for gonorrhoea) are advised to report any conjunctival discharge from their infant's eyes at once.

If local circumstances make it desirable to use prophylactic eye treatment, tetracycline 1 per cent ointment is the drug of choice.

### Vitamin K

Most newborn babies develop vitamin K deficiency by the third day of life. Lack of vitamin K predisposes the baby to a bleeding diathesis caused by depression of clotting factors II, VII, IX and X. Clinically affected babies may bleed from the gastro-intestinal tract, the umbilical cord or from skin punctures. Recently a late-onset variety of vitamin K deficiency has been reported. This affects exclusively breast-fed babies who were not given vitamin K at birth. It manifests as gastro-intestinal haemorrhage or, more seriously, as intracranial haemorrhage, and occurs between 4 and 6 weeks after birth. To prevent these problems all neonates should be given vitamin $K_1$ (phytomenadione) 1mg intramuscularly or 2mg orally (if available) at birth or with the first feed.

# MANAGEMENT OF THE THIRD STAGE

The placenta separates within 3 minutes of birth when uterine contractions, added to the marked retraction which occurs after the child is expelled, diminish the size of the decidual plate of the placenta. The separation is aided by the spread through the decidua of the extravasated blood. Since the vessels supplying the placenta are large, haemorrhages from the veins would be marked were it not for the structure of the myometrium. The vessels pass through a lattice of interdigitating muscle fibres, and the marked retraction of this twists and occludes the vessels at several places forming 'living ligatures' (Fig. 13/6). Beyond and between the 'ligatures' the blood clots.

The efficiency with which the placenta separates and with which haemorrhage is controlled is an index of myometrial function. The more active the uterus the less the blood loss. Anything which interferes with the normal process of the third stage may cause haemorrhage.

Two methods of management of the third stage are presently available. In the first, a marked uterine contraction is produced by the use of an oxytocin; in the second the traditional 'watchful expectancy' is followed.

The active management of the third stage of labour is followed by: (1) one-fifth the incidence of post-partum haemorrhage; (2) a reduction in the mean length of the third stage to 5 minutes; (3) a slightly increased rate of retained placenta, and (4) if the drug is given with a second twin in utero, it may be trapped in a tonically contracted uterus and die. The advantages outweigh the disadvantages, provided that the patient is delivered in a place where manual removal of the placenta can be performed with a delay of less than 1 hour.

### The active management of the third stage

As the head of the baby is being born an intramuscular injection of 0.5ml of Syntometrine is given (or if the woman has hypertension, an intraven-

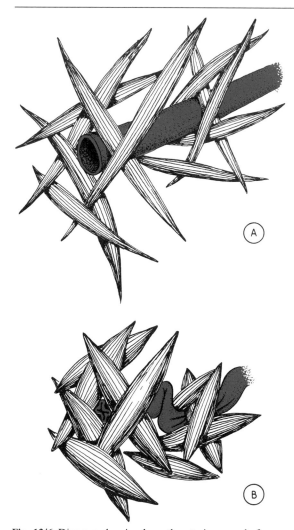

**Fig. 13/6** Diagram showing how the uterine muscle forms a 'living ligature' to occlude blood vessels

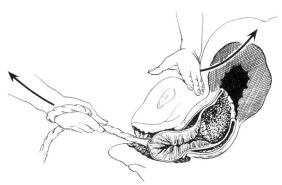

**Fig. 13/7** Controlled cord traction

ous injection of 10 units of Syntocinon is given with the birth of the anterior shoulder of the baby). The remainder of the delivery is slow and deliberate, 1 minute being taken. The cord is severed between clamps a minute after birth. The oxytocic effect of the drug occurs $2\frac{1}{2}$ minutes from the time of injection, and this contraction is awaited. As it occurs, the ulnar border of the left hand is placed on the uterus suprapubically and used to push the uterus upwards towards the umbilicus. At the same time the right hand, grasping the cord as it emerges from the vulva, pulls the placenta out of the vagina in a controlled manner (Fig. **13/7**). The membranes are stripped intact by drawing them out with sponge forceps or by twisting them into a rope by rotating the placenta. In 1 to 2 per cent of cases the placenta will be retained, but no blood loss will occur. After a 10-minute delay further controlled cord traction should be practised, and if the placenta is not delivered by this means, it should be removed manually.

The routine adminstration of an oxytocin in the third stage of labour reduces the risk of postpartum haemorrhage (> 500ml blood) by 40 per cent. Syntometrine appears to be the safest and most effective oxytocic.

**The traditional management of the third stage**

In this method the placenta is allowed to separate, and to descend into the vagina without any interference. The ulnar border of the hand is placed on the abdomen just above the globular uterus, and the signs of the placental descent are awaited. These are: (1) a gush of blood occurs; (2) the umbilical cord lengthens; (3) the fundus rises and becomes spherical; and (4) traction upwards of the fundus fails to draw the cord up with it. No attempt is made to hurry the appearance of the signs, the desire to 'fiddle with the fundus' is resisted, unless haemorrhage occurs, when a contraction must be 'rubbed up'. About 20 minutes usually pass before the signs of placental descent appear.

Once the placenta has descended into the upper vagina a contraction is obtained by 'rubbing up' the fundus and the entire uterus is pushed downwards towards the pelvis by the ulnar border of the hand, so that it acts as a piston in expelling the placenta from the vagina. The expelled placenta is grasped and twisted round and round with continuing traction so that the membranes are stripped intact.

The uterus is now massaged once again to obtain

a contraction to expel any contained clots, and is drawn up towards the umbilicus for a moment to reduce the myometrial congestion. An injection of ergometrine, 0.5mg, is given intramuscularly.

**Inspection of the placenta and membranes**

A careful inspection of the placenta should be made whilst the obstetrician is still scrubbed up. The placenta is held up by the umbilical cord and the fetal surface is examined and the completeness of the membranes is ascertained. Any vessels running to the edge of the membranes are noted as these may indicate a placenta succenturiata. The hole in the membranes is round if the membranes are complete.

The maternal surface is now exposed and cleaned by swabbing off the blood clot with gauze or running water. Holding the placenta in both hands each maternal cotyledon is inspected, and they are fitted together to ensure that none is missing. The maternal surface is covered with the greyish decidua.

The absence of a cotyledon, or evidence of a succenturiate lobe in the uterus, or very ragged membranes demands that the obstetrician explore the uterus.

**Inspection of the genital tract for injuries**

Following the delivery of the placenta, uterine bleeding ceases. The episiotomy wound should now be repaired, and the vagina inspected for injuries. If the delivery has been by a difficult forceps operation, the cervix must be inspected in a good light, and the lower uterine segment palpated.

The patient should remain in the delivery room for 1 hour, the degree of contraction of the uterus being noted frequently, the amount of bleeding recorded, and any clots present expelled from the uterus.

During this time the woman and her partner celebrate the birth of their baby. Vital signs, including uterine contraction and blood loss are checked at intervals.

Before returning to the ward the attendant must be sure (1) that the mother is in good general condition, with a normal pulse and blood pressure; (2) that the uterus is well contracted and contains no clots; (3) that the perineum has been repaired and that there is no bleeding from internal lacerations; (4) that the placenta and membranes are complete and have been checked; (5) that the bladder is empty; and (6) that the infant is in good condition and has been checked for congenital malformations.

## Chapter 14

# The Physiology of the Puerperium

The puerperium is that period of time in which the genital organs return to their pre-pregnant condition, and this takes from 6 to 8 weeks. The retrogressive changes are termed involution.

**Endocrine changes after childbirth**

With the expulsion of the placenta, the secretion of HCG, HPL and the sex steroids falls rapidly. HCG is undetectable in the urine of a puerperal woman, whose renal function is normal, within 7 to 10 days of delivery whilst HPL becomes undetectable in plasma within 2 days. The fall in oestrogen and progesterone is equally dramatic.

By three days after the expulsion of the placenta the blood levels of oestrogen and progesterone have fallen significantly and by the seventh day have reached basal levels. If the woman chooses to breast-feed, the levels remain low, because of high prolactin levels in her blood. If she decides not to breast-feed, oestradiol levels begin to rise 14 to 21 days after childbirth, indicating a resumption of ovarian follicular development and later ovulation.

Prolactin levels increase in the blood of lactating women, the level depending on the number of suckling episodes which occur each day, and remain high throughout lactation. Amongst non-lactating women the levels decline to reach the normal range within 14 to 21 days.

**Involution of the uterus**

At the end of the third stage the contracted uterus is the size of a 20-week pregnancy and weighs about 1000g. It rapidly becomes smaller and by the end of the 1st week weighs 500g and by the end of the 2nd week 350g. It involutes more slowly over the next 6 weeks, at the end of which time it is only slightly larger than its pre-pregnant size. Abdominal examina-

tion shows that involution reduces the size of the uterus by about 1.6cm (a finger-breadth) a day, and by the 12th puerperal day it has sunk behind the symphysis.

Involution is due to the withdrawal of the oestrogen stimulation of RNA (and consequently protein) synthesis by the myometrial cells and by the activity of proteolytic enzymes breaking down the cytoplasm into soluble end products which are removed by the bloodstream. At the same time phagocytes invade the collagen fibres between the myometrial cells and remove fat from the area. The thrombosed blood vessels also disappear by autolysis and new vessels grow through the thrombus. Involution is never complete, and a parous uterus is not identical with that of a nulliparous woman. With each pregnancy, the muscle weight and collagen content of the uterus increase by about 20 per cent. At the same time elastin is deposited in the uterus, mainly around blood vessels. In this way the uterus of the high multigravida contains relatively more collagen and elastin, and is a less efficient container for a pregnancy, so that malpresentations, postpartum haemorrhage and spontaneous uterine rupture are more likely to occur.

**Involution of the placental site**

Following expulsion of the placenta the placental bed contracts rapidly and measures 7.5cm on the 1st day. Invasion of the placental bed by lymphocytes, macrophages and polymorphs occurs and a cellular 'barrier' forms beneath it, and in the decidua of the remainder of the uterine cavity to a lesser extent. All the tissues superficial to the cellular barrier are shed and new epithelium covers the area. Except for the placental bed the re-epithelization of the uterine cavity is complete within 10 days. By this day the area of the placental bed has been reduced to 2.5cm but from now on its disappearance, and the growth of covering epithelium, is slower and fragmentary pieces of trophoblast continue to be shed for a further 4 or 5 weeks.

### The lochia

This is the discharge from the genital tract during the first 4 or 5 weeks of the puerperium. For the first 3 or 4 days it consists mainly of blood which comes from the placental site. As the thrombosed veins become organized, the character of the lochia changes and it now contains blood, leucocytes and decidua and the exfoliated pieces of trophoblast-covered villi which are shed from the placental site. For the first 8 to 12 puerperal days its colour is reddish-brown but after this time, when only the placental bed has not been covered with epithelium, it changes to a yellowish colour. The quantity of the lochia varies from day to day and is increased if the placental site has been large, as in multiple pregnancy, or if portions of the membranes or placenta are retained.

The uterus continues to contract during the puerperium, particularly after suckling, and this causes increased amounts of lochia to be lost. Occasionally the organized thrombi obstructing the mouths of vessels separate and red lochia returns for a while. Persistent bright red lochia for more than 10 days, or the passage of clots, means that the placental site is not involuting properly, and the administration of an oxytocic, or even curettage, to remove placental debris may be required. In the uterine cavity the lochia is sterile but it becomes contaminated in the vagina with organisms, and develops a characteristic heavy smell. The vaginal organisms multiply in the lochia and invade the uterine cavity by the 5th day. By this time the cellular 'barrier' has formed and infection rarely occurs. However, if the resistance of the tissues forming the placental bed is low, or labour has been traumatic, more virulent organisms can penetrate the barrier and produce puerperal infection (see Chapter 48).

### The cervix

Immediately after delivery the cervix is patulous, flabby, bruised, purple in colour and the os admits two or three fingers. Within 48 hours it has diminished in volume (by loss of the contained fluid) and the bruised appearance has gone. The cervical os now admits one or two fingers.

### The vagina and the vulva

Immediately after delivery the vaginal wall is swollen, bluish and pouting, but it very rapidly regains most of its tonicity. The mucosa remains delicate for the first few weeks, and submucosal venous congestion persists even longer. For this reason surgery on the puerperal vagina is complicated by marked capillary oozing. Small lacerations heal quickly in the mucosa but larger ones must always be sutured. The hymen disappears except for some small tags called carunculae myrtiformes.

The perineum, immediately after delivery, has either been torn; or had an episiotomy performed; or has been stretched, and at the vulval ring small lacerations may be seen. With amazing rapidity healing and absorption of collections of blood and serum occurs, so that by the 5th puerperal day the perineum looks relatively normal.

### The urinary tract

In the first few hours after delivery micturition may be difficult, partly because of reflex suppression of detrusor activity and sphincter spasm from irritation of the levator ani muscles during delivery, and partly due to oedema of the bladder base which occurs in labour. During the first 1 or 2 days a marked diuresis occurs, because of a fall in progesterone content of the blood and the alteration of cell metabolism to the non-pregnant state. The physiological dilatation of the urinary tract clears within 6 weeks in 95 per cent of patients and in all by the 12th week after childbirth.

### Blood changes

In the last 4 weeks of pregnancy, a significant rise occurs in the levels of fibrinogen, plasminogen and factors II, VII, VIII and X. During the first few days after delivery a rapid fall occurs in the fibrinogen, plasminogen and factor VIII levels, whilst at the same time there is a rise in the level of circulating fibrin degradation products, probably due to the lysis of fibrin deposited in the placental bed. These changes have reverted by the 14th puerperal day, and the blood coagulation-lysis factors return to normal levels. However, in the first 2 weeks of the puerperium, the coagulability of the blood is increased and an increased risk of thrombosis is present.

The blood loss at delivery reduces the red cell

mass from its raised pregnant levels, but a further slow decline to non-pregnant levels occurs during the puerperium. Non-pregnant levels are reached by the 40th day.

### Restoration of ovulation and menstruation

Women who breast-feed exclusively, and suckle 'on demand' are likely to delay ovulation and menstruation for a considerable period. The more frequently a woman suckles, the higher is the plasma prolactin level and the longer ovulation is delayed. However, in a proportion of lactating women, especially those who only partially breast-feed, ovulation may occur, and subsequently pregnancy, without any menstrual episode. Ovulation is unusual amongst lactating women for about 20 weeks. Menstruation may start earlier, 10 per cent of breast-feeding women menstruate by the 10th week after childbirth, 40 per cent by 20 weeks and 60 per cent are menstruating by 30 weeks.

Amongst women who choose not to breast-feed, 80 per cent menstruate by the 10th week after childbirth, and ovulation is likely to occur from this time onwards.

*Chapter 15*

# Conduct of the Puerperium

Until recently a puerperal woman was treated as an ignorant, idle, ill woman who required careful discipline so that she would not damage herself, and who was expected to obey orders and fit into the hospital routine with humility and without question. She was confined to bed, as to get up would undoubtedly cause a prolapse, and in consequence was unable to pass urine and became constipated, which confirmed the nurses' opinion that she was a sick woman. On the 7th day or later after the confinement she got out of bed for the first time, and since she had not used her muscles whilst in bed, her first steps were faltering, again confirming the nurses' opinion that she was ill. Some women are emotional after birth, and this is a normal psychological reaction to the process of reproduction, but again the emotional instability confirmed that the woman was ill. For the convenience of the hospital her baby was kept in a nursery and at regular intervals was produced in a production line manner for breast feeding. The patient's perineum was painful, her emotions affected, her psyche dominated by an attitude that nurse knows best.

Today a new approach has been adopted by health professionals. In essence, this philosophy is that the puerperal woman is a healthy, intelligent individual who has just achieved a memorable event: she has given birth to a live healthy individual; she is a person who must be treated with understanding; she is a person who is anxious to see and touch her child and to co-operate in caring for it.

If this attitude prevails amongst the doctors and nurses attending the patient, the first few days of the puerperium can be a time of rest and of education for the responsibility of caring for the baby after discharge from hospital, and also one of emotional enhancement and of a sense of achievement.

## REST

Immediately after the birth of the baby, the mother and her partner need to be able to spend a quiet time with their baby, celebrating its birth and bonding with it. After this, the woman may wish to sleep. Occasionally a patient will ask for sedation as she is 'too excited to sleep' but most fall into a natural sleep and waken refreshed. When she awakes she will want to see her baby again, and when possible rooming-in should be practised from this time on. The patient may get out of bed whenever she likes, but some prefer to stay in bed for about 24 hours and to walk about after that time. Early ambulation has much to commend it, provided it is done at the patient's speed and not for the convenience of the nursing staff. If the patient walks about she does not lose the tone of her muscles and the drainage of lochia is improved. Admittedly, the puerperal woman requires more rest, but this can be ensured by insisting on at least 2 hours in bed after the midday meal. At other times she is free to walk and talk with her neighbours, to go to the toilet and to shower herself. If a continuous catgut suture is used to repair episiotomy wounds she will not be inconvenienced and swabbing rounds can be eliminated.

## 'ROOMING-IN'

'Rooming-in' implies that for all, or most, of the time the child remains in a cot beside the mother's bed. 'Rooming-in' has many advantages over the alternative method of keeping the baby in the nursery from which it is brought out at fixed times to be fed. First, the mother is psychologically attached to her child and rooming-in enables her to become accustomed to its behaviour and to interpret its cry at a time when more experienced help is available to reassure her. If the baby is kept in the nursery the mother is inexperienced when she leaves hospital with her child. Secondly, by treating mother and child as a 'unit' cross-infection is reduced to a minimum. Thirdly, it makes it possible for the mother to care for her child, thus relieving the nursing staff, and to feed the baby 'on demand'. It is necessary to provide nursery accommodation for fractious babies and for those of ill mothers, but apart from these two classes the babies can 'room-in' at all times.

## ROUTINE CARE

The temperature and pulse are taken and charted twice daily; the perineal wound is inspected; the character of the lochia is noted, and if clots are present after the 3rd day or recur later in the puerperium, ergometrine 1mg is given orally twice or thrice daily for 2 or 3 days. Apart from this the routine use of oxytocics is not recommended. Some patients, particularly multigravidae, feel that the 'uterus flops about inside' and are more comfortable wearing a girdle.

### Care of vulva

With early ambulation and the 'continuous suturing' of perineal wounds, toilet of the vulva is reduced to a minimum. If the mother has an oedematous, painful perineum, or is not permitted to go to the shower room because of pre-eclampsia or cardiac disease, then vulval swabbing should be performed, preferably by jug douching with a dilute antiseptic solution, so long as she remains in bed. In all other cases the mother can attend to her own vulval hygiene by taking a shower as often as she wishes.

If the perineum has been badly lacerated and has required an extensive repair, reactionary oedema may make it very painful. The patient should be given analgesics, and infra-red irradiation applied to the perineum is often helpful. With severe tears, it is usual to order a low residue diet, in order to reduce the need of the patient to defaecate. However, if she has a need to do this, she should be encouraged to open her bowels, and if it is thought that the faeces may be 'hard', one tube of Micralax (or some similar substance) should be injected into the rectum.

### Micturition

It has been noted that micturition is often difficult in the first 24 hours after delivery. If the patient is ambulant, difficulty of micturition is less likely to occur than if she is confined to bed. Should she be unable to pass urine, catheterization may be required. After catheterization 60ml of 1:5000 chlorhexidine solution should be instilled into the bladder before removing the catheter.

### Bowels

The ambulant patient rarely has any difficulty in defaecation but if the perineal wound is large and the patient is constipated, a rectal suppository of bisacodyl may be given on the 3rd or 4th day. Alternatively Senokot may be given by mouth.

### Afterpains

The uterine contractions continue after delivery and tend to be particularly painful in some multigravidae especially during feeding. The discomfort should not be ignored and analgesics, such as tabs. codeine co. or in some cases pethidine, may be required.

### Breast-feeding

This is fully discussed in Chapter 16.

### Visitors

Provided the patient has had a normal delivery and is not unduly tired she should be allowed to see as many visitors as she wishes. There should be no restriction on the visits of her partner (subject to ward routine which in most hospitals can be considerably reduced) but other visitors should be given specific times when they may visit. It was usual to prevent other children from seeing their mother as it is said they are likely to introduce infection. This is extremely doubtful provided no child with obvious infection is allowed to enter the hospital, and when practicable the mother should be able to see her other children. In a properly designed hospital this can take place in the day room if there is anxiety about children coming into a ward.

### 'Third day blues'

A number of women become temporarily depressed between the third and fifth day after childbirth. The cause of the depression has not been established. Speculation about its aetiology includes hormonal imbalance (although none has been identified), reaction to the excitement of childbirth, and uncertainty by the mother about her ability to care for her dependent child. Another factor in our culture may be the expectation that a mother immediately loves her baby, when in reality, mother-love is a learned behaviour. The condition called 'third day blues' leads to bursts of crying, to irritability and in some cases to general depression. The management is for one of the medical or nursing staff to talk with the woman, explaining what is occurring, and if the woman wishes, to restrict visitors. There is some evidence that 'third day blues' are less likely to occur if maternal-infant bonding has occurred and if rooming-in is practised. 'Third day blues' is a misnomer as the inability to adjust to parenthood, with feelings of inadequacy, tiredness, reduced sexuality, emotional liability and, in a small proportion of women, severe depression, may persist for weeks or months.

### Adjustment to parenthood and puerperal depression

Few doctors understand that adjustment to parenthood is difficult for most women. Women have been brought up to believe that they should be good housekeepers, excellent lovers and experienced mothers all at the same time. Yet on return home after childbirth, the persistent demands of the new born baby on the energy, the time and the emotions of a woman may cause considerable stress. This stress is aggravated by the nuclear family and the tendency for young people to live at some distance from their close relatives, who in other cultures, are readily available to offer help and consolation. The stress becomes intensified as the mother realizes that she has the sole responsibility for a small, unpredictable infant who needs attention by day and night. She had not realized that the baby would cry so much, for so little apparent cause. Her sleep is constantly broken and fatigue is added to her feelings of maternal inadequacy. Her relationship with her husband requires adjustment; and this can be emotionally disturbing, particularly if he does not do his share of parenting. As the baby occupies so much of her time, the mother finds that she cannot keep the house as clean as she would wish, and feels guilty that she is not the efficient housewife she believed she was.

The fatigue induced by the demands of the baby, the emotional re-adjustment in her marital relations, the guilt experienced over her untidy house and the lack of a helpful counsellor, often induces depression. In about 5 per cent of women the depression becomes so severe that medical help is sought, usually between the 2nd and 7th week of the puerperium. The presenting symptoms are mainly changes in mood: tearfulness, feelings of inadequacy and inability to cope predominating. These changes are labile, and depression is worse towards evening, when associated psychosomatic complaints of fatigue, anorexia and nausea may occur. Doctors all too frequently offer sedation or psychotrophic drugs, when explanation, reassurance and advice would be even more useful. It is also important to tell patients of community-based helping organizations such as the La Lèche League in Britain and the USA, and the Nursing Mothers Associations and Play Groups in Australia. These organizations provide 24-hour home counselling and home visiting when needed. Their activities in helping women adjust to parenthood can be of great value in reducing the incidence of puerperal depression.

### Sexuality

Problems of adjusting to parenthood, and tenderness in the episiotomy scar reduce the sexual desire and activity of many puerperal women. Other women have increased sexual desire.

Traditionally, doctors have forbidden coitus until the postnatal check-up, but there is no medical reason for this. Couples should be told that they may resume coitus whenever the woman finds it comfortable, and can, of course, use non-coital methods of sexual pleasuring whenever they wish.

The frequency of complaints about the episiotomy repair make it mandatory for doctors to perform and to repair the incision with skill.

## PERINATAL BEREAVEMENT

About 14 babies in every 1000 are either stillborn or die in the first 28 days of life. They constitute the perinatal deaths (see p. 425). Many of these babies are born preterm, are of low birth-weight and about 25 per cent have severe congenital malformations. Parents whose baby dies in the perinatal period have grief reactions similar to those which follow the loss of any loved person. At first the mother (and often the father) feels numb and 'shocked'. After a few days the reaction changes to a desire to understand why the baby died, or to expressions of anger or guilt about events in pregnancy or during labour. Over the next 2 or 3 months many parents are likely to review the event surrounding the baby's death, often repeatedly. More than 50 per cent of mothers suffer from depression and anxiety which may last for months, but at last, the couple adjust, often embarking on a new pregnancy.

The severity and duration of the bereavement reaction may be reduced if the parents are given the opportunity to talk with the attending medical staff soon after the baby's death. Most want to understand what has gone wrong, explained in clear, simple language. A few become angry, blaming the staff for the child's death. The person should listen to the parents with sympathy and understanding and explain as clearly as possible the events surrounding the death. A parent who wishes to see her dead child (even if malformed) so that she may mourn the loss, should be given the opportunity. Before the parents see the baby they should be told how the infant will look. If deformities are present, they should be described (perhaps with a photograph). The baby is presented to the parents clothed and wrapped, and when they become accustomed to him or her, the baby is undressed by them. This procedure is often emotional, and support from a health professional may be invaluable. The parents should be told that they can spend as much time as they wish with the baby, and should be encouraged to name the child. Many parents wish to have a photograph of their dead baby. When the mother leaves hospital it is important to suggest that she makes contact with her family doctor (or health visitor) and should be told about community-based helping organizations in her area.

One woman in every five whose baby is stillborn or who dies in the neonatal period will suffer severe symptoms of bereavement (sleeplessness, depression and withdrawal). Women who have little or no support from husband, partner or family, who have insensitive health professionals, and who lack a caring environment are more likely to be affected severely. These women, particularly, need help from sympathetic health professionals who listen, communicate and counsel.

There is some evidence that parents cope better, psychologically, with the next pregnancy if conception is delayed for a few months, but the decision has to be made by the couple, rather than imposed by a doctor. During the pregnancy, continuity of care is important and supportive, communicating, sympathetic health professionals help reduce possible mothering difficulties and puerperal problems.

### Child abuse

Women who find difficulty in coping with their baby, or who have strange, disturbed behaviour whilst in hospital, are more likely to abuse the baby after discharge. The prevalence of child abuse before the age of 3 is not known, exactly, but it is probable that at least 6 per 1000 live-born children are abused. Mothers who have social problems, who have no supportive partner or relative, or who have marital problems are more likely to abuse their child. It is possible, by simple observation in the puerperium, to identify some 'vulnerable' women, and this is part of postnatal care. Preventive intervention by family doctors, paediatricians and social workers has been shown to reduce the prevalence of child neglect and abuse.

## TIME OF DISCHARGE

In Asia because of shortage of maternity beds patients who have had a normal labour are usually discharged from hospital after 24 hours. Provided the woman can be visited at home and the routine carried out this has not proved harmful. In the most affluent countries it has been usual to keep the patient in hospital for 5 to 10 days, probably because of a biblical injunction entering the culture. There is no need for the patient without complications to remain in hospital so long and most women are anxious to go home 3 to 5 days after delivery. The time of discharge should be arranged to suit the individual and not be made a routine for all.

### At home

Readjustment on return home is required and the patient should, and usually does, adjust her activities to fit her own needs. Two points need stressing. First, the baby is often fractious in the first 24 to 36 hours after returning home and requires more cuddling and care. Secondly, should heavy lochia or bright bleeding recur the woman should notify her doctor. In general she need not limit her activities beyond realizing that if she is breast-feeding she requires extra rest.

# Chapter 16

# The Breasts and Breast-feeding

During pregnancy the breasts develop considerably. This development is consequent on the increased circulating oestrogen and progesterone, and is probably influenced by human placental lactogen (HPL) secreted by the syncytiotrophoblast. Oestrogen leads to an increase both in size and number of the duct system, whilst progesterone appears to increase the number of alveolar cells. HPL also stimulates the development of the cells lining the acini or alveoli, and probably initiates the changes in the cell structure leading to the synthesis of casein, lactalbumin and lactoglobulin. Prolactin levels also rise in pregnancy and remain at high levels.

Fat is deposited around the lobules, with the result that the size of the breasts increases. The deposition of fat is under the influence of the female sex hormones, particularly progesterone.

Despite this marked activity of cellular development, lactation does not occur during pregnancy, although limited amounts of colostrum are secreted.

The function of prolactin is to induce the alveolar cells of the breast to secrete milk, yet during pregnancy, lactation is unusual despite raised plasma prolactin levels. The reason is that the high circulating levels of oestrogen (and probably progesterone) act directly on the alveoli of the breasts, occupying binding sites on the epithelial cells, which prevent them responding to the lactogenic effects of prolactin.

Prolactin is secreted by the galactophore cells of the anterior pituitary gland. Its synthesis and secretion is controlled by a prolactin-inhibiting factor (PID). PID, which is mainly dopamine, is released by the hypothalamus and reaches the pituitary via the hypophyseal portal vessels. Its release is influenced, in turn, by a number of behavioural and physiological factors.

Following childbirth and placental expulsion, the oestrogen levels fall within 3 days, permitting prolactin to act on the alveoli to initiate lactation. Lactation will continue if the mother suckles her baby, as this reflexly encourages prolactin secretion and release from the pituitary, thus maintaining lactation (Fig. **16/1**).

The quantity of prolactin released depends on the frequency the mother suckles her baby. If a mother exclusively breast feeds her baby on demand, higher levels of prolactin will be maintained than if she feeds it to a fixed time schedule and adds supplements early in its life. During exclusive breast-feeding amenorrhoea is usual. Endocrine studies have shown that maternal blood concentrations of FSH are in the high normal range, those of LH are in the low normal range but without pulsatile activity, and the hypothalamic release of GnRH is reduced. Oestrogen levels are low, suggesting that prolactin prevents ovarian follicular development. This oversimplifies a complex control system, and many details are still obscure. For example, there is no doubt that emotions can reduce the supply of milk, presumably acting through the hypothalamus; and for the maintenance of lactation suckling is essential, as are normal levels of ACTH, adrenocortical hormones and possibly growth hormone, thyroid hormone and insulin. It may be that prolactin-inhibiting factor is always present in the hypothalamus, and that the effect of suckling, the emotions, and certain hormones is to inhibit the tonic release of the factor, thus releasing the adenohypophysis from control, and permitting prolactin release.

By the second day after childbirth, the levels of oestrogen and progesterone have fallen sufficiently to permit prolactin to act on the alveolar cells and milk secretion begins.

The first secretions from the breast are mainly colostrum, a thickish yellowish fluid which has a high

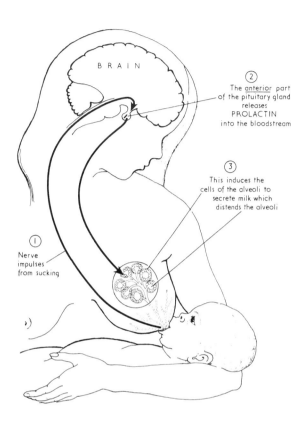

Fig. 16/1  The prolactin reflex

② The anterior part of the pituitary gland releases PROLACTIN into the bloodstream

③ This induces the cells of the alveoli to secrete milk which distends the alveoli

① Nerve impulses from sucking

content of anti-infective substances (including 10⁷ maternal lymphocytes per ml, providing passive immunity) and higher zinc and sodium levels than 'mature' milk.

Mature milk, which is secreted following the release of prolactin inhibition, is thin and bluish in colour. The milk distends the mammary alveoli, and the breasts become 'engorged ' by about the 3rd or 4th postpartum day. Clinically the engorged breasts are heavy and tense. Turgid veins can be seen beneath the skin, and the milk ducts can be felt as tender, irregular, hard strings coursing through the breast tissue. Engorgement is due to secretion of milk in the absence of its ejection along the ducts. This is effected by the 'milk ejection' reflex.

By the 7th puerperal day, engorgement has ceased and lactation is fully established (Fig. **16/2**).

### Antenatal breast (nipple) discharge

A few women develop a reddish, brown or chocolate coloured discharge from one or both nipples during the antenatal period. The cause of this is unknown. The condition is not painful and usually disappears when lactation is established, and milk is flowing. If the breast discharge occurs, the woman should avoid antenatal breast expression, and a breast examination should be made, especially if the discharge is unilateral.

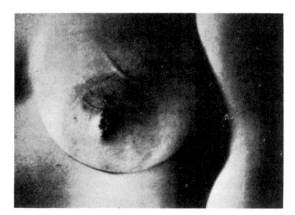

**Fig. 16/2** Lactating breast. Photograph taken on the 7th puerperal day. Note the engorged veins, the larger nipple and the larger and more heavily pigmented areola (from Lockhart, R.D., *Living Anatomy*, 7th edition. Faber and Faber, London, 1974)

### THE MILK EJECTION REFLEX

The milk secreted by and filling the alveoli is largely unavailable to the infant until the myo-epithelial cells (Fig. **16/3**), which surround the alveoli and smaller ducts contract in response to a reflex initiated by suckling, and the milk is propelled along the ducts to the small reservoirs (lactiferous sinuses) lying beneath the areolae. The milk ejection reflex, which is of a neuro-endocrine nature, is mediated via the hypothalamus and the neurohypophysis, and leads to the release of oxytocin (Fig. **16/4**). The oxytocin causes contraction of the myo-epithelial cells, and ejection of milk from the alveoli. It is also thought to stimulate further prolactin secretion in the adenohypophysis, and to inhibit further release of the prolactin-inhibiting factor by the hypothalamus, so that milk production is maintained.

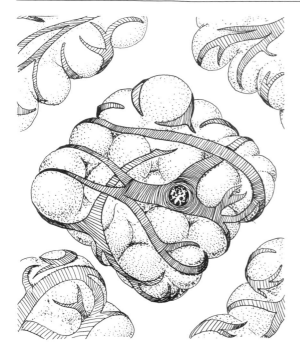

**Fig. 16/3** Myo-epithelial cells surrounding a partially filled villus (redrawn from Richardson, K. C., *Proc. Roy. Soc.*, Series B. 1949, **136**, 30)

Emotional and physical stress can reduce the milk ejection (or 'let-down') reflex to a considerable extent. Stress is thought to operate by increasing the release of noradrenaline in the midbrain. This, in turn, reduces the 'firing rate' of neurones which release oxytocin from the neurohypophysis.

The first 'milk' produced is the thick yellow colostrum which has filled the alveoli in late pregnancy. Within 2 days of birth the biochemical composition of the colostrum has changed into 'transitional milk', which in turn becomes mature milk by the 5th day after childbirth. Mature breast milk varies in composition from hour to hour and from day to day, but on average contains 87 per cent water, 7 per cent sugar, 4 per cent fat, 1 per cent protein and 1 per cent salts.

## THE MAINTENANCE OF LACTATION

It can be appreciated that the maintenance of lactation is a complex affair, and many factors are involved; for example, the emotions can affect lactation considerably, as can extreme starvation. The most important factor in maintaining lactation is regular suckling, so that both the prolactin reflex and the milk ejection reflex are initiated frequently, and abnormal distension of the alveoli by milk is prevented. If the latter happens, the alveolar cells are unable to secrete milk efficiently, and at the same time suckling is avoided because of pain. For these reasons the reflex which prevents the release of the prolactin-inhibiting factor is lost, and the inhibiting factor reduces prolactin release so that alveolar activity diminishes, with further reduction of milk secretion.

Although many medications are given to increase milk secretion, most operate only by a placebo effect. The exception is metoclopramide 10mg given three times a day, for about 2 weeks.

## PREPARATION FOR BREAST-FEEDING

During pregnancy the obstetrician should discuss breast-feeding with the expectant mother. He should point out the benefits of breast milk as the most balanced, convenient food for human babies, and

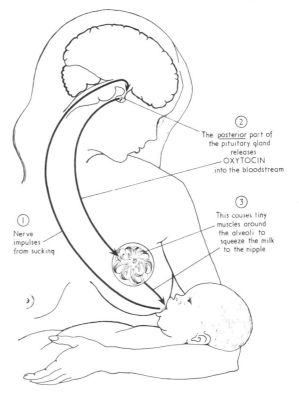

**Fig. 16/4** The milk ejection reflex

the advantages of breast-feeding in maternal-infant bonding. If a woman chooses not to breast-feed, for whatever reason, he should avoid making her feel guilty and should discuss the importance of preparing formula milk precisely in accordance with the manufacturer's directions. He should also stress the importance for the future health of the baby by avoiding the introduction of 'solids' until about the 5th month of life.

If the woman chooses to breast-feed, the obstetrician should determine if her nipples are protractile, pseudo-protractile or inverted. This can be ascertained by placing the thumb on one side of the base of the areola and the index finger on the other and squeezing towards the nipple. Normally, protractile nipples project, whilst pseudo-protractile nipples tend to retract into the breast tissue. Inverted nipples remain inverted.

Pseudo-protractile nipples are thought to be due to adhesions which 'anchor' the nipple to the tissues underlying the areola. Exercises should be started, in the second half of pregnancy, to break the adhesions. Several times each day, the woman places her thumbs on the opposite sides of her nipples at the areolar margin, first in a horizontal plane and then in a vertical plane, and draws the thumbs apart. If the nipples are truly inverted and fail to project with these exercises, plastic nipple shields worn under the brassière should be used.

Some obstetricians advise that women should massage their breasts, pressing from the periphery towards the nipple, five or ten times each day in the second half of pregnancy. The exercise is believed to 'condition' the prolactin and 'let-down' reflexes, although there is some doubt about its value. In late pregnancy some drops of colostrum are usually expelled from the nipples during the exercises.

Nipple care is important during pregnancy. The nipples should be washed each day with water, to remove any crusts, and anhydrous lanolin may be applied. Soap, and toughening or abrasive agents should not be used as they damage the epithelium and predispose to 'cracked' nipples after childbirth.

In late pregnancy, it helps to expose the nipples to the air, and, when possible, to sunbathe.

In the past ten years there has been a modest but significant return to breast-feeding. The reasons for this are not clear, but there is some evidence that an important factor has been the activity of community-based women's groups such as La Leche League International in the USA, The Nursing Mothers' Association in Australia and The National Childbirth Trust in Britain. These organizations provide information and counselling services for mothers who have questions about, or problems with breast-feeding. They, and other groups such as The Childbirth Education Association have been active in inducing obstetricians and hospital staff to alter outdated hospital practices.

## ESTABLISHMENT OF BREAST-FEEDING

It will be realized that the establishment of successful breast-feeding has three elements. First, milk secretion within the alveoli must occur. Second, and more important, the milk-ejection reflex must operate to propel the milk from the alveoli through the ducts to collect in the sub-areolar 'reservoirs'. The milk-ejection reflex is affected by the emotions, and is stimulated by suckling. Third, the mother must be motivated to breast-feed.

There is now evidence that many hospital practices are detrimental to the establishment of lactation and breast-feeding. These include the separation of mother and baby at birth; keeping the baby in a nursery, instead of 'rooming-in'; 'routine' 4-hourly feeds; giving the baby water (or, even worse, glucose-water) in the days before lactation is established.

Breast-feeding is most successful if the following conditions apply. (1) The mother and baby 'bond' as soon after birth as possible and the baby suckles during this time. (2) The baby 'rooms-in' with the mother from birth. (3) The baby is suckled frequently for short periods of about 5 minutes from soon after birth to 'bring the milk in'. This technique, which can replace 'scheduled' breast-feeding, does not cause damage to the nipple. (4) Once the milk flow is established the baby is demand fed, including during the night. In the first 2 days of life only colostrum is obtained by the baby, but this provides immunoglobulins and may have a laxative function. (5) No supplemental feedings (of water or glucose-water), or complementary feedings (of formula milk) should be given without the express permission of the woman and her doctor.

It is now known that failure of the milk ejection reflex is the main reason for unsuccessful lactation. The milk-ejection reflex is stimulated by frequent suckling and enhanced if the mother is relaxed, unhurried and confident of her ability to breast-feed.

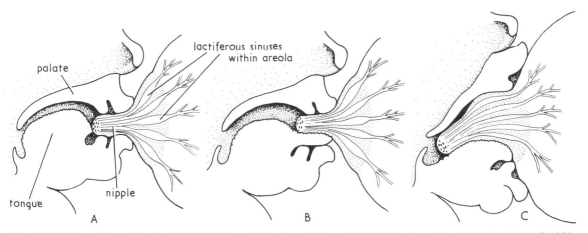

**Fig. 16/5** Ideal position of nipple in the infant's mouth. In A and B the nipple is being chewed; in C the nipple is well within the baby's mouth

This psychological state is induced by helpful supportive medical and nursing attendants.

The mother should be made comfortable during breast-feeding, and may suckle sitting in a chair, in bed with a back-rest, or lying with the baby beside her. Since the mother and child have to form a harmonious relationship, instruction in feeding should be sympathetic and unhurried, or psychological factors will inhibit prolactin and possibly oxytocin release. In order to avoid damage to the nipples, the nurse–midwife should supervise the early attempts of breast-feeding, and ensure that the nipple is well within the infant's mouth and not being nibbled by its hard gums (Fig. **16/5**).

Both the doctor and the nurse–midwife have a duty to help the mother establish breast-feeding. This demands a kindly unhurried approach, and the realization that many mothers have no idea what to do. The mother must be shown how to stroke the mouth of her infant with her nipple so that it may open its mouth to grasp the nipple. This is called the 'rooting reflex' in the USA. The mother must be shown how to grasp her breast behind the areola with her forefinger and middle finger, so that the nipple becomes more prominent, and the baby grasps the areola and not the tender nipple. This technique also enables the baby to breathe when feeding, as its nose is no longer pressed into the breast substance (Fig. **16/6**). The mother must also be shown how to detach the baby when she wants to 'burp' him. This is not done by dragging the baby away from the nipple, but by inserting the little finger into the corner of the baby's mouth to break the suction before he is pulled off the nipple (Fig. **16/7**).

As soon as possible, and certainly once the milk is flowing freely, feeding should be 'on demand', the baby being put to the breast when it is awake and hungry, irrespective of the time interval between feeds. Women in the undeveloped countries do this by habit, and the 'scheduled' feeding introduced in developed lands 30 years ago was more for the convenience of the hospital than the physiological needs of the mother and child.

Very few babies managed in this way require additional fluids in the first 3 or 4 days of life, but if

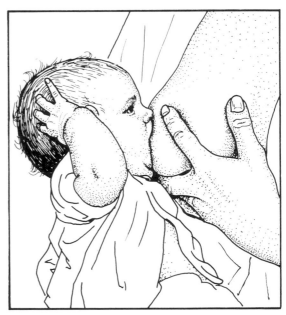

**Fig. 16/6** The technique of breast-feeding

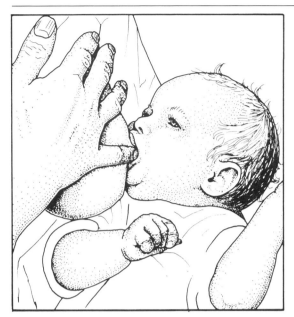

Fig. 16/7 How the mother releases her nipple from the baby's mouth

dehydration is observed, the baby should be given water (with added lactose if desired) by a dropper or a spoon following the nursing session. A bottle should not be used as it may disturb the infant's learning to suck properly at the breast.

### Engorgement of the breasts

Adjustment between supply of milk and demand takes time, as does the establishment of the milk ejection reflex, and during this period engorgement of the breasts may occur, usually on the 3rd to 4th day of the puerperium. Engorgement is less common and less marked if the regimen suggested to establish lactation is adopted. Engorgement can be prevented, in most cases, by making sure that the breasts are emptied after each feed, by manual expression of any remaining milk, and by keeping the intervals short between feeds.

If the breasts become engorged they become turgid and tender, the veins are distended and prominent, and the skin tense and hot. Some patients develop pyrexia and, unless the milk is ejected, further secretion is reflexly inhibited, with failure of lactation.

Many nurses claim success in reducing engorgement by applying hot and cold packs, alternately, to the breasts before the feed is due. These stimulate blood flow through the engorged areas of the breasts. If the engorgement is more severe, the milk ejection reflex can be stimulated by using an electric breast pump (the Egnell pump).

If the engorgement is very severe, it may be reduced by giving small doses of the prolactin antagonist, bromocriptine, for 24 to 48 hours.

Since the failure of the milk ejection reflex is the main cause of engorgement, and this is activated by suckling, the infant should continue to be breast-fed from the engorged breasts, and indeed should be put to the breast at more frequent intervals if this is not too painful.

## THE INHIBITION OF LACTATION

A large number of women today do not wish to breast-feed their infants. The reasons are complex, and the influences of cultural patterns of behaviour and the mass media are considerable. This change is noticeable both in the developed and developing countries, and amongst all classes of society; but it is more usual amongst affluent urban dwellers. Investigations have shown that in Britain, for example, one-third of women elect not to breast-feed, and a further one-third abandon breast-feeding within 14 days of childbirth.

These women require to have lactation inhibited or suppressed. Inhibition of milk secretion before lactation has begun is generally accomplished more easily than suppression of lactation. Whilst it is true that milk production will diminish and finally cease if suckling is avoided, the engorged breasts are particularly painful for a few days. If this method is adopted, the breasts should be well supported, but there is no need for tight binding. Fluids should not be restricted, and the use of purgatives is to be condemned.

Because of the discomfort, and often pain associated with this method, many obstetricians choose drugs to inhibit or suppress lactation. Dopamine agonists are the principal medication available.

### Dopamine agonists

Bromocriptine, pergolide and cyclofenil are dopamine receptor agonists. In the body they act directly on the galactophores in the anterior pituitary gland, inhibiting prolactin secretion. Bromocriptine in a dose of 2.5mg twice daily, given for 14 days, effectively inhibits lactation. None of the drugs alter blood coagulation factors or liver function tests, but cyclofenil has a more sustained effect on prolactin secretion, and there is less likelihood of a recurrence of lactation after ceasing medication. The drugs are expensive, and their use may be associated with an early return of ovulation, so that some form of contraception is indicated if the couple wish to avoid pregnancy.

### Cracked nipples

Aggressive suckling by the baby allied to over-filling of the breasts can lead to fissures in the mucosa of the nipples (cracked nipples). These can be very painful, and if infected can lead to the development of acute mastitis. The nipple should be treated with hexachlorophane or chlorhexidine cream during the day, compound tincture of benzoin being applied at night. A nipple shield should be used to protect the abraded area during feeding.

### Failing lactation

A number of women find that on returning home lactation begins to fail. The reasons for this are little understood. Treatment is to give helpful support and, perhaps, to prescribe metoclopramide.

### Contraception

Although exclusive breast feeding, especially when on demand, reduces considerably the chance that ovulation will occur, this event may happen. In consequence many lactating women seek contraceptive advice. If hormonal contraceptives are chosen, combined oral contraceptives are best avoided, as the oestrogen content may reduce lactation, and the progestogen-only pill (the mini-pill) is to be preferred.

## BREAST PROBLEMS DURING LACTATION

Lactating women presenting with inflammatory conditions of the breast may have milk stasis ('caked breast'), non-infectious inflammation or infectious mastitis. *Milk stasis* tends to occur early in lactation and to be associated with, or to follow breast engorgement. It is due to pressure on a main duct by milk engorged alveoli. This leads to a tender, lumpy area in the breast. It has a short duration. *Non-infectious breast inflammation* is usually the result of severe or persistent milk stasis. It is believed that the pressure in the alveoli may cause some to become damaged, with the result that milk seeps into the breast tissues, setting up a non-inflammatory reaction. The signs and symptoms are those of milk stasis, only more severe. *Mastitis* follows the introduction of micro-organisms into the duct systems of the breast.

Infection may be introduced into the duct system of the breasts, or into the breast issue, through cracked nipples, or may be carried in the blood stream in puerperal infection. The majority of women are infected by their own babies, whose skin, umbilical or nasopharyngeal areas harbour colonies of staphylococci or streptococci within a few days of birth. Evidence for this comes from a study in which the incidence of acute mastitis was reduced from 2.5 per cent to 0.2 per cent by applying hexachlorophane, chloroxylenol or chlorhexidine cream over the entire body of the babies at birth, and on alternate days, for 10 days.

The symptoms of acute mastitis rarely appear before the end of the 1st week of the puerperium, and frequently not until the end of the 3rd week. Marked engorgement is followed by hard, red, tender breasts, and associated with chills and elevation of the pulse and temperature. The patient complains of severe pain in the affected breast.

In cases where the diagnosis is in doubt, a milk sample should be taken for leucocyte count and culture. If there are less than $10^6$ leucocytes and $< 10^3$ bacteria per ml of milk, acute mastitis can be excluded.

### Treatment

The three conditions will occur less frequently if breast-feeding is established early and occurs often so that engorgement (due to stagnation of milk in the alveoli) is reduced.

*Milk stasis:* The baby should be breast fed more often, and the breasts emptied manually after each feed. The application of hot and cold towels to the swollen area before feeding is said to help, and the use of a vibrator is claimed to be effective.

*Non-infectious inflammation:* The treatment is that for milk stasis. Analgesics may be needed.

*Mastitis:* Analgesics are required and antibiotics started. The breasts should be emptied regularly. As most infections are due to staphylococci, flucloxacillin is preferred.

If possible, breast-feeding should continue, unless pus is expressed from the nipple. In such cases, which are uncommon, lactation should be suppressed using bromocriptine or oestrogens.

If suppuration occurs, as shown by a clearly defined fluctuant area surrounded by induration, incision and drainage under anaesthesia is necessary. The incision should be made radially to avoid the milk ducts, and locules in the breast should be broken with the fingers. A drainage tube may be required for 48 hours. Infra-red heat often hastens healing of breast abscesses.

### Prophylactic measures

As has been noted, cleansing of the skin of the baby with hexachlorophane cream has reduced the incidence of acute mastitis. Further reduction can be effected by rooming-in of babies and treating the mother and baby as a single unit. Cracked nipples require proper attention. Engorgement, or incomplete emptying of the breasts after feeding, leaves milk stagnant in the duct system. This is an excellent growing medium for introduced bacteria. The breast should therefore be emptied completely after each feed.

### 'ARTIFICIAL FEEDING'

Despite the advantages of breast-feeding, many mothers are currently reluctant to breast-feed. Studies in many developed countries show that by 6 weeks after delivery, less than 30 per cent of women still breast-feed their infant. Whether this is due to changed cultural patterns, to persuasive advertising of formula milks, or to imitation of other mothers, is uncertain, but the fact remains that many women prefer not to breast-feed.

In these circumstances, the medical attendant must have some knowledge of 'formula feeding'. Cow's milk is the ingredient used in 'formula feeding', and this is often modified to make it as much like human milk as possible. Table **16/1** shows the difference between cow's milk and human milk. It can be seen that cow's milk contains more protein (mainly casein) and less sugar. The quantity of casein is important, as this tends to make the curd of cow's milk lumpy and less easily digested. If a formula milk is used, and if bottle-feeding is made as personal and intimate an affair as possible, then artificial feeding as practised today is most satisfactory. To make bottle-feeding simulate breast-feeding as nearly as possible, the baby should be cuddled and fondled during the process, and not fed by having the bottle

| Biochemical substance | Human milk | Cow's milk |
|---|---|---|
| Water per 100ml | 87.1 | 87.3 |
| Total solids g/100ml | | |
| Protein | 0.9 | 3.3 |
| Casein % of total | 20 | 82 |
| Whey % of total | 80 | 18 |
| Fat | 4.5 | 3.7 |
| Milk sugar–lactose | 6.8 | 4.8 |
| Minerals mg/100ml | | |
| Calcium mg | 34 | 125 |
| Phosphorus mg | 14 | 96 |
| Sodium mmol/litre | 7 | 25 |
| Vitamins per 100ml | | |
| vitamin A iu | 190 | 100 |
| vitamin $B_1$ iu | 16 | 44 |
| vitamin $B_2$ iu | 36 | 175 |
| vitamin B iu | 150 | 950 |
| vitamin C mg | 43 | 11 |
| Energy provided kcal/100ml | 75 | 69 |

**Table 16/1** Composition of human milk and cow's milk

stuck into its mouth as it lies in the cot. The proper way to bottle-feed should be taught to the mother whilst she is in hospital, as should the preparation of the milk and its storage.

### Breast-milk substitutes (formula milks)

A variety of breast-milk substitutes are available, and in general any one is as good as any other, provided it has been modified to resemble human milk biochemically. Most modified milks have sugar and vitamins added, whilst evaporated milks generally require the addition of 5 to 10 per cent of carbohydrate. It seems unimportant which carbohydrate is chosen, whether cane sugar, brown sugar, dextrose, lactose, maltose or corn syrup; one being as good as the other, and none having fewer or more side-effects. To a large extent the mother should be given the opportunity to choose the breast-milk substitute she prefers.

### Evaporated milk

If evaporated milk is chosen, a convenient way of keeping the milk sterile is to wash and scald the top of the can. It is then perforated with a scalded beer-can opener, and a plastic cover is placed over the top of the can. The can is then placed in the refrigerator.

| Age of infant (days) | Evaporated milk | Boiled water | Cane sugar |
|---|---|---|---|
| | Quantities per day | | |
| 1 9 | 90ml (3oz) | 540ml (18oz) | 50g (4 level tblsp) |
| 10–20 | 150ml (5oz) | 450ml (15oz) | 25g (2 level tblsp) |
| 21 | 210ml (7oz) | 450ml (15oz) | 25g (2 level tblsp) |

**Table 16/2** Formula feeding using evaporated milk

When milk is required, the appropriate amount of milk is poured into a clean (but not necessarily sterile) feeding-bottle, boiled water is added, together with carbohydrate. The strength of the 'formula-milk' mixture depends on the age of the child (Table **16/2**). The baby is preferably 'demand fed', but may be fed 3 to 4-hourly if desired. At each feed, 120 ml are offered, and the baby takes as much as it wishes. Feeding is not *forced*. The amount per feed is increased if the baby finishes the bottle and is still hungry.

### Dried milk

A bewildering variety of full-cream and half-cream dried milks are available, many of which have been adapted to resemble human milk. If a 'full-cream' milk is chosen, it is generally wise in the first 10 days to give it at half the strength recommended, with an addition of 50g (4 level medicinal tablespoonsful) of cane sugar or milk sugar. Between the 10th and 21st days, the strength is increased to three-quarters of that recommended and 25g (2 tablespoons) of sugar are added. After the 21st day, the infant is given full-strength full-cream milk.

The schedule of feeding and quantity offered at each feed are identical to those described if evaporated milk is used.

### Sweetened condensed milk

Except for certain premature babies, sweetened condensed milk should not be used for formula feeding, as it is deficient in protein and has carbohydrate excess. This leads to poor muscular development, and a fat flabby baby.

## PROBLEMS IN FEEDING

These are discussed in more detail in my book *'Breast Feeding'* (Faber, 1983), but two matters require discussion.

### Underfeeding and overfeeding

It should be remembered that it is very difficult to overfeed a baby, and underfeeding is more likely. An overfed baby becomes irritable, tends to vomit, and to pass loose, green, curdy stools through excoriated buttocks. An underfed baby cries a lot, fails to gain weight, and passes small amounts of dark yellowish stools. If underfeeding is suspected, the baby should be 'test-fed' for 24 hours. It is weighed before and after feeding, the difference indicating the quantity of milk taken. If underfeeding is diagnosed, complementary feeds to make up the amount required (i.e. 230ml per kg per day) should be given.

### 'Burping'

In American and British child care practice, it is considered essential to 'wind' or 'burp' the baby during or after a feed. This is done because it is believed that unless the baby brings up wind he will not settle after the feed and will develop 'colic'. This custom is being questioned, as it has been observed that in most countries burping is never practised, and x-ray investigations have shown that all babies swallow air, but only a few refuse to settle after a feed. In an investigation in Australia, of 110 mothers, 20 per cent believed burping essential, 25 per cent never found it necessary to 'burp' the baby, although several had burped previous babies. The remaining 55 per cent of mothers adopted a modified burping technique when changing the baby from one breast to another (or during a formula feed). They sat the baby upright and talked and played with him for a while. During this period most babies burped, but if no wind came up, the mother continued feeding. The ritual back-slapping or pounding was not used. A few mothers preferred to hold the baby over their shoulder and stroke his back.

## Chapter 17

# The Postnatal Examination

The pregnant uterus takes about 6 weeks to return to its non-pregnant size and weight and during this involutionary period the lochia is diminishing, finally to cease in the 4th or 5th week. Since an objective of antenatal care is to ensure that the mother is healthier at the end of pregnancy than at the beginning, a postnatal examination 6 to 8 weeks after confinement should be offered to all women. The woman and her baby should both be seen (unless she has access to a paediatrician) and the opportunity taken to discuss her adjustment to parenthood, her need for information about child care, her sexual relationships and contraception. In addition the doctor examines the woman physically to make sure that her genital organs have reverted to the non-pregnant state.

The patient should be seen in pleasant surroundings and enquiries should be made regarding the duration and character of the lochia, whether menstruation has returned, if there is a vaginal discharge and whether breast-feeding continues.

The examination takes place next. If the patient had hypertensive disease during pregnancy, or pyelonephritis or bacteriuria, the blood pressure and urine are examined. The abdomen is palpated and a vaginal examination is performed first with a speculum and then bi-manually to determine the size, position and mobility of the uterus. This gynaecological examination may reveal several abnormalities.

## THE VAGINA AND VULVA

Gaping of the vulva, prolapse of the vaginal walls and the quality of healing of the episiotomy wound and the perineal muscle tone are sought. As mentioned earlier, many women complain of discomfort or pain in the area of the episiotomy for weeks, and in over 30 per cent sexual intercourse is painful or impossible for up to 4 months. These matters should be discussed with the woman. If the vagina is lax, exercises can be given which will increase the vaginal tone. In essence these exercises consist of contracting the levator ani muscles, and can be best described as 'trying to draw in the anus to make it touch the chin without using the abdominal muscles'. The exercise should be repeated about 100 times a day, and in addition to strengthening the vaginal muscle and its supports it will reduce, or cure, stress incontinence if this is present. If a vaginal discharge is noticed a swab should be examined and treatment prescribed according to the findings.

## THE CERVIX

This is first inspected with a speculum and a smear is taken for exfoliative cytological examination if this has not been done previously. In many cases persisting ectopic columnar epithelium will be present on the portio. This is called a cervical 'erosion', which is a misnomer as there is no discontinuity of the epithelium: a more correct term is a cervical eversion (or ectropion). Unless this is causing a marked vaginal discharge it should not be treated at this time, as 70 per cent of 'erosions' disappear spontaneously in the next 16 weeks. Provided the cervical exfoliated cells show no abnormality, the cervix should be left untouched and the patient seen again 16 weeks later.

If the eversion persists at this second visit and is associated with an annoying, severe vaginal discharge, it may be cauterized, using either an electric cautery or using cryosurgery. Cryosurgery freezes the area. The refrigerated tip is applied to the cervix for at least 3 minutes, until the 'ice-ball' extends 2mm beyond the edge of the eversion. No anaesthesia is required.

If heat cautery is used, fairly deep linear strokes with the cautery should be made. The strokes start within the cervical canal and extend into the native cervical epithelium, three to four burns being required on each lip. To do this properly either local anaesthesia using 10 per cent cocaine hydrochloride, or a paracervical nerve block, or preferably, intravenous thiopentone anaesthesia is required. The common practice of dabbing the 'erosion' with a blunt cautery at the first postnatal visit is to be condemned as unnecessary interference.

## THE UTERUS

Pelvic examination is made to determine the size, and the position of the uterus. If the uterus is bulky (subinvoluted) and red lochia persists, it may be necessary to prescribe tablets of ergometrine for 3 days. If bleeding continues a curettage may be necessary. The curettage should be examined by a histologist, to exclude the rare malignant trophoblastic tumour, choriocarcinoma. Occasionally the uterus is found to be retroverted. This is of no consequence although some obstetricians antevert the uterus.

### The back

Backache is frequently complained of and is due to a variety of causes, usually muscular. It is aggravated by incorrect posture and much stooping to wash diapers. In recent years the frequency of this complaint is decreasing, perhaps due to better and more widespread antenatal care and greater mobility in the puerperium.

At the end of the physical examination the woman should have the opportunity of talking to the doctor so that she may be able to discuss any problems regarding the care of her infant which have arisen and about her relationship with her partner. The doctor should have discussed, before she left hospital, when she might resume sexual intercourse, but as many doctors fail to do this, the matter should be raised at the postnatal visit. It is important to remind women that pregnancy may occur if contraceptive precautions are not taken. This is discussed in the next section.

Another enquiry is when the first period may be expected. If the patient is not lactating this usually occurs 6 to 10 weeks after confinement and is often heavy. If the patient is lactating, great variations occur and 70 per cent of women do not menstruate until they stop breast-feeding. The other 30 per cent menstruate during lactation. Lactation does not necessarily prevent ovulation and pregnancy is possible during the period of breast-feeding.

# CONTRACEPTIVE ADVICE

An important reason for the postnatal visit is that this is an appropriate time to discuss contraception with the mother. Information about the various methods available should be given so that she can choose which one she thinks is most suitable for her.

Data from several industrialized developed nations indicate that today, the majority of couples seeking family planning advice choose either hormonal contraceptives or the intra-uterine device (the IUD). Increasing numbers of women prefer to use a vaginal diaphragm (together with a spermicidal cream), or their partner chooses to use a condom. Those whose religion does not permit any of these methods choose to use one of the methods of 'periodic abstinence'.

Contraceptive technology is discussed at greater length in *Fundamentals of Obstetrics and Gynaecology, Volume II, Gynaecology*. For these reasons, only a summary of those methods most often chosen will be given in this chapter.

## HORMONAL CONTRACEPTIVES

Hormonal contraceptives have been used since the mid-1950s. Two main forms are available. These are the oral hormonal contraceptives (the Pill) and the injectable hormonal contraceptives.

### The 'Pill'

The combined oral hormonal contraceptive contains two steroids. The first is oestrogen, usually in the form of ethinyl oestradiol, or its 3-methyl ether, mestranol. Following an epidemiological investigation which suggested that the oestrogen content of the Pill was a factor in the development of thrombo-embolism, the majority of oral contraceptives now contain $50\mu g$ of ethinyl oestradiol or less. Oestrogen in this dosage by 'feedback' to the hypothalamus-pituitary usually (but not always) prevents the release of the surge of LH, which is a necessary precursor for ovulation to occur. If only oestrogen is given, the subsequent withdrawal bleed tends to be prolonged, or heavy, and unwanted pregnancies may occur.

These unwanted incidents can be avoided if a progestogen is given as well as oestrogen. When the two hormones are given, the withdrawal bleed occurs at a predictable time and is usually not excessive. Progestogens supplement the contraceptive effect of oestrogen, as they alter the character of the cervical mucus so that it is relatively impenetrable by spermatozoa. The hormone also affects the endometrium so that it becomes 'out of phase', should ovulation occur despite the oestrogen. This prevents the fertilized egg from implanting.

The progestogens in currently available oral contraceptives are: norgestrel, norethisterone, norethisterone acetate and ethynodiol diacetate. Norgestrel is the most potent progestogen, being three times as potent as norethisterone and six times as potent as the other two progestogens. These facts are recognized in the dose of the progestogen in various formulations of the Pill.

The complementary effects of oestrogen and progestogen in the Pill make it a most efficient method of birth control. Provided the Pill is taken daily as directed pregnancy is very unlikely to occur. The number of pregnancies per year amongst women taking the Pill as prescribed is less than 0.05 per cent.

Unfortunately, certain 'side-effects' occur, although it is difficult to determine how many of these are due to the hormones, and how many are induced by anxiety or guilt. The common side-effects attributed to the Pill are listed in Table 17/1.

In the present state of our knowledge, the Pill should not be prescribed to women (1) who have previously developed thrombo-embolism or cerebrovascular insufficiency; (2) have liver disease; (3) have blood dyscrasias; (4) have severe migraine—especially focal migraine; (5) have severe hypertension, unless the woman agrees to regular blood-pressure checks. Apart from such women, the Pill is the method of postpartum birth control chosen by about 75 per cent of women.

### The 'progestogen-only' contraceptive

When the combined oral hormonal contraceptive is contra-indicated, the 'progestogen-only' pill may be prescribed. It is also known as 'the Mini-Pill'. Unfortunately, the progestogen-only pill has a pregnancy rate of about 2.5 per cent in the first year of use, and its use is associated in some 30 per cent of women with irregular, unpredictable bleeds.

### The 'injectables'

Because of the problems believed (by some) to be associated with the need for a woman to take a pill each day, the use of a long-acting, slow-release progestogen, given at 3- or 6-month intervals has been

| Oestrogen effects | Progestogen effects | Combined effects |
|---|---|---|
| Nausea and vomiting | Premenstrual depression | Tiredness |
| Fluid retention (i.e. transient weight gain) | Appetite increase | Irritability |
| | Weight gain | Breast fullness |
| Premenstrual tension | ? Leg cramps | ? Decreased libido |
| Headache | Reduction in menstrual flow | Vaginitis |
| Cervical 'eversion' | | |
| Vaginal discharge | Disturbance in menstrual cycle | |
| Increase in menstrual flow | Acne | |
| Venous thrombosis | Greasy hair | |

**Table 17/1** The side-effects of oral contraceptives

recommended. The pregnancy rate at the end of one year's use is about 1.5 to 2.5 per cent. However, as with the progestogen-only contraceptive, about 30 per cent of women have irregular bleeds, and a similar number develop amenorrhoea. These two side-effects limit the acceptability of the method.

## THE IUD

The intra-uterine device, no matter what its shape, prevents pregnancy by provoking an allergic response in the endometrium, with the infiltration of plasma cells and macrophages. It is believed that these cells render nidation unlikely, although in about 2.5 per cent of women who use the IUD for a year, unwanted pregnancy occurs. The larger the device, the lower is the pregnancy rate, but the higher are the unwanted side-effects of uterine cramps and heavy prolonged menstruation. Two innovations have been made to the IUD. The first is to cover part of the device with fine copper wire. The metal induces a greater allergic response in the endometrium. This permits a smaller device to be used, with no increased unwanted pregnancy rate. The smaller device (such as the Copper 7) is easier to introduce into the uterus. The introduction is made without anaesthesia or analgesia and is almost painless. The second innovation is to make a device of silastic impregnated with a progestogen which is released slowly over the subsequent year or so (a vaginal ring is also available). The older IUDs could remain in the uterus for long periods, but the newer ones require to be replaced at shorter intervals because the copper ionizes and the progestogen diffuses.

The IUD is contra-indicated in cases of pelvic infection, and if the shape of the uterine cavity is distorted by myomata.

## MECHANICAL BARRIERS—THE CONDOM AND THE VAGINAL DIAPHRAGM

Despite the advantages of the Pill and the IUD, many couples choose to use condoms or vaginal diaphragms for family planning. Modern condoms are siliconed so that they are easy to draw on to the erect penis. They are bought in individual sealed packets so that they have a long shelf-life. Used properly, condoms are associated with an unwanted pregnancy rate of less than 2 per cent if used for a year. Vaginal diaphragms, used with a spermicidal cream, have a similar pregnancy rate. Both are without unwanted side-effects, and usually are not noticeable to the sexual partner. However, many couples consider them unaesthetic.

## PERIODIC ABSTINENCE
(natural family planning)

Couples whose beliefs prevent the use of contraceptives avoid pregnancy by practising sexual abstinence, or by making use of one of the methods of determining the 'safe period', that is the time in the menstrual cycle which is at least 3 days before or after ovulation. Using one or other method of calculating the 'safe period', a pregnancy rate of about 20 per cent over a 12-month period is reported, except amongst highly motivated couples who have infrequent sexual intercourse, and consequently a lower chance of an unwanted pregnancy.

A woman who breast feeds at least five times every 24 hours, the baby suckling for at least 10 minutes, is effectively using breast-feeding as a contraceptive, as pregnancy is unlikely to occur. However, as an additional precaution breast-feeding women may be prescribed the progestogen-only contraceptive. This will not reduce the quantity of milk secreted.

## PERMANENT BIRTH CONTROL METHODS

The contraceptive methods listed so far permit the couple to space their children. However, many couples desire a permanent method of birth control, when they have had the number of children they wish. In recent years increasing numbers of men choose to have a vasectomy performed, and more women choose to have a tubectomy (tubal ligation) performed.

Evidence is now appearing which shows that women who have a tubal ligation performed immediately after childbirth are less satisfied with the operation than women who have it some time later. This fact should be recognized, and postpartum tubal ligation avoided in the early puerperium unless it is established that the woman is completely certain that she wants a permanent method of birth control.

*Chapter 18*

# Pain Relief in Labour

The pain associated with labour varies very considerably. A few women have relatively painless labours; most women have moderate pain which is usually forgotten in the joy of holding the newborn baby, and to a few women labour is a prolonged and painful ordeal remembered with horror. Apart from her desire for a healthy infant, adequate relief from the pain of labour is the next most important desire of all labouring women, and every doctor practising obstetrics must have a wide knowledge of the various drugs and techniques that may be used to achieve safe and effective pain relief.

While a good doctor will never give powerful drugs unnecessarily, it is not good obstetrics to allow a labouring woman to suffer when adequate relief is available. One of the problems facing obstetricians is the difficulty of adequately assessing the severity of the patient's pain. A woman who is silently suffering may be having much more pain than a noisy woman in the next room, but often the silent one is overlooked and gets inadequate relief. A survey of postnatal patients in Sydney revealed that more than 20 per cent were seriously disappointed by the lack of effective pain relief.

A patient who has knowledge of the physiological events of labour, who has received antenatal instruction and who has confidence in her medical attendants, will approach labour well adjusted psychologically and willing to co-operate in the process of birth. The mental preparation for labour will help her to put up with discomfort and may, in some women, result in a reduction of the drugs required. This prenatal preparation must be complemented by enthusiastic encouragement by all medical and nursing staff during labour, because a patient quickly senses any attitude of indifference and becomes disheartened. The psychoprophylactic method of 'prepared childbirth' is discussed on page 68.

The ideal obstetric analgesic or anaesthetic should

(1) do no harm to the mother or her baby; (2) not prevent the patient's co-operation, particularly in the second stage of labour; (3) not alter uterine activity, and so prolong labour or predispose to postpartum haemorrhage.

## SEDATION IN EARLY LABOUR

In early labour the uterine contractions are not particularly painful and analgesia is usually not required. However, some women are apprehensive, and their fear may be suppressed by prescribing tranquillizers, provided that the woman requests medication.

The currently preferred tranquillizers in labour are promazine, diazepam or lorazepam. The latter two drugs reduce the need for pethidine, when this is required. However, diazepam crosses the placenta readily and accumulates in the fetus leading, occasionally, in the newborn baby to hypotonia, difficulty in temperature regulation and respiratory depression. Lorazepam, which has a shorter half-life (12 hours) and is metabolized to an inactive glucuronide, is to be preferred, if one of these tranquillizers is chosen.

## ANALGESIA AND ANAESTHESIA IN THE FIRST STAGE OF LABOUR

Because of the widely different cultural and psychological attitudes to labour, and to the perception of pain by different women, there is no single way of relieving pain in labour. Three main approaches are possible, and each should have been discussed with the patient during pregnancy so that she may know what is available and make an initial choice of the approach she hopes will suit her. The first approach is the use of the psychoprophylactic method. The second is the use of intermittent injections of pethidine, or some other injected analgesic in early established labour, with intermittent inhalational analgesia in the late first stage and the second stage. The third approach is to start an epidural nerve block once active labour is established and to give supplemental injections to maintain analgesia until delivery has occurred. Often a combination of one or more methods may be chosen. For example, pethidine injections are given in early labour, and later an epidural nerve block is established; or a patient uses psychoprophylaxis but requests supplementary inhalational analgesia in the late first stage of labour.

Again it must be stressed that analgesic medication should not be given routinely. It should be offered to the woman and its benefits (and disadvantages) discussed with her, so that she may make an informed choice, whether or not to accept the offer.

## Analgesics given by injection

### PETHIDINE

Pethidine is a synthetic analgesic drug which depresses the respiratory centre to some extent, the degree being similar to that produced by morphine. Pethidine can be given intramuscularly or intravenously. If the latter route is chosen the dose should be well diluted with normal saline and given slowly, or vomiting and respiratory depression may occur. After intramuscular injection, pethidine takes effect in 20 minutes and the duration of the effect varies from 2 to 3 hours. The initial dose should be 100 to 150mg and the drug can be repeated as needed during the first stage. An average woman will require no more than 300mg. The analgesic effect of pethidine is increased if lorazepam (2mg) has been given orally at the onset of established labour. Since pethidine produces some degree of respiratory centre depression in the infant, an antagonist may be required if the drug has been given to the mother late in labour. The antagonist, naloxone, 0.01mg/kg body-weight is given to the baby by intramuscular injection, or, if he is severely depressed, half the dose is given intravenously and half intramuscularly. All premature babies should receive the injection as soon as possible after birth; mature babies, who are depressed at birth and who after normal resuscitation measures have a 1-minute Apgar score of less than 5, should be given the injection at 1 minute.

### MEPTAZINOL

Meptazinol may be used in place of pethidine in similar doses. Meptazinol is as effective an analgesic as pethidine but depresses the neonate less, and produces less fetal acidosis than pethidine.

## Inhalational analgesia—self-administration

The contractions of the late first stage and those of the second stage can be painful and many patients require further analgesia. Unless an anaesthetist is available to administer inhalational anaesthesia or epidural anaesthesia, self-administration of gases can be very helpful. One problem of the method is that unless the level of the inhaled drug reaches analgesic levels quickly its effects are minimized. This implies that intelligent supervision and attention to the timing of the inhalation are of great importance. If the supervision is negligent, satisfactory pain relief is unlikely. Currently two inhalational analgesics are used. These are trichloroethylene and nitrous oxide–oxygen.

### TRICHLOROETHYLENE

Trichloroethylene (Trilene) is a cheap, transparent, volatile liquid with a sweet smell. In concentrations of less than 0.6 per cent the vapour is safe, fairly effective and non-irritant to the skin. Trichloroethylene should only be administered in special apparatus (Emotril or Tecota Mark 6), which have control devices to ensure that the concentration of the inhaled vapour remains constant. The patient is instructed to breathe the gas in deeply during the incremental and peak phases of a contraction, and to discard the mask between contractions. Inhalations should not be continued for more than four hours as 50 per cent of inhaled trichloroethylene is not exhaled but is degraded in the liver to a number of products which themselves have a minor depressant action. The products are readily soluble so that they accumulate progressively and may cause a sleepy mother and baby.

A recent suggestion is that trichloroethylene may be replaced by another inhalational analgesic drug, methoxyflurane, which is probably a more effective agent.

### NITROUS OXIDE AND OXYGEN

Mixtures of nitrous oxide in air produce reasonable levels of analgesia, but the oxygen level is unacceptably low. For this reason, a machine which delivers nitrous oxide (up to 70 per cent) and oxygen (30 to 100 per cent) intermittently is preferred. The patient inhales the mixture during a contraction and discards the mask between contractions.

No adequate comparative studies of effectiveness between trichloroethylene inhalers and nitrous oxide–oxygen machines have been made and such evidence as there is indicates that neither is better than the other and that both are of value in obtaining relief in the late first and second stages of labour. The advantage of the trichloroethylene apparatus is that it is light and foolproof; the gas–oxygen machine is cumbersome and care must be taken that the cylinders (particularly the oxygen cylinder) are not empty.

**Epidural anaesthesia**

The introduction of an anaesthetic agent into the peridural space in the lumbar region will cause blockage of most nerve impulses up to the tenth dorsal segment if an appropriate dose is used. Since the sensory fibres from the uterus reach the spinal cord either in the sacral segments or via the nerves reaching the cord at T11 or T12, the elimination of the pain of labour will be obtained. Whether the approach to the space is made via the sacral hiatus (caudal block) or at the second lumbar interspace (epidural block) is of secondary importance (Fig. **18/1**).

In recent years increasing numbers of anaesthetists have received training in performing epidural puncture, and this form of analgesia is being offered to increasing numbers of women in labour. The block should not be started until labour is established and the cervix at least 3cm dilated, and the patient should labour at a tilt of 15°, preferably lying on her side. In Sydney hospitals, between 40 and 60 per cent of all women receive an epidural nerve block when in established labour. The use of epidural nerve block is associated with some side-effects, of which the most serious are transient hypotension and respiratory paralysis due to inadvertent subarachnoid injection. The chance of severe hypotension is minimized if the woman has an intravenous infusion of 500ml normal saline before the anaesthetic is injected. Epidural anaesthesia fails to relieve the pain completely in 10 per cent of patients. One woman in five complains that the epidural is associated with 'shivers and shakes' or with nausea.

Because of the reduced uterine activity and the difficulty some women have in correlating their expulsive efforts with the painless uterine contractions, the length of the second stage of labour is increased, and the frequency of forceps deliveries rises. Low forceps deliveries increase up to 10-fold, and midforceps (following rotation of the fetal head) is required six times as frequently as amongst women who do not have epidural analgesia.

In spite of these problems most patients are satisfied with the relatively or completely painless labour.

The need for a skilled anaesthetist to establish the block, the need to monitor the patient's response and the increased frequency of forceps delivery, limits the use of epidural analgesia to properly equipped hospitals.

**Paracervical nerve block**

In areas where it is impossible to offer epidural analgesia, labour may be made less painful by supplementing pethidine injections with paracervical nerve block. The method is based on the physiological finding that direct infiltration of the paracervical area will anaesthetize the great cervical plexus (Frankenhauser's plexus) and will consequently eliminate the pain of cervical dilatation, although the pain of uterine contractions may still be felt and the discomfort due to perineal stretching is not affected. This limits the use of the method, although it may be supplemented by pudendal nerve block or perineal infiltration. The injection can be given when the cervix is 5cm or more dilated and the fetal head engaged. As the anaesthesia lasts only about 3 hours it has to be repeated. A special guide is used through

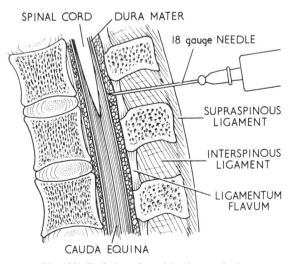

SPINAL CORD    DURA MATER

18 gauge NEEDLE

SUPRASPINOUS LIGAMENT

INTERSPINOUS LIGAMENT

LIGAMENTUM FLAVUM

CAUDA EQUINA

**Fig. 18/1** Technique for epidural anaesthesia

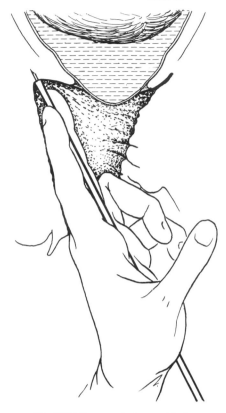

**Fig. 18/2** Paracervical nerve block

which the needle projects a distance of 7mm. The guide, with the needle withdrawn, is placed against the paracervical tissues in the lateral vaginal fornix at between 8 and 9 o'clock on the right and 3 and 4 o'clock on the left, and the needle advanced as far as it will go. Five to 10ml of 0.25 per cent bupivacaine is injected on each side (Fig. **18/2**).

The disadvantages of the method are its limited area of anaesthesia and its short duration of action. It is most useful in the multigravida whose labour is advancing rapidly. Since 15 per cent of infants develop bradycardia, which correlates with the level of the anaesthetic in the fetal circulation, the method should not be used to produce analgesia if placental dysfunction is present or the baby is at 'high risk'.

## ANALGESIA IN THE SECOND STAGE OF LABOUR

In the second stage of labour, various choices for pain relief may be offered to the patient. If effective analgesia has been obtained in the first stage of labour by psychoprophylactic methods or by pethidine injections, all that may be needed are inhalations of $N_2O/O_2$ mixture when uterine contractions occur, or the establishment of a pudendal or perineal nerve block so that the pain associated with the actual birth of the fetal head is eliminated. Of course, if an epidural nerve block has been set up in the first stage of labour its use should be continued, or, if not, it may be started in the second stage of labour.

### Pudendal and perineal nerve blocks

#### NERVES OF THE FEMALE VULVA

The female vulva is innervated mainly by branches of the pudendal nerve. The pudendal nerve, derived from S2, S3 and S4 leaves the pelvis medial to the sciatic nerve through the greater sciatic foramen. It then crosses the external surface of the ischial spine and re-enters the pelvis through the lesser sciatic notch and, passing along the lateral wall of the ischio-rectal fossa, divides into branches which supply most of the perineum (Fig. **18/3**). Further sensory branches to the skin of the perineum are derived from the ilio-inguinal nerve, the pudendal branch of the posterior femoral cutaneous nerve and the genital branch of the genito-femoral nerve (Fig. **18/4**).

#### PERINEAL INFILTRATION

Using a 7.5cm, 22 gauge needle, and 20ml of 0.5 to 1 per cent lignocaine, the perineum is infiltrated in a fan-like manner, the base being the posterior fourchette at the midline. Three lines of infiltration are required, one medially as far as the anal sphincter and midway between the skin and the vaginal mucosa, and two others at 45° to block the nerves as they reach the perineum (Fig. **18/4**). Perineal infiltration enables the delivery to be made with little discomfort, permits the making and repair of episiotomy wounds and, if Trilene inhalations are used in addition, permits outlet forceps to be performed relatively painlessly. The analgesia is effective in about 3 minutes and lasts between 45 and 90 minutes. It should be tested by pricking the skin with a sharp needle before any procedure is begun.

#### PUDENDAL NERVE BLOCK

A 10cm, 20 gauge needle and, if available, a needle director are required. Two fingers are introduced

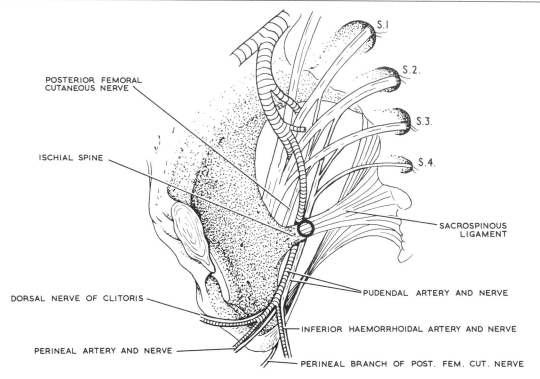

**Fig. 18/3** The course of the pudendal nerve. The area in the circle which lies just medial to and below the tip of the ischial spine is the area into which the local anaesthetic is infiltrated

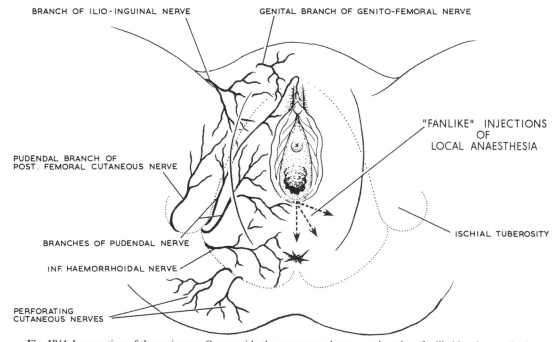

**Fig. 18/4** Innervation of the perineum. On one side the nerves are shown, on the other 'fanlike' local anaesthesia

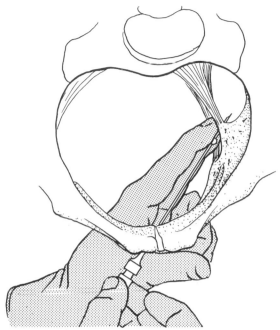

**Fig. 18/5** Transvaginal pudendal nerve block shown diagrammatically (from Klink, E. W. *Obstet. and Gynecol.* 1953, **1**, 137)

into the vagina and palpate the ischial spine, the guide containing the needle is introduced in the groove between the index and middle finger to impinge on the spine. It is then directed to lie just medial to, and below, the ischial spine and the needle is advanced 1cm beyond the guide (if no guide is available the needle is introduced between the fingers to the same site) and pushed through the sacrospinous ligament (Fig. **18/5**); 10ml of 0.5 per cent lignocaine is injected behind each ischial spine, and a further 10ml is used to make a perineal infiltration. Anaesthesia should be effective within 5 minutes when it should be tested. The lower vagina and perineum becomes insensitive to pain. The use of pudendal nerve block is not without problems. The needle may be difficult to introduce accurately in a relatively mobile patient, particularly when the fetal head is deeply engaged.

## ANALGESIA IN DYSTOCIC LABOUR

When the normal triple descending gradient of uterine activity does not occur, but is replaced by reversed gradients, or by inco-ordinate uterine action, labour can become extremely painful and distressing to the patient. In this situation an epidural nerve block will relieve the pain, but in many cases a skilled anaesthetist is unavailable and the method cannot be used.

An alternative is to use a *pethidine infusion*. The method is simple and can be set up and supervised by the nursing staff. An intravenous infusion containing 400 to 600mg pethidine and 50mg of promazine in 1000ml of 5 per cent dextrose is started. Initially the infusion is run rapidly to obtain good analgesia and sedation, and once the patient is sleeping (usually after 100 to 150ml) the rate is adjusted by the attending medical staff to maintain the analgesia.

## ANAESTHESIA FOR MID-FORCEPS OPERATIONS

The degree of anaesthesia obtained by pudendal nerve block is adequate for most low forceps and a few mid-forceps deliveries. But it is insufficient for almost all forceps rotations and all manual rotations of the head arrested in the transverse diameter of the mid-pelvis, and epidural anaesthesia should be established.

If expert anaesthetic care is unavailable local anaesthesia can be supplemented by intravenous anaesthesia in these cases or other methods described in the next section can be used. The supplementation is to give an intravenous injection of pethidine 100mg and promazine 25mg. (More correctly, pethidine 2mg, and promazine 0.4mg per kg body-weight.) The drugs are mixed with 20ml of normal saline and injected slowly over a period of 3 minutes. About 10 minutes after the injection the patient will be asleep and although she stirs during manipulations, does not resist or remember them. After a pudendal nerve block has been introduced, Kielland's forceps rotation or manual rotation of the head can be performed. The patient sleeps for 1 to 2 hours after delivery.

The method may be associated with marked (although transient) hypotension especially if the patient is dehydrated. It should only be used if an anaesthetist is not available and after the patient has been properly rehydrated which may require 20ml/kg normal saline or Hartmann's solution. If an anaesthetist is available he may choose to establish an epidural nerve block or a spinal nerve block or to give a general inhalational anaesthetic. These are discussed in the next section.

## ANAESTHESIA FOR DIFFICULT OPERATIVE DELIVERIES

### Epidural anaesthesia

Because of the side-effects of subarachnoid (spinal) anaesthesia it has been replaced by epidural anaesthesia for caesarean sections and mid-forceps deliveries. Epidural anaesthesia is being used increasingly for difficult operative deliveries. Caesarean section under epidural anaesthesia is associated with less postoperative pain, pyrexia, gastro-intestinal stress and coughing than general inhalational anaesthesia. A further benefit of epidural anaesthesia is that the mother can see (and cuddle) her baby immediately after birth, which may be important for maternal–infant bonding.

### General anaesthesia

The alternative is to use general anaesthesia, the main hazard of which is that vomiting may occur during induction of anaesthesia. The regurgitated vomit and acid stomach juices may be inhaled causing immediate obstruction and asphyxia, or a chemical pneumonitis which may be fatal. Every year obstetric patients are killed in this way. These deaths are preventable, provided that the anaesthetic is given by a trained anaesthetist. In some hospitals vomiting is induced by giving an injection of apomorphine prior to administration of the anaesthetic, or by giving intravenous cimetidine or by emptying the stomach using a nasogastric tube.

The aim in using general anaesthesia is to induce anaesthesia rapidly without the patient vomiting, and since all the agents traverse the placenta, to use as small an amount as is compatible with effectiveness, safety and satisfactory operating conditions.

When a trained anaesthetist is available several techniques are used but most are variants of the following method. After premedication with atropine 0.6mg, anaesthesia is induced with thiopentone 100 to 250mg, given as 4 to 10ml of a 2.5 per cent solution. A rapidly acting muscle relaxant, such as succinylcholine is given in a dose of 50 to 100mg to enable a cuffed endotracheal tube to be passed. The intubation is preceded by inflation of the lungs with pure oxygen with the patient flat and supine. A properly instructed assistant applies pressure backwards on the patient's cricoid cartilage with a finger and thumb as soon as she is unconscious. This will compress the oesophagus and prevent any passive regurgitation of gastric contents. This cricoid pressure should always be employed at the induction of anaesthesia when the stomach is not known to be empty and it must be maintained until the endotracheal tube is in place and the cuff inflated. Anaesthesia is maintained using $N_2O$ and $O_2$. Halothane is contra-indicated as it induces myometrial relaxation and possible postpartum haemorrhage, whilst cyclopropane has a depressant action on the fetus if given to the mother before it is delivered.

## SELECTION OF ANAESTHESIA AND ANALGESIA

Different obstetric situations require the use of different agents or combinations of agents. In Table **18/1** a suggested scheme is laid out. In each section the method of choice is listed first.

1. *Dystocia* – especially minor disproportion and inco-ordinate uterine action
   Epidural nerve block
   Pethidine and phenothiazine infusion
   Paracervical nerve block

2. *Intra-uterine manipulations*
   General anaesthesia

3. *Mid-forceps delivery*
   Epidural anaesthesia
   Pudendal nerve block, supplemented by intravenous pethidine 100mg and chlorpromazine 25mg diluted in 10ml of normal saline, and injected slowly
   General anaesthesia

4. *Low forceps delivery, episiotomy repair*
   Perineal infiltration
   Pudendal nerve block

5. *Breech delivery*
   (a) Assisted: Pudendal nerve block supplemented by intravenous thiopentone with birth of fetal abdomen; or epidural anaesthesia
   (b) Extraction: General anaesthesia using $N_2O/O_2$

6. *Caesarean section*
   Epidural anaesthesia (supplemented by a light general anaesthetic)
   General inhalational anaesthesia

   **Table 18/1** Anaesthesia and analgesia in obstetrics

## DANGERS OF ANAESTHESIA IN OBSTETRICS

### Local anaesthesia

If an excessive dose of a local anaesthetic agent is given or if the drug is injected intravenously in error, toxic manifestations may occur. The maximum single injection of lignocaine is 20ml of a 1 per cent solution although in special circumstances this may be exceeded. The toxic manifestations initially are drowsiness and cerebral depression or mental confusion. These may be followed by muscular twitching and convulsions, with cardiac and respiratory failure as terminal events. Treatment is to maintain high oxygenation, and if convulsions occur to control them with intravenous suxamethonium or thiopentone, and ventilate the patient's lungs with oxygen.

### Epidural anaesthesia

As a few patients develop hypotension after epidural anaesthesia, a prophylactic intravenous infusion should be set up and about 500ml infused before starting the procedure. The episode is usually brief, and responds to positioning the patient on her side and to elevating the foot of the bed. If these measures fail to restore the blood pressure to normal the drip is turned up and a rapid infusion of 200 to 1500ml of Hartmann's solution given. A few patients complain of backache, and rarely post-spinal headache occurs if the dura is inadvertently punctured.

### General anaesthesia

Apart from overdosage, which should never occur if the anaesthetic is given by trained staff, the great hazard of general anaesthetic agents in obstetrics is inhalation of regurgitated vomit. Statistics in Australia between 1964 and 1975 indicate that one woman in every 100 000 delivered dies from this cause and the condition accounts for 2 per cent of all maternal deaths.

Two types of accident can occur: (1) the obstructive type due to blockage of the main bronchus by solid food particles; and (2) the pneumonitic type due to aspiration of acid stomach contents into the small bronchioles which causes a marked allergic bronchiolar spasm.

Aspiration of solid vomitus causes immediate signs of anoxia, whilst the onset of symptoms from inhalation of acid stomach contents may be immediate or delayed for some hours. The patient becomes acutely ill with respiratory distress, bronchospasm, cyanosis, tachycardia and pulmonary oedema. The syndrome only occurs if the pH of the aspirate is 2.5 or less.

As soon as vomiting is recognized the patient should be placed head down and the mouth and pharynx aspirated with a sucker. Oxygen is given and intermittent positive pressure ventilation may be necessary. If it is thought that solid food particles have been inhaled, a bronchoscope is passed and suction of the bronchial tree carried out, but the procedure is not without hazard, particularly in the anoxic patient. Hydrocortisone 1g intravenously and a wide spectrum antibiotic are administered in an attempt to combat shock and prevent infection. Recent studies show that effects of aspirating acid stomach contents into the lungs (Mendelson's syndrome) may be prevented by giving an intravenous injection of 50mg ranitidine before inducing general anaesthesia.

# Chapter 19

# Medical Imaging in Obstetrics

Following the radiological investigations of pelvic architecture by Caldwell and Molloy and Thoms in the 1930s, routine radiological pelvimetry came to be considered an essential investigation, the omission of which rendered the obstetrician liable to a charge of neglect or malpractice. In the post-war years the dangers of indiscriminate radiation have become increasingly obvious, with the result that radiological investigations in pregnancy are now used less frequently and with much greater discrimination. This has occurred particularly with the introduction of ultrasound as a diagnostic tool.

A major reason why radiological investigations have diminished in frequency is the awareness of the possible dangers of radiation to the embryo and fetus. Most mammalian cells, including those of man, are susceptible to radiation damage and possible genetic mutation, particularly at a time of rapid frequent mitosis. In the human embryo organogenesis occurs most rapidly during the 1st to 10th week of the gestation interval and continues in lesser degree until delivery. It follows that no period of intra-uterine life is free from radiation hazard, but this is most marked in the first 6 to 8 weeks after fertilization. For this reason no female who might be pregnant should undergo any pelvic radiological investigation in the second half of the menstrual cycle, or during pregnancy, unless there is a good reason. Gene mutation is cumulative and related to dosage in a linear fashion, so that care should be taken at all times before recommending radiological investigations and this applies particularly in pregnancy when two individuals are at risk.

The development of highly efficient, relatively cheap ultrasound machines, has meant that to a large extent radiology has been replaced in obstetric practice by ultrasound (Table **19/1**). The potential dangers of radiation are eliminated, and ultrasound (in the amounts used) has no dangers to the fetus.

*Weeks*

| | |
|---|---|
| 0–10 | Detection of pregnancy, blighted ovum or empty sac |
| | ? Detection of ectopic gestation |
| 11–20 | Estimation of fetal maturity |
| | Detection of multiple pregnancy |
| | Detection of some neural tube defects (NTD) |
| | Diagnosis of fetal death |
| 21–30 | Detection or diagnosis of multiple pregnancy, fetal defects and fetal death |
| 31–40 | Placental localization |
| | Detection of possible fetal growth retardation |
| | Diagnosis of multiple pregnancy |
| | Detection of retroplacental clots |
| | Diagnosis of fetal death in utero |

**Table 19/1** Indications for ultrasound imaging in pregnancy

The principle underlying ultrasound is that sound waves are reflected from the interfaces between different tissues. The amount of reflected energy varies directly with the differences in acoustic impedances of tissues that lie close to each other.

The sound is generated by a crystal enclosed in a probe, and the sound is emitted at 1.5 to 10 megaHertz (MHz). It is usually pulsed at 600 pulses a second. Because air bubbles between the probe and the skin can reflect sound, the probe and the skin are kept in contact by a thin film of oil, or a waterbag, so that acoustic coupling is obtained. If a machine using a water-bag is chosen the woman lies prone upon the water-bag. The probe is moved either longitudinally from the xiphisternum to the symphysis or transversely from one flank to the other. The reflected sounds are visualized as echoes on a long persistence cathode ray display tube and can be photographed.

Four forms of ultrasonic scanning are used in obstetrics. The first and oldest method is for a sound

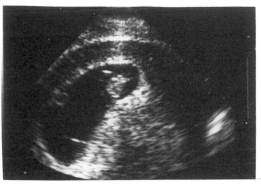

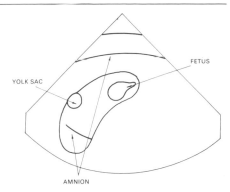

Fig. 19/1 Ultrasound scan showing yolk sasck and amnion

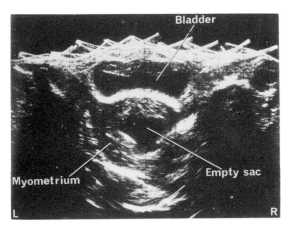

Fig. 19/2 The echogram shows an empty amniotic sac at 11 weeks' gestation. The patient aborted one week later

to be emitted which is reflected and returned to the oscilloscope as an echo. The echo is recorded as a spike, the amplitude of which represents the strength of the echo, and its position on the display the depth of the interface. This is the amplitude mode (*A-scan or A-mode*).

The second method is the bi-dimensional (brightness) mode (*B-scan or B-mode*). In this technique the strength and position of the echoes determines the position of dots on the display. Using a scanning arm and a storage technique, tissues or organs appear as a series of dots which together form a picture (in much the same way as a newspaper picture). In the display, the shapes of reflecting surfaces are recorded as white (echoes) on a black background (no echoes).

More recently, it has become possible to record the strength of the echoes as shades of grey (stronger echoes appearing as brighter dots) using a develop-

ment of television technology. *Grey-scale ultrasound* enables the observer to evaluate the shape, location and the acoustic texture of tissues, which makes the interpretation more precise.

The fourth method is to produce moving images of fetal structures as they are actually occurring using a complex technology. This is *real-time scanning* as the movements of the fetal heart or its body are seen as they occur. The apparatus is compact and can be used for many examinations which are currently done by a B-scan or a grey-scale apparatus.

## ULTRASOUND IN EARLY PREGNANCY

Echoes from the fetus and conception sac can be identified as early as the 6th week of pregnancy, and in cases of threatened or incomplete abortion, the presence of a blighted ovum or an empty sac may be detected (Figs **19/1** and **19/2**). With real-time scanning, the pulsations of the fetal heart can be detected and fetal life established from about the 7th week of pregnancy. With combined A-mode and B-mode techniques fetal life can be detected as early as the 6th week of pregnancy (Figs **19/3** and **19/4**).

Ultrasound is helpful in establishing the presence, or absence, of a benign trophoblastic tumour – a hydatidiform mole. The numerous small hydropic villi create a 'honeycomb' of echoes, which only appear at a high sensitivity, and of course no fetal echoes are seen (Fig. **19/5**). Ultrasound enables the obstetrician to establish the presence of, or exclude, hydatidiform mole, earlier and with greater accuracy than any other method (see Chapter 34).

In the second quarter of pregnancy, ultrasound is

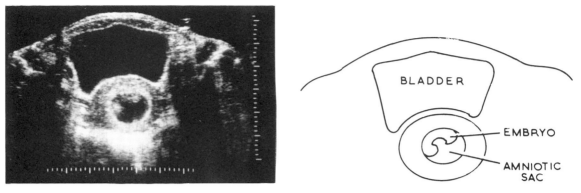

**Fig. 19/3** Early intra-uterine pregnancy (9 weeks) (transverse scan). Line drawing shows identification of relevant points

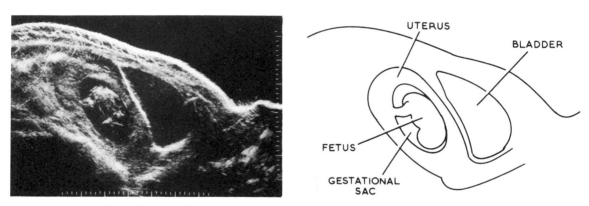

**Fig. 19/4** Twelve-week fetus (sagittal scan). Line drawing shows identification of relevant points

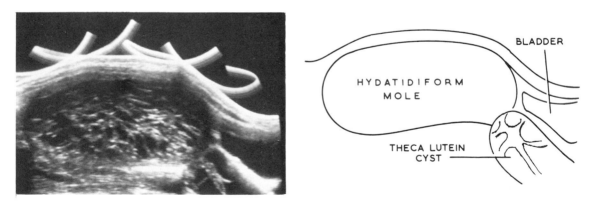

**Fig. 19/5** Benign trophoblastic disease (hydatidiform mole), 24 weeks' gestation. The honeycomb appearance is found using grey-scale ultrasound. Line drawing shows identification of relevant points

used, prior to diagnostic amniocentesis, to determine the position of the placenta, so that this can be avoided by the needle.

Ultrasound, using the grey-scale method, is helpful in examining the fetus for neural tube defects if amniocentesis shows a raised amniotic alphafeto-protein level.

Between the 10th and 13th week measurement of

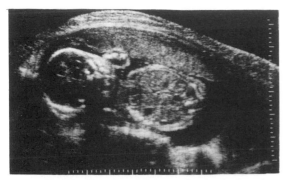

**Fig. 19/6** Breech at 24 weeks' gestation (sagittal scan)

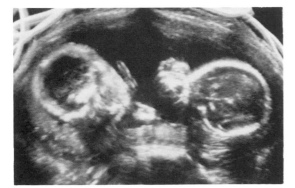

**Fig. 19/7** Twin pregnancy, 26½-weeks' gestation (transverse scan)

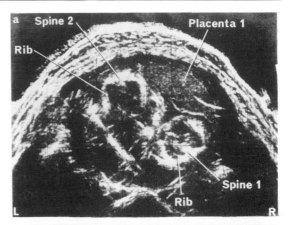

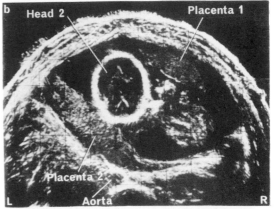

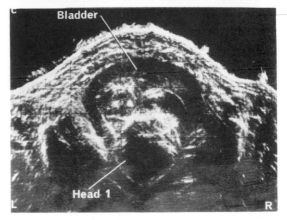

**Fig. 19/8** Three echograms showing a multiple pregnancy (transverse sections at different levels)

the crown–rump length of the fetus is accurate in determining gestational age to within 4 days in 95 per cent of cases. After the 13th week varying flexion of the fetal trunk makes the measurement less reliable, but the measurement of the biparietal diameter between the 16th and 20th week predicts the estimated date of delivery to within 10 days in 90 per cent of cases. Ultrasound at this time will also detect a multiple pregnancy and some fetal abnormalities.

## ULTRASOUND IN LATE PREGNANCY

In the last quarter of pregnancy, ultrasound is used to diagnose abnormal fetal presentations (Figs **19/6–19/19**), to confirm the presence or absence of a multiple pregnancy, and to detect gross fetal abnormalities not detected earlier. Ultrasound is also useful in determining the position of the placenta and in identifying its margins in relation to the cervix, whether it is situated on the anterior or posterior wall of the uterus, and its thickness (Fig. **19/13**).

It may be that transvaginal ultrasound will prove more accurate than current transabdominal technique. Ultrasound has value in cases of abruptio placentae in determining the position and volume of the retroplacental clot.

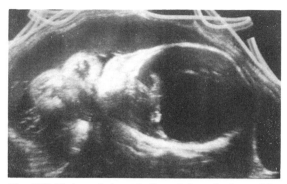

**Fig. 19/9** Hydrocephaly with distended cerebral ventricles and disturbances of the midline structures. The placenta is anterior (transverse scan)

Ultrasound may be used to help determine the rate of fetal growth and to diagnose fetal growth retardation. Between the 20th and 30th week the fetal skull grows at about 2.8mm per week (with a small standard deviation), and from 31 to 40 weeks it grows at about 1.5mm per week (but with a wider standard deviation). As mentioned earlier, measurement of the fetal biparietal diameter between the 12th and 22nd week in patients whose period of gestation is uncertain can give an accurate estimate ( ± 7 days) of fetal maturity.

In the last quarter of pregnancy, fetal maturity and fetal growth retardation (FGR) are more difficult to determine. The most exact method is to measure

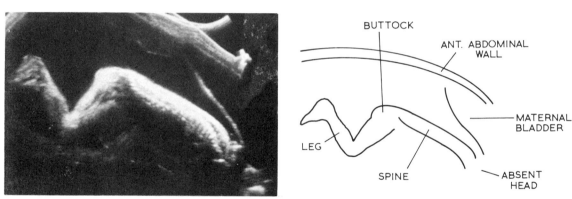

**Fig. 19/10**  Ultrasound scan showing an anencephalic fetus. Line drawing indicates relevant landmarks

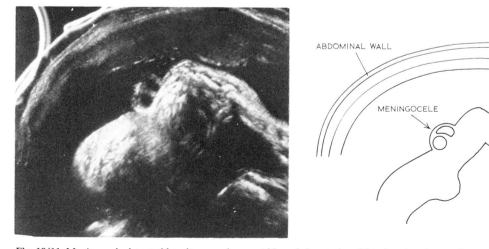

**Fig. 19/11** Meningocele detected by ultrasound scan at 30 weeks' gestation. Line drawing shows relevant landmarks

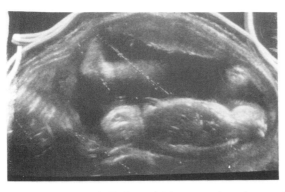
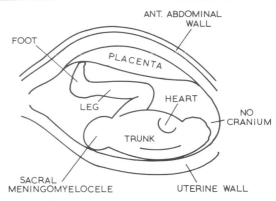

**Fig. 19/12** Anencephalic fetus with large sacral meningomyelocele detected by ultrasound scan. Line drawing shows relevant landmarks

the biparietal diameter (Fig. **19/14**), the abdominal circumference and the length of the femur. These measurements are related to nomograms; however an error of + or − 7–10 days must be accepted. A number of obstetricians routinely screen pregnant women at 32 weeks' gestation for the presence of fetal growth retardation. If FGR is found, a further ultrasonic examination is made at 34 or 36 weeks' gestation.

## RADIOLOGY IN OBSTETRICS

As has been mentioned, with the development of more sophisticated ultrasound machines and their increasing availability, the place of radiology in obstetric care had diminished. However, in certain countries, radiology may be the only available method to confirm the presentation of the fetus (Figs **19/16–19/18**) or to establish that the patient has a multiple pregnancy (Fig. **19/19**). Radiology

should not be used to diagnose pregnancy, as immunological tests and ultrasound are less hazardous and more accurate. Nor should radiology be used to determine fetal maturity as it is neither accurate nor safe. If ultrasound is not available and the obstetrician suspects that a fetal abnormality such as anencephaly (Fig. **19/20**) or hydrocephaly (Fig. **19/21**) is present, radiology will confirm or deny the diagnosis. In the past radiology was used to confirm the diagnosis of fetal death in utero (p. 190), but this investigation is rarely needed today with the development of real-time ultrasound.

Radiology has retained its place for determining the size of the bony pelvis and in the investigation of suspected cephalopelvic disproportion. The procedure is called radiological pelvimetry. This term is unfortunate because the information obtained concerns not only the pelvic measurements but delineates the architecture of the bony pelvis and the size of the fetal head or breech.

Radiological pelvimetry has severe limitations as

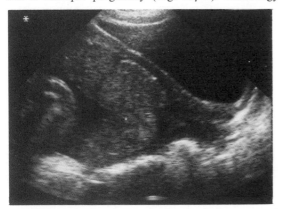
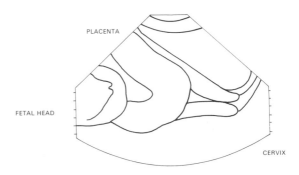

**Fig. 19/13** Sagittal section, major degree of placenta, previa in fourth quarter. Cervix and vagina on right

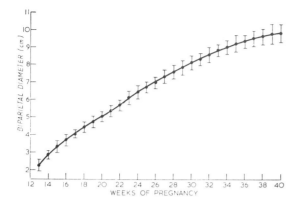

**Fig. 19/14** Fetal biparietal diameter measured by ultrasound related to gestational age. (Source: Campbell, S. J. *J. Obst. Gynaecol. Brit. Cwlth.* 1968, **75**, 568)

it cannot predict the outcome of labour. But it gives the obstetrician an additional source of information to make an assessment.

**Radiological pelvimetry**

The indications for radiological pelvimetry are listed in Table **19/2**, and the most important is the non-engagement of the fetal head (or breech) by the 38th week of pregnancy, in primigravidae. In pregnancy radiological pelvimetry should not be made until a clinical pelvic assessment has been made and the 38th week of pregnancy has been reached, but following difficult labour, pelvimetry can be satisfactorily performed in the puerperium and the patient told of the probable method of delivery in her next pregnancy.

*1. Obstetric History*
a. Difficult or prolonged labour ending with a difficult forceps delivery or a caesarean section
b. Previous unexplained intra-uterine fetal death in labour or the neonatal period

*2. Obstetric Examination*
a. Pelvis. Promontory reached; prominent ischial spines with a sacrospinous ligament accepting less than 2 fingerbreadths; narrow subpubic angle or outlet
b. Fetal. Non-engagement of the fetal head in the primigravid pelvis after the 37th week of gestation, and certainly in labour
c. Breech presentation in a primigravida which on clinical examination indicates a large baby

**Table 19/2** Indications for radiological pelvimetry

Many obstetricians have reduced still further the use of radiological pelvimetry, claiming that the information obtained when the indication was an unengaged fetal head at the 38th week did not contribute to the management of the labour; other obstetricians dispute this opinion.

TECHNIQUES

Many different techniques have been devised to overcome the distortion which is inevitable when an object which has three dimensions is projected on to a two-dimensional plate. Since the various pelvic diameters lie in different planes their projection on to the film will be at differing magnifications, and allowance for this must be made before the film is

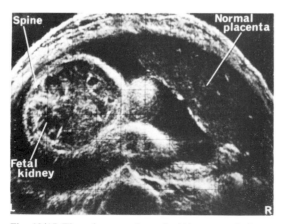

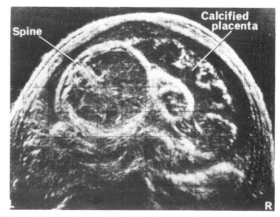

**Fig. 19/15** The echogram shows in (A) a normal placenta at 39 weeks' gestation and in (B) a degenerative placenta with areas of calcification. Note the reduced volume of amniotic fluid. The fetus was dysmature

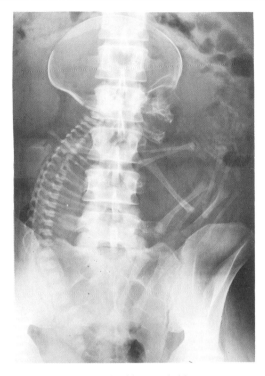

**Fig. 19/16**  Breech with extended legs

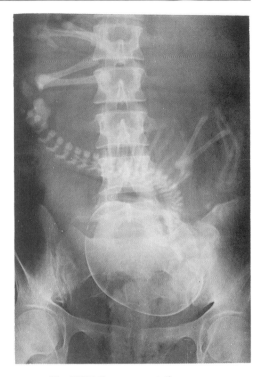

**Fig. 19/17**  Brow presentation

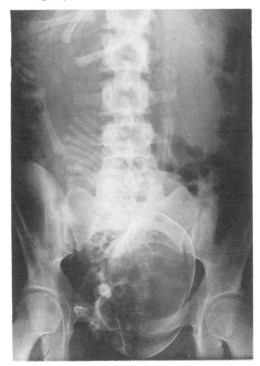

**Fig. 19/18**  Face presentation

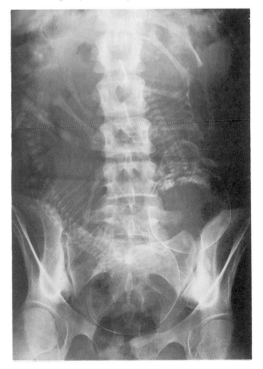

**Fig. 19/19**  Multiple pregnancy

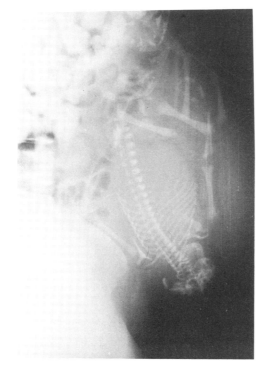

**Fig. 19/20**  Anencephalic fetus – lateral view

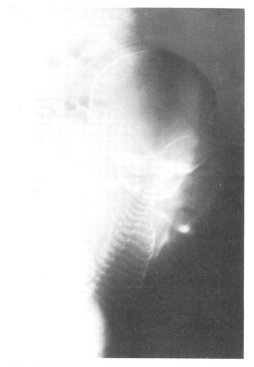

**Fig. 19/21**  Hydrocephalic fetus, breech – lateral view

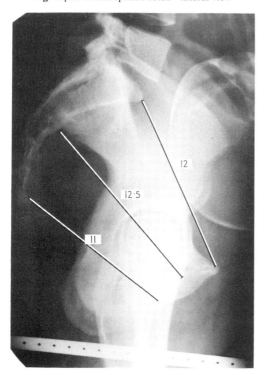

**Fig. 19/22**  Lateral view of pelvis

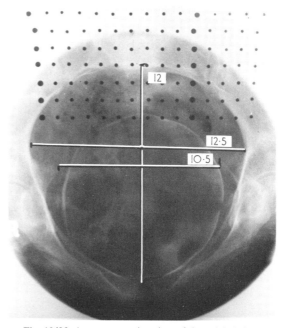

**Fig. 19/23**  Antero-posterior view of the pelvic brim

interpreted. These matters are properly the province of the radiologist, and most techniques have overcome them and can give measurements of ±0.5cm.

Two views are essential, the lateral and the antero-posterior of the pelvic brim, and a third, the outlet, is indicated in special cases. In labour the lateral film gives the most information and is attended by the least radiation hazard.

*1. Lateral view of the pelvis.* This is carried out preferably with the patient erect. An isometric scale is secured in the cleft of the buttocks and since this is on the same plane as the diameters required, a direct measurement can be obtained. The tube is centred on the greater trochanter of the femur and a tube film distance of 90cm is adopted. If the patient is positioned correctly the film will show a superimposition of the two acetabular notches.

In the lateral view the following information can be obtained: (1) the antero-posterior diameter (AP) of the pelvic inlet, the midpelvis and the outlet; (2) the pelvic architecture as shown by the shape of the anterior surface of the sacrum, the ischial spines and the greater sciatic notch, and (3) the presentation, position and station of the fetal presenting part (Fig. **19/22**).

*2. Antero-posterior view of the pelvic brim.* It is this view which requires correction because of the divergent distortion of the different pelvic levels. The use of a special isometric scale, or stereoscope projections or of calculations will give the required information. The patient lies supine with the shoulders supported at an angle of 30° above the horizontal. This has the effect of making the pelvic brim roughly parallel to the film. The x-ray tube is centred on the midpoint between the anterior superior iliac spines, and a tube film distance of 90cm is used.

The antero-posterior film will show the shape of the pelvic inlet, the AP and transverse measurements (Tr) of the brim, and by calculation the interspinous diameter can be found (Fig. **19/23**).

*3. Outlet view.* This view is only required in those cases where outlet contraction is suspected on clinical examination. Two methods are used: (1) the patient sits on the cassette, leaning well forward with the legs apart, and a postero-anterior view of the tuberosities and pubic rami is obtained on a small film, or (2) the patient lies supine with her legs apart and a marker pressed between the ischial tuberosities. The tube is directed at the pubic arch at an angle of 45° and an antero-posterior view taken.

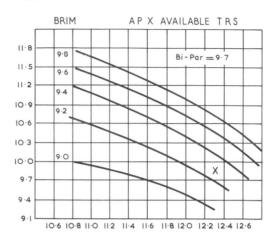

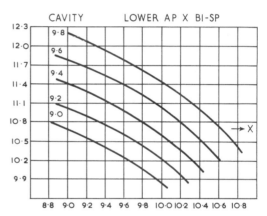

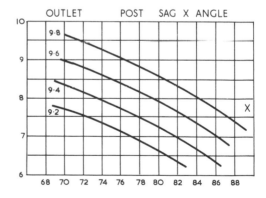

**Fig. 19/24** Example of Moir's forecast graphs. Primigravida with obstetric conjugate measuring 9.8cm, and an estimated biparietal diameter of the fetal head of 9.7cm. Graphs show decided disproportion at brim level (none at other levels). A trial of labour (indicated on clinical grounds) was allowed but was unsuccessful. Caesarean section was performed; the baby weighed 3.3 kg

## INTERPRETATION OF THE FILMS

As was pointed out, the assessment of pelvic contraction from a single measurement may be misleading, and several mathematical approaches have been introduced:

*1. The brim area.* This is calculated from the formula

$$\pi \times \frac{AP}{2} \times \frac{Tr}{2}.$$

If the brim area is more than $100cm^2$ and the pelvic architecture favourable no difficulty in vaginal delivery need be anticipated. If the brim area is less than $85cm^2$ vaginal delivery is unlikely.

*2. Forecast graphs and reconstruction charts.* In Moir's method the fetal biparietal diameter and pelvic diameters at the inlet, narrow midplane and outlet are correlated and plotted on a graph in order to give some indication of the outcome of labour. The graphs have been prepared from the pelvic measurements of patients delivering normally. If the measurements of the unknown pelvis are plotted above the line indicating the normal, then a vaginal delivery may be expected (Fig. **19/24**).

All the calculations necessarily ignore the importance of uterine contractions and maternal fortitude as factors in determining the outcome of labour and can only be a guide, therefore the obstetrician must never base his treatment on the forecast of the radiologist alone. He must assess all the information available to him for each individual case. Ultimately the responsibility for obtaining a live, healthy baby without damage to the mother, is his. Radiology is a valuable adjunct to prognosis but it should not be used as an excuse by the lazy or inadequate obstetrician for resorting to unnecessary caesarean section.

*Part Three*

# ABNORMAL PREGNANCY

*We must not suppose that all pregnant women
are in good health. There are some with the
itch, some with venereal disease and a large
number with fever and other maladies.*

Tenard (1788)

## Chapter 20

# 'Minor' Disturbances of Pregnancy

The physiological changes which occur in pregnancy may have consequences which cause distress or discomfort to the pregnant woman. Although these changes may be perceived as 'minor' by the obstetrician, they are often anything but minor in the opinion of the patient. Nausea and vomiting occurring in early pregnancy is the most common disturbance. This is dealt with first and is followed by mention of other common complaints dealt with in alphabetical order.

## NAUSEA AND VOMITING

Vomiting in pregnancy may be a symptom of general disease such as pyelonephritis, duodenal ulcer or hiatus hernia, or may be due to pregnancy itself. Whilst the vomiting due to incidental disease can occur at any time during the 40 weeks, nausea and vomiting due to pregnancy usually begin by the 6th week and cease by the 12th week but may persist throughout pregnancy. About 50 per cent of pregnant women complain of the symptoms.

Vomiting is mediated by two centres in the brain. One, the emetic centre, is activated by impulses from higher brain centres and by afferent impulses from the gastro-intestinal tract. The other, the chemoreceptor trigger zone (CTZ), is stimulated by central acting emetics, and induces vomiting by then activating the emetic centre. Stimulation of the emetic centre first induces nausea, and vomiting follows.

### Aetiology

The vomiting which is so common in early pregnancy appears due to the effect of rising oestrogen levels or to high levels of HCG on the CTZ. Once the body has become 'habituated' to the new hormonal climate, the vomiting diminishes and ceases. In cases of severe vomiting, the induced ketosis further stimulates the CTZ, which induces further vomiting. The importance of psychological factors in vomiting in early pregnancy is not clear, but they undoubtedly play a part, acting on the emetic centre via the cerebral cortex.

### Symptoms and signs

Three groups can be distinguished, but one tends to merge into the next, and the incidence of the severe type (hyperemesis gravidarum) is low.

#### MILD

Nausea and occasional vomiting usually occur in the morning, but may be provoked by travel or by emotional stress at any time of the day. If morning vomiting occurs, it is of the overnight accumulation of gastric secretions. The mild form affects 45 per cent of pregnant patients.

#### MODERATE

In 5 per cent of pregnant women the vomiting is more marked and may occur at any time of the day. The patient feels miserable and since she does not eat, often becomes slightly dehydrated, and acido-ketones appear in the urine.

#### SEVERE (HYPEREMESIS GRAVIDARUM)

In rare cases (less than 2 in 1000 pregnancies) the nausea and vomiting become continuous with increasing dehydration and acidoketosis. If treatment is not instituted quickly, liver damage may result. In the final stages, the lack of vitamin $B_1$ may lead to polyneuritis and encephalopathy, but this is extremely rare. Patients dying show pathological changes in the organs identical with those found in patients dying from extreme malnutrition. The condition is more common amongst women carrying multiple pregnancies, and those who have a history of unsuccessful pregnancies. One-quarter of women who develop hyperemesis have a recurrence in a subsequent pregnancy.

### Diagnosis and treatment

Although uncommon, the incidental causes of vomiting must be eliminated before a diagnosis of vomiting due to pregnancy is made. Treatment can be started whilst investigations are proceeding. These consist of obtaining a full history, examination of haemoglobin and haematocrit, and urine analysis, including a mid-stream specimen to exclude urinary tract infection. The subsequent management depends on the degree of vomiting. For example, when vomiting is severe, serum electrolyte estimations will aid in assessing the degree of dehydration and electrolyte imbalance.

Drug therapy of nausea and vomiting is to use antihistamines which act mainly on the emetic centre, or one of the phenothiazides, which act mainly by 'damping' the CTZ, but also act on the emetic centre.

### MILD TYPE

An explanation that this disorder will settle should be given, and the patient advised to eat frequent small dry meals (up to six a day), to take fluids in between meals and to avoid fatty and spicy foods. As a central sedative, one of the antihistamines such as cyclizine (50mg) or meclozine (25 to 50mg) twice or three times a day may be prescribed. Promethazine 25mg morning and evening is probably more effective, but produces quite marked sleepiness which limits its value. Therapy is unsatisfactory on the whole, as evidenced by the large number of drugs and regimens which are available, and treatment must be adjusted to each patient.

### MODERATE TYPE

The treatment suggested for the mild type applies, but if ketosis persists the patient should be admitted to hospital where visitors should be restricted. Sedation should be increased, and prochlorperazine (Stemetil) 5 to 10mg twice or three times a day or metoclopramide HCl 10mg three times a day have proved helpful. Dehydration and ketosis must be corrected and, if oral feeding fails, an intravenous infusion of 500 to 1000ml of 5 per cent dextrose containing promethazine (25 to 50mg) may be necessary. If treatment of the moderate type is aggressive, the patient will not pass into the severe group.

### SEVERE TYPE

The patient must be admitted to hospital, and visitors are prohibited. The pulse rate is recorded 4-hourly and the blood pressure twice daily. The urine is checked twice daily for acetone, bile, sugar and specific gravity. Plasma electrolytes are measured, and low potassium or sodium corrected by intravenous therapy. The intake and output of fluids are measured, and a positive fluid balance obtained. Dehydration and ketosis are corrected by an intravenous infusion of 1 litre of 5 per cent dextrose, followed by 1 litre Hartmann's solution, if an electrolyte disturbance is found. Over a 24-hour period the woman should receive 3 to 4 litres. If vomiting persists promethazine 25mg or metoclopramide 10mg may be given intramuscularly as needed. The infusion is continued until hydration and electrolyte balance are normal, and the patient has no further nausea. During this time, nothing is given by mouth, but ice may be sucked. Once vomiting has ceased, the patient is treated as in the moderate type. In the past therapeutic abortion was sometimes required to prevent deterioration of the severe type of hyperemesis, but this is rarely necessary today.

The patient may be discharged when the vomiting has ceased for 2 days and she is gaining weight.

## BACKACHE

This is especially common in the last trimester and is felt over the sacro-iliac joints. It is usually worse at night and may prevent sleep. Backache is due to relaxation of the ligaments and muscles supporting the joints. Treatment should begin in early pregnancy when the patient should avoid wearing high-heeled shoes when possible, and given instruction in posture. The increasing weight of the uterus causes a woman to correct her balance by drawing her shoulders back, with increasing strain on the lower lumbar spine. She should be taught to straighten her whole spine, rather than the upper part only.

# CONSTIPATION

Constipation is usual in pregnancy and is due to the lowered muscle tone of the gut, aggravated in late pregnancy by the pressure of the enlarged uterus. Treatment is by increasing the fluid intake, by eating wholemeal bread in place of white bread, by re-establishing the normal habit of defaecation after a meal, and by the use of purified senna (Senokot) or the contact laxative bisacodyl.

If drugs are required hydrophilic bulking agents or stool softeners (dioctylsulphosuccinates) which are relatively free from side-effects should be tried first, and if they fail to relieve the patient, the irritant laxatives, bisacodyl or purified senna (Senokot) may be prescribed.

# DYSPNOEA

About 25 per cent of women are dyspnoeic on exertion by the 15th week of pregnancy. The proportion increases to 50 per cent by the 20th week and 75 per cent by the 30th week. The condition is probably due to a lack of adaptation to progesterone induced hyperventilation. It is without significance to the health of the woman or her fetus, but can be anxiety-provoking unless the woman is reassured of its 'normality'.

# HEARTBURN

Relaxation of the cardiac sphincter (possibly due to progesterone) permits the regurgitation of stomach contents causing irritation of the lower oesophagus. A recent study also implicates relaxation of the pyloric sphincter in the aetiology of heartburn. This permits the reflux of bile into the stomach which then irritates the lower end of the oesophagus. Symptomatic relief is all that can be offered, and a variety of drugs has been given with varying success. Frequent small meals, avoidance of spices and cigarettes, and the use of antacid tablets will help in most cases. Antacids not only neutralize the regurgitated acid stomach contents but provoke gastrin secretion. This hormone appears to increase the tone of the cardiac sphincter. If antacids fail to relieve heartburn, 'floating' antacids, such as a sodium alginate, sodium bicarbonate mixture (Gaviscon) may be tried; or metoclopramide, which increases the pressure of the oesophageal sphincter, may be prescribed.

Paradoxically if antacids do not relieve the symptoms, dilute hydrochloric acid or prostigmine may help. Extra pillows, so that the patient sleeps propped up, may also be of value.

# HEADACHES, PALPITATIONS AND FAINTING

These are common in pregnancy and are due to the altered cardiovascular dynamics, and the introduction into the vascular system of the placental bed. The patient must be reassured that she has no organic lesion. Owing to the hypervolaemic circulation, soft systolic murmurs may be heard in pregnancy over the precordium. They have no sinister significance. A mild sedative may be required for the anxious patient, but when possible drugs should be avoided in pregnancy.

# INSOMNIA

Many pregnant women find that they are unable to sleep, particularly in the last trimester when the uterus is large, leg cramps common and backache usual. There is no harm in giving hypnotic drugs to these women.

# LEG CRAMPS

The cause of leg cramps in pregnancy is not known but there is evidence which suggests that they are due to the sudden involuntary pumping of blood out of distended venous sinuses into the calf muscles. The cramps tend to occur more frequently in the second half of pregnancy, usually at night. Of the various prophylactic and remedial methods suggested, none can be said to be specific, but recently it has been reported that the cramps occur less frequently if the foot of the bed is raised about 25cm.

# MICTURITION

## Frequency

This is common in the early weeks of pregnancy when it is due to the supra-normal excretion of water by the kidney, and in the last weeks when pressure of the fetal head engaging in the pelvis causes direct irritation of the trigone.

### Incontinence

During pregnancy, over 50 per cent of women develop stress incontinence of urine. Following 'stress' such as a cough or laughing, a small amount of urine is voided, before the woman can voluntarily suppress the loss. Most women with stress incontinence do not find it troublesome. The condition disappears in the early puerperium.

## OEDEMA

Oedema, particularly of the legs, in the absence of hypertension, is a physiological adaptation to the pregnant state. The cause is water storage in the ground substance of connective tissue. Due to the greatly increased secretion of oestrogen in pregnancy, the ground substance alters from a colloid-rich, water-poor matrix to a colloid-poor, water-rich matrix. In addition, in late pregnancy increased mechanical obstruction to the venous return from the lower limbs by the relatively high velocity venous blood coming from the uterus adds a small moiety to leg oedema. About one woman in three develops oedema in pregnancy without any evidence of hypertension or proteinuria, which strongly suggests the physiological nature of the oedema.

In general, oedema of the ankles and legs appearing towards evening is of no significance. It is more common in hot weather, in hot climates and in obese women. Treatment is to sit with the feet elevated, and there is generally no place for the use of diuretics.

On the other hand, there is a clear association between oedema and pregnancy-induced hypertension, and over 90 per cent of women who develop hypertension and proteinuria have oedema. Initially the oedema may only be manifested by an abnormally high weight gain. A weight gain in excess of 1kg per week, which does not respond to dietary measures, is due to fluid retention and is followed in 40 per cent of patients by oedema. It is a warning of the possible onset of pregnancy-induced hypertension (see Chapter 25).

## PLACIDITY AND DROWSINESS

These common symptoms are due to the increased circulation of progesterone and apart from explanation no treatment is required.

## PELVIC OSTEO-ARTHROPATHY

In a few women abnormal relaxation of the ligaments of the pubic joint occurs, with the result that the pubic bones move upon each other during walking (Fig. **20/1**). This also throws a strain on the sacro-iliac joints. The patient complains of pubic pain and backache, which may be very severe. Examination shows tenderness over the pubis. Treatment is to put the patient to bed and to nurse her on one or other side. A firm binder around the pelvis reduces discomfort in the ambulant patient.

## SWEATING AND 'FEELING THE HEAT'

Owing to the increased peripheral circulation, and vasodilatation, pregnant women sweat more and 'feel

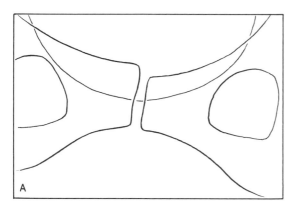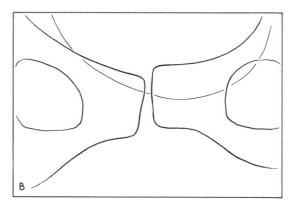

Fig. 20/1 Pelvic osteo-arthropathy. The patient was 39 weeks pregnant. The sliding movement of the symphysis is shown when (A) the patient stands on her right leg; (B) the patient stands on her left leg (redrawn from radiographs)

the heat' in late pregnancy. No treatment is available, but patients should avoid excessive exertion and take frequent rest periods, and cold showers on hot days. Fluid intake should be increased.

## VARICOSE VEINS

The reasons for the increased incidence of varicose veins in pregnancy have been given in Chapter 3.

Patients with varicose veins should sit with their feet elevated whenever possible. If the discomfort is great, nylon elastic stockings should be put on in the morning before the woman gets out of bed. A few surgeons inject isolated segments of the veins with sodium tetradecyl, but in general such treatment is best deferred until after the puerperium. Very occasionally deep vein thrombosis occurs in pregnancy, and is treated with heparin, all other anticoagulants being contraindicated, as these cross the placenta (see p. 375).

## Chapter 21

# Abnormalities of the Genital Tract Complicating Pregnancy

## ABNORMAL POSITIONS OF THE UTERUS

### Retroversion

Normally the uterus lies in an anteverted and anteflexed position, but in at least 10 per cent of women it is retroverted or retroflexed. The mobile retroverted uterus is without clinical significance and does not cause infertility, nor is it a cause of abortion.

In about 10 per cent of pregnant patients, the initial vaginal examination will show that the uterus is retroverted. Unless the retroverted uterus is fixed, which is unlikely, there will be no symptoms and the uterus can be expected to rise up out of the pelvis spontaneously by the 12th week of pregnancy. Apart from avoidance of constipation, and regular voiding, no treatment is required, but the patient should be examined vaginally at about the 12th week to confirm that spontaneous anteversion has occurred. If it has not, the position of the uterus should be corrected by bimanual manipulation between the 12th and 14th week. The vaginal fingers are first placed in the anterior fornix and the cervix is pushed backwards. At the same time the hand on the abdomen presses down into the pelvis in an attempt to reach behind the uterine fundus. Because of the projection of the sacral promontory the uterus should be manipulated to one or other side of the midline. If this manoeuvre does not succeed, the vaginal fingers are placed in the posterior fornix and the fundus is pushed up until the external hand can be pressed down behind the erect uterus. The vaginal fingers are then transferred to the anterior fornix and used to push the cervix backwards. This has the effect of further anteverting the fundus.

### Incarceration

In rare instances, usually because of adhesions, the retroverted gravid uterus becomes incarcerated in the pelvis. Incarceration occurs between the 12th and 14th week and the earliest symptoms are frequency of micturition and dysuria. If the displacement is not corrected the symptoms increase in severity and eventually there is complete retention of urine. In these advanced cases the bladder becomes enormously distended and finally retention with overflow occurs.

The difficulty in micturition and the retention are caused by the pressure of the cervix on the bladder neck which results in reflex suppression of detrusor activity. The urethra is not obstructed by the cervix, but with increasing distension of the bladder it becomes elongated and the external meatus may be slit-like and difficult to find. If not treated, oedema of the bladder and infection of the retained urine is certain and generalized infection and sloughing of the bladder may occur as a terminal event. Today such an outcome would be exceptional.

Examination shows a firm, tender, cystic abdominal tumour arising from the pelvis which may be mistaken for the uterus. On vaginal examination a soft pelvic tumour is detected which is the pregnant uterus, but which may be mistaken for an ovarian tumour or a myoma. The passage of a catheter will clear up the confusion and will relieve the symptoms. A medium-sized plastic catheter should be used and the bladder decompressed slowly. Once the bladder is empty, the uterus usually becomes upright or anteverts spontaneously, and only rarely requires manipulation.

Since renal tract infection is usual, appropriate investigations should be made before the manipulation is performed.

### Anteversion – pendulous abdomen

Separation of the recti abdominis and frequent child-bearing may so weaken the muscular abdominal wall that little support is offered to the uterus in late pregnancy, so that it becomes pathologically anteverted – the pendulous abdomen. In late pregnancy the condition may cause abdominal discomfort, and occasionally pain. During labour dystocia may arise as the axis of the uterus is acutely angled to that of the pelvis, and engagement of the presenting part is delayed. Since the patient is usually a 'high multigravida' malpresentations are common (Fig. 21/1). Treatment in pregnancy is to wear a corset or some other support. In labour a binder should be applied, and the patient nursed on her back. With each contraction the patient should draw her uterus upwards.

### Uterovaginal prolapse

In the developing countries, particularly, uterovaginal prolapse complicating pregnancy is not uncommon. The prolapse precedes the pregnancy but becomes more obvious in the first 12 weeks, partly because of the weight of the pregnant uterus and partly because of the hormonal relaxation of the pelvic tissues. As the pregnancy advances the uterus becomes an abdominal organ and the pressure is largely relieved so that the prolapse is less obvious, but occasionally a swollen infected cervix may protrude through the vulva. The treatment in pregnancy is to bring the patient into hospital, to replace the cervix inside the vagina and to keep it there with packs soaked in chlorhexidine solution or cream. Surprisingly, prolapse causes little trouble during labour and cervical dilatation is rapid. Rarely the head of a preterm fetus is pushed through the vulval ring still inside a prolapsed uterus. Treatment is to incise the cervix and deliver the fetus by forceps.

### PREGNANCY AFTER A VAGINAL REPAIR OPERATION

If the repair operation has included a suburethral suspension to cure a stress incontinence, or a high amputation of the cervix, delivery should be by elective caesarean section at the 38th week.

In all other cases the decision may be delayed until late pregnancy. If the repair was vaginal, and the cervix was not amputated, a vaginal delivery following an episiotomy may be anticipated. If the cervix was amputated, the degree of scarring and chances of dilatation can be assessed, and a separate decision made for each case.

## CERVICAL CONDITIONS

### Cervical eversion

The increased secretions of oestrogen and progesterone in pregnancy soften the ground substances of the cervix and increase the hygroscopic qualities of the connective tissue. The resulting swelling and softening of the cervix draws the endocervical

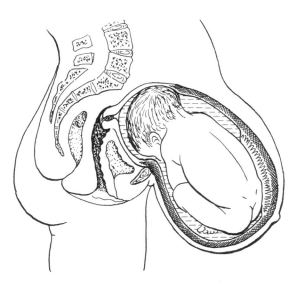

**Fig. 21/1** Pendulous abdomen. The patient was Indian, aged 36, gravida 4

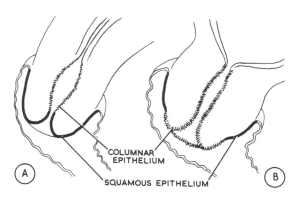

**Fig. 21/2** The cervix. (A) In a virgin; (B) in pregnancy. The softening of the collagen and imbibation of liquid increases the cervical size with the result that the endocervical columnar cells 'pout' and are visible as a circumoral 'erosion'

columnar epithelium out of the canal so that it forms a zone around the external os (Fig. **21/2**). This has been called a 'cervical erosion', but since there is no loss of epithelium, is better termed an eversion. The eversion is covered by columnar epithelium which excretes mucin and consequently the pregnant patient may have a heavy 'vaginal' discharge. As this is a normal secretion no treatment is required. On occasion the columnar epithelium may form a polyp, which may bleed in pregnancy. Should a polyp be found it should be removed by torsion, and examined microscopically.

**Oedema of the cervix**

This may occur in pregnancy, particularly if the cervix is prolapsed. The cause is an obstruction to the venous return and the oedema is aggravated by infection.

Treatment is to replace the cervix in the vagina and to apply gauze soaked in chlorhexidine solution or cream. In rare cases the cervix is so distended that small incisions are necessary to reduce its volume.

Oedema of the cervix may arise in labour from a combination of the same causes, and may be increased because the patient 'pushes' before the cervix

is fully dilated. The anterior lip is most affected and may precede the head as a swollen bluish haemorrhagic tumour. With each contraction the anterior lip of the cervix becomes more prominent, and can delay the delivery of the head. Provided that only the anterior lip is palpable, the rest of the cervix having dilated fully, it may be pushed up above the head with two fingers in the vagina. The manipulation is best made during a contraction and the fingers should be kept in the vagina for two or three contractions to ensure that the cervix does not prolapse again between contractions. Once the cervix has been displaced above the head, delivery is rapid.

## MALFORMATIONS OF THE UTERUS AND VAGINA

The uterus and vagina are formed by the fusion of the two Mullerian ducts and the subsequent ablation of the joining septum. Abnormalities may occur if only one Mullerian duct is present, or if the fusion of the two ducts is abnormal, or if the joining septum fails to be absorbed. About 3 per cent of women have some abnormality of the genital tract and many

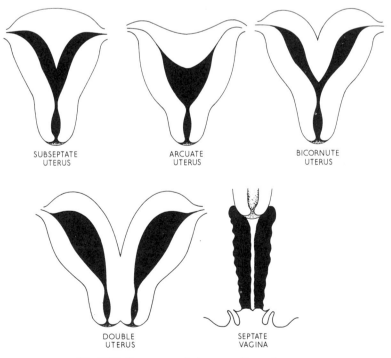

Fig. 21/3 Common genital tract malformations

become pregnant. The commonest abnormalities are the arcuate uterus, the subseptate uterus and the bicornute uterus (Fig. **21/3**).

Abortion and premature labour are four times as frequent when the uterus is malformed but the majority of patients go to term. If the uterus is arcuate or subseptate, transverse lie or breech presentation is often found, and the recurrence of one of these malpositions in several pregnancies suggests that a uterine malformation is present.

Vaginal delivery occurs in 80 per cent of cases and caesarean section is required in 20 per cent. The incidence of retention of the placenta is increased. Labour in these patients should be supervised with great care.

The 'pregnancy wastage' in women with uterine abnormalities is greatest if the uterus is septate or bicornute. If a woman with a uterine abnormality repeatedly aborts or has premature labour, metroplasty may be indicated and is usually followed by the birth of a mature baby in a subsequent pregnancy. The delivery must be by caesarean section and uterine rupture may occur in pregnancy so the operation should be reserved for women who have had 'unsuccessful' pregnancies.

If a longitudinal vaginal septum is found on vaginal examination, it should be left and only removed if it causes delay in the second stage of labour, as the descending fetal head usually displaces it to one side or other.

## VAGINAL DISCHARGES IN PREGNANCY

The vagina is self-sterilizing and this property is due to its acidity (pH about 4.5) in which organisms are unable to grow. The acidity is due to the presence of Döderlein's bacillus acting upon the glycogen in the exfoliated vaginal cells. The glycogen in turn is dependent upon the activity of oestrogen on the cells, causing their growth and maturation. During pregnancy, because of increased oestrogen production, the vaginal acidity potential is increased, but this is largely offset by the increased alkaline mucoid discharge which comes from the ectopic columnar epithelium of the cervix. Thus, although the vagina is too acid for significant bacterial growth the patient notices a vaginal discharge. The discharge is a mixture of mucoid secretion and a glairy whitish discharge which forms when the mucus coagulates in

its passage down the vagina. This is an exaggeration of the normal 'vaginal' secretion and requires no treatment beyond reassurance. Some patients are particularly sensitive to the presence of a vaginal discharge and for them the vaginal instillation of an acid jelly (Acijel) or any one of a variety of acid vaginal pessaries may be prescribed. Vaginal douching should be prohibited.

Two organisms which are widely distributed and are largely resistant to acidity, grow preferentially in the moist, high carbohydrate atmosphere of the pregnant vagina. These are *Trichomonas vaginalis* and *Candida albicans*.

### Trichomonas vaginalis (Fig. 21/4)

This small flagellated protozoon lives in the folds of the vaginal mucosa and causes a greenish-yellow offensive discharge, which consists of trichomonads, leucocytes and contaminating saprophytes, the last causing the odour.

In severe neglected cases the vagina is reddened and tender, and may show punctate reddened spots. In most cases, however, the clinical findings are non-specific for the infestation. The patient complains of an intense pruritus and itching just inside the vaginal introitus. It may be so severe as to prevent sleep, and because the patient scratches she may cause secondary staphylococcal ulcers to form on the inner surfaces of the labia minora. The diagnosis is made by examining a drop of the vaginal discharge

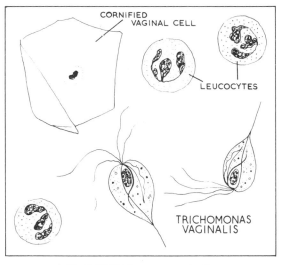

CORNIFIED VAGINAL CELL

LEUCOCYTES

TRICHOMONAS VAGINALIS

Fig. 21/4 Trichomonas vaginalis

mixed with a drop of warm saline, under a microscope, when mobile trichomonads will be seen. For
greater accuracy, a sample of the discharge is added
to a test tube of Kupferberg's medium and incubated.
Treatment is to give oral tablets of metronidazole
200g three times a day for 7 days.

About 8 per cent of pregnant women have vaginal
trichomoniasis but the flagellate causes symptoms in
only a few of them.

### Candidiasis or moniliasis (Fig. 21/5)

Vaginal fungal infection with *Candida albicans* is
even more common in pregnant women, and over 20
per cent harbour the fungus, although it causes symptoms in only a few. The reason for the high incidence
in pregnancy is because of the higher glycogen content of the vagina. The main symptom of candidiasis
is an intense vulval or vaginal irritation which is
usually associated with a vaginal discharge. In most
cases examination of the vagina merely confirms
that an increased discharge is present but, in severe
infections, the discharge is 'cheesy', thick, and tends
to form adherent patches on the vaginal wall.

The diagnosis is made by examining a smear made
from the discharge after staining it with 10 per cent
potassium hydroxide or 1 per cent methylene blue,
when the long branched filaments of hyphae will be
seen. Greater accuracy in diagnosis is obtained in
doubtful cases if swabs from the posterior fornix are
cultured on Sabouraud glucose-agar medium, or on
Nickerson's medium.

Several drugs are available to treat vaginal candidiasis. No one seems superior to any other. Because of problems of patient compliance, the trend
has been to reduce the duration of the course of
treatment. Most of the drugs are imidazole derivatives. They include clotrimazole, econazole, is-
oconazole and micronazole. They are given as a
vaginal pessary or a cream (using an applicator)
placed high in the vagina. The duration of treatment
is a single application; or a 3- or a 6-day course
depending on the doctor and patient preferences.
The imidazole derivatives have largely replaced
nystatin pessaries which needed to be used for at
least 7 days, and messy gentian violet (2 per cent in
water) vaginal paintings. As the intestinal tract is
the source of re-infection, women should pay attention to hygiene. They should wipe the area from
front to back after defaecation and should avoid

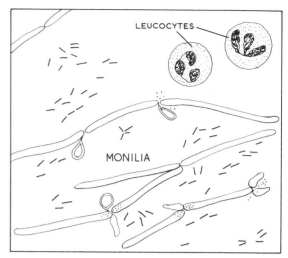

**Fig. 21/5** Monilia or Candida albicans

introducing a finger into the vagina which may be
contaminated by anal touching.

### Amine vaginosis

This is due to the interaction of a normal vaginal
contaminant, *Gardnerella vaginalis* and anaerobes in
the vagina. Symptoms are an offensive 'fishy', thin,
greyish, vaginal discharge with occasional vaginal
irritation. Anaerobic vaginosis is diagnosed by examining a vaginal smear. A drop of the smear is
added to a drop of saline on a slide. When examined
through a microscope, vaginal cells with serrated
edges, called 'clue cells', may be seen. A Gram stain
made from the same swab will show coccibacilli
attached to vaginal cells, giving a 'pepper and salt'
appearance. Treatment is the same as that for trichomoniasis.

### Genital warts

Genital warts are caused by the human papilloma-
virus (HPV), a sexually transmitted disease. During
pregnancy, warts often increase in size, and spread.
It is also possible that HPV may infect the baby
during childbirth, leading to laryngeal warts. Isolated
vulval warts may be left, but vaginal warts should
be treated by using $CO_2$ laser or electrocoagulation
in late pregnancy. Podophyllin probably should not
be used in pregnancy as it may be absorbed into the
fetal circulation.

# Chapter 22

# Abortion

Abortion means the expulsion of a fetus before it reaches viability. The World Health Organization has recommended that a fetus shall be considered viable when the gestation period is more than 22 completed weeks, or the fetus weighs 500g or more. Australia, and several states in the USA, have adopted this criterion, but Britain and most other nations continue to contend that viability occurs at the 28th week of pregnancy or if the fetus weighs 1000g or more. In Australia, it is held that if the expelled fetus weighs less than 400g it is an abortus; if between 400 and 999g it is an 'immature infant'. Occasionally the euphemism miscarriage is used, particularly by non-medical people as synonymous with abortion, the latter term implying (to them) a 'criminal' abortion.

## FREQUENCY

Most textbooks claim that between 10 and 15 per cent of clinically diagnosed pregnancies end as an abortion. Recent investigations in which pregnancy was diagnosed within 21 days of conception by measuring beta HCG and an ultrasound examination was made at 8 weeks' gestation, indicate that the abortion rate is higher, probably about 33 per cent, but 22 per cent occur before the pregnancy can be diagnosed clinically, so that the *clinical* abortion rate is 11 per cent.

Abortions occur more frequently as the woman grows older. Among women aged > 30 years about 3 per cent abort; the rate doubles if the woman is aged 30 to 34 and trebles if she is 35 or older. Abortion also increases with increasing gravidity. About 6 per cent of first or second pregnancies terminate as an abortion; with third and subsequent pregnancies the abortion rate increases to 16 per cent.

Of clinically diagnosed pregnancies 65 per cent of abortions occur between the 6th and 10th week of pregnancy.

Abortion is not the only cause of bleeding in early pregnancy, although it accounts for 95 per cent of cases. Rarer causes are ectopic gestation (1 per cent), cervical eversion (1 per cent), endocervical polyp (1 per cent), hydatidiform mole (0.1 per cent), and cervical carcinoma (0.05 per cent).

## AETIOLOGY OF SPONTANEOUS ABORTION

The causes of abortion can conveniently be divided into three groups – ovo-fetal, maternal and paternal (Table **22/1**). In the early weeks (0 to 10) of pregnancy, when most abortions occur, ovo-fetal factors predominate, but in the later weeks (11 to 19) maternal factors become more common and the fetus is often born fresh and apparently normal, although too immature to survive.

### Ovo-fetal causes

Careful studies of abortuses show that in about 60 per cent of cases the ovum is defective and has failed to develop, or the fetus is malformed (Fig. **22/1**). In

| Fetal or ovular | Percentage |
|---|---|
| Defective ovo-fetus | 60 |
| Defective implantation | 15 |
| *Maternal* | |
| Uterine abnormalities | 8 |
| General disease | 2 |
| ?Psychosomatic | 15 |

Table **22/1** Aetiological factors in 5000 abortions

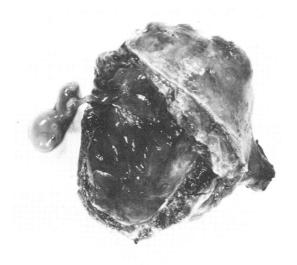

**Fig. 22/1** Blighted ovum

many cases the defect occurs at the time of conception. Chromosome studies of abortions occurring before the 15th gestational week show that at least 35 per cent have chromosomal abnormalities. As the defect affects all parts of the ovum, the trophoblast does not implant adequately, and fetal development is impaired. The earlier the abortion the higher is the proportion of those with chromosomal defects.

### Maternal causes

*General maternal disease*, especially acute fevers, favours abortion perhaps by the transplacental passage of viruses or bacteria, or perhaps due to the general metabolic effects of pyrexia and diminished oxygen release through the placenta.

*Local disorders of the genital tract*, such as retroversion, myomata and developmental defects were, at one time, considered to be important causes of abortion. It is now known that only when the retroverted uterus is fixed in the pelvis, or when the myomata distort the uterine cavity do these conditions increase the risk. Developmental defects are relatively uncommon, and of them a bicornuate uterus may cause abortion, especially after the 12th week of pregnancy. Another cause of late abortion is cervical incompetence which may be due to a congenital weakness, but is usually due to previous rough dilatation of the cervix. Cervical incompetence

accounts for no more than 1 per cent of all abortions, and is considered further on page 188.

### Psychosomatic causes

It is known that environmental stress operating through the cerebrum affects the secretion of substances by the medial eminence of the hypothalamus. This area is richly supplied with nerves which are in intimate connection with the pituitary portal vessels. These carry the substances which regulate the release of pituitary hormones, which in turn affect uterine function. Stress may affect uterine activity, and may lead to abortion. This is most clearly seen in some patients who habitually abort, and the only common factor in the success of the many treatments offered is the interest shown in the patient by the obstetrician.

### Paternal causes

Since the paternal spermatozoon gives to the ovum half of its chromosomes, defects may result in abortions, particularly if both partners share many common HLA antigen sites.

## MECHANISM OF ABORTION

The immediate cause of the abortion is the separation of the ovum by minute haemorrhages in the decidua. The altered uterine environment stimulates the onset of uterine contractions, and the process of abortion begins.

Before the 8th week the ovum, covered with villi and some attached decidua, tends to be expelled en masse. If the internal os dilates but the external os of the cervix fails to dilate, the sac may be retained in the cervix (cervical abortion).

Between the 8th and the 14th week, the mechanism may be as described, or, more commonly, the membranes rupture expelling the defective fetus but the placenta is only partially separated and protrudes through the cervical os into the vagina or remains attached to the uterine wall (incomplete abortion). This type of abortion is attended by considerable haemorrhage.

After the 14th week, the fetus is usually expelled, followed by the placenta after an interval. Less commonly, the placenta is retained. Bleeding is not marked and the process of abortion resembles a 'miniature labour'.

# VARIETIES OF ABORTION

For descriptive purposes the abortion is classified according to the findings when the patient is first seen, but obviously one kind may change into the next with the passage of time. The following clinical types are recognized (Fig. **22/2**):

threatened abortion
inevitable abortion
incomplete abortion
complete abortion
missed abortion.

Any of the above types, but usually the inevitable or incomplete types, may be complicated by infection, when the term *septic abortion* is used.

*Recurrent abortion* indicates that the woman has had three or more known successive abortions, and *therapeutic abortion* indicates that the pregnancy was terminated legally for a specific medical indication. Induced or *criminal abortion* indicates that the abortion was induced illegally for social reasons.

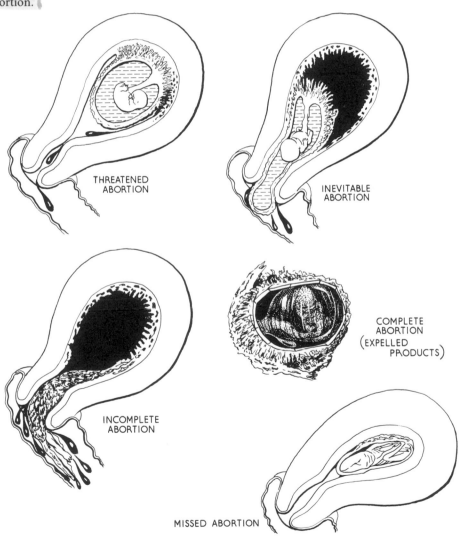

**Fig. 22/2** The types of abortion which may be seen

## THREATENED ABORTION

An abortion is presumed to threaten when a woman who is known to be pregnant develops vaginal bleeding during the first 20 weeks of pregnancy, whether this bleeding is associated with uterine contractions or not. Threatened abortion affects about 10 per cent of all pregnancies. A few patients bleed slightly the time of the first missed period when the trophoblast is implanting deeply, and this is called implantation haemorrhage. It may be difficult to distinguish this type of bleeding from threatened abortion, but in the former the amount is slight, the colour bright red, and the bleeding settles quickly.

Threatened abortion is diagnosed by (1) determining that the patient is pregnant; (2) determining that the bleeding is coming from inside the cervix; (3) deciding that the uterine contractions, if present, are only slight and that the cervix is not dilated. It is sometimes advised that a speculum or bimanual examination should not be carried out on a patient threatening to abort, as this may precipitate the abortion or introduce infection. This is bad advice, and provided the examination is done gently no harm will result, and an occasional mistake in diagnosis will be avoided. To avoid infection the speculum should be passed and the bimanual examination performed with attention to aseptic technique.

If possible an ultrasound examination (using a modern sector or curvilinear transducer) should be made, particularly if the pregnancy has reached the 7th gestational week. The echogram may show (1) a normal-sized sac and a fetus whose heart is pulsating, (2) an empty sac (Fig. 22/3), (3) a missed or an incomplete abortion. Examination of the adnexae may show a mass indicative of a tubal (ectopic) pregnancy, particularly if a transvaginal probe is used.

### Treatment

Traditionally a woman who is threatening to abort and whose fetus is alive is put to bed, although there is no objective evidence that bed rest has any value. Nor are drugs, hormones or sedatives of any value except as a placebo. If the echogram shows a normal-sized sac (for gestational date) and a live fetus, the pregnancy will continue in 97 per cent of cases, and the woman can be reassured. However, about 5 per cent of the pregnancies will be curtailed and a preterm baby will be delivered. If the echogram shows an incomplete or a missed abortion, curettage should be performed.

## INEVITABLE ABORTION

The abortion becomes inevitable if, in addition to the signs described in threatened abortion, the uterine contractions become increasingly painful and strong, and lead to dilatation of the cervix. The patient complains of severe colicky uterine pain, and vaginal examination shows a dilated os with some part of the conception sac bulging through. This sequence may follow signs of threatened abortion, or, more commonly, may occur without warning, the whole process being speeded up. Quite soon after the onset of the symptoms, the abortion occurs, either completely, when all the products of conception are expelled, or incompletely when either the pregnancy sac, or placental tissue remains in the uterine cavity or distends the cervical canal. This last can produce considerable shock, even in the absence of marked haemorrhage.

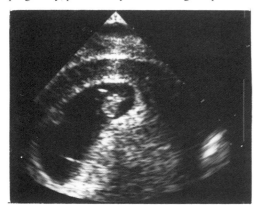
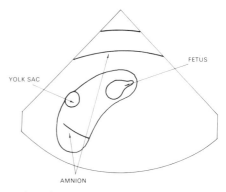

**Fig. 22/3** Ultrasound scan showing yolk sac and amnion

## INCOMPLETE ABORTION AND COMPLETE ABORTION

The majority of patients present with an incomplete abortion. The amount of bleeding may have been considerable, associated with cramp-like uterine contractions and the patient claims that she has passed 'something'. This may mean that all the products of conception have been passed and the uterus is empty (complete abortion) or it may mean that only part has been passed (incomplete abortion). If the obstetrician has not had the opportunity to examine everything that has been expelled, he should consider the abortion to be incomplete and curette the uterus. However, an empty uterus, as shown by ultrasound, obviates the need for this invasive procedure.

### Treatment

Unless the patient has aborted completely when seen, or the abortion is imminent, she should be transferred to hospital. Whilst waiting for the arrival of the ambulance, morphine 15mg or pethidine 100mg should be given if the patient is in pain. A sterile vaginal examination must be made, as placental tissue distending the cervix can cause considerable shock. Any tissue in the cervix should be removed with finger or sponge forceps, and if there is any degree of haemorrhage, ergometrine 0.5mg should be given intramuscularly. Once this has been done, the patient's condition usually improves and evacuation of the uterus can be completed by curettage in a calm and deliberate way when convenient.

In hospital, treatment is conservative only if the abortion is proceeding quickly and with minimal blood loss. On admission, the general condition is assessed and compatible blood obtained. A vaginal examination is carried out and if products of conception are distending the cervix, these are removed with sponge forceps or the finger. Pethidine 100mg or morphine 15mg is given to relieve the pain, and ergometrine 0.25mg intravenously to control bleeding.

If the entire products of conception are not rapidly expelled, active intervention is required and the sooner the uterus is emptied the better. Evacuation of the pregnant uterus should be done with care as in unskilled hands damage can easily occur. Under general anaesthesia the patient is examined, and if the cervix is sufficiently dilated to admit a finger, this is used to detach any remnants of placental tissue. It is by far the safest instrument!

In cases in which the cervix is insufficiently dilated to admit a finger, the suction curette or sponge forceps and sharp curette may be used. If the sponge forceps is chosen it is introduced into the uterus until the tip reaches the endometrium at the fundus, and then the two jaws are opened and closed again whilst rotating the forceps (Fig. 22/4). In this way products of conception are grasped without danger to the myometrium. Finally the uterine cavity is curetted. A large sharp curette, used gently, is safer than a blunt curette used roughly. Towards the end of the operation ergometrine 0.25mg is given intravenously and intramuscularly.

After a complete abortion (or one which has been completed by curettage) the bloody discharge diminishes and ceases in about 10 days. When placental remnants have been left in the uterus, bleeding continues beyond this time and varies in severity from day to day, and may be accompanied by periodic uterine cramps. Examination shows a bulky uterus, with a patulous os. Careful curettage should be performed in these cases, and all tissue examined histologically in case the rare choriocarcinoma is present.

Following an incomplete or a complete abortion a woman who is Rhesus negative should be given an injection of anti-D immunoglobulin, and a Kleihauer test should be performed to determine the amount of fetal blood in her circulation (see p. 258).

## INDUCED (CRIMINAL) ABORTION

Many cases of inevitable and incomplete abortion have been induced by a variety of people, using a variety of methods, in a variety of places. The common factor is that the operation has generally been hurried, little attention has been paid to asepsis and infection is likely. The treatment is that described for active intervention in incomplete abortion, but since infection is likely, high doses of antibiotics should be given before operating.

## SEPTIC ABORTION

Infection of the uterus may occur with any abortion, but is usually found in association with incomplete abortion and most frequently after an induced abortion. The incidence of septic abortion varies considerably, depending on the kind of patient treated, and figures varying from 6 to 38 per cent of all abortions have been reported, the mean being 12 per cent.

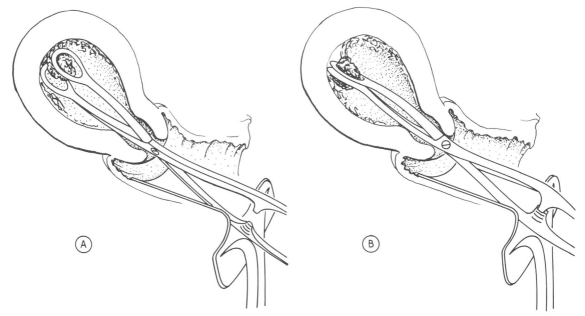

**Fig. 22/4** The use of sponge forceps for clearing placental tissue from the uterus

In countries which have 'liberalized' their laws on abortion, the number of septic abortions has fallen considerably suggesting that most of those reported in the past occurred following induced abortion inexpertly performed with poor control of infection.

**Pathology**

In 80 per cent of cases the infection is mild and is localized to the decidua. The organisms involved are usually endogenous, and are most commonly anaerobic streptococci, staphylococci or *E. coli*. Their virulence is low. In 15 per cent of cases the infection involves the myometrium with spread to the tubes and pelvic cellular tissues or pelvic peritoneum. In 5 per cent of cases there is generalized peritonitis or vascular collapse. These cases are most often due to the release of endotoxins by *E. coli*, or to the growth of *Clostridium welchii*.

**Clinical features**

The first sign is pyrexia, the degree of which may not be related to the severity of the infection. Associated with this is a tachycardia. If the pulse rate is faster than 120 per minute, spread beyond the uterus has usually occurred. In infections localized to the endometrium an offensive vaginal discharge is common, but this is less marked in spreading infections. Examination shows a boggy tender uterus and evidence of extra-uterine spread may be apparent. Diagnosis is by finding in a case of abortion, whether threatened, incomplete or complete, two of the following: a temperature in excess of 37.8°C (100°F); a foul-smelling pink discharge; a leucocytosis in excess of 15 000 or extra-uterine spread of infection.

**Investigations**

A high vaginal, or cervical, smear is taken and if the temperature exceeds 38.4°C (101°F) a blood culture is also made. In severe infections, urinalysis, serum electrolyte and fibrinogen studies are also undertaken.

**Treatment**

Antibiotics are given to combat the infection. The precise antibiotic chosen will depend on knowledge of the prevalence of bacterial resistance in the area and on the result of the bacteriological examination of the smears. As about 60 to 70 per cent of pathogens are Gram-negative, amoxycillin 500mg three times a day, and metronidazole 1g 12-hourly (for 2 doses) should be given. An alternative is to give cefoxitin 2g, 6-hourly.

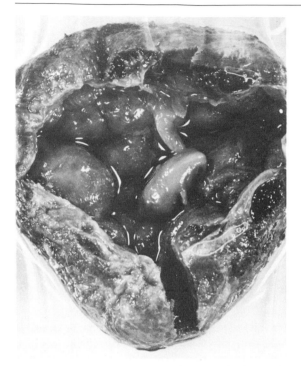

**Fig. 22/5** Carneous mole – a small fetus can also be seen in the centre

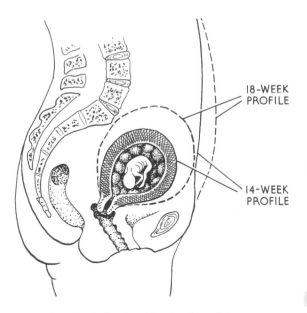

**Fig. 22/6** Missed abortion. The duration of the pregnancy is 18 weeks but the uterus has failed to enlarge beyond the size of a 14 week gestation. Note that the abdomen is flat

18-WEEK PROFILE

14-WEEK PROFILE

## MISSED ABORTION

In a few cases the dead embryo and placenta are not expelled spontaneously, and a condition of missed abortion occurs. If the embryo dies in the early weeks, it is likely to be blighted and multiple haemorrhages occur in the chorio-decidual space. These bulge in mounds into the empty amniotic cavity, whilst on the maternal side layers of blood clot are deposited. This condition is known as a carneous mole (Fig. **22/5**). When the fetus dies at a later period of pregnancy, and is not expelled, it is either absorbed or becomes mummified and thin, the liquor amnii is largely absorbed and the placenta becomes thin and adherent.

### Clinical aspects

The patient usually has a history of a threatened abortion which settles down, but the symptoms of pregnancy disappear and the uterus fails to enlarge or may become smaller (Fig. **22/6**). Sooner or later an intermittent brown discharge recurs. An immunological test for pregnancy will remain positive so long as placental tissue survives, but eventually all the trophoblast dies and the test becomes negative. The diagnosis is not usually confirmed for 21 days or so, by which time most cases will have terminated by a spontaneous abortion. The diagnosis can be established earlier if ultrasound is available, as a distinct pattern appears in cases of missed abortion.

### Treatment

There is no urgency in treating missed abortion, but if after a reasonable time spontaneous abortion of the products of conception has not occurred, treatment may be instituted. If the size of the uterus is less than 12 weeks' gestation, evacuation is made per vaginam with a suction curette or with sponge forceps and curette after cervical dilatation. The operation is messy and laborious, and should continue until the uterus is empty. Blood loss can be reduced by setting up an oxytocin infusion before starting the dilatation of the cervix. If the uterus is larger than 12 weeks in size it should be stimulated to expel the fetus by giving the patient an intravenous infusion of prostaglandin $F_{2\alpha}$ or $E_2$, or by using pharmacological doses of oxytocin infused intravenously (see Chapter 49).

An alternative is to insert vaginal pessaries of

prostaglandin $E_2$(20mg) high up the vagina every 3 to 6 hours, depending on the strength of the uterine contractions.

The side-effects of prostaglandin are nausea and vomiting in 80 per cent of women and diarrhoea in 70 per cent.

## RECURRENT ABORTION

Only a few women have the misfortune to abort successively. It has been calculated that after one abortion the risk of another abortion is 20 per cent, after two abortions 25 per cent and after three abortions about 30 per cent.

A woman who has three or more successive abortions is referred to as a 'recurrent aborter'. She has a 30 per cent chance of aborting the next pregnancy. Recurrent aborters are also said to be at greater risk of delivering a preterm baby (before the 37th week) if they escape aborting once again. If the abortions occurred in the first quarter of pregnancy, there is no increased risk of delivering a preterm baby. Women who have recurrent second quarter abortions, and those whose next pregnancy reaches 20 weeks, have a 30 per cent chance of delivering a preterm baby.

The aetiological factors in recurrent abortion vary with the population surveyed and to some extent with medical fashion. Two series of over 100 recurrent aborters reported from the USA and Norway offer some idea of the aetiology (Table **22/2**), and indicate possible approaches to investigation and treatment.

### Investigation of recurrent abortion

A full medical and obstetrical history may disclose systemic disease or suggest cervical incompetence. A vaginal examination may show uterine myomata, or evidence of cervical incompetence. A hysterogram should be performed to exclude uterine malformations (bicornuate uterus, a subseptate uterus or submucosal myomata). If endometrial infection is considered to be a factor, endometrial tissue cultures should be set up for the isolation of urealyticum and *Toxoplasma gondii*. Not all workers believe that endometrial infection is a cause of recurrent abortion. Endocrine dysfunction, for example hypothyroidism, should be excluded, and in certain cases chromo-

### RECURRENT ABORTERS

| *Possible aetiology* | *Per cent of abortions occurring* | |
|---|---|---|
| | ⩽12 weeks | >12 weeks |
| Unknown | 55 | 35 |
| Uterine malformations or abnormality | 10 | 10 |
| Cervical incompetence | 3 | 30 |
| Chromosome abnormality | 5 | 4 |
| ? Endometrial infection | 15 | 15 |
| Endocrine dysfunction | 3 | 3 |
| Systemic disease | 1 | 1 |
| ? Sperm factors | 3 | 1 |
| ? Immune factors | ? | 1 |

**Table 22/2** The aetiology of recurrent abortion

somal studies made on both parents, although the value of this has not been established.

On page 27 it was noted that if the two parents shared several HLA sites, the fetus might provide an insufficient stimulus for the mother to produce blocking IgG. This antibody is thought to be a major factor in preventing the fetus from being rejected. Some women who have recurrent abortions lack circulating blocking IgG antibodies, as measured by a mixed lymphocyte reaction test. If these women are injected with allogenic (paternal) leucocytes or compatible leucocyte-rich erythrocyte transfusions (obtained from a donor or the husband) prior to the woman's becoming pregnant, abortion may not occur and a viable infant may be born.

Conversely, a strong blocking antibody response may be found in women who have an autoimmune disease, especially systemic lupus erythematosus (SLE). SLE must be excluded before donor leucocytes are injected or transfused, as the autoimmune disease may be aggravated. If SLE is identified, small doses of aspirin (75mg a day) or corticosteroids may permit the pregnancy to continue to fetal viability. In these women, pregnancy complications, especially pregnancy-induced hypertension, are more likely than in other pregnant women. Immunotherapy must still be considered experimental until long-term follow-up of mothers and their babies has been undertaken.

### Cervical incompetence

About 20 per cent of recurrent aborters will be found to have cervical incompetence. This is diagnosed by evaluation of the following criteria: (1) a

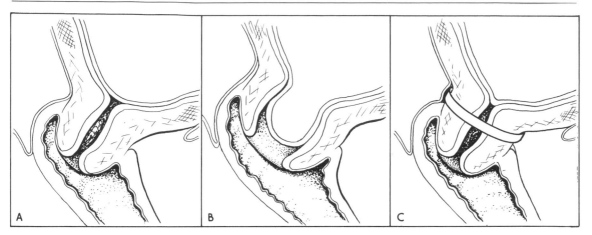

**Fig. 22/7** Cervical incompetence. (A) Normal cervix at 16 weeks; (B) Incompetent cervix at 16 weeks; (C) 'Circlage' with an unabsorbable suture

history of two or more abortions, occurring after the 14th week of pregnancy and usually starting with painless leaking of liquor amnii; (2) the easy passage through the cervix of a Hegar sound, size 8, when the patient is non-pregnant, and the absence of internal os 'snap' on its withdrawal; (3) the finding in pregnancy of a gradual and painless dilatation of the internal os until it is more than 3cm dilated; (4) its detection by ultrasound.

Recently ultrasound has been shown to enable the obstetrician to make the diagnosis at an earlier stage than the clinical finding described in (3), and should be used increasingly in these cases.

When cervical incompetence is thought to be the cause of the habitual abortion, a soft unabsorbable suture, such as Mersilk 4, is placed around the cervico-vaginal mucosa, or submucosally, at the level of the internal os and this is tied (Fig. **22/7**). The patient remains in bed for 3 to 5 days and then can go home, but should rest adequately through the remainder of the pregnancy. The use of progesterone during and after the operation has no valid basis. The operation should not be done if there is infection or if the membranes have ruptured. Should abortion become inevitable despite the suture, it must be cut; otherwise it is left until about 7 days before term when it is divided and the patient permitted to deliver vaginally.

### The treatment of recurrent abortion

If a specific cause for recurrent abortion is found treatment can be given. Uterine myomata may be

extirpated by myomectomy; cervical incompetence treated as described; endometrial infection treated with doxycycline or trimethoprim-sulphamethoxazole. Chromosomal abnormalities are untreatable but over half of the patients will subsequently deliver a live child. The use of injections of donor leucocytes has been mentioned.

Women with diagnosed SLE may produce a viable infant if treated during pregnancy with corticosteroids or aspirin, although the results are unimpressive. If the woman is found to have an apparent immunological cause for recurrent abortion, pre-pregnancy treatment with paternal or donor leucocytes may be effective, but this approach is still experimental.

In over 50 per cent of patients, no aetiological cause is found. For these patients 'tender loving care' and supportive psychotherapy is associated with the birth of a live baby in over 80 per cent of cases.

In all cases the patient should be given an adequate diet, cease smoking and once she becomes pregnant should avoid all travel, discontinue coitus and should go to bed for 2 hours each afternoon. The results from this regimen are as good as those following the use of hormones, vitamins, metallic chemicals, thyroid extract or acupuncture, and are far less expensive and time-consuming.

### THERAPEUTIC ABORTION

In the past 20 years, legally induced abortion has

become possible in many countries, although the regulations permitting legal abortion vary considerably. In some countries abortion may be performed legally in the first 28 weeks of pregnancy; in others the operation may only be performed in the first 20 or 24 weeks. In addition, in countries where abortion is illegal, large numbers of women obtain an 'illegal' abortion. The purpose of legalizing abortion was to enable all women, irrespective of social or economic status, to obtain an abortion performed by a trained health professional in hygienic surroundings; and to obtain counselling before and after the operation. To a large extent these objectives have been met.

The indications for therapeutic abortion are listed in Table **22/3**. Over 95 per cent of abortions are performed for social or psychiatric reasons. Most of these could have been avoided if one or other of the couple had used a reliable (or any) contraceptive.

**The sequelae of induced abortion**

If the abortion is performed in a well-equipped clinic or hospital by a trained surgeon, complications are few. Less than 1 per cent of women develop infection or post-abortal haemorrhage requiring a curettage. The mortality from induced abortion is less than 1 per 100 000 (when abortion is performed before week

* *Social*
* *Psychiatric:* severe neuroses, psychoses
* *Medical*
    Severe cardiac disease, heart failure
    Severe chronic renal disease, renal failure
    Malignant disease, especially breast or uterine
        cervix
* *Fetal*
    Viral infections
    Haemolytic disease
    Genetic defects
    Congenital defects incompatible with normal life
        (e.g. anencephaly, spina bifida)

**Table 22/3** Indications for therapeutic abortion

13) and rises to 12 per 100 000 (when the abortion is performed after the 13th gestational week).

**The effect of abortion on future fertility and obstetric success**

Provided the abortion is performed in an appropriate place by a skilled gynaecologist and, preferably, before the 12th week of pregnancy, it is not associated with any reduction in fertility or any increase in spontaneous abortion, preterm birth or fetal loss in a subsequent pregnancy. However, recurrent induced abortions may increase the risk of fetal loss in a subsequent pregnancy.

# INTRA-UTERINE DEATH OF THE FETUS

**Before the 20th week**

Death of the fetus may occur in the early weeks of pregnancy when it usually leads to an abortion, although in a few patients the dead fetus is retained in utero and the condition is one of missed abortion. In these cases sufficient placental tissue survives to produce progesterone which damps down the tendency of the uterus to expel the contained conceptus. Clinically the patient complains of a dirty brown discharge which initially is thought to be due to a threatened abortion, particularly as the pregnancy test is positive. However, the vaginal discharge continues and subsequent confirmation of the fetal death may be obtained by noting that the uterus fails to

increase in size, or by making a real-time ultrasound examination to detect if the fetal heart is beating.

**After the 20th week**

It is usual for fetal movements to become apparent to the mother by the 20th week, and intra-uterine fetal death after this time may be suggested by the cessation of fetal movements. This symptom is only suggestive, as even in normal pregnancy fetal movements may not be felt for periods of up to 3 days. Auscultation may reveal the absence of a fetal heart beat, but once again this finding is only suggestive as the fetal heart may be difficult to detect, particularly in obese patients.

The diagnosis of intra-uterine fetal death can be confirmed by using real-time ultrasonic scanning or by applying a fetal heart detection machine to the patient's abdomen. The absence of fetal heart movements using real-time ultrasonic scanning or the absence of heart sounds using a fetal heart detector confirms the diagnosis. Both machines can detect fetal heart activity as early as the 12th gestational week.

Apart from the psychological upset if an expectant mother knows she has a dead fetus, medical problems are unlikely, at least in the first 3 weeks after intra-uterine death. During this time, labour starts spontaneously in between 70 and 90 per cent of cases and a macerated fetus is expelled.

Three to four weeks after fetal death, an increasing risk of hypofibrinogenaemia occurs and this may have serious consequences. If spontaneous delivery of the fetus does not occur within 3 weeks of its death, or within a week of diagnosis, measures to induce labour should be started.

## Treatment

When both fetus and placenta die, the uterus contracts to expel the foreign body. When the fetus dies, but the placenta continues to produce progesterone, the establishment of spontaneous uterine activity is prevented. Uterine activity leading to the expulsion of the dead fetus can be established by the use of prostaglandins or by an intravenous oxytocin infusion, but most authorities prefer to use prostaglandins. Prostaglandins may be given by the intra-amniotic, the extra-amniotic or the vaginal route. The last is the least invasive and avoids the risk of infection. Prostaglandin $E_2$ in a 'Tylose' gel is used. The dose depends on the duration of the pregnancy. Before the 30th week PGE 15mg is advised; after the 30th week PGE 5mg is sufficient. If expulsion is not in progress 12 to 18 hours after the insertion, an oxytocin infusion is set up. The mean time for expulsion is 15 hours; and about 80 per cent of women require an oxytocin infusion. Gastro-intestinal side-effects occur in about 20 per cent of women.

In cases of prolonged intra-uterine death of the fetus, frequent checks must be made to detect maternal hypofibrinogenaemia, either by observing the clotting time of venous blood or by using the 'Fibrindex' test which estimates the actual fibrinogen level. If the blood fails to clot within 10 minutes, or the clot forms poorly and soon dissolves, or if the serum fibrinogen level is less than 100mg per 100ml, fibrinogen 2 to 6g must be given intravenously.

## Chapter 23

# Ectopic Gestation (Tubal Pregnancy)

Ectopic gestation is the condition when the fertilized ovum fails to reach the uterine cavity and becomes implanted in some part of the oviduct (the Fallopian tube) or rarely, in the ovary. The incidence of ectopic pregnancy has increased in the developed countries from 1 in 250 conceptions to 1 in 150 conceptions and now equals that in the developing countries. The reason for the increase is not clear, but may be due to an increase in pelvic inflammatory disease, or to earlier diagnosis using ultrasound. The latter is suggested as between 15 and 50 per cent of ectopic gestations spontaneously abort or are resorbed. There is no evidence that induced abortions or the use of an IUD as a contraceptive are factors.

The right and left tubes are involved with equal frequency, and rarely a tubal pregnancy may occur in both tubes.

## AETIOLOGY

Despite many theories the aetiology of tubal pregnancy remains unknown. Implantation can only occur when the zona pellucida has been partially or completely shed. This usually takes place in the uterine cavity but in tubal pregnancy it must occur earlier. This could be because (1) an ovum released just prior to menstruation is impregnated and its passage down the tube is delayed by the back flow of menstrual blood; or (2) the progress of the fertilized ovum down the tube is delayed by mechanical

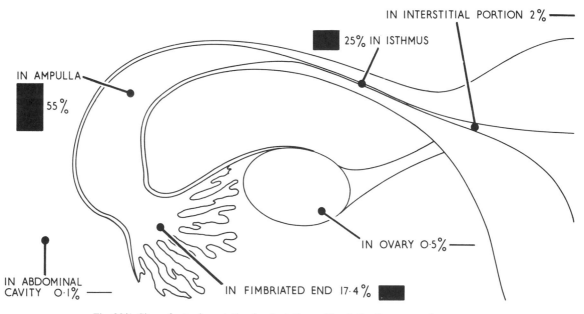

IN INTERSTITIAL PORTION 2%

25% IN ISTHMUS

IN AMPULLA

55%

IN OVARY 0·5%

IN ABDOMINAL CAVITY 0·1%

IN FIMBRIATED END 17·4%

**Fig. 23/1** Sites of ectopic gestation implantation, with relative frequency of occurrence

factors such as increased tortuosity or agglutination of the tubal endothelium caused by previous low-grade infection.

## PATHOLOGY

Implantation may occur in (1) the fimbriated end (17 per cent); (2) the ampulla (55 per cent); (3) the isthmus (25 per cent); (4) the interstitial portion (2 per cent); and rarely (5) the ovary (0.5 per cent); or (6) the abdominal cavity (0.1 per cent) (Fig. **23/1**).

Under the influence of hormones synthesized by the corpus luteum and the invading trophoblast, the uterus enlarges and a complete decidua is formed. In the tube only a slight decidual reaction occurs with enlargement of the stromal cells of the tube wall, and some hypertrophy of the tubal muscle fibres and blood vessel walls. The further sequence of

events depends upon the site of implantation, as the degree the weakened tube can distend before it ruptures varies with the calibre and thickness of the part of the oviduct involved and the degree of tropho-blastic activity.

If the ovum implants in the fimbriated end or ampulla of the tube, the trophoblast initially erodes capillaries supplying the convoluted epithelial covered folds of mucosa. The resulting haemorrhage is usually slight, but may be sufficient to separate the ovum from its attachment to the mucosa leading to a tubal abortion. More active trophoblastic invasion maintains the viability of the ovum but causes repeated episodes of haemorrhage from deeper vessels of the tube wall at the implantation site, and some of this blood gravitates from the tube lumen into the peritoneal sac. As the ovum grows the tube becomes progressively distended and trophoblastic invasion through the muscularis further weakens this

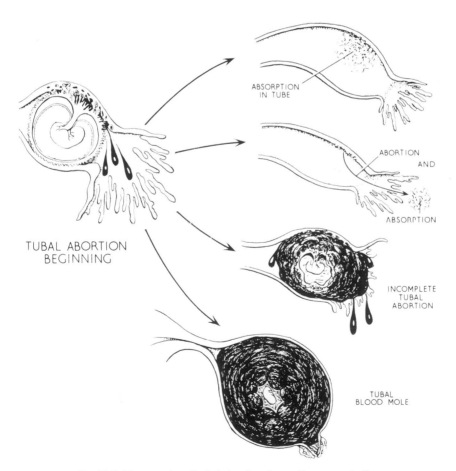

ABSORPTION
IN TUBE

ABORTION
AND
ABSORPTION

INCOMPLETE
TUBAL
ABORTION

TUBAL ABORTION
BEGINNING

TUBAL
BLOOD MOLE

**Fig. 23/2** The sequelae of tubal abortion shown diagrammatically

layer with more episodes of bleeding. The gradual penetration of the tubal wall finally leads to a small rupture. This is usually sealed at once by blood clot, but repeated episodes lead to a peritubal haematoma. If the rupture is larger, part of the ovum is extruded through the rent by the peristalsis of the tube, and bleeding persists which covers the surface of the ovum with clots or gravitates to the pouch of Douglas. In both of these cases a marked local peritoneal reaction occurs and the mass is covered by exudate, adherent omentum and bowel. In time a thick layer of exudate covers the blood in the pouch of Douglas, which is now called a 'pelvic haematocele'. Should the invading trophoblast erode a large vessel at the time of tubal penetration, severe internal haemorrhage into the peritoneal cavity, or between the layers of the broad ligament occurs (a pelvic haematoma) with the sudden collapse of the patient.

If the implantation is in the isthmus, where the mucosa is thinner and the vessels larger, penetration of the muscularis and tubal rupture occurs earlier and internal haemorrhage is usually severe, whilst if the implantation is in the interstitial portion of the oviduct, rupture is often delayed as the myometrium surrounds the growing conceptus; but eventually it does occur and is attended by severe haemorrhage.

## OUTCOME FOR THE PREGNANCY

In most cases the pregnancy terminates between the 6th and 10th week of pregnancy in one of several ways.

### Tubal abortion

This occurs in 65 per cent of cases and is the usual termination in fimbrial and ampullary implantation. Repeated small haemorrhages from the invaded area of the tubal wall separate the ovum, which dies, and is either (1) absorbed completely; or (2) aborted completely through the tubal ostium into the peritoneal cavity; or (3) aborted incompletely so that the clot-covered conceptus distends the ostium; or (4) forms a tubal blood mole (Fig. 23/2).

### Tubal rupture

This occurs in 35 per cent of cases, and is more common when the implantation is in the isthmus.

Whilst rupture of the ampulla usually occurs between the 6th and 10th week, rupture of the isthmus occurs earlier, frequently at the time of the first missed period. The trophoblast burrows deeply and eventually erodes the serosal coat of the tube, the final break being sudden or gradual. Usually the ovum is extruded through the rent and bleeding continues. If the rupture is on the mesenteric side of the tube, a broad ligament haematoma will form (Fig. 23/3).

### Secondary abdominal pregnancy

Very rarely the extruded ovum continues to grow as sufficient trophoblast maintains its connection with the tubal epithelium and later the trophoblast covering the ovisac attaches to abdominal organs. A few of these pregnancies advance to term and in a few the fetus dies early and is converted into a lithopaedion (mummified).

## CLINICAL ASPECTS

The possibility of an ectopic gestation should always be considered in a woman of childbearing age. The history is of greater importance than the physical signs, as these can be equivocal. Usually there is a short period of *amenorrhoea*, although in 20 per cent of cases this may not be present. The *pain* is lower abdominal in site, but not distinguishable from that of abortion. However, in ruptured ectopic gestation, fainting is usual although this may only be momentary. Vaginal bleeding follows the pain and may be mistaken for bleeding due to a delayed menstrual period or an abortion. The bleeding is slight, brownish in colour and continuous, and clots are rarely present (Table 23/1).

Two clinical patterns occur, and are due to the extent of the damage to the tube wall by the invading trophoblast. The first is subacute, the second acute.

|  | *Percentage* |
|---|---|
| Abdominal pain | 90 |
| Amenorrhoea | 80 |
| Vaginal bleeding | 70 |
| Adnexal tenderness | 80 |
| Abdominal tenderness | 80 |
| Adnexal mass | 50 |

Table 23/1 Symptoms and signs in ectopic gestation

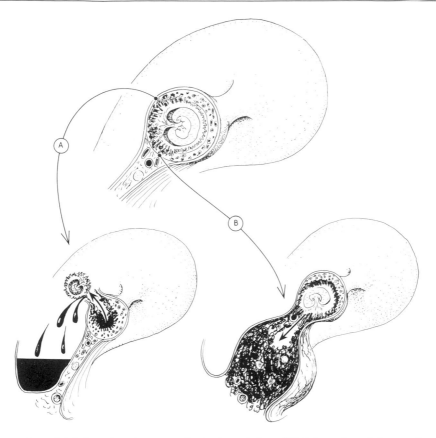

**Fig. 23/3** The sequelae of tubal rupture in cases of ectopic gestation. (A) Intraperitoneal haemorrhage and pelvic haematocele; (B) broad ligament haematoma

**Subacute**

After a short period of amenorrhoea, the patient complains of some lower abdominal discomfort, which may be so mild that she considers it due to normal pregnancy. Occasionally there is an attack of sharp pain and faintness, due to an episode of intraperitoneal bleeding, and if these symptoms are marked she will seek advice, particularly if the episode is followed by slight bleeding. Examination may reveal tenderness in the lower abdomen, and vaginal examination may show a tender fornix, or a vague mass, but the signs may be insufficient to make a diagnosis. If the patient is observed, further episodes of pain will occur, and the vaginal bleeding, usually brown in colour, continues until acute collapse supervenes (indicating tubal rupture or incomplete tubal abortion) or the symptoms cease (indicating complete abortion with or without pelvic haematocele).

**Acute-dramatic**

Sudden collapse with little or no warning is more common when the implantation is isthmal, but is not the most frequent event. It is more usual for the acute tubal rupture to supervene upon the subacute, but the mild symptoms of the latter may have been thought to be normal occurrences in pregnancy and ignored.

As the tube ruptures the patient is seized with a sudden acute lower abdominal pain, sufficiently severe to cause fainting. The associated internal haemorrhage leads to rapid collapse, with pallor, a weak pulse with a rising rate and a falling blood pressure. Usually the condition improves after a short time, as the haemorrhage diminishes or ceases, but abdominal discomfort persists and pain is felt in the epigastrium and referred to the shoulder. A further episode of haemorrhage and collapse is likely, and continued bleeding can be suspected from increasing pallor and a falling haemoglobin level.

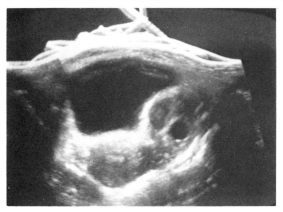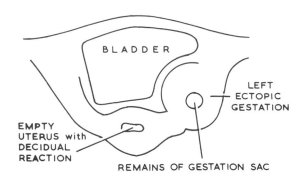

**Fig. 23/4** Ectopic gestation (transverse scan). Line drawing shows identification of relevant points

On examination the patient is shocked, the lower abdomen is tender with some fullness and muscle guarding. Vaginal examination, which should only be carried out in hospital, shows extreme tenderness in the fornices and marked tenderness on movement of the cervix from side to side.

## DIAGNOSIS

Although in acute cases the presence of internal bleeding is obvious and the diagnosis not in doubt, in subacute cases it can be extraordinarily difficult. Laboratory tests may help, but in most instances are not particularly informative. In ectopic gestation, an immunological pregnancy test is positive in 75 per cent of cases which is not very specific. However, if facilities are available for a radio immunoassay for the beta sub-unit of HCG, the accuracy of the procedure is increased. A negative result (<1ng/ml) indicates that the woman is not pregnant, and ectopic gestation can be excluded. If the ßHCG test is positive, a pelvic ultrasound examination should be made, preferably using a transvaginal probe. If this shows an empty uterus (Fig. **23/4**), and particularly if it shows a sac and fetus in the Fallopian tube the diagnosis is certain and a laparotomy should be made. On the other hand, if ultrasound shows an intra-uterine pregnancy, a concurrent ectopic pregnancy is extremely unlikely. If the diagnosis remains in doubt a laparoscopy will clear the matter up.

If ultrasound is not available, or is equivocal, the presumptive diagnosis may be confirmed by laparoscopy.

Diagnosis of suspected ectopic gestation is summarized in Table **23/2**.

## TREATMENT

Whenever tubal pregnancy is suspected the patient must be transferred to hospital, *without a vaginal examination*, provided she is not in shock. If she is, this must be treated first by adequate, rapid blood transfusion if this service is available. If it is not, the patient should be laid flat, morphine or pethidine given to reduce the pain, and an intravenous infusion of saline or a plasma expander given. With this first-aid treatment the patient's condition usually improves sufficiently for her to be taken to hospital.

As soon as the diagnosis of ectopic gestation is made in hospital, laparotomy should be performed *at once*, even if the patient is collapsed. Blood transfusion should be started as soon after admission as possible and continued throughout the operation. When donor blood is not available, auto-transfusion using the blood sucked from the peritoneal cavity can be used. This is collected into bottles containing 200ml sodium citrate per litre and retransfused intravenously.

After opening the abdomen through a sub-umbilical midline incision, the uterus is grasped and brought up into the wound, and the ruptured tube isolated. Before deciding on further treatment the other tube and ovary should be inspected. Partial salpingectomy, by clamping the tube on each side of the damaged area and excising the wedge, or total salpingectomy is the preferred treatment and can be performed rapidly. If the patient desires further children and the implantation is fimbrial or ampullary, the other tube being absent or damaged, salpingostomy is possible. This will give her a 5 per cent chance of a further pregnancy, and in selected patients may be the operation of choice. If the implanta-

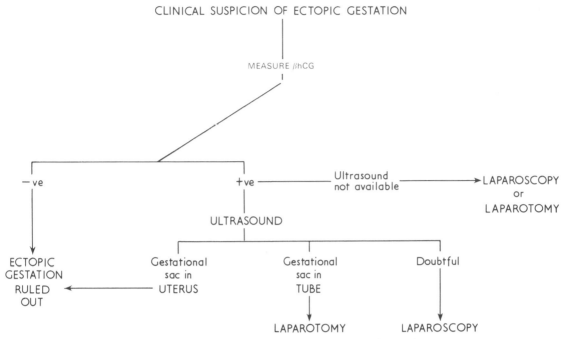

CLINICAL SUSPICION OF ECTOPIC GESTATION

MEASURE βhCG

−ve

+ve ——————— Ultrasound → LAPAROSCOPY
not available          or
LAPAROTOMY

ULTRASOUND

ECTOPIC
GESTATION
RULED   ←   Gestational    Gestational    Doubtful
OUT         sac in          sac in
            UTERUS          TUBE

            LAPAROTOMY    LAPAROSCOPY

**Table 23/2** Algorithm for diagnosis of suspected ectopic gestation

tion is interstitial, the damaged cornual area of the uterus must be excised and sutured with haemostatic sutures. Occasionally the damage to the uterus may necessitate hysterectomy, and the operation may also be required if there is uterine pathology and the patient is able to tolerate the more extensive procedure.

In cases of intraligamentary bleeding, the broad ligament is opened after salpingectomy and the contained blood clot evacuated. Where the bleeding was intraperitoneal all the free blood and clots should be removed before closing the abdominal wall. This makes for a smoother convalescence and a reduced risk of damage to the remaining tube.

Recent developments using laparoscopic lasers have enabled experienced surgeons to remove the gestation sac from the Fallopian tube and to save the tube in many cases of ectopic gestation.

## PROGNOSIS

Only 60 per cent of patients who have had an ectopic gestation become pregnant again. Of the women who do not have a further pregnancy, 75 per cent avoid pregnancy voluntarily, and 25 per cent are involuntarily infertile. The risk of a second ectopic gestation is about 10 per cent, as compared with 0.4 per cent in other women. The chance of delivering a term baby is about 50 per cent. Patients who have previously had an ectopic gestation therefore require additional care during pregnancy.

# Chapter 24

# Antepartum Haemorrhage

In about 3 per cent of pregnancies significant bleeding from the birth canal occurs after the 20th week of gestation and this is referred to as antepartum haemorrhage. The adjective 'significant' is used to distinguish this form of bleeding from the 'show' which occurs at the onset of labour, although it must be admitted that in certain cases when the show is heavy, no distinction can be made. All the conditions causing antepartum haemorrhage may operate before the 20th week of pregnancy and may cause abortion, so the division is arbitrary, merely indicating that after the 20th week there is a chance of fetal survival.

The main forms of antepartum haemorrhage are: (1) placenta praevia; and (2) accidental haemorrhage or abruptio placentae. They were distinguished originally in 1775 by Edward Rigby in Norwich. Bleeding may also occur from local conditions of the cervix, such as cervicitis, cervical polyps or carcinoma, but the last is rare.

The incidence of the types of antepartum haemorrhage can be seen in Table **24/1**, and it should be noted that two important principles govern the management of all forms of antepartum haemorrhage. These are: (1) do not examine the patient vaginally before admission to hospital; and (2) do not treat the patient in a hospital which has no blood transfusion service and is not equipped for all obstetric operations.

|  | Proportional percentage | |
|---|---|---|
| Placenta praevia | 18 | |
| Abruptio placenta | 80 | 2–3 per cent |
| Mild* | 55 | of |
| Moderate | 20 | all |
| Severe | 5 | pregnancies |
| Cervical bleeding | 2 | |

Table **24/1** The relative prevalence of various types of antepartum haemorrhage (source: Hospital reports)

* Many of these cases are classified as 'antepartum haemorrhage of unknown aetiology', in some hospital reports

# PLACENTA PRAEVIA

In this condition the placenta is either wholly, or partially, implanted in the lower uterine segment, and therefore lies before (praevia) the presenting part. It occurs in 0.5 per cent of all pregnancies and accounts for 20 to 40 per cent of all cases of antepartum haemorrhage. It is twice as common in multigravidae (incidence 1 in 90 deliveries) as in primigravidae (incidence 1 in 250 deliveries). Apart from this association no definite aetiological factor has been found.

## CLASSIFICATION

The greater the proportion of the placenta lying in the lower uterine segment, the greater is the likelihood of complications and for this reason various classifications have been suggested.

### Minor (20 per cent of all cases)

The edge of the placenta dips into the lower part of the uterus but does not reach the internal os.

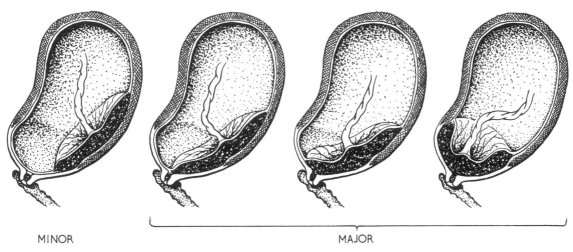

MINOR                                          MAJOR

**Fig. 24/1** Types of placenta praevia

**Marginal (30 per cent of cases)**

The edge of the placenta reaches the margin of the internal os. Two types can be differentiated: one when the placenta is implanted mainly upon the anterior uterine wall, and the other when the implantation is mainly on the posterior wall.

**Major (50 per cent of cases)**

The placenta covers the internal os either partially or completely.

Today, as cases of marginal and major placenta praevia are treated by caesarean section, the classification may be amended to the two groups, *minor* and *major* (Fig. **24/1**).

## CAUSE OF THE BLEEDING

The growth of the placenta both in size and weight slows down after the 30th week of pregnancy, yet at this time the lower segment is increasing in length. Shearing stresses between the placental trophoblast and the maternal venous blood sinuses may occur, leading to an episode of bleeding. Bleeding may also be initiated by coitus, the movement of the penis against the fornices causing damage to thin walls of the venous sinuses of the placental bed.

The first episode of bleeding may occur at any period of gestation and in one series studied personally, it occurred between the 28th and 31st week in 10 per cent, between the 32nd and 35th week in 30 per cent and after the 36th week in 60 per cent of cases. The cases in which bleeding occurs before the 36th week require the greatest degree of clinical judgement for proper treatment.

## SYMPTOMS AND SIGNS

1. The bleeding is painless, causeless and recurrent, and although the first episode is usually slight this is not invariable, and in a few cases the bleeding coincides with the onset of labour, so that confusion may arise.

2. The presenting part is usually high and often not central above the pelvic brim. Contrary to the usual view, malpresentations are not more frequent in cases of placenta praevia, particularly when the period of gestation at which the first bleed occurs is taken into account.

## DIAGNOSIS

Clinical confirmation of the diagnosis can only be made by seeing that the placenta is praevia at operation, or by feeling placental tissue on vaginal examination. The latter examination should never be performed when placenta praevia is suspected except in a fully equipped operating theatre with everything in readiness for an immediate caesarean section should torrential bleeding be provoked by the examination.

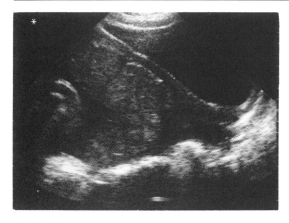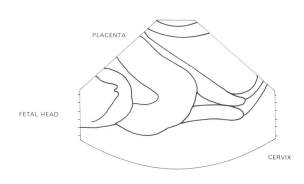

**Fig. 24/2** Sagittal section, major degree of placenta, previa in fourth quarter. Cervix and vagina on right

Today with the availability of ultrasound, placenta praevia can be confirmed soon after the patient's admission to hospital by arranging for an ultrasound picture. Ultrasound identifies the position of the placenta, its thickness and its relationship to the cervix (Fig. **24/2**). When a placenta praevia of major degree is identified by ultrasound, a vaginal examination should not be made, as delivery will be by caesarean section.

## MANAGEMENT

### At home

A patient with antepartum haemorrhage should be transferred to hospital as soon as possible, so that a diagnosis may be made and treatment instituted. On no account should a vaginal examination be performed. If the bleeding is slight or has ceased prior to the arrival of the doctor, the general condition of the patient should be checked, the abdomen palpated gently, a sedative given and the patient transferred to hospital. If bleeding is heavier and continuing, a blood transfusion should be given before the transfer.

### In hospital

Examination of the patient will determine her condition, and that of the fetus, whether bleeding is continuing or whether labour has started. In all cases the patient's haemoglobin must be ascertained and blood loss replaced. Extra blood of a suitable group should be reserved and kept readily available should a further haemorrhage occur.

The object of treatment is to prolong the pregnancy until the 37th week so that a more mature fetus can be born (provided this can be done without additional risk to the mother). This is accomplished by a regimen of 'expectant treatment'.

## EXPECTANT TREATMENT

About 40 per cent of the patients with placenta praevia will be admitted before the 36th week, and in this group expectant treatment should be practised provided the baby is alive and vaginal bleeding ceases soon after admission. The patient is confined to bed. No vaginal examination is performed, but a general assessment of her condition is made. A blood transfusion is given if indicated. With this regimen bleeding usually ceases quickly but bed rest is continued for 5 to 7 days. During this time an ultrasound examination is made and, when appropriate, the cervix is inspected with a vaginal speculum to make sure that a local condition is not the cause of the bleeding. This examination is made whether bleeding has ceased or not. Expectant treatment is continued until the 37th week provided that no further severe haemorrhage occurs and the fetus remains alive. In many patients further episodes of slight bleeding occur and are treated with sedation and blood transfusion if required.

If the diagnosis of placenta praevia is confirmed by ultrasonic examination or suspected clinically, the patient is kept in hospital, and often in bed, until the 37th week. At this time she is taken to the operating theatre, anaesthetized and either examined vaginally and labour induced by amniotomy or she is operated upon without prior vaginal examination, depending on the certainty of the diagnosis and the degree of placenta praevia. The 37th week is chosen as at this period of gestation the fetal loss is no greater than at term, and continued expectant treatment may lead to a further episode of haemorrhage.

## ACTIVE TREATMENT

If the patient is admitted on or after the 37th week expectant treatment has no place and delivery should be effected as soon as possible.

The method of delivery will depend upon the degree of placenta praevia. If the degree is minor amniotomy is usually sufficient to control the blood loss and initiate labour. After amniotomy, the fetal head descends into the pelvis and presses upon the damaged venous sinuses preventing further blood loss. If the placenta is marginal and implanted posteriorly, pressure by the fetal head may lead to a reduced oxygen exchange as the placenta is compacted between the bony sacral promontory and the bony skull, and for this type lower segment caesarean section is recommended. Placenta praevia of major degree is treated by caesarean section, even if the baby has died in utero. Except in areas remote from adequate medical aid, and then only rarely, there is no place for penetrating the placenta with the fingers, seizing and bringing down a fetal leg to act as a haemostatic.

## COMPLICATIONS OF PLACENTA PRAEVIA

In pregnancy the haemorrhage can be severe, and lead to intra-uterine death from anoxia. This is more common when the mother is anaemic. Following delivery, owing to the erosion, by trophoblast, of the poorly supported veins of the lower uterine segment, postpartum haemorrhage may occur. This should be anticipated and oxytocics given as the baby is delivered. In a few cases haemorrhage will continue despite treatment and caesarean hysterectomy may be required. For these reasons placenta praevia should only be treated by obstetricians qualified to cope with these complications and in a well-equipped hospital: it is not a case for the occasional obstetrician.

## MATERNAL AND FETAL MORTALITY

In good hands, and provided no vaginal examination has been performed before admission, the *maternal mortality* should be very low. Unfortunately, these conditions are not always met, and the mortality varies between 0.1 and 3 per cent. Deaths are due to haemorrhage, particularly postpartum, infection, and trauma from unskilled intra-uterine manipulations.

The *fetal mortality* varies between 5 and 15 per cent and the principal causes of fetal death are intra-uterine death from hypoxia due to placental separation and maternal anaemia; prematurity, and fetal abnormalities. Prematurity can be avoided by expectant treatment, which is the reason for the method; but fetal abnormalities are twice as common in cases of placenta praevia as in normal cases.

# ABRUPTIO PLACENTAE

In abruptio placentae the bleeding follows separation of a normally implanted placenta. Rigby differentiated this type of bleeding from the 'inevitable' bleeding of placenta praevia and wrote that 'the separation of the placenta must be owing to some accidental circumstance, to violence done by blows or falls, to some peculiar laxity of the uterine vessels from badness of habit or fever, or to some influence of passion of mind suddenly excited such as anger, fear, etc.'

## INCIDENCE AND CLASSIFICATION

Abruptio placentae, or accidental haemorrhage, occurs in 2 per cent of pregnancies, and accounts for about 60 per cent of all cases of antepartum haemorrhage. The older classification, in which the haemorrhage was divided into revealed, concealed or mixed, has now been replaced by a clinical classification which depends on the degree of placental separation and on the assessment of certain signs and

| | Mild | Severity of bleeding | |
| --- | --- | --- | --- |
| | | Moderate | Severe |
| Pulse | No change | Raised | Raised |
| Blood pressure | No change | Lowered | Lowered |
| Shock | None | Often | Always |
| Oliguria | Rare | Occasionally | Common |
| Hypofibrinogenaemia | Rare | Occasionally | Common |
| Uterus | Normal | Tender | Tender and tense |
| Fetus | Alive | Usually dead | Dead |
| Blood loss in pints (litres) | Less than one (2) | 1–3 (2–6) | 3–6 (6–12) |

**Table 24/2** Comparison of the clinical picture in the various grades of accidental haemorrhage

symptoms. In this, cases are divided into the groups of mild, moderate and severe placental separation, and the amount of haemorrhage parallels the degree of separation. About 70 per cent of cases are classified as mild, 25 per cent as moderate and 5 per cent as severe abruptio placentae (Table **24/2**).

Ultrasound is helpful in confirming the diagnosis and may help to establish the size of the retroplacental clot objectively. In cases of mild separation serial weekly ultrasound will establish whether further retroplacental bleeding has occurred, but the cost-benefit of this procedure is questionable.

## AETIOLOGY

The aetiology of abruptio placentae is obscure, and the only relevant association is with high multiparity. In a personal series the incidence amongst primigravidae was only 0.7 per cent, but amongst patients pregnant for the sixth time or more it was 3.0 per cent. Hypertensive disease or pregnancy-induced hypertension is found in association in about 15 per cent of cases, and the more severe the haemorrhage the higher is the incidence of hypertension. In a few patients (about 3 per cent) trauma, either due to external version or injury, is a cause.

## PATHOLOGY

The cause of the bleeding is damage to the walls of the maternal venous sinuses in the placental bed. The uterine vessels of the high multigravida contain a larger proportion of fibrous and elastic tissue amongst the muscle bundles, and perhaps this leads

to vascular dysfunction at the decidua–placental interface, with subsequent rupture. The hypertensive episodes in pregnancy-induced hypertension would add to the risk of rupture, and this could account for the higher incidence of pregnancy-induced hypertension amongst the severe group.

The bleeding separates the placenta to a greater or lesser degree, and the blood eventually escapes into the vagina by separating the membranes. When the haemorrhage is severe, and the intra-uterine tension high, some of the blood is forced outwards from the placental bed, between the muscle fibres towards the serosal coat of the uterus. In extreme cases the damage is marked and the uterus has the appearance of an oedematous, bruised organ with splits in the serosal coat. The condition was first described by Couvelaire as *apopléxie utéroplacentaire*.

The extravasation of blood into the placental bed and between the uterine muscle fibres may have three further effects, but these are unusual except in cases of severe abruption. They are: (1) shock; (2) blood coagulation defects; and (3) oliguria or anuria.

### Shock

The shock is due to hypovolaemia and to the effects of the distraction and separation of the muscle fibres. It is analogous to that found in crush injury. An additional factor may be the profound changes resulting from the release of thromboplastins from the damaged decidua–placental interface into the general systemic circulation. It is important to remember that the degree of shock is often much greater than would be expected from the blood lost through the vagina.

## Blood coagulation defects

These result from the release into the systemic circulation of large quantities of thromboplastins following the retroplacental clotting and its associated damage to the decidua and placenta. This results in widespread intravascular coagulation. The fibrin microthrombi are rapidly dissolved by circulating fibrinolysins (mainly plasmin which is released from its inert precursor, plasminogen).

Lysis of fibrin results in the release of fibrin degradation products (FDP). FDP prevent platelet aggregation, the polymerization of fibrin monomers and act as thromboplastins. Since the conversion of maternal fibrinogen into fibrin takes place more rapidly than the liver is able to synthesize fresh fibrinogen, a progressive deficiency occurs, with clinical hypofibrinogenaemia. At the same time there is a decrease in plasminogen levels, platelet disturbance, a fall in factors II, V and VIII, and increased levels of FDP. The result is a tendency to haemorrhage in many organs of the body if they are traumatized. The coagulation defects are rare except in severe abruptio placentae.

If this postulated sequence of events is correct, treatment with fibrinogen or fibrinolysin inhibitors is, in general, undesirable. Infused fibrinogen will immediately be converted into fibrin and will be lysed immediately, which leads to an increase in FDP levels. Similarly, the administration of fibrinolytic inhibitors may be hazardous as vascular occlusion from small fibrin deposits may occur.

The multifactorial nature of the coagulation disturbance suggests that adequate transfusion of *fresh* whole blood (which is also needed to correct the hypovolaemia) is the most rational method of treatment, and the rapid restoration to normal of the coagulation defects following vaginal delivery without trauma emphasizes that therapy is rarely required.

## Oliguria and anuria

Oliguria is initially due to the effects of hypovolaemia but may be aggravated by the intravascular microthrombi and the altered platelet adhesiveness occasioned by the fibrin degradation products. Several recent studies have shown that in conditions of intravascular microthrombosis and platelet aggregation, the microthrombi and the platelets are deposited on the endothelium of the vessels of the glomerular tufts in the kidney, and may occlude

them. If the occlusion is marked and sufficient glomerular capillaries are involved, the blood supply to the tubules may be diminished or eliminated, with resulting ischaemia and acute tubular necrosis. This explanation of the oliguria is more likely than the previous belief that oliguria was due to spasm of the interlobular arterioles of the kidney due in turn to the utero-renal reflex. If the ischaemia is of short duration, no changes occur; if of longer duration, reversible tubal necrosis may arise; and when of long duration irreversible cortical necrosis is likely.

## SIGNS AND SYMPTOMS

The degree of haemorrhage, of shock, and the incidence of complications is related to the amount of placental separation and, as has been noted, patients can be divided into three groups. These are shown in Table **24/2**.

### Mild separation

The amount of placental separation and of haemorrhage is slight (less than 500ml having been lost), and is not accompanied by any disturbance of the maternal or fetal condition. The patient is not shocked, the baby is alive and the uterus is not tender. Non-stress fetal monitoring (p. 278) establishes that his condition is good. With so little disturbance the condition may be indistinguishable from placenta praevia, or bleeding due to cervical conditions unless an ultrasound picture is made. Mild separation accounts for about 60 per cent of cases of abruptio placentae.

### Moderate separation

At least one-quarter of the placenta has been separated and at least 1000ml of blood has been lost to the circulation in cases in this group. Some of the blood will escape vaginally, and some will infiltrate between the uterine muscle fibres. The patient is often shocked with a low blood pressure and a raised pulse rate, but in 5 per cent of cases the pulse rate is normal until after delivery when it rises precipitately. The patient complains of abdominal pain and the uterus is tender owing to the blood infiltration. Pregnancy-induced hypertension is associated in 24 per cent of cases. The fetus is rendered hypoxic by the separation, signs of fetal distress are usual, and intra-uterine fetal death frequent.

### Severe separation

This degree of separation constitutes an obstetric emergency, as at least two-thirds of the placenta will have been separated and at least 2000ml of blood will have been lost to the body. Some of this blood is forced between the muscle fibres, more is retained behind the placenta as a retroplacental clot and only a moderate amount escapes vaginally. The patient is always shocked, and the degree of shock cannot always be related to the amount of blood seen externally. Since pregnancy-induced hypertension is present in 36 per cent of cases, the blood pressure may be normal despite other evidence of severe shock. The uterus is tender and tense because of the amount of haemorrhagic infiltration, and abdominal pain may be marked. The fetus is almost always dead. Coagulation defects and oliguria are most frequently found in association with this group.

## TREATMENT

### Mild haemorrhage

If the patient is not in labour, and pregnancy has not reached the 37th week treatment is expectant. If bleeding ceases and placenta praevia has been excluded by ultrasound, the patient may go home, but should return if bleeding recurs. Patients admitted after the 37th week are examined by ultrasound, and if placenta praevia is excluded, are examined vaginally. If conditions are suitable, amniotomy is performed. Should bleeding continue despite amniotomy, or fetal distress arise, caesarean section should be performed.

### Moderate haemorrhage

The aim is to restore blood loss and deliver the patient with the least delay. At least 1500ml of blood should be obtained and 1000ml run in rapidly, the first 500ml being given in about 10 minutes. If possible, the actual quantity needed to restore the blood volume should be monitored by estimating the central venous pressure. If the patient is in severe pain, morphine 15mg should be given and repeated as needed.

The condition of the fetus should be monitored. If signs of fetal distress are found, which persist, urgent action should be taken to deliver the fetus, usually by caesarean section. In other cases, the decision has to be made, once 1000ml of blood has been transferred, whether to perform a caesarean section (in the absence of signs of fetal distress) or to rupture the membranes. The membranes may be ruptured, whether shock is present or not, and the procedure seems to reduce the degree of shock. Uterine contractions usually begin soon after amniotomy.

Labour usually starts soon after this, but if there is any delay an oxytocin infusion is set up. Should bleeding continue despite the oxytocin infusion, as shown by an increase in the height of the fundus, or should fetal distress be diagnosed, caesarean section may be necessary, and is sometimes required. At the time of the amniotomy, a catheter is inserted into the bladder and the urine output assessed by releasing it every 2 hours and measuring the urine. Oliguria may persist until delivery, when a diuresis is usual.

Venous blood should be examined every 2 hours for evidence of hypofibrinogenaemia or excessive fibrinolysis and, if the clotting time exceeds 10 minutes, fibrinogen and fibrinolysin estimations should be made. As has been noted, treatment is only needed if a clotting defect is present and the clinical condition of the patient indicates that bleeding is continuing. If this occurs, 5 to 10g of fibrinogen, or 5 to 15g of epsilon aminocaproic acid may be administered intravenously, but in most cases correction of the coagulation disturbance is only required if caesarean section is contemplated or if the defect persists after delivery.

### Severe haemorrhage

The treatment of severe haemorrhage follows the principles outlined for moderate haemorrhage, but at least 2500ml of blood must be obtained, and 1500ml given rapidly before amniotomy is performed. Once again, monitoring the central venous pressure is a considerable help in determining the adequacy of the transfusion. Once the blood has been given and the membranes have been ruptured, the condition of the patient improves and labour is usually rapid. Should any delay occur an oxytocin infusion will stimulate contractions. Postpartum haemorrhage is frequent and oxytocics should be given to prevent this, an injection of 0.5mg ergometrine being given intravenously, or an ampoule of Syntometrine being given intramuscularly, with the birth of the baby.

|  | Placenta praevia | Abruptio placentae | |
| --- | --- | --- | --- |
|  |  | Mild | Moderate and severe |
| Visible blood loss | Usually slight at first episode. Tends to recur. Symptoms proportionate to visible blood loss | Slight, does not usually recur. Symptoms proportionate to visible blood loss | Moderate, continuing haemorrhage. Symptoms out of proportion to visible blood loss |
| Pain | None | Rare | Usual |
| Pregnancy-induced hypertension | Rare | 10 per cent | 25 to 35 per cent |
| Uterus | Normal | Normal | Tense and tender |
| Fetus | Presenting part high, often eccentric. Pressed down into pelvis it recoils. Fetus always alive and unaffected | Presenting part often engaged in the pelvis Fetus usually alive, and unaffected | Fetus difficult to palpate Usually dead |

**Table 24/3** Differential diagnosis of the main causes of antepartum haemorrhage

To summarize, the treatment of moderate and severe abruptio placentae is:

1. Fairly rapid blood transfusion, at least 1500ml being given in moderate cases, and 2500ml in severe cases. If blood is not readily available, dextran-70, 500ml, may be infused while waiting for the blood to arrive. Central venous pressure monitoring is important to determine the adequacy of the transfusion as the blood lost is frequently not seen externally and is usually underestimated.

2. Rupture of the membranes, even if shock is present and irrespective of the tenseness of the uterus. The uterus is not inert, it is overdistended, and function will be restored by amniotomy. It can be further stimulated by an oxytocin infusion.

3. Anuria is prevented by rapid tranfusion of adequate quantities of blood. Coagulation defects are usually prevented: (1) by giving adequate blood transfusion; and (2) by early amniotomy and rapid delivery, preferably per vaginam. If a coagulation defect occurs, an attempt should be made to find if it is due to hypofibrinogenaemia or hyperfibrinolysis, and then treated appropriately. But if the clinical condition of the patient is good, it is probably better to withhold treatment until after delivery, as in most cases the clotting defect is corrected spontaneously.

4. Caesarean section is required: (1) when haemorrhage cannot be controlled by more conservative measures, (2) if the fetus is alive and monitoring indicates 'fetal distress', and (3) when labour is prolonged and oliguria persists.

## DIFFERENTIAL DIAGNOSIS

The diagnosis of the main causes of antepartum haemorrhage can be difficult and distinguishing points are shown in Table **24/3**.

Severe accidental haemorrhage constitutes an obstetric emergency and in the differential diagnosis acute appendicitis, ruptured uterus, volvulus of the bowel, retroperitoneal haematoma and rectus muscle haematoma must be considered. All these require laparotomy which should be avoided in severe abruptio placentae.

## MATERNAL AND FETAL LOSS

The *maternal mortality* will depend on the time of diagnosis and the rapidity with which treatment, particularly adequate blood transfusion, was initiated. Delay in transfusing predisposes to renal ischaemia which, if severe, leads to irreversible cortical necrosis. The hazards of the coagulation defects can be reduced by adequate transfusion and by amniotomy. Postpartum haemorrhage can lead to death in a woman already partially exsanguinated, and should be anticipated and prevented.

The fetal loss depends on the degree of placental separation. In mild cases it is slightly increased, but in moderate and severe cases, if the fetus is alive, an emergency caesarean section may save the baby; but often the fetus is dead when the mother is admitted.

## RENAL FAILURE OF OBSTETRIC ORIGIN

Acute renal failure may be defined as occurring when, despite a normal blood volume, insufficient urine is filtered through the glomeruli and tubules to prevent rising blood levels of nitrogenous products. Generally less than 20 to 30ml of urine/hour is secreted, but occasionally renal failure can be present with a higher urinary output.

In obstetrics, 60 per cent of cases follow a self-induced abortion, or one performed by a 'back-street' abortionist; and 40 per cent of cases follow severe abruptio placentae, severe postpartum haemorrhage or severe pregnancy-induced hypertension and eclampsia.

In recent years the incidence has fallen to a low level, because of the increasing acceptance of legal abortion, with adequate, early blood transfusion in abruptio placentae and severe postpartum haemorrhage, and with the efficient treatment of severe pregnancy-induced hypertension. In many major obstetric hospitals few, or no cases are treated each year.

The pathological lesion in the kidney is a diffuse tubular necrosis in most cases, although cortical necrosis may occur in late pregnancy. It is likely that the two lesions are facets of a single cause, arteriolar spasm. The more prolonged and severe the spasm the greater is the chance that cortical necrosis will develop.

Should renal failure develop, and the oliguria fail to respond to the restoration of the blood volume and the use of mannitol, treatment is required. Treatment is to limit the fluid intake to balance the insensible fluid loss in sweat and transpiration, to restrict the protein intake, to provide adequate calories in the form of glucose, and to monitor the electrolyte balance with great care. If, despite this, the blood urea rises to over 150mg per 100ml, or is increasing at more than 30mg per 100ml per day, the patient should be transferred to a special renal unit for probable renal dialysis.

## Chapter 25

# Hypertensive Disease in Pregnancy (Toxaemias of Pregnancy)

In the past the term *toxaemia of pregnancy* has been used to include three distinct disease entities, which have a similar triad of the signs of hypertension, proteinuria and oedema, and which, in certain circumstances, may progress to fits and coma (eclampsia). Since there is no evidence that any of the conditions is due to a toxin, the term is inaccurate. It is retained only to emphasize the clinical similarity of the three conditions, which can be classified as follows:

1. *Pregnancy induced hypertension* (PIH) (*Pre-eclampsia*)
   a. Mild
   b. Moderate
   c. Severe
2. *Essential hypertension* (see Chapter 26)
   a. Uncomplicated
   b. With superimposed pre-eclampsia
3. *Chronic nephritis* (see Chapter 27)
   a. Uncomplicated
   b. With superimposed pre-eclampsia
4. Each of the above may predispose to: *Eclampsia.*

The most important clinical criterion is hypertension, proteinuria being a later event and one which indicates a worsening of the disease. It is known that there is a circadian variation in the blood pressure. Studies have shown the highest systolic and diastolic pressures occur in the afternoon and evening and the lowest between 3 a.m. and 7 a.m. Because of this, care should be taken in making the diagnosis. Oedema is now considered to be non-specific to the diagnosis but, if gross, indicates a worsening of the disease entity.

Between 5 and 8 per cent of all pregnancies are complicated by hypertension. Pre-eclampsia or pregnancy-induced hypertension (PIH) is unusual amongst multigravidae. Hypertension in such women is more likely to be the manifestation of latent essential hypertension or of renal disease.

When the proportional incidence of the conditions is examined, PIH accounts for 80 per cent, essential hypertension for 18 per cent, chronic renal disease for 2 per cent and eclampsia for about 0.1 per cent. The final diagnosis is frequently impossible to make during pregnancy, but with further assessment at about 6 months after delivery, the above proportions were obtained.

# PREGNANCY-INDUCED HYPERTENSION (PRE-ECLAMPSIA)

Pregnancy induced hypertension, or pre-eclampsia, may be, as its second name implies, the precursor of eclampsia. Eclampsia occurred frequently in the past, but with increasingly careful attention to the early signs of pre-eclampsia, the incidence of eclampsia has diminished markedly, and in many countries the disease is rarely seen.

Pregnancy-induced hypertension is more likely to occur in the primigravid patient, and especially in the older woman. It is more common in obese patients of the lower socio-economic groups, although this may merely be due to the less careful prenatal supervision of such patients. The disease only occurs after the 20th week of pregnancy and is uncommon before the 30th week.

## CLASSIFICATION

There is no generally accepted classification of the degree of severity of PIH. This causes considerable difficulty in comparing the results of treatment in different hospitals. However, in all studies the risk of eclampsia increases and the danger to the mother and to the fetus increases proportionately with the severity of the disease.

### Potential PIH

Potential pre-eclampsia is diagnosed if a rise occurs in the diastolic blood pressure of 15 points or more, over the basal blood pressure recorded in early pregnancy. In this and in subsequent groups, it is understood that the diastolic blood pressure is taken after the patient has rested for at least 10 minutes. A weight gain of more than 1kg per week, or oedema of the legs may also be present. These two findings are not diagnostic.

### Mild PIH

This condition is diagnosed when a rise in the diastolic blood pressure occurs in a woman whose blood pressure was less than 90mmHg up to the 20th week of pregnancy. The diastolic blood pressure (after rest) is found to be between 90 and 99mmHg, and the elevation observed on at least two occasions separated by 6 hours during a 24-hour period. Oedema of the legs may be present, but no protein is found in the urine.

### Moderate PIH (pre-eclampsia)

The blood pressure lies in the range 140–170/100–110, confirmed on two occasions after 10 minutes rest, 24 hours apart. Proteinuria may be present in the range > 30– < 300mg/dl, in the absence of urinary tract infection. Oedema of the legs or hands may be found.

### Severe PIH (pre-eclampsia)

The blood pressure exceeds 170/110; proteinuria is present, usually exceeding 300mg/dl and oedema is usually detected.

### Imminent eclampsia

In addition to the signs of severe PIH, the patient complains of severe headaches, blurring of vision or gastric pain, and her nervous responses are hyperactive.

## INCIDENCE

Pregnancy-induced hypertension complicates 3 to 8 per cent of all pregnancies, and 5 to 10 per cent of pregnancies in primigravid women. The risk of recurrence of PIH in a subsequent pregnancy is low, less than 5 per cent, and its presence is usually indicative of an underlying essential hypertension or renal disease. During the past 20 years, there has been a gradual decline both in the absolute incidence of PIH and in the relative incidence of the severe form. The reduction has been most marked in the latter. Despite this, PIH constitutes the main indication for admission to hospital during pregnancy.

## PHYSIOLOGICAL ALTERATIONS IN PIH

In PIH generalized vasoconstriction occurs. Many of the physiological alterations found in the disease depend upon the degree and distribution of the vasoconstriction, becoming increasingly obvious with increasing severity of the disease. There is a reduction of *uterine blood flow* of up to 50 per cent with evidence of alteration in the structure of the trophoblast of the placental villi, and occlusive vascular lesions in the placental bed. The *placental alterations* are due to the hypoxia caused by the reduction of blood flow through the spiral arteries of the decidua. They include hyperplasia of both syncytio- and cytotrophoblast, with the appearance of increased numbers of syncytial sprouts on terminal villi, swelling of the microvilli, and thickening of the basement membrane. These changes are attempts to correct the placental dysfunction which results from the hypoxia. Both the degree of the changes and the reduction of the placental function vary considerably in cases studied, but tend to be more marked as the PIH becomes more severe. In the *kidney*, vasospasm of the afferent arteriole causes decreased renal blood flow, a decreased glomerular filtration rate, and a lowered glomerular filtration fraction. The hypoxaemia leads to a reversible swelling of the cytoplasm of the endothelial cells of the capillaries in the glomerular tuft. It also increases the permeability of the glomerular basement membrane, so that albumin molecules filter through and appear in the urine. These alterations have the effect of reducing the glomerular and renal tubular blood flow. They may be the cause of the increase of total body water found in PIH, and it appears that a relatively greater proportion of this extra fluid is retained *within* the cells. This would aggravate the effect of tissue hypoxia, particularly in the brain. Sodium retention also occurs in PIH, but the quantity of sodium retained is not excessive.

Either, because of the loss of albumin in the urine, or for some other reason, hypo-albuminaemia occurs. The reduced concentration of plasma albumin lowers the plasma osmotic pressure and predisposes to a loss of fluid from the vascular compartment. This leads to tissue oedema and contributes to the reduced *plasma volume haemoconcentration* and hypovolaemia characteristic of PIH.

The *cardiac output* decreases with increasing severity of PIH and capillary permeability increases, which may contribute to the hypovolaemia. The hypovolaemia and increased blood viscosity found in PIH may reduce tissue and organ perfusion aggravating the tissue hypoxia. Occasionally pulmonary oedema develops, probably due to a combination of pulmonary hypertension, increased cardiac output and increased capillary permeability. The blood flow through the cerebral arteries is unaltered unless eclampsia occurs, when it is reduced, but in all cases of PIH there is some increase in cerebrovascular resistance, indicating some degree of cerebral vasospasm. The blood flow through mesenteric vessels, the muscles and peripheral vessels is unaltered. *Hepatic function* is not disturbed, and no alterations in liver cells are found when liver biopsy is performed; however, areas of periportal haemorrhage and necrosis are found in some patients dying from severe PIH or eclampsia. The distribution of these lesions suggests an intense vasospasm in the hours preceding death, and that they are caused by the disease rather than that they are its cause.

## BIOCHEMICAL CHANGES

These are variable and in general not particularly helpful in establishing a diagnosis. Once again, the greatest alterations are found in the most severe form of the disease. There is an increase in the haematocrit (indicating haemoconcentration); the serum urate is raised, due to increased tubular reabsorption of urate (not to liver damage). In spite of initial enthusiasm that a rising plasma urate in pregnancy was predictive of the later onset of PIH more recent studies indicate that the rest is unreliable. However, once PIH has supervened, a rapidly rising plasma urate may indicate a deterioration of the hypertensive process, although other signs are usually present.

Thrombocytopenia occurs in between 30 and 50 per cent of patients who have severe PIH. Its cause is unknown. In severe PIH and in eclampsia, an increase in circulating fibrin degradation products is found in many patients. There are no consistent differences between normal pregnancy and PIH levels in any of the enzymes investigated, in serum protein and protein electrophoretic patterns, or in other blood investigations performed.

## AETIOLOGY

The aetiology of PIH is unknown, and all of the many theories so far advanced have failed to be substantiated. Recent investigations suggest that PIH may be an immunological disorder in which paternal and maternal HLA and other antigens are close so that the production of blocking antibody is reduced (p. 27). This may lead to an alteration in the metabolism of trophoblast, which secretes a vasoconstrictor substance or leads to an alteration in the ratio between the vasodilator prostanoids (prostacyclines) and the vasoconstrictor prostanoids (thromboxane $A_2$ and prostaglandin). Studies have shown that in PIH, thromboxane levels are higher and prostacycline levels are lower than in nonaffected pregnant women. The predominance of vasoconstrictor substances acting upon alpha receptors in the walls of uterine arterioles reduces placental blood flow and causes a fall in $pO_2$ tension. The action of the vasoconstrictor prostanoids may be direct or may increase vascular sensitivity to other vasoconstrictor substances, such as angiotensin II. It is unclear whether the deficiency in vasodilator prostaglandins acts directly, or by increasing vascular sensitivity to other vasoconstrictor substances.

The placenta responds to the relative hypoxia by trophoblastic proliferation of the villi so that a larger area of syncytium is presented to the less well oxygenated maternal blood. These syncytial sprouts are likely to become detached, to embolize into the general circulation and to be carried to the lungs where they are destroyed with release of thromboplastin. This in turn may cause some degree of disseminated intravascular coagulation. The kidneys attempt to excrete the resulting fibrin-like compound, but fail to do so, so that it accumulates in the glomerular epithelial cells. The generalized vasospasm causes a reduced renal plasma flow and relative hypoxia in the glomeruli, the epithelial cells of which swell, further reducing the glomerular filtration rate. Concurrently sodium retention occurs, with a possible shift of sodium into the arterial walls which may be a factor in their increased responsiveness to pressor substances.

The generalized vasospasm accounts for the symptom of hypertension; the renal glomerular lesion for the sign of proteinuria; the sodium retention and reduced glomerular filtration for the oedema.

The reduced uteroplacental blood flow reduces placental function, and diminishes placental transport mechanisms so that fetal malnutrition, or death, results.

## PREVENTION OF PIH

Although it is doubtful if PIH can be prevented, the incidence appears to be reduced if the patient restricts her weight gain to about 0.5kg per week in the second half of pregnancy, if she limits her intake of excessively salty foods, and if she regularly attends for antenatal examinations, when the blood pressure is estimated and the urine examined for the presence of protein.

If the theory of increased release of thromboxane is true, aspirin should suppress proaggregatory vasoconstrictor platelet thromboxane $A_2$. In a preliminary study small daily doses of aspirin (60mg) have been shown to reduce the incidence of PIH in primigravidae.

If the patient persistently continues to gain more than 0.5kg per week, she should be given dietary instruction, and should limit her carbohydrate intake. But provided her salt intake is not excessive, salt intake need not be limited. Oedema in a pregnant woman, with no associated hypertension or proteinuria, is of no consequence, unless she has the oedema on waking. Diuretics should only be given if the oedema is causing marked discomfort.

If diuretics are used, the patient should be seen after an interval of 3 days as persisting oedema requires further investigation. The diuretics should not be used for periods exceeding 5 days.

The main criterion for diagnosis is a rise in the diastolic blood pressure to 90mmHg.

## CLINICAL COURSE

In general, PIH is a disease of slow onset and steady progression, but occasionally it may arise quite suddenly and develop into eclampsia in a few days. For this reason the early signs must be sought at each visit.

Three signs are usually considered to indicate the development of PIH. These are (1) hypertension, (2) proteinuria, and (3) oedema.

### Hypertension

A diastolic blood pressure of 90mmHg is considered diagnostic, subject to the provisos mentioned earlier. If the diastolic blood pressure exceeds 110mmHg severe PIH is diagnosed, and if it exceeds 120mmHg, urgent action to reduce its level is indicated.

### Proteinuria

This is a sign that moderate or severe PIH has supervened. It indicates that renal vasospasm is marked. Small amounts of proteinuria (<300mg per litre) may be found in normal pregnancy, but until PIH, chronic nephritis and renal tract infection have been excluded, the finding must be treated seriously. A more exact method is to estimate the amount of protein in a 24-hour urine specimen. Excretion of 300mg to 2000mg of protein per 24 hours usually indicates pre-eclampsia, whilst less than 300mg may be normal, because of the slightly increased permeability of the glomerular basement membrane in pregnancy. However, collecting a 24-hour sample of urine is inconvenient and unreliable. A more convenient method is to measure urinary protein and creatinine using the following formula:

$$\frac{\text{protein mg/l}}{\text{creatinine mmol/l} \times 10} \times \frac{(140 - \text{age in years})(\text{wt in kg})}{5000} \times 0.85$$

The result is the 24-hour protein excretion rate.

## Oedema

Recent research has shown that dependent ankle oedema is a normal condition in pregnancy, but oedema of the ankles which is present in the morning, or oedema of the legs, hands or face should be considered pathological and is a sign of PIH. The cause of the oedema remains obscure, but it is likely that more than one cause is involved. Attempts to prevent the onset of PIH by preventing oedema are illogical and ineffective. For this reason the administration of prophylactic diuretics to pregnant women should be avoided.

## TREATMENT

Since the cause of PIH is unknown, treatment can only be symptomatic. Bedrest is the main modality used, although its value has not been assessed adequately. The patient should either be propped up in bed, or lie on her side, as in the supine position uterine blood flow is diminished.

The management of PIH is to control the patient's blood pressure and to monitor the growth and well-being of the fetus (see Chapter 36).

### Hypertension

The generalized vasospasm leads to the development of hypertension, which is often labile, suggesting the influence of emotional factors.

The treatment of *mild and moderate PIH* remains controversial. Some authorities insist on admission to hospital, strict bed rest and the administration of sedatives. Nearly all agree that there is no need to restrict the patient's salt intake and that diuretics should be avoided because of the hypovolaemic state. Bed rest is thought to improve placental blood flow, and sedatives are believed by some obstetricians to control the blood pressure, although no well-designed clinical trial has been made. In fact, one observer has suggested that the sedative might benefit the doctor more than the patient!

The treatment of PIH with antihypertensive drugs is controversial. The most experience is with using methyldopa, but recently some obstetricians have used labetalol or beta-antagonist drugs, such as atenolol, pindolol or oxprenolol, in cases of mild or moderate PIH. The reasons for choosing labetalol or one of the beta-blockers is (1) that the drugs are effective hypotensive agents and some patients can be treated as outpatients; and (2) the drugs may increase the plasma volume and the uteroplacental blood flow, thus (theoretically) reducing fetal growth retardation.

There is no conclusive evidence that any of the drugs mentioned is superior to any other in terms of fetal outcome, method of delivery, birth-weight or the head circumference of the neonate. However, the beta-blockers have adverse effects and should probably be avoided if the hypertensive patient has asthma, diabetes or incipient cardiac failure. They may also produce disturbed sleep, vivid dreams, hallucinations and depression. The latter group of side-effects is least common if a poorly lipid-soluble beta-blocker, such as atenolol, is prescribed.

Labetalol has theoretical advantages over beta-blockers as it decreases peripheral resistance without changing cardiac output or producing tachycardia.

It should be mentioned that few double-blind randomized trials of these drugs have been made so that the benefit of using them in mild and moderate PIH may be no greater than bed rest alone.

If the blood pressure rises to merit a diagnosis of severe PIH, additional treatment is needed.

*Severe PIH* (> 170/110–115) especially if proteinuria is present requires urgent treatment to reduce the risk of left ventricular failure or a cerebrovascular accident. Intravenous labetalol (0.5–1.0mg/kg/hour), increasing to a maximum of 3.0mg/kg/hour, or diazoxide should be given (see p. 215). In *very severe PIH* (*imminent eclampsia*) the treatment is that for eclampsia.

Details of treatment are summarized in Table **25/1**.

### Proteinuria

There is no treatment for this sign, but it indicates that the vasospastic process is marked, and that the fetus is at greater risk.

### Oedema

The effect of bed rest is to improve renal blood flow, and this alone will reduce oedema to some extent.

Diuretics should be avoided in the management of oedema associated with the other signs of PIH, as hypovolaemia already exists. This is likely to be aggravated by the additional loss of sodium and water if a diuretic is given. The diuretics do not alter the disease process, nor do they reduce the fetal loss.

| Classification | Nursing responsibilities | Obstetrician's treatment |
|---|---|---|
| 1. Potential PIH | Report significant rise in blood pressure, or excessive weight gain, to obstetrician | Usually no treatment required. See patient in 7 days |
| 2. Mild PIH | Report rise in blood pressure or excessive weight gain to obstetrician | Possible admission to hospital, depending on socio-economic conditions. If not admitted, see patient in 3 days. ?Atenolol 100mg each evening |
| 3. Moderate PIH | *In hospital:*<br>1. Four-hourly recording of the blood pressure<br>2. Twice-daily urine testing for protein<br>3. Regular observation of the patient's condition, including fluid intake and output<br>4. Bed rest but toilet privileges allowed | 1. Probably admit to hospital<br>2. Sedation (if indicated)<br>3. Labetalol (starting) 100mg b.d. or atenolol (starting) 100mg in evening or oxprenolol (starting) 20mg t.d.s. or methyldopa, (starting) 250mg t.d.s. |
| 4. Severe PIH | 1. Two-hourly blood pressure recording for 6 hours, then 4-hourly<br>2. Urine testing for protein and acetone twice daily<br>3. Fluid intake and output recorded<br>4. Careful observation of the patient for the signs of imminent eclampsia<br>5. Complete bed rest for 24 hours, thereafter possible toilet privileges | 1. Admit to hospital<br>2. Depending on the severity of the illness:<br>  (a) labetalol intravenously or orally<br>  (b) diazoxide 30mg intravenously every 60 seconds until BP <90, then diazepam 10–20mg parenterally or orally<br>3. ?Intravenous frusemide 20mg or stable plasma protein substitute (SPPS), if gross oedema present<br>4. ?Caesarean section |
| 5. Imminent eclampsia | The patient requires careful systematic observation and accurate recording of the findings as eclampsia is a possible outcome. The blood pressure requires frequent estimation at intervals determined by the obstetrician. Fluid intake and urinary output must be measured meticulously, and the urine tested quantitatively for protein | 1. Diazoxide 30mg intravenously every 60 seconds until BP <90, then diazepam 10–20mg parenterally or orally<br>2. Labetalol intravenously (see p. 216)<br>3. ?Caesarean section |

Table 25/1 Summary of the management of pregnancy-induced hypertension

By contrast, side-effects may occur, and the abuse of diuretics may mask the progress of the disease. The only place for diuretics in pre-eclampsia is to relieve severe discomfort due to massive oedema.

## DURATION OF TREATMENT

The aim of treatment is to permit the continued growth of the fetus in utero until it is sufficiently mature to survive, or until it is estimated that the danger of intra-uterine death exceeds that of premature extra-uterine existence. For this reason the duration of treatment and the time of termination of pregnancy will depend on: (1) the severity of the PIH; (2) the duration of the pregnancy; and (3) the response to treatment.

Prior to the 34th week of pregnancy the object is to keep the fetus in utero if possible. If the patient does not respond to treatment or if there is deterioration in the severity of the PIH and this fails to respond, termination of pregnancy must be considered. Even if the PIH is controlled or at least does not deteriorate, the fetus may die in utero at any stage. A sinister sign is slow fetal growth despite good response to treatment. In all cases of PIH, the health of the fetus requires to be assessed at least three times a week. The biophysical methods of fetal movement counts, non-stress cardiotocography and possibly ultrasound assessments should be chosen. These are discussed on pages 278.

Regular serum urate measurements may also give an indirect index of fetal well-being. A rising serum urate suggests increased fetal risk. If the level exceeds 0.35mmol/litre (6mg/dl) (on 3 consecutive readings), in the presence of severe PIH, urgent delivery is indicated. Not all observers agree, because other, non-specific, factors may alter the serum urate level.

If the risk to the fetus in utero is considered serious, labour is induced either by amniotomy followed by oxytocin infusion (or by prostaglandin infusion); or by caesarean section. The choice is determined by the severity of the illness and the state of the uterine cervix. If there is a rapidly deteriorating PIH and the cervix is 'unfavourable' (i.e. is firm, uneffaced and less than 1 cm dilated), caes-arean section is advisable, unless the obstetrician has experience with intravenous infusion of prostaglandins. In all other situations amniotomy is to be preferred, as the uterus is very sensitive to stimuli and labour is rapid. The art of obstetrics is to determine from clinical and laboratory data when the risk of intra-uterine fetal death is greater than the risk of premature birth.

If PIH occurs after the 36th week of pregnancy and is mild, there is no indication for the induction of labour and the pregnancy is permitted to continue to term. The majority of patients will enter labour spontaneously. It is not wise to allow the pregnancy to continue beyond term as the combined risk of post-maturity and PIH is hazardous to the baby. If moderate or severe PIH supervenes, termination of the pregnancy is recommended when adequate control of the hypertension has been obtained. Once again each case must be considered on its own merits, but on average about 40 per cent of patients with PIH require induction of labour by artificial rupture of the membranes or delivery by caesarean section.

After delivery the patient's blood pressure should be monitored 4–8 hourly for seven days, as an increase in blood pressure may occur. Hypotensive drugs may be required.

# ECLAMPSIA

The term eclampsia is derived from the Greek words meaning 'like a flash of lightning'. It was introduced when it was believed that fits and coma in pregnancy appeared without any pre-existing disorder. It is now known that eclampsia occurs extremely rarely unless there have been pre-existing symptoms, although the duration of the episode may be short. For this reason careful and frequent observation in the antenatal period by detecting and treating pre-eclampsia should reduce markedly, or even eliminate, eclampsia.

Eclampsia is characterized by convulsions and coma supervening upon hypertensive disease in pregnancy and hence may occur in patients with pregnancy-induced hypertension, or in patients who have pre-eclampsia superimposed upon essential hypertension or chronic nephritis (Fig **25/1**).

## PHYSIOPATHOLOGY

In eclampsia there is an intense vasospasm with tissue hypoxia. The uterine blood flow is considerably reduced, as is the renal plasma flow, and consequently the glomerular filtration rate is decreased by at least 25 per cent and urinary output falls. The cerebral vascular resistance is markedly increased, cerebral oxygen consumption falls and cerebral oedema may occur. (In conditions of relative cerebral hypoxia, the incidence of cerebral dysrhythmia increases and this may be the cause of the convulsions.) The capillary walls become more permeable with increasing tissue waterlogging. Simultaneously there is an increased water retention in the cells which impedes cellular metabolism. The blood viscosity increases with a rise in fibrinogen levels

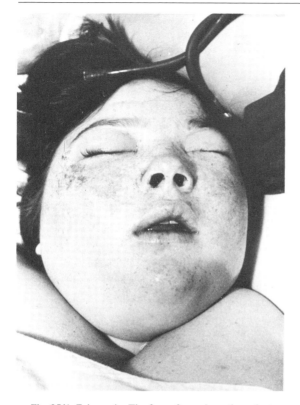

**Fig. 25/1** Eclampsia. The face of an eclamptic patient

and in fibrin degradation products so that there is an increased tendency to the intravascular dissemination of fibrin deposits. These are considered by some to account for the variable visceral lesions found in fatal cases. Blood platelet levels fall. The liver may show patchy periportal haemorrhagic and necrotic areas with deposition of fibrin and thrombosis of vessels. These changes are not usually found in liver biopsies of patients surviving eclampsia and are probably terminal in nature. The kidney lesions are those found in pregnancy-induced hypertension but, occasionally, cortical necrosis occurs.

## INCIDENCE

The incidence of eclampsia varies from country to country and is an index of the availability and acceptance of antenatal care, the provision of adequate prenatal accommodation in hospital, and the training of the doctors who deal with obstetric patients. In Britain and Australia the incidence amongst public patients is about 1 in 1500, amongst private patients even less; in the developing countries the incidence is higher.

## PREVENTION

These facts indicate that eclampsia can be prevented if:

1. Properly staffed antenatal clinics are made available to all patients in areas convenient to their homes.
2. All pregnant women are induced to attend the clinics regularly from early pregnancy.
3. The first signs of PIH are sought, recognized and treated adequately.
4. Sufficient prenatal beds are available so that early treatment can be instituted.

## SYMPTOMS AND SIGNS

Usually the convulsion is preceded by a period of deterioration in the severity of PIH, with drowsiness, headache, and dimness of vision (imminent eclampsia). If this period is not recognized and treated, fits may ensue. A particularly dangerous time is during labour. In about 50 per cent of cases the initial convulsion is antepartum, in 30 per cent intrapartum and in 20 per cent postpartum.

The convulsion is preceded by a preliminary stage when the patient become disassociated from her surroundings, her eyes roll, her hands twitch, her respiration becomes spasmodic, and within 30 to 60 seconds she passes into the tonic stage of the convulsion. During this stage, which lasts about 30 seconds, there is general muscular rigidity and the whole body goes into a tonic spasm. The back arches, the hands clench, the features are distorted by a grimace, the tongue may be bitten, breathing ceases and the patient becomes cyanosed. She then passes into the clonic stage, in which the tonic spasm is replaced by spasmodic episodes of muscular contraction and relaxation. The body jerks uncontrollably, the limbs flail, the mouth opens and shuts convulsively, the breathing is stertorous and frothy saliva fills the mouth. This stage lasts from 1 to 4 minutes and the patient passes into coma which may last hours or may be replaced by a further series of convulsions, without consciousness being regained.

## TREATMENT

The aims of treatment are: (1) to relieve the generalized vascular spasm and so permit a better blood flow to the brain, the kidneys and the uterus; (2) to decrease the sensitivity of the brain to external and internal stimuli; (3) to reduce the high blood pressure to the normal range for the patient; (4) to aid in the elimination of the retained water and electrolytes; (5) when the above are satisfactorily dealt with, to deliver the baby.

### General management

The prime consideration is to prevent the occurrence of further convulsions, since the danger of the additional hypoxia from this cause is considerable. Once the convulsions are controlled, and adequate oxygenation obtained, termination of pregnancy will result in improvement of the generalized vasospasm.

### Nursing care

Each patient should have a doctor or trained nurse–midwife in constant attendance. The duties of the attendant are to detect any change in the condition of the patient presaging the recurrence of convulsions, to protect her from injury during a fit, to maintain a clear airway, especially following a fit, and to note changes in blood pressure, temperature, pulse rate and urinary output as these have prognostic significance. If possible the patient should be nursed in a single room, although this is not absolutely necessary. The patient is nursed on her side and her head and shoulders are raised. A gag (a well-padded metal spatula is useful) is available to prevent her biting her own tongue during a convulsion. Oxygen is administered continuously to improve tissue oxygenation. Suction is employed to clear the nose and pharynx of frothy secretions. To prevent infection, a broad spectrum antibiotic is administered intramuscularly. Because the blood volume is depleted, intravenous fluid replacement should be started, and the quantity required monitored by estimating the central venous pressure.

Some authorities recommend that one unit of stable plasma protein substitute (SPPS) should be infused initially to restore the blood volume and to encourage renal perfusion.

The presence of oedema should be ignored, as a considerable diuresis usually follows delivery. However, if there is evidence of cardiac failure, frusemide 20mg may be given intravenously. As hypovolaemia is usual in severe PIH and eclampsia it must be given with care. The alternative is to give an intravenous infusion of an osmotic diuretic such as 15 per cent mannitol.

## LABORATORY TESTS

A platelet count and a blood coagulation profile should be made as soon after diagnosis as possible.

## SPECIFIC TREATMENT

Since eclampsia is most frequently encountered in areas where obstetric care is most needed any complicated regimen is bound to fail, and episodes of severe hypotension are as dangerous as those of marked hypertension. Several methods are currently recommended, none appears to be superior to any other. The three most suitable are the use of (1) diazoxide/diazepam (Valium), (2) diazepam with a short-acting hypotensive agent, or (3) magnesium sulphate (in the USA).

### Diazoxide/diazepam

Diazoxide is a non-diuretic benzothiazide derivative which has a marked and rapid hypotensive effect when injected intravenously. This hypotensive effect is apparently due to the ability of the drug to relax the smooth muscle of the peripheral arterioles. Simultaneously cardiac output is increased, the heart rate is increased and the circulation time is reduced. The main side-effects are an increase in nausea, dryness of the mouth, and transient hyperglycaemia, which apparently does not have any adverse effect on the fetus or neonate, provided the drug is used for a period not exceeding 24 hours at any one time.

In extremely severe PIH, imminent eclampsia and in eclampsia, diazoxide is very effective in reducing the blood pressure. An intravenous line is set up and 30mg of diazoxide is injected every 60 seconds. The blood pressure is measured each minute, and when the desired level has been obtained, the injections are stopped. This method reduces the quantity of diazoxide needed.

Diazoxide produces an immediate and marked fall in the diastolic blood pressure which lasts, on average, 4 to 6 hours but may persist for longer. The blood pressure is monitored at 1-minute intervals for 10 minutes, every 15 minutes for the next hour, and then hourly for 18 to 24 hours. Should the hypertensive crisis recur, a further injection of diazoxide is given. The degree to which the diastolic pressure falls is very variable, but an average fall of $35 \pm 20mmHg$ is reported. Should profound hypotension occur, it is reversed by a rapid infusion of 500ml of a 5 per cent dextrose, rather than by giving intravenous metaraminol which may cause marked hypertension. Diazoxide may reduce uterine activity, and if amniotomy is performed, an oxytocin infusion should be set up at once. If the patient is not relaxed, and has hyperactive reflexes, intermittent doses of diazepam 10 to 20mg may be given intravenously or intramuscularly at about 4-hourly intervals.

### Diazepam

An initial dose of 10 to 20mg of diazepam is given intravenously, slowly, so that the patient becomes drowsy. An intravenous infusion of diazepam 40mg in 500ml of Hartmann's solution is set up. The rate of the drip is adjusted to keep the patient sleeping, and the diastolic blood pressure below 100. If required, extra doses of diazepam are injected intravenously via the drip tube. The side-effects of the method are minimal, and good control appears fairly easy to obtain, but there is a tendency for the infant to become hypothermic in the first hours of life, and this requires to be anticipated.

In the past hydralazine was recommended if diazoxide failed to reduce the blood pressure to the normal range. Current opinion is that hydralazine should be avoided as it produces headaches, flushes, tachycardia and hyper-reactive reflexes in some women. Its use may be followed by the lupus syndrome.

In some centres, chlormethiazole in a 0.8 per cent concentration is given intravenously (40mg per 500ml 5 per cent dextrose) in place of diazepam. The rate of the infusion is governed by the patient's response, a deeply sedated patient with an active cough reflex being sought. In other centres, labetalol is being evaluated.

### Labetalol

Labetalol may be used in place of diazoxide. An intravenous infusion of 200mg of labetalol in 5 per cent dextrose is given initially at 0.5mg/kg/hour. The dose is increased by 0.5mg/kg/hour every 20 minutes to a maximum of 3.0mg/kg/hour to achieve a diastolic pressure of 85–90mmHg. When this has been obtained the infusion is continued at the concentration for 10 to 24 hours.

### Phenytoin

Some clinicians attempt to reduce the number of fits by giving a loading dose of phenytoin (15mg/kg intravenously over 20 to 30 minutes) and follow this with oral phenytoin for 5 days after the acute phase has passed.

### Magnesium sulphate ($MgSO_4$)

In the USA, magnesium sulphate is the standard treatment for eclampsia. Magnesium sulphate, 4g, is given intravenously at a rate of no more than 1g per minute, followed immediately by 10g of a 50 per cent solution, half given into each buttock. If fits recur, an additional 2g of $MgSO_4$ is given intravenously, and repeated once if required.

Intramuscular $MgSO_4$, 5g in a 50 per cent solution, is given 4-hourly after checking that magnesium intoxication is not present. This is continued for 24 hours after childbirth.

If the hypertension is severe (diastolic $> 120$) hydralazine is given in 5 to 10mg doses at 20–30-minute intervals, until the diastolic pressure is 90–100 torr.

Fluid (5 per cent dextrose in Hartmann's or lactated Ringer's solution) is given at 60 to 150ml per hour.

## OBSTETRICAL MANAGEMENT

As soon as good blood pressure control and adequate sedation have been obtained the obstetrical management of the patient can be initiated. If she is not in labour, but the baby is viable, the cervix 'ripe' and no contra-indication to vaginal delivery exists, amniotomy is performed and uterine activity stimulated with a dilute oxytocin infusion. If the cervix is firm, elongated and rigid, and amniotomy is not possible, the patient should be delivered by caesarean section, provided the fetus is alive and viable. Caesarean section will not be required in more than 20 per cent of cases.

Occasionally with a very small baby, pregnancy may be allowed to continue provided the convulsions and hypertensive crisis are controlled but it is rare for such babies to survive.

## PROGNOSIS IN PIH (PRE-ECLAMPSIA) AND ECLAMPSIA

### Fetal

In mild PIH the perinatal mortality is only raised slightly above that for 'normal' pregnant women, varying from 20 to 60 per 1000 depending upon the community attended. The perinatal loss in severe PIH is higher, varying from 100 to 300 per 1000, and in eclampsia it rises to between 400 and 600 per 1000. About half of the fetal deaths occur in utero, a stillborn baby being delivered. The other half occur in the neonatal period, most babies dying being premature at birth. However, if the baby survives the neonatal period, no deleterious effects on his mental or physical development have been observed up to the age of 8 years.

### Maternal mortality

Mild PIH is not a cause of maternal death, but once the disease becomes severe some patients will die. The cause of death is usually a cerebrovascular accident involving a congenital aneurysm, or else hypertensive heart failure. Deaths from PIH are extremely rare in the developed countries, but in the developing countries, where anaemia is an additional complication, they are encountered more frequently.

The development of eclampsia is an obstetric catastrophe, and the maternal mortality ranges from 3 to 20 per cent depending on the speed with which treatment is instituted and the quality of obstetric care. Death is due to cardiorespiratory failure, following the intense vasospasm, in 25 per cent; to cerebral haemorrhage in 50 per cent; to renal failure in 10 per cent; to infection in 5 per cent; to hepatic failure in 5 per cent and to miscellaneous causes in 5 per cent of cases.

### Maternal morbidity

This is more difficult to assess. PIH and eclampsia do not cause chronic renal disease, nor do they cause a permanent hypertension, although they may bring to light a latent essential hypertension at an earlier stage in the patient's life. Alternatively those patients who were destined to become hypertensive, are more likely to develop PIH, which brings out their latent hypertension. It has been suggested that the longer the duration of the PIH the greater the risk of the development of permanent hypertension, but this cannot be substantiated. Some of the confusion in the past has been due to inadequate follow-up. This is because the hypertension may take more than 3 weeks to settle after delivery, although it usually does so within 7 days. Proteinuria may persist even longer, even up to the first postnatal examination 6 weeks after delivery. Neither of these findings is necessarily indicative that PIH has caused permanent damage.

The final diagnosis can only be made after a full vascular and renal assessment 6 months after delivery. If this disease is confirmed to have been PIH, the patient can be told that she may embark upon a further pregnancy as soon as she wishes. The superimposition of eclampsia on PIH does not alter this advice.

## Chapter 26

# Essential Hypertension in Pregnancy

Essential hypertension is a disease which is probably of hereditary origin, but the course of which is considerably influenced by emotional and environmental factors. The disease runs a long and relatively benign course, and the initial change is a generalized arteriolar spasm, which is manifested clinically by an elevation of the blood pressure. Much discussion has occurred as to what constitutes the upper limit of a normal blood pressure, and any definition is complicated by the fact that the blood pressure is a quantity which varies from hour to hour, from day to day, and shows a slow but steady upward progression with increasing age. Consequently in pregnancy, essential hypertension is encountered most commonly in women over the age of 30. By convention, hypertension is defined amongst women of the fertile age group as a blood pressure exceeding 140/90 which persists after rest and is found on two or more occasions before the 20th week of pregnancy. During the reproductive years, essential hypertension is considered mild if the initial blood pressure is less than 160/100; and severe if it equals or exceeds this level. In young women, severe hypertension is occasionally secondary to chronic pyelonephritis, and rarely to coarctation of the aorta, renal artery stenosis (nodular arteriosclerosis) or phaeochromocytoma. These conditions should be excluded before a diagnosis of essential hypertension is confirmed. As the usual cause of secondary hypertension is chronic pyelonephritis, investigation of the patient's past history for renal involvement and the examination and culture of a midstream specimen of urine are essential. Coarctation of the aorta may be suspected if palpation of the femoral arteries fails to elicit pulsation.

## DIAGNOSIS

The mean blood pressure of women who have essential hypertension decrease in the first half of pregnancy; and the diastolic level is 10 to 15mmHg lower than when the woman was not pregnant. This may make the diagnosis of essential hypertension difficult unless the woman's pre-pregnant blood pressure is known. However, in the absence of a secondary cause of hypertension, a raised blood pressure ($\geqslant$ 140/90) which is present prior to pregnancy or detected before the 20th week of pregnancy, and persisting after rest, may confidently be diagnosed as essential hypertension. A patient who has no history of essential hypertension and who does not present before the 20th week of pregnancy may be found to be hypertensive at the first visit. The hypertension may be pregnancy-induced or may be essential hypertension. In these cases the firm diagnosis must await confirmation at least 12 weeks after delivery, when a persistently raised blood pressure is usually diagnosed as essential hypertension, provided the secondary causes of hypertension have been excluded.

The onset of the malignant phase of essential hypertension is rare in women of childbearing age, and is determined by the presence of an excessively high blood pressure, failing vision, due to bilateral retinopathy, and later, renal damage. Retinopathy may be found in the benign phase, but is uncommon and the lesions are reversible. When present, they consist of small sharply defined white patches on the retina.

## INCIDENCE

Essential hypertension complicates 0.5 to 2.5 per

cent of all pregnancies, generally amongst older women, and accounts for 10 to 20 per cent of all cases of hypertensive disease in pregnancy.

## PHYSIOLOGICAL CONSIDERATIONS

The main physiological alteration is an increase in peripheral resistance consequent upon the arteriolar spasm. To counterbalance the increased peripheral resistance, cardiac work increases as shown by an increased stroke-volume and, to a lesser extent, by an increase in the heart rate. This maintains the normal blood flow to most body organs, with one important exception – the uterus. In normal pregnancy, uterine blood flow increases, but radio-isotope studies have shown that in patients with essential hypertension the increase is small, and it is probable that the higher the blood pressure, the less is the uterine blood flow. The reduced blood flow affects the placental bed particularly, and is associated with proliferation of the intima of the spiral arteries which supply the decidua and placental lake. As a consequence of this, placentation may be affected and placental dysfunction and retardation of fetal growth are likely to occur. The effect of essential hypertension on renal function is minimal in most women in the reproductive era, but paradoxically excess sodium excretion occurs in pregnancy.

### The effect of pregnancy upon the disease

In 60 per cent of hypertensive women, a rise of blood pressure occurs in pregnancy, and in 30 per cent proteinuria also occurs (usually after the 30th week), so that the condition is indistinguishable from severe PIH. This condition is classified as essential hypertension, with superimposed proteinuria. In one-third of these patients, pregnancy is followed by a permanent deterioration of the hypertension, but in all the others pregnancy has no permanent effect on the disease process.

### The effect of the disease upon pregnancy

In the mild forms, the maternal mortality is unaltered, but in the severe forms the onset of proteinuria and abruptio placentae (in 5 per cent) add to the maternal risk. Pregnancy complicated by malignant hypertension is rare and rapidly fatal, although there is no clear evidence that the progress of the disease is altered by the pregnancy. However, if the condition is detected early in the pregnancy, therapeutic abortion should be performed.

The fetal prognosis varies with the degree of hypertension. When the blood pressure remains less than 160/100, the perinatal loss is between 30 and 60 per thousand births, which is double that amongst non-hypertensive women. If the blood pressure exceeds 160/100, the perinatal loss doubles again, and if proteinuria appears it trebles. In prognosis, the diastolic reading is of more significance than the systolic. Although the incidence of abortion is not increased in essential hypertension, one-quarter of the fetal loss is of infants weighing between 500 and 999g, or of 20 to 28 weeks' gestation.

## TREATMENT

The aims of treatment are: (1) to obtain and maintain as good a blood supply as possible to the uterus, especially during placental formation; (2) to control the hypertension and prevent the superimposition of proteinuria; and (3) to induce labour if the condition deteriorates markedly, or if the fetus is failing to grow adequately, provided it is sufficiently mature to survive.

### 1. Maintenance of uterine blood supply

It is possible that the newer hypotensive drugs increase uterine blood flow, but it is important for the patient to have physical and mental rest. If the condition has been diagnosed before pregnancy and is mild, the patient should rest each afternoon, and spend 10 hours in bed at night, particularly in the first 12 weeks of pregnancy. If the essential hypertension is severe, or if the patient has a history of unsuccessful pregnancies, she should be admitted to hospital for rest and assessment, and may require to remain in hospital throughout the pregnancy.

The importance of rest, which is known to improve uterine blood supply, must be stressed, but the patient must not be made into a 'blood-pressure invalid' by an inadequate physician, or an officious nurse.

### 2. Control of hypertension and avoidance of pregnancy-induced hypertension

The decision when to use hypotensive drugs, and when hospital admission is required, can only be arrived at by frequent and careful supervision of the pregnant patient. She must be seen at 2-weekly intervals until the 28th week of pregnancy, and thereafter weekly. Before considering specific therapy, the patient must be instructed in how to regulate her life and to obtain adequate rest. If she is overweight, a reducing diet must be ordered. Even if her weight is normal, she should limit her carbohydrate and fat intake, and gain no more than 0.5kg every 2 weeks. Her salt intake should probably be restricted, but commonsense must be applied, particularly as an increased urinary loss of sodium occurs. The routine use of diuretics is contra-indicated, and hypertensive pregnant women who were receiving the drugs before pregnancy should cease to take them. Diuretic therapy reduces uteroplacental blood flow, reduces plasma volume and increases the perinatal mortality. When the blood pressure is less than 160/100 medication is usually not required, but anxious women may benefit by being given mild sedation.

When the blood pressure lies between 160/100 and 170/110, hypotensive drugs are usually prescribed although their value in reducing perinatal loss has not been established. Several drugs are available; none has been shown to be significantly superior to any other.

*Beta-blockers and labetalol.* These drugs increase plasma volume and hence uteroplacental blood flow, thus theoretically reducing fetal growth retardation. They cross the placenta and may cause fetal bradycardia and fetal hypoglycaemia, although other factors are more likely to be the cause. It does not seem to matter which drug is used although one study suggests that if labetalol is chosen, the mean birth-weight of the baby is greater than if atenolol or oxprenolol is chosen. If the chosen drug fails to control the blood pressure, methyldopa or other hypotensive agents (e.g. prazosin or diazoxide) may be added to the regimen.

*Methyldopa.* The experience using methyldopa in pregnancy is greater than that using beta-blockers or labetalol. Most physicians recommend starting with 750mg daily and increasing to a maximum of 4000mg. The objective is to reduce the blood pressure to 140–150/80–90. Methyldopa is slow to affect the blood pressure so increases in dose should not be made at less than 3-day intervals.

*Hydralazine.* Hydralazine should not be used alone because of side-effects (tachycardia, increased intracranial pressure, headache, flushing, nausea, postural hypotension). If hydralazine is chosen it should be used with a beta-blocker.

### 3. Induction of labour

Since placental dysfunction is common in cases of severe essential hypertension, and since the fetal mortality is no greater at the 38th week than it is at term, induction of labour at the time is recommended. Unfortunately, in some cases fetal growth is noted to be slow or stationary before this time, and a 'small-for-dates' baby is likely to die in utero. Should clinical evidence of retarded fetal growth be present, or should proteinuria superimpose upon the essential hypertension, biophysical tests for fetal wellbeing should be started, so that the optimal time for delivery can be determined. The decision must take into account the history of previous pregnancies, the height of the blood pressure, the response or otherwise to treatment, and the estimated size and growth-rate of the fetus. As a principle, it is wiser to induce early than late, as the superimposition of proteinuria increases the perinatal loss. Induction by amniotomy, supplemented by an oxytocin infusion, is generally all that is required, but selected patients (for instance, older primigravidae with a history of infertility) are better delivered by caesarean section.

## PROGNOSIS FOR FURTHER PREGNANCIES

This will depend upon the height of the non-pregnant blood pressure and no opinion can be given until 3 months after delivery. If there is no evidence of renal damage and other causes of hypertension have been excluded, and if the diastolic blood pressure is less than 100, the patient can be told she may embark on another pregnancy. If the diastolic blood pressure exceeds 100, pregnancy is associated with an increased risk of development of proteinuria and a higher fetal mortality. Provided the patient attends her physician as early as possible after becoming pregnant and is prepared, if required, to spend time in hospital during pregnancy, the chance of delivering a live child are good. If the diastolic blood pressure exceeds 100, and the patient also has impaired renal function, the chance of a successful outcome to the pregnancy is reduced considerably.

Since all patients with essential hypertension have to learn to live with the disease, each hypertensive pregnant woman should be made an active, knowledgeable participant in her own care throughout pregnancy and the puerperium, and indeed throughout her life.

## Chapter 27

# Renal Tract Diseases in Pregnancy

## SYMPTOMLESS BACTERIURIA

The prevalence of significant bacteriuria (more than 100 000 bacteria per ml of urine) in sexually active women is about 2 per cent, but in pregnancy, because of the hormonally induced dilatation of the renal pelvis and ureters and the increased stasis of urine in the bladder, it increases to between 3 and 5 per cent. Symptomless bacteriuria is of some consequence, as 30 per cent of affected women develop clinical renal tract infection in pregnancy; the perinatal mortality is $2\frac{1}{2}$ times that of non-infected women, the incidence of low birth-weight and hypertension is doubled; and the incidence of PIH is slightly increased. These complications can be avoided by early detection of symptomless bacteriuria and its adequate treatment. In over 80 per cent of cases the infective agent is *Escherichia coli*, and in the remainder, *Klebsiella*, coagulase negative *Staphylococci*, *Proteus mirabilis* or *Streptococcus faecalis* are most likely to be encountered.

Because of the sinister significance of symptomless bacteriuria in pregnancy, routine examination of a fresh midstream specimen of urine from every pregnant woman should be made in the first 10 weeks. There is good evidence that pyuria is an inaccurate basis for the diagnosis of symptomless bacteriuria, and it should not be used as a screening device. For this reason a clean midstream specimen is examined by some form of chemical test (such as the Uritest, the nitrate test, the 'blotting paper' test or the triphenyl tetrazolium chloride test); or by the more accurate dipslide, 'streak plate' or 'pour plate' methods. A positive finding is an indication for a further midstream specimen to be examined by culture but bladder aspiration is not usually needed in pregnant women, particularly as bladder puncture can only be performed when the bladder is distended. This has the effect of reducing the number of bacteria in each ml of urine.

If the urine specimen shows significant bacteriuria, treatment should be given. Over 80 per cent of urinary tract infections are due to *E. coli*, and 15 per cent to *Klebsiella spp*, *Proteus* or *Staphylococcus saprophyticus*. Depending on the organism, a 5-day course of amoxycillin or cephalexin will cure over 95 per cent of patients. (Some clinicians prefer a single dose of amoxycillin 3g or cephalexin 2g.) If either of these regimens fails to eliminate the bacteria, a longer course of antibiotics is indicated.

A midstream specimen of urine is re-examined 7 days after completion of treatment. If no bacteria are grown, no further treatment is needed, but midstream specimens should be examined every 2nd week for the remainder of the pregnancy. Persisting infection or new infection requires further treatment either with antibiotics, nitrofurantoin 50mg 8-hourly or nalidixic acid 500mg 8-hourly for 7 to 14 days.

Since about 25 per cent of women with symptomless bacteriuria have abnormalities of the renal tract, it is wise to consider performing an intravenous pyelogram about 10 weeks after confinement if re-infection has occurred in pregnancy.

## PYELONEPHRITIS IN PREGNANCY

Thirty per cent of women with pre-existing bacteriuria, and 3 per cent of women whose urine is sterile at the first visit, develop pyelonephritis in pregnancy. The condition arises from infection of the stagnant urine in the upper renal tract by bacilli lurking in the urethra and bladder, or it may be introduced into the bladder in pregnancy by coitus or by catheterization. The disease usually begins at or after the 20th week of pregnancy, and is common in the puerperium.

The sequence is urethritis → cystitis → oedema of the ureteric sphincter → reflux of infected urine → pyelonephritis. Haematogenous infection is rare. In one-fifth of patients, and particularly those who have recurrent infection, abnormalities of the renal tract will be found.

The infecting agent is *E. coli* in 90 per cent of cases, and mixed infection of *Ps. pyocyanea*, *Staph. aureus* and *Klebsiella aerogenes* in the remainder.

### Symptoms

The disease may be mild or severe, the mildest form of the disease being when only symptomless bacteriuria is found. In other cases, malaise and urinary frequency may be the only symptoms, and in early pregnancy these may be confused with the common nausea and frequency of micturition. The latter is due to the increased urinary excretion of water at this time, and laboratory investigation of the urine is essential to differentiate the two conditions.

The severe form of pyelonephritis starts abruptly with chills and rigors, vomiting and pyrexia which is frequently high, the pulse rate being proportionately raised. Pain in the renal area, frequency of micturition and dysuria follow. Without treatment, the patient becomes dehydrated and toxic.

### Diagnosis

If the urine is examined, diagnosis is easy; but confusion may occur with acute appendicitis or severe accidental haemorrhage (Table 27/1).

### Treatment

Bed-rest and adequate fluids are required early in the disease, and if there is persistent vomiting, intravenous fluids may be necessary. Bacterial sensitivity tests should be made and, pending the result, the patient should be given trimethoprim 200mg twice daily for 7 days or amoxycillin 500mg 6-hourly. As so many patients with severe pyelonephritis are nauseated, or are vomiting, it may be necessary to give ampicillin intramuscularly. The intramuscular injections are continued for 2 to 3 days, and once there is symptomatic relief, may be replaced by oral therapy for a further 5 days. Should symptomatic relief fail to occur, or should bacterial sensitivity tests reveal resistance to amoxycillin, the appropriate drug is substituted.

On completion of the course of treatment, urine specimens are taken for culture at 2-weekly intervals throughout pregnancy. The occurrence of bacteriuria or of further attacks of overt pyelonephritis is an indication for a further course of the appropriate antibiotic. The persistence of infection, recurrence, or infection with a new organism is an indication that a full renal tract investigation should be made 10 weeks after confinement.

| Symptoms and signs | Renal tract infection | Appendicitis |
|---|---|---|
| *Symptoms* | | |
| Week of onset | After 20th week | Any time |
| Pain | In renal area | In lower right quadrant |
| Urinary symptoms | Frequency, dysuria | None |
| *Findings* | | |
| Temperature | Frequently high (above 39°C), fluctuating | Rarely over 38°C |
| Pulse | Above 100 | Below 100 |
| Tenderness | In loin | In right lower quadrant |
| *Laboratory* | | |
| Leucocytes | Often over 18 000/ml | Rarely over 18 000/ml |
| Urine | Pus cells present | Usually normal |

Table 27/1  Differential diagnosis of renal tract infection in pregnancy

# RENAL DISEASES IN PREGNANCY

About 0.2 per cent of pregnant women and 5 per cent of those with hypertensive disease in pregnancy will be found to have an underlying chronic renal disease. Classification of chronic renal disease is not satisfactory. Even with percutaneous renal biopsy an accuracy of only 60 per cent can be obtained. The procedure is not without danger in pregnancy and is of doubtful prognostic value. As far as pregnancy is concerned, it is the glomerular and tubular function, not the histopathological disturbance to structure, which is of importance from the therapeutic and prognostic points of view.

## DIAGNOSIS OF RENAL DISEASE IN PREGNANCY

A history of acute glomerulonephritis or of attacks of acute pyelonephritis prior to pregnancy should alert the physician to the possibility of the presence of chronic glomerulo- or pyelonephritis. However, in at least half of patients no antecedent history is detected. Much help would be obtained if every pregnant woman attended in the first 10 weeks of pregnancy, when her urine should be tested for the presence of bacteriuria and protein. Abnormal findings in any of these tests demands full investigation, particularly creatinine clearance (as an index of the glomerular filtration rate) and examination of the fundi of the eyes. Although there are technical problems in measuring the creatinine clearance in pregnancy, the test should be made in cases of renal disease. The problems are (1) the woman may not empty her bladder completely during the 24-hour test period, and (2) the clearance rate (ml/min) falls in late pregnancy.

However, such early assessment is uncommonly performed, and the patient who presents later in pregnancy with hypertension and proteinuria may have a chronic renal condition, which cannot be accurately diagnosed until after pregnancy.

When the diagnosis of chronic renal disease is possible, three forms can be delineated clinically. These are:

1. The nephrotic syndrome.

2. Glomerulo- or pyelonephritis with no impairment of renal function.
3. Glomerulo- or pyelonephritis with impairment of renal function.

## NEPHROTIC SYNDROME

The patient presents with oedema and proteinuria, and electrophoresis of the blood shows a hypoproteinaemia. There is usually no history of acute glomerulonephritis, and there are no other symptoms. The syndrome is the result of a variety of preceding diseases, and the histological manifestations in the kidneys are various and not informative. Most frequently, biopsy will show evidence of patchy or focal thickening of the endothelial cells of the capillary walls in the glomeruli. Despite this, renal function tests, blood urea nitrogen, and serum creatinine levels are normal.

### Prognosis

Pregnancy in no way affects the course of the disease, but the disease affects the pregnancy. There is an increased risk of abortion, and the perinatal mortality rate is about 100 per 1000, unless pre-eclampsia supervenes when it rises to 300 per 1000. Pre-eclampsia occurs in about one-third of patients, so that the overall fetal mortality is 15 per cent.

### Treatment

The patient is encouraged to rest in early pregnancy, and a high protein diet is prescribed ( > 3g/kg bodyweight). Oedema usually increases during pregnancy but diuretics should be avoided, in general, as they may decrease the blood volume and compromise placental perfusion. As urinary tract infection is a hazard, the patient should be screened for symptomless bacteriuria, each month from 20 weeks gestation. The patient should be examined at 2-weekly intervals until the 24th week, and weekly thereafter when evidence of hypertension is sought. If hypertension develops, or the growth of the fetus is slow, bed-rest in hospital should be advised.

## CHRONIC NEPHRITIS WITH NO IMPAIRMENT OF RENAL FUNCTION

The patient may have a history of acute nephritis, or persistent proteinuria may be found at routine antenatal visits. The blood pressure is usually raised slightly, but only rarely exceeds 180/110. In some cases anaemia is present. Renal function tests show no alteration and the serum creatinine is less than 0.09mmol/litre (1mg/dl). Lupus erythematosus cells should be sought in the peripheral blood.

### Prognosis

It is doubtful if renal function amongst patients with well-compensated disease is adversely affected by pregnancy, but in at least 40 per cent of cases the blood pressure rises above normal pregnant levels. There is an increased risk of abortion in early pregnancy, the babies are frequently small, dry and wizened at birth ('dysmature'), and the perinatal mortality is about 40 per cent.

### Treatment

The patient requires additional bed-rest throughout pregnancy. She should be seen in consultation with a renal physician at frequent intervals. Fetal growth rate should be assessed by serial ultrasound examinations starting in the second quarter of pregnancy. Renal function should be checked regularly, and a rising serum creatinine or a falling creatinine clearance are of concern. Bacteriuria should be sought each month and if found treated. If hypertension occurs it should be treated (see p. 211).

Evidence of increasing renal failure (a falling creatinine clearance and a rising serum creatinine) and the finding of fetal growth retardation requires either delivery or dialysis, although the latter is associated with an increased risk to the fetus. If LE cells are found, prednisone 30 to 60mg daily may improve the prognosis.

## CHRONIC NEPHRITIS WITH IMPAIRMENT OF RENAL FUNCTION

About 25 per cent of patients with chronic renal disease will have evidence of impaired renal function at the initial visit. When renal failure is advanced, pregnancy is unusual; and when lesser degrees of impairment exist, abortion is common. If pregnancy continues, it is likely to diminish the life of the patient, but no absolute evidence is available. Most of these women are anaemic, their blood pressure usually exceeds 180/110, and evidence of renal decompensation may be marked. If the serum creatinine exceeds 0.12mmol/litre (1.4mg/dl), at the initial visit, it is unlikely that a live baby will be born.

### Prognosis

Over 70 per cent of patients in this group will show deterioration in pregnancy; in some this reverts after delivery, but in others it is progressive. The fetal loss is over 60 per cent.

### Treatment

If the patient is seen in early pregnancy and has all the children she wants, or has evidence of severe renal impairment, therapeutic abortion should be discussed. If she chooses to continue the pregnancy, bed rest in hospital should be advised, or she should be seen at weekly intervals. The treatment is that described in the last section.

The problem is to determine when the risk to the fetus in utero exceeds that to the infant in a neonatal intensive care nursery. As well, many fetuses die unexpectedly in utero or at a stage when delivery is associated with a high perinatal loss and a high risk of handicap in the survivors (pregnancy <26 weeks, fetus less than 750g weight).

Following childbirth the question of further pregnancies should be discussed, and contraception or a permanent method of birth control suggested.

## GENERAL POINTS IN MANAGEMENT OF CHRONIC RENAL DISEASE

1. Examination of a midstream specimen of urine for bacteria, protein and casts should be performed at the first visit.
2. The presence, or suspicion, of renal disease is managed as follows:
   (a) The patient must be seen throughout pregnancy at intervals of no more than 2 weeks.
   (b) Admit the patient to hospital if increasing hypertension, a rising serum creatinine (or blood urea), or slow fetal growth is detected.
   (c) If the patient has signs of renal impairment in

early pregnancy, continuation of pregnancy is contra-indicated, except in special circumstances.

(d) A serum creatinine about 0.18mmol/litre (2mg/dl), with evidence of poor fetal growth, is an indication for renal dialysis or induction of labour, depending on the duration of the pregnancy.

(e) In general, labour should be induced at the 37th week in patients with chronic renal disease.

(f) As all forms of renal disease may be associated with (or lead to) fetal growth retardation, regular assessment of fetal growth (by serial ultrasound), and fetal well-being (see Chapter 36) should be made from about the 25th week of pregnancy.

## ORTHOSTATIC PROTEINURIA

This is a relatively uncommon disturbance in which protein appears in the urine, usually in a concentration of less than 100mg/dl when the patient stands erect and lordotic. It disappears when the patient lies down or puts her shoulders forward. It is believed to be due to renal venous congestion. The importance of orthostatic proteinuria is that it must be differentiated from the proteinuria of glomerulonephritis. In the latter the protein does not disappear from the urine when the patient lies down. In cases of doubt, the patient should micturate late at night without getting out of bed, and again in the morning before rising. If protein is absent in the morning specimen, orthostatic proteinuria is the probable diagnosis.

## Chapter 28

# Haematological Disorders in Pregnancy

Of the various haematological disorders which may occur in pregnancy, anaemia is the most common. Even in the developed countries, many women enter pregnancy with depleted body stores of iron, and in the developing lands this depletion is marked. Anaemia is closely related to social and economic status: the lower the status the greater is the incidence of anaemia, and in each social group the degree of anaemia is always greater in women than in men.

## IRON METABOLISM IN WOMEN

The absorption of iron from the intestine is a function of the mucosal epithelial cells of the small gut, the most important factor being the mucosal cell iron content. A precise interplay occurs between the iron content of the cell when formed and the iron which enters the cell during its absorptive period. Thus the greater the amount of iron fixed in the cell during its differentiation, the less it can absorb during its life. Since the cells have a short life, at any one time only 10 to 30 per cent of iron available to the mucosa can be absorbed, the percentage depending on the presence or absence of anaemia. The lower the haemoglobin level of the individual, the greater is the amount of iron absorbed. Any iron which is absorbed is very rapidly transferred through the cells to the plasma. In the plasma it links with transferrin and is transferred in this way to the body stores where it is stored in the form of ferritin and the insoluble haemosiderin. Iron is released from ferritin to the bone marrow for incorporation into the erythrocytes and the enzyme systems.

A mature woman has a total body iron content of between 3500 and 4500mg. Of this, 75 per cent is held in the erythrocytes as haemoglobin, 20 per cent in the body stores, mainly in the bone marrow and reticuloendothelial system as a ferritin complex, and the remaining 5 per cent is held in muscles and in enzyme systems, mainly in the form of myohaemoglobin.

The iron content is not static, and that portion in the erythrocytes, particularly, is in constant flux. This is because the average life of an erythrocyte is 100 to 120 days. Each day erythrocytes die and disintegrate, and new erythrocytes are formed. The disintegrating erythrocytes release about 27mg of iron, and approximately 1mg is lost to the body through cells shed from the gastro-intestinal tract, the skin, hair, nails and genito-urinary tract. Since the developing erythrocytes require about 27mg of iron daily, a deficit of 1 mg results. Iron is also lost each month by women in the menstrual flow (mean 30mg, or 1mg daily). Thus the non-pregnant woman needs to absorb 2mg of iron a day to maintain iron balance, and to keep her body stores full.

A non-anaemic woman absorbs between 14 and 20 per cent of the iron available in food, provided the diet is the 'mixed' diet usually eaten in the developed nations; when the diet is predominantly cereal in nature, very much less iron is absorbed. Thus to obtain the 2mg required daily, a woman eating a diet containing 25 per cent of animal food, needs 12mg of dietary iron; while a woman eating a cereal diet needs between 20 and 28mg of dietary iron each day.

Pregnancy imposes additional demands for iron. Although menstruation ceases in pregnancy and lactation, the increased red cell mass and additional muscle formation (including that of the uterus) requires about 425mg of iron spread out over the 40 weeks of pregnancy; the fetus requires 300mg and the placenta about 25mg. Most of the fetal requirements are in the last 10 weeks of pregnancy, relatively little iron being needed before this.

Pregnancy thus places an additional demand for

| | Over period | | Daily needs | |
| | | | | |
| Week | Net maternal needs[1] | Fetoplacental needs | Total daily need | Daily intake required[2] |
| | mg | mg | mg | mg |
| 1–9 | 90 | 40 | 2.3 | 10–12 |
| 10–19 | 112 | 65 | 2.5 | 10–12 |
| 20–29 | 112 | 120 | 3.3 | 14–16 |
| 30–39 | 112 | 200 | 4.5 | 18–22 |

Notes

1. The net maternal needs are calculated from:

| | |
|---|---|
| Replacement of iron lost from epithelial cells | 1mg/day |
| Increase in red cell mass and muscle development | 1.6mg/day |
| *Less* Savings due to amenorrhoea | 1mg/day |
| Net daily needs | 1.6mg/day |

2. Assumes a daily utilization rate of 20 to 25 per cent of dietary elemental iron.

**Table 28/1** Iron requirements in pregnancy

iron on the mother of 750mg, less the 250mg 'saved' by the cessation of menstruation, a total of 500mg of iron being needed. Although the red cell mass and muscle needs occur evenly throughout pregnancy, the fetal demand for iron is only marked after the 30th week, so that the daily amount of iron needed varies. In the first 29 weeks the total daily iron intake required is about 2.5mg, and in the last 10 weeks the quantity needed daily rises to 4.5mg (Table **28/1**). About 20 to 30 per cent of the iron presented to the intestinal mucosa is absorbed, the larger percentage occurring in the last quarter of pregnancy. For this reason the diet of the pregnant woman needs to contain 15 to 20mg of elemental iron (Table **28/1**). If, as is common in the tropics, the woman has hookworm infestation, which can cause a considerable loss of blood in the stool, considerably more iron is needed.

Should iron needs exceed iron intake, as may occur in pregnancy, iron is mobilized from the iron stores held in the bone marrow, the liver and the spleen.

Depletion of iron stores can be detected clinically by measuring serum ferritin. If the serum ferritin is below 10μg/litre the iron stores are depleted. The lower the serum ferritin, the greater the depletion.

Depletion of iron stores increases during pregnancy, even if oral iron is given, and in the last quarter of pregnancy over 50 per cent of women have depleted stores. Clinical anaemia (Hb < 10.5g) only appears after considerable depletion of the stores.

Depleted iron stores may be a physiological change associated with pregnancy, or may be an indication for giving supplemented iron. The issue remains controversial. For this reason the place of iron medication in pregnancy is uncertain. Most women in the higher socio-economic groups in the developed nations eat a diet providing an adequate amount of iron and need no supplementation, or, at most, a daily tablet containing 85mg of elemental iron from about the 26th week of pregnancy. Underprivileged women in the developed nations and most pregnant women in the developing nations need iron supplementation in larger amounts. The WHO recommends a supplement of 120 to 240mg per day, and in addition the women should receive 500μg of folic acid daily in the second half of pregnancy.

# ANAEMIA IN PREGNANCY

The haematological changes which occur in pregnancy were described on page 37, and will only be summarized (Fig. **28/1**). The plasma volume increases proportionately more than the red cell volume, so that an apparent hydraemia occurs with a fall in haemoglobin concentration to about 12g/dl after the 20th week of pregnancy. However, the total red cell mass is greater than in the non-pregnant woman, and there is adequate oxygen-carrying capacity to meet the needs of mother and fetus.

Anaemia can result from: (1) inadequate iron in the diet; (2) malabsorption; or (3) excessive iron loss (in menstruation, pregnancy or hookworm infestation). Initially the body stores become depleted, but later anaemia becomes apparent. In tropical countries where the diet often contains insufficient iron, where pregnancy is frequent and hookworm infection common, the average female has a mean haemoglobin concentration of 10.5g/dl as compared with one of 13.5g in women of the higher socio-economic groups of the developed countries.

## THE EFFECTS OF MATERNAL ANAEMIA

The effect of severe anaemia was studied in 2250

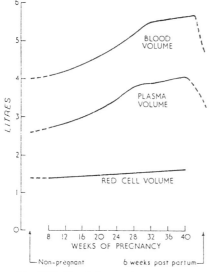

Fig. **28/1**  Blood changes in pregnancy

women in Malaysia. The *maternal* mortality amongst anaemic women was five times that of non-anaemic women (Table **28/2**). The effect on the *fetus* was even greater, the stillbirth rate being six times as high as in the non-anaemic patient (Table **28/3**).

| Mothers | Anaemic | Non-anaemic |
|---|---|---|
| Died | 35 | 248 |
| Lived | 2215 | 70 550 |
| Total (73 048) | 2250 | 70 798 |
| Maternal death rate (per 1000) | 15.5 | 3.5 |

**Table 28/2**  The effect of severe anaemia (haemoglobin less than 6.5g/dl) on the maternal mortality rate (1953–62)

## THE DIAGNOSIS OF ANAEMIA

Most cases of anaemia in pregnancy are due to iron deficiency, but in areas where migrants from southern Europe, Africa or SE Asia live, thalassaemia or sickle cell anaemia may be the cause. For these reasons it is recommended that where facilities exist, the following minimal investigations are made. Anaemia is present if one or more of the following are found:

| | |
|---|---|
| Haemoglobin | < 10.5g/dl |
| Haematocrit | < 0.30 |
| MCV | An MCV of < 70fl indicates possible beta-thalassaemia. If found, an estimation of haemoglobin $A_2$ and haemoglobin electrophoresis should be made |
| MCH | < 28pg |
| MCHC | < 32g/dl |
| Serum ferritin | A level of < 50µg/l indicates a strong possibility that anaemia will develop, whilst a level < 10µg/l indicates severe depletion of iron stores. In this case iron tablets should be prescribed, irrespective of the haemoglobin level. Some authorities estimate serum ferritin at 24, 30 and 36 weeks to ensure that iron deficiency does not occur. |

|  | Infants born of mothers who were | |
|  | Anaemic | Non-anaemic |
|  | Hb < 6.5g | Hb > 6.5g |
| Fetal loss | | |
| Premature | 215 | 2 358 |
| Mature | 85 | 1 555 |
| Fetal survival | | |
| Premature | 202 | 1 775 |
| Mature | 1795 | 66 308 |
|  | 2297 | 71 996 |
| Premature rate (per cent) | 18.1 | 5.7 |
| Fetal loss – overall (per cent) | 13.1 | 6.8 |
| Mature babies only (per cent) | 4.5 | 2.3 |
| Premature babies only (per cent) | 51.6 | 57.0 |
| Stillbirth rate (per 1000) | 91.0 | 15.7 |
| Neonatal death rate (per 1000) | 43.1 | 40.3 |

**Table 28/3** Fetal maturity and loss related to maternal anaemia ('premature' indicates a birth-weight between 500 and 1999g)

## IRON DEFICIENCY ANAEMIA

The majority of cases of anaemia in pregnancy are due to iron deficiency in the diet, or to lack of absorption from the intestine. The former is the more important. A routine haematological examination should be made at the first visit, at the 30th week, and again at the 36th week of pregnancy. If the haemoglobin is less than 10.5g, anaemia should be diagnosed. The packed cell volume should be determined and a peripheral blood film examined. The majority of patients with mild anaemia will be asymptomatic, although as the haemoglobin level falls, pallor, dyspnoea and oedema become increasingly common. Severe anaemia is potentially dangerous, as circulatory changes occur when the haemoglobin level falls below 6.5g. The changes are compensatory to maintain adequate tissue oxygenation, and consist of a rise in cardiac output and right atrial pressure, and a fall in the red cell mass. Symptoms of tachycardia and dyspnoea therefore become increasingly frequent.

### Treatment

Treatment depends upon the length of time available between diagnosis and expected date of delivery, and upon the degree of anaemia.

If anaemia is detected before the 36th week, it can be safely treated with oral iron provided the haemoglobin concentration is greater than 6.5g/dl. The iron salt used is unimportant, for all are equally absorbed and none gives a greater incidence of gastro-intestinal upset, provided the total dose of soluble elemental iron is the same. The amount of iron absorbed depends on the degree of the anaemia, and the condition of the intestinal tract. The average person cannot tolerate more than the equivalent of 600mg of ferrous sulphate daily which provides about 200mg of elemental iron. The amount of iron absorbed depends on the severity of the anaemia, but on average 25 per cent will enter the bloodstream. If the haemoglobin level is less than 10.5g/dl, this amount of elemental iron will lead to a daily increase of haemoglobin of about 0.15g/dl. Ferrous succinate 650mg or ferrous glucinate 900mg provide approximately the same amount of elemental iron as ferrous sulphate 600mg.

In the developed countries a daily dose of more than 200mg of elemental iron per day does not significantly improve haematological responses. However, in developing nations the high phytic acid content of the diet and the possibility of impaired intestinal absorption may make it necessary to double the daily iron dose to obtain a good response.

Treatment should be started with one-third of the dose required, and increased gradually to lessen gastro-intestinal upsets. The chosen iron salt should be given 8-hourly so that absorption may occur throughout the entire 24 hours of the day. If a patient is unable to take a particular salt, another should be substituted, but there is no evidence that compound tablets with trace elements have any additional value. The response to oral iron should be noticed within 21 days.

If the patient is unable to take oral iron, if the time between instituting treatment and delivery is short, or if the anaemia is marked, parenteral iron should be substituted for oral therapy. Two forms, iron dextran (Imferon) and iron-citrate-sorbitol (Jectofer) are available. Iron dextran given intramuscularly is slowly released from the depot site. Skin staining is common, but there is no evidence that the drug is carcinogenic in the human. Iron-citrate-sorbitol given intramuscularly is more rapidly mobilized, and oral iron should not be given at the same time, as there may be insufficient transferrin available to bind the iron in the plasma and reactions from free iron may occur. The drug also has a provocative effect on latent renal infection, and should be avoided if there is a history of pyelonephritis.

The dose (in mg) of parenteral iron is calculated from the formula:

mgFe =
[weight in kg × (15 − Hb deficit in g) × 4.4] + 500

Although daily injections of 2 to 5ml (100 to 250mg iron) can be given in alternate buttocks until the total dose has been given, the preferred method is to give the entire iron required in a single total dose infusion. The method is as follows:

1. The calculated dose is diluted in normal saline to make a solution not exceeding 5% (w/v iron dextran or iron sorbitol). If more than 50ml are needed, the infusion is divided and given on two separate days.
2. An oral antihistamine (such as promethazine 25mg) is given 30 minutes before starting the infusion.
3. The infusion is started at 10 drops a minute, and increased to the standard rate of 45 drops a minute if there are no reactions within 30 minutes.
4. Hidden folic acid deficiency may be unmasked and folic acid should be given orally for at least 10 days. No oral iron should be given after the infusion.

### Treatment of severe iron deficiency anaemia

The patient must be admitted to hospital, and if the

pregnancy is less than 38 weeks' gestation the anaemia is treated by parenteral iron, the total dose infusion method being preferred. Blood transfusion is the alternative, but is not recommended except in special circumstances because (1) transfusion reactions may occur; (2) the transfusion itself may precipitate cardiac failure; (3) blood is scarce and should be reserved for the treatment of haemorrhage.

If the pregnancy has advanced beyond the 38th week, the choice lies between total dose infusion of iron dextran and blood transfusion, using packed cells. But if the latter is employed and the patient's haemoglobin is less than 4g/dl, an exchange transfusion should be given, or ethacrynic acid 50mg added to the packed cells to produce a simultaneous diuresis, thus preventing circulatory overload.

A number of these patients have a concurrent folate deficiency which is 'masked' by the severe iron deficiency anaemia. Patients with severe anaemia should be given 5 to 10mg of folic acid daily for 20 days from the time of diagnosis to prevent the development of oral folate deficiency.

## MEGALOBLASTIC ANAEMIA

Folic acid is necessary in all body cells as it controls the synthesis of DNA precursors. During pregnancy when fetal cell growth is great, additional folic acid is required, and unless additional intake occurs, folic acid deficiency will arise. The clinical manifestations take some time to arise (Fig. 28/2), but by the 32nd week most pregnant women have a low serum folate. Megaloblastic anaemia is a late manifestation of folic acid deficiency and is frequently associated with an iron deficiency anaemia. In the developed countries the disease is relatively uncommon, and only 0.2 to 2 per cent of anaemic patients will show the disorder. In tropical countries the disease is more common and about one-third of patients with severe anaemia have a megaloblastic marrow in addition, and the more severe the anaemia, the greater the proportional incidence of megaloblastic marrow (Table 28/4).

| Haemoglobin concentration | Per cent megaloblastic |
|---|---|
| 0   to 2.49g | 40.0 |
| 2.5 to 4.99g | 49.0 |
| 5.0 to 6.5g | 24.4 |

Table 28/4 The incidence of megaloblastic anaemia in patients who were investigated fully (1066 severely anaemic patients, Malaysia, 1953–62)

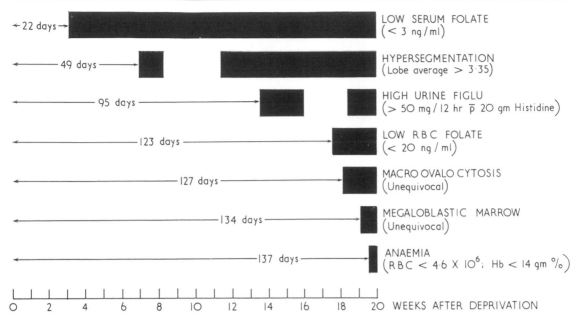

**Fig. 28/2** Development of megaloblastic anaemia in a man deprived of all folic acid (redrawn Herbert, V. *Proc. Roy. Soc. Med.* 1964, **57**, 377)

The symptoms are the same as those of iron deficiency anaemia, but the disease may develop with extreme rapidity as the folic acid deficiency becomes manifest. It may also be suspected if a patient with apparent iron deficiency anaemia fails to respond to adequate iron therapy.

The diagnosis can only be established by examination of a stained bone marrow film for megaloblasts, but may be suspected if more than 7 per cent of the neutrophils examined in a stained film have hypersegmentation of the lobes of the nucleus. Five or more lobes indicate hypersegmentation. In addition, a serum iron of above 26.8μmol/litre (150μg/dl) in the presence of severe anaemia is suggestive of megaloblastic anaemia. Examination of the leucocyte buffy coat has not proved helpful in our laboratory.

Treatment of megaloblastic anaemia is by oral folic acid in doses of 5 to 10mg daily. If absorption problems are present (as in tropical sprue or coeliac disease) and the anaemia fails to respond to oral therapy, the folic acid should be given parenterally. Since iron deficiency frequently accompanies the folate deficiency, iron should be administered simultaneously. In cases of severe anaemia it is advisable to give the iron by total dose infusion, but in other cases oral iron may be given initially and parenteral iron given only if there is no response to oral therapy.

## PREVENTION OF ANAEMIA IN PREGNANCY

It is customary for obstetricians in the developed countries to prescribe iron tablets routinely for all pregnant women without regard to the individual woman's needs. Recent investigations reviewing the use of iron given prophylactically have found no benefit either to mother or to the fetus.

Low iron stores in pregnant women do not have the same significance as in non-pregnant women, and in most women the stores are restored within twelve weeks of childbirth.

If women are healthy, are eating a good mixed diet and their haemoglobin level exceeds 10.5g/dl, prophylactic iron tablets are probably unnecessary, are wasteful, and may cause gastro-intestinal side-effects. Many physicians feel that iron tablets should be prescribed in the second half of pregnancy. Most of the side-effects are avoided if the doctor instructs the patient to take no more than 80mg of elemental iron each day (the amount contained in a 270mg tablet of ferrous sulphate, for example).

It is also uncertain if prophylactic folic acid is necessary, at least for affluent women in the developed nations. However, many doctors prescribe folic acid to pregnant women from the 20th week of pregnancy when fetal demands for the enzyme are great. This is particularly so when the patient carries a multiple pregnancy, as such women are invariably deficient in folic acid. The dose required to prevent megaloblastic change is low, and no more than 1mg per day is required.

## HAEMOLYTIC ANAEMIAS

### The thalassaemias

The thalassaemias are a genetically determined group of blood disorders, characterized by a reduced production of one or more of the globin chains which make up haemoglobin. Consequently haemoglobin synthesis is impaired. Normal adult haemoglobin is made up of two α-chains and two β-chains. Four genes control α-chain formation and two genes control β-chain formation. In α-thalassaemia one or more of the genes is deleted. In β-thalassaemia no gene deletion has been detected, but the β-chains are unstable.

All forms of thalassaemia are inherited as an autosomal recessive trait. If all four α-controlling genes are inherited, a stillborn hydropic baby is born. If three α-controlling genes are inherited, the baby is live-born but is severely anaemic because of ineffective erythropoiesis: and most of these children die in childhood. If two α-controlling genes are inherited, hypochromic anaemia is common, which is compatible with adult life and with reproduction. If one α-controlling gene is deleted the person is a clinically undetectable carrier.

Beta-thalassaemia may be homozygous or heterozygous. In homozygous β-thalassaemia both β-controlling genes are affected but α-chain production is unimpaired.

The α-chains accumulate and eventually precipitate, leading to severe haemolysis, a condition called Cooley's anaemia, or β-thalassaemia major. The affected person becomes severely anaemic, requires blood transfusions every 3 to 6 weeks and death occurs by the age of 30. In heterozygous β-thalassaemia, the normal β-gene permits developing red cells to produce about 75 per cent of the normal complement of haemoglobin, so that anaemia is usual but life is not markedly affected.

Thalassaemia is found throughout the world, but is concentrated in the Mediterranean countries, in Central Africa and in parts of Asia. β-thalassaemia is about twice as common as α-thalassaemia and affects between 5 and 10 per cent of Mediterranean peoples.

Thalassaemia in pregnancy can be excluded if the MCV is greater than 80fl. If an MCV of less than 80fl is found, iron studies should be performed. A serum iron greater than 50mg/dl ($8.95\mu$mol/litre) and a saturation greater than 15 per cent indicates iron deficiency anaemia. If the iron studies are normal, the $HbA_2$ level is determined by electrophoresis. A level greater than 3.5 indicates a β-thalassaemia trait, whilst a level less than 3.5 suggests that the person has α-thalassaemia.

If α- or β-thalassaemia is diagnosed, the father of the child is evaluated by a complete blood count and electrophoresis. If this shows he is a carrier of a like thalassaemia trait, or of another haemoglobinopathy, the situation is discussed with both parents. Thalassaemia can be detected in the fetus in early pregnancy by chorionic villus sampling and DNA probes (see p. 56). In the second quarter of pregnancy it can be diagnosed by sampling the fetal blood in the umbilical cord under ultrasonic guidance, or by introducing a fetoscope into the amniotic sac and obtaining cord blood under direct vision. If these tests show that the fetus is affected, termination of pregnancy may be offered to the parents.

During pregnancy, anaemia (Hb < 10.5g/dl) occurs in 30 per cent of thalassaemic women, and urinary tract infection is equally common. Pregnancy-induced hypertension occurs about twice as frequently as amongst women of equivalent parity.

Urinary tract infection should be sought, and if present, treated adequately. The anaemia also requires further consideration; iron preparations should only be given if studies on blood indicate iron deficiency; in other cases blood transfusion should be made available, should bleeding occur during childbirth, or if a haemolytic crisis occurs in pregnancy or labour.

## OTHER ABNORMAL HAEMOGLOBINOPATHIES

The inheritance of a defective gene which alters the locus on the chromosome responsible for haemoglobin synthesis leads to the production of abnormal haemoglobins. Erythrocytes containing abnormal haemoglobin have a greatly reduced life (2 to 15 days as opposed to 100 to 120 days in normal erythrocytes), and episodes in which destruction (sequestration) of the erythrocytes increases may occur suddenly, causing a profound anaemia. This may be associated with infarction, especially in bones, because of sludging of the erythrocytes in the capillaries.

These clinical effects are seen in individuals who are homozygous for the gene or heterozygous for two genes at the same locus. The most common abnormal haemoglobin is sickle cell (S) haemoglobin. This originated in the Middle East and has spread to Central Africa, Southern Europe and India, the highest incidence being in Uganda where 45 per cent of the population are affected. Another abnormal haemoglobin, C, is found in Ghana, and both haemoglobin S and C have reached the United States, the Caribbean and South America with slave migrants. In South-East Asia, particularly Thailand, haemoglobin E is found.

The effect of abnormal haemoglobins upon pregnancy varies with the particular haemoglobinopathy.

### Sickle cell disease (haemoglobin S and C)

Although fertility is not lowered and the incidence of abortion is not increased, the diseases cause a considerable morbidity and mortality in pregnant women, particularly if sickle cell anaemia develops. The anaemia, which is haemolytic, may develop with extreme rapidity in pregnancy (particularly if the patient also has malaria) and is accompanied by a megaloblastic erythropoiesis in many cases, as insufficient folic acid is available for the needs of the fetus and the rapid erythropoiesis. It can largely be prevented by administration of folic acid during pregnancy and, if it occurs, is more likely in the last 10 weeks. If the destruction of the erythrocytes is exceptionally rapid, it may be followed by enlargement of the liver and spleen (which are distended by the damaged sickle cells) and by sludging in the capillaries leading to the acute bone pain crisis. The sludging is due to the fact that haemoglobin S crystallizes when the $O_2$ content of the erythrocyte decreases, which causes the erythrocyte to alter its shape to that of a sickle. The sickling is reversible, but when present increases the viscosity of the blood. This in turn causes local stasis and transient vascular occlusion. Sludging is enhanced by hypoxia, by dehydration, by acidosis and by trauma, and is therefore more common in labour. The main danger of the

infarction in bone, which occurs distally to the occlusion of the capillaries, is fat embolus.

### Haemoglobin E

This abnormal haemoglobin causes fewer abnormalities but is a cause of refractory megaloblastic anaemia in pregnancy. If the trait affects the baby, haemolysis of fetal cells may occur in utero with the birth of a hydropic stillborn infant, and a large oedematous placenta. The findings resemble those of Rhesus iso-immunization, but the latter is very rare amongst the peoples of South-East Asia.

### Treatment

In areas where sickle cell disease and thalassaemia are common, or if patients come from such areas, antenatal care should be directed to early detection of the disorder, and particularly of anaemia. Folic acid should be prescribed for all patients, and frequent haemoglobin estimations made. If the haemoglobin falls below 6g/dl a direct or an exchange transfusion is required, and this may need to be repeated during pregnancy. Recently it has been suggested that prophylactic transfusions of packed cells will suppress marrow production of sickle cells and dilute the number of sickle cells in the circulation. The objective of the transfusions is to maintain the HbA levels greater than 60 per cent and the haematocrit greater than 25 per cent.

Infection (especially renal infection) should be treated vigorously and prophylactic antibiotics should be given during childbirth and the early puerperium.

Should a bone pain crisis develop, the haemoglobin level must be estimated every 4 hours and a drop of more than 2g indicates the need for exchange transfusion. Heparin, given to maintain the clotting time at more than 20 minutes, appears to reduce the severity of the bone pain and the incidence of emboli. If transient hypertension and proteinuria develop during an episode of bone pain, urgent delivery is recommended.

Oral contraceptives may be prescribed safely in the puerperium.

## Chapter 29

# Cardio-respiratory Complications in Pregnancy

## CARDIAC DISEASE

The slowly progressive nature of most forms of cardiac disease reduces the life expectancy of the patient and each pregnancy places an additional strain on the heart. It is the duty of the obstetrician to minimize the effects of this strain and to prevent any reduction of cardiac reserve due to pregnancy.

### PHYSIOLOGICAL CONSIDERATIONS

It will be recalled that owing to the hormonal alterations of pregnancy various changes occur in the cardiovascular system. These are a reduction in peripheral resistance, an increase of blood volume and of cardiac output which have the effect of an arteriovenous shunt (Table **29/1**). The result of this is to increase the work load of the heart both by a rise in heart rate and in stroke volume. The additional burden on the heart starts at about the 8th week, reaches a maximum between the 28th and 32nd week and is then maintained to term. Rises occur with each uterine contraction in labour, and the burden on the heart persists, although reduced, for the first 10 days of the puerperium.

| | A-V Shunt | Pregnancy |
|---|---|---|
| Heart rate | ↑ | ↑ |
| Pulse pressure | ↑ | ↑ |
| Cardiac output | ↑ | ↑ |
| Blood volume | ↑ | ↑ |
| Blood pressure | ↑ | ↓ |
| Central A-V $O_2$ difference | ↓ | ↓ |

**Table 29/1** Comparison of circulatory alterations associated with arteriovenous shunts and pregnancy

### INCIDENCE

In the North Atlantic countries and Australasia, between 0.2 and 0.5 per cent of pregnant women have heart disease. The incidence is dropping in all nations because of better control of streptococcal infections and rheumatic fever in children. In both areas the condition is of rheumatic origin in 60 per cent of the patients, the rest being congenital (40 per cent), or due to hypertension, thyrotoxicosis or anaemia.

### PHYSIOPATHOLOGY OF CARDIAC DISEASE IN PREGNANCY

Mitral stenosis is the most common pathological disorder in women of childbearing age who have rheumatic heart disease. The narrowing of the mitral valve obstructs the flow of blood passing from the left atrium to the left ventricle during diastole. To maintain the flow at normal levels, the pressure in the left atrium increases, which also leads to an increased back pressure in the pulmonary veins and capillaries, but which is usually well compensated.

In pregnancy, this system is liable to be disturbed. The increased blood volume is distributed in the systemic and pulmonary vessels, and there is consequently an increase in the pulmonary hypertension. The increased cardiac output demands a greater and more rapid filling of the left atrium, which can only be effected by increasing the pressure in the pulmonary vascular bed. Finally the increased heart rate reduces the diastolic interval so that the flow of blood into the left ventricle through the stenosed mitral valve can only be maintained by further increase of pressure. The overall effect is to increase the likelihood of pulmonary congestion. This is due not to myocardial insufficiency, but to a mechanical obstruction caused by the damaged heart valve.

The main lesions of congenital heart disease are atrial septal defect, patent ductus arteriosus, ventricular septal defect and pulmonary stenosis. In the first three conditions, an increase in pulmonary hypertension is likely, whilst in pulmonary stenosis right ventricular failure may occur because of the increased return flow to the heart.

## CLASSIFICATION

Irrespective of the anatomical lesion, the efficiency of the heart as a pump will depend on the ability of the myocardium to force oxygenated blood through the arterial tree. The functional capability of the heart is most important in determining how the patient will fare in pregnancy. Four classes are recognized.

*Class I.* The patient has no symptoms, although signs of cardiac damage are present. She is able to engage in all normal physical activities.

*Class II.* The patient is comfortable at rest but ordinary physical exertion leads to fatigue, palpitations and occasionally dyspnoea.

*Class III.* Less than ordinary physical exertion causes dyspnoea and fatigue, although the patient is comfortable at rest.

*Class IV.* The patient has symptoms of cardiac insufficiency even at rest. She is unable to engage in any physical activity without discomfort.

Classes I and II account for over 80 per cent of all cardiac patients and although the additional burden of pregnancy may place the patient in a higher class, in general this can be avoided by careful attention from early pregnancy. The haemodynamic response of pregnant women who have cardiac disease, even of Class I severity, is less than normal. At rest, the cardiac output is lower, and the response to exercise is impaired. This could also account for the lower mean average birth-weights of infants born to mothers with heart disease. The observation is important, for it emphasizes the need for increased rest in pregnancy, as a means of improving uteroplacental blood flow.

## DIAGNOSIS

The heart of every pregnant woman should be auscultated at the first visit, and any suspicious signs, particularly a diastolic or loud systolic murmur, require further investigation, preferably by a cardiologist. At the same time the past history of the disease is assessed and the present functional capacity of the heart determined. In many cases electrocardiography and echocardiography (and, occasionally, exercise tolerance and respiratory gas exchange tests) may be needed to assess cardiac reserve.

It is particularly important to assess the patient's heart in early pregnancy as, in the second half of pregnancy, cardiac assessment becomes increasingly difficult. As pregnancy advances dyspnoea and slight oedema are relatively common, and the unwary physician may feel that these symptoms suggest heart disease. In normal women the heart appears enlarged transversely; heart murmurs, due to the hyperdynamic circulation, are fairly common, and a change in lead III in an electrocardiogram often occurs, so that the diagnosis of heart disease may be difficult.

## MANAGEMENT

The aim of management of patients with diagnosed heart disease is to prevent heart failure. To achieve this the full, intelligent co-operation of the patient is essential. At the initial visit her daily activities should be evaluated, and advice given to lighten the burden of household duties. Since the early signs of cardiac decompensation are dyspnoea and cough the patient should be instructed to report at once if these occur. Anaemia must be sought and treated, and the onset of infection, particularly of the respiratory tract, requires urgent aggressive treatment. Overactivity must be avoided and the patient should restrict her activities to some extent. The degree and type of restriction can only be determined by considering the degree of cardiac malfunction and the patient's social background and living patterns. The obstetrician must determine these factors before giving advice, as overtreatment can create a cardiac cripple and do more harm than good. Indeed anxiety, by increasing the heart rate, may in itself precipitate heart failure. As a general statement it can be said that the patient should try to rest each afternoon for at least 2 hours, and spend 10 hours in bed at night.

The sinister warning of dyspnoea should be stressed and the patient instructed to contact her obstetrician at once should this arise. Weight gain must be regulated and, if necessary, diets ordered.

In order to anticipate signs of failure the patient should be seen at intervals of no more than 2 weeks in the first 28 weeks and thereafter weekly until delivery occurs. At each visit the patient is interrogated to find out if increasing breathlessness on exertion has arisen, or whether she has a cough or orthopnoea. These symptoms may indicate pulmonary venous congestion and are the first signs of impending failure. The lung bases must be auscultated at each visit to detect râles. The presence of these signs and symptoms is usually an indication for admission to hospital. Further treatment will depend on the functional grade, and this must be assessed at each visit:

*Grade I.* No additional treatment is needed.

*Grade II.* Most patients in this grade do not require any additional therapy, but should make sure that they avoid undue exertion, particularly between the 28th and 32nd week when the strain on the heart is maximal. Unfavourable social conditions, or any signs of deterioration in cardiac reserve, require that the patient be admitted to hospital.

*Grade III.* In general these patients are best admitted to hospital for the duration of pregnancy and, certainly, from the 28th week. Digitalis is generally required.

*Grade IV.* Patients in this grade (only 5 per cent of the total) are at grave risk and must be in hospital throughout pregnancy.

Should any patient develop heart failure she must be admitted to hospital and remain there until delivered.

## DIGOXIN

The use of digoxin as a prophylactic measure to improve cardiac output is under discussion and no agreement has been reached. Since the main physiopathological disorder is not myocardial failure, but a mechanical obstruction, digoxin is only indicated in patients in whom it will decrease the heart rate and so permit a longer time for blood to flow into the left ventricle. If the pulse rate is less than 90, there seems no reason to use the drug, but it is of obvious value in atrial fibrillation secondary to mitral stenosis. Some authors recommend prophylactic use of digoxin if investigations show left atrial enlargement.

## PROPHYLACTIC ANTIBIOTICS

Controversy persists whether prophylactic antibiotics are advisable in pregnancy. The protagonists note that although active rheumatic fever is rare, it may arise without warning. The antagonists instance the rarity of the episodes, and stress that unless patient motivation is high, the drugs are often omitted. If antibiotics are prescribed, the relatively cheap sulphadiazine (0.5g twice daily) is as useful as amoxycillin or ampicillin.

## Heart failure

The increased work load of the heart in pregnancy may lead to heart failure because of impaired myocardial contraction, but is usually consequent on increased pulmonary venous congestion in patients whose myocardial action is not impaired but whose mitral valve is markedly stenosed. The first form leads to low output heart failure and the second to high output failure. In the unsupervised patient or the patient who does not reduce her activities despite warning, failure may develop suddenly and dramatically. The treatment of the condition does not differ from that of the non-pregnant woman; complete rest in the Fowler position, oxygen, aminophylline, digoxin and rapid, short-acting diuretics being prescribed. Should labour start the prognosis is much worse.

The majority of cases of failure occur in patients with mitral valve disease. Patients with non-cyanotic congenital heart disease usually pass through pregnancy without much disability.

## Cardiac surgery

Selected patients in Grade III and IV may benefit by cardiac surgery during pregnancy, although the operation is better performed prior to conception. When failure occurs in early pregnancy the choice may lie between surgery and therapeutic abortion. If surgery is chosen the best results are obtained between the 16th and 20th week, before pregnancy puts the maximum strain on the heart.

## Therapeutic abortion

With increasing sophistication of cardiac surgery, the need for therapeutic abortion has been reduced. The method should be reserved for those women in the first 20 weeks of pregnancy who remain in Grade III or IV despite medical treatment, and who are assessed as unsuitable for surgery. Termination may be indicated if the patient has cyanotic congenital heart disease, primary or secondary pulmonary hypertension or Eisenmenger's syndrome. This is because the maternal mortality is high ($>40$ per cent if the patient has Eisenmenger's syndrome) as is the fetal loss ($>20$ per cent). Before the 12th week the operation should be by the vaginal route and after that time intra-uterine injection of prostaglandin $F_{2\alpha}$ or E is preferred to dilatation and curettage. In most cases hysterotomy is contra-indicated.

## MANAGEMENT IN LABOUR

The majority of patients with heart disease have an easy spontaneous labour. During labour the additional strain on the heart is intermittent and in total is less than that imposed upon the heart at the end of the third quarter of pregnancy. There is no indication for premature induction of labour or caesarean section in the management of cardiac disease, although these methods may be required for the management of other obstetric complications in the cardiac patient.

The pattern of labour does not differ from that of normal obstetric patients and the management is similar, but because of the known cardiac lesion the pulse rate should be checked at frequent intervals. Any rise above 110 between uterine contractions in the non-digitalized patient, indicates possible decompensation and the patient should be 'digitalized' rapidly with intravenous digoxin 0.5 to 0.75mg or lanatoside C 1.5mg. Patients in the severer grades should be kept propped up in the semi-Fowler position, and oxygen should be administered if cyanosis occurs.

If the second stage is delayed or if the patient becomes distressed, delivery should be effected by forceps, a preliminary pudendal nerve block having been established.

Analgesics should be given in the first stage, pethidine being preferred. If self-administered analgesia is required Trilene is preferable to nitrous oxide and oxygen, because the latter reduces the oxygen saturation in the blood. Epidural analgesia is preferable to both provided the patient is placed in the left lateral position, to prevent hypotension.

The third stage of labour is conducted in the same way as for normal patients. Because of the theoretical danger of a sudden increase in blood volume due to blood expelled from the uterus after intravenous ergometrine, this should be withheld, but the active management of the third stage using intramuscular Syntometrine is safe.

## MANAGEMENT IN THE PUERPERIUM

The burden on the heart continues into the puerperium, and for the first 24 hours after delivery constant observation for signs of decompensation is required in patients in Grade III and IV. The pulse must be checked hourly, the semi-Fowler position maintained, oxygen kept available and sleep encouraged. If failure does not occur in the first 24 hours, it is unlikely to occur later.

Puerperal infection is a hazard as circulating bacteria may infect the damaged heart valve and lead to subacute bacterial endocarditis. For this reason many authorities recommend the prophylactic administration of sulphonamides or ampicillin from the onset of labour and during the first puerperal week. The value of this has not yet been determined.

Although the cardiac patient is said to be most likely to develop thrombophlebitis and thromboembolic phenomena, the evidence for this is not clear, especially if antenatal care of the patient has been good. The prophylactic use of anticoagulants is to be deprecated.

The cardiac patient should remain in hospital for at least 7 and preferably 10 days and arrangements must be made to ensure that she will receive continued care from a physician after discharge.

### Future pregnancies

If the patient wants more children she can safely become pregnant again provided that she is in Grade I or II and that her heart is well compensated. Patients in Grade III and IV should be discouraged from becoming pregnant, until cardiac surgery has been performed.

If the patient desires no further children, contraceptive measures should be made use of, or tubal ligation performed. The latter may be performed in the puerperium, but in general is better left until later, when the patient has had time to weigh the implications and when the additional strain on the heart imposed by pregnancy is no longer present.

## PROGNOSIS

### Maternal

Pregnancy has no permanently damaging effect upon the cardiac function provided it is properly supervised and the hazard of cardiac failure avoided.

However, each new child requires to be reared and since cardiac disease is progressive, this attention may impose an additional strain on the heart and shorten the patient's life. For this reason the size of the family should be limited.

**Fetal**

Unless heart failure develops, cardiac disease does not alter the perinatal mortality.

# PULMONARY COMPLICATIONS

The majority of respiratory diseases do not affect the course of pregnancy and are not affected by pregnancy. Two conditions which require further consideration are pulmonary tuberculosis and asthma.

## PULMONARY TUBERCULOSIS

Although the incidence of pulmonary tuberculosis is very low in Australia and low in Britain and the USA, it is a common disease in the developing countries of the world where campaigns have been mounted to control its spread. An indirect effect of these campaigns has been to detect an increasing number of pregnant women suffering from pulmonary tuberculosis. Fortunately advances in antibiotics and chemotherapy, and surgery, have altered the prognosis for patients and the present emphasis is increasingly upon early detection and treatment of patients and their contacts. In the developing countries the emphasis is away from the institutional to the domiciliary handling of most of these patients.

It is now known that pregnancy has no adverse effect upon pulmonary tuberculosis, and tuberculosis has no effect upon the course of pregnancy. The social problems of the extra activity and reduced nutrition of the mother in the puerperium and afterwards now cause most concern: child rearing, rather than child bearing, affecting the patient adversely.

### Diagnosis

In countries where pulmonary tuberculosis is common, unless a pregnant woman has been screened for pulmonary tuberculosis by chest x-ray and/or a Mantoux test within the previous 12 months, this should be arranged by the attendant physician. Because of the possible danger of radiation to the fetus the examination should be delayed until the 16th week and a single large film should be taken.

### Management

#### ACTIVE TUBERCULOSIS

If the condition is diagnosed pregnancy should be avoided until the disease has become inactive, and remains inactive for 12 to 24 months. Should the patient become pregnant, despite advice, or if the disease is first detected in pregnancy, treatment is instituted and continued throughout pregnancy and for 6 months postpartum, or until the disease is arrested. Although regimens vary from place to place, most workers use two, or more, of isoniazid 300mg daily orally, rifampicin 450mg daily or ethambutol, 1.0 to 1.5g daily. Streptomycin should be avoided because of the potential danger of toxic damage to the eighth cranial nerve of the fetus.

#### INACTIVE TUBERCULOSIS

This requires little additional care in pregnancy apart from careful surveillance which should include at least three sputum analyses. If the social conditions of the patient are poor, assessment by a qualified social worker should be obtained.

#### SURGERY IN PREGNANCY

With the introduction of chemotherapy in treatment, there is almost no place for the therapeutic abortion, the exception being the patient who is unable to tolerate the drugs because of excessive vomiting.

Occasionally thoracic surgery may be contemplated. In general this is to be avoided in pregnancy and medical management adopted. If surgery is undertaken it should never be performed after the 32nd week of pregnancy.

#### OBSTETRIC MANAGEMENT

Labour in no way differs from that experienced by

the normal woman, and the conduct is identical. However, since the aim is to avoid fatigue, prophylactic low forceps may be used to facilitate the second stage, although most women do not require this assistance.

### THE PUERPERIUM

The patient with inactive tuberculosis may breast-feed her baby if she wishes and, apart from advising extra rest, no restrictions need be placed upon her activity. A chest x-ray should be made at the time of the postnatal examination.

The patient with active open disease should avoid close contact with her baby until the disease is quiescent. For this reason lactation should be suppressed and when possible the baby cared for by relatives. The baby should also be vaccinated with BCG as soon after birth as practicable.

The patient with active tuberculosis requires additional rest in the postpartum period and discussions should take place with the chest physician regarding further management before she is discharged from the obstetric ward.

### ASTHMA

The effect of pregnancy upon asthma is variable. The majority of patients experience less frequent attacks (probably due to the increased production of corticosteroids in pregnancy) but a few experience more attacks. Asthma has no effect on the course of pregnancy, or labour, or on the birth-weight of the fetus. In acute asthmatic attacks beta-adrenoreceptor agonist aerosol preparations such as salbutamol or terbutaline may be used. In severe attacks corticosteroid drugs (such as beclomethasone dipropionate as an aerosol) may be added, or prednisone may be given orally. Theophylline should only be added if beta-adrenoreceptor agonists or corticosteroids fail.

If recurrent severe asthmatic attacks persist in spite of the above treatments, maintenance treatment with oral or inhaled corticosteroids may be needed.

## Chapter 30

# Endocrine Disorders in Pregnancy

## DIABETES MELLITUS

Diabetes is a hereditary disorder in which insufficient or absent circulating insulin, or insensitivity to insulin, leads to high blood sugar levels, diminished glucogenesis, and the use of fat oxidation to produce energy.

Diabetics may be divided into two distinct groups. The first type '*insulin dependent diabetes mellitus*' (IDDM) usually appears in childhood or adolescence. The patient is thin, and has little or no endogenous insulin to convert blood sugar into muscle glycogen because of the destruction (probably due to auto-immune disease) of most of the islets of the pancreas. Because of this, fat is oxidized to provide energy, but the oxidization is incomplete and ketosis develops. Coma is common. The second type '*non-insulin dependent diabetes mellitus*' (NIDDM) also called mature diabetes, usually develops in middle age. The patient is fat, due to excessive carbohydrate intake over a long period of time. The disease is largely insulin resistant, and large doses are required for its control. Ketosis is rare, and diet alone often controls the glycosuria.

The aetiology of diabetes has not been fully elucidated. The current view is that the disease is due to an inherited defect in the ability of the beta-cells of the pancreas to synthesize and/or release insulin. The defect is most severe in juvenile diabetics, and less severe in mature onset diabetes where the defect may be mainly an inability of the beta-cells to release the synthesized insulin. Clinically, in the most severe cases, the expression of the defect is by a minimal insulin release in response to a glucose challenge. In less severe cases, the insulin response is sluggish and delayed. In such cases the defect may only become apparent with advancing age, with obesity, in acromegaly and in pregnancy. In constitutionally pre-disposed individuals it is also possible that antagonists to the biological activity of insulin exist, and that these accelerate the appearance of clinical diabetes.

It has been estimated that between 1 and 3 per 1000 women of childbearing age have diabetes, and a further 15 to 25 per 1000 develop impaired glucose tolerance (gestational diabetes) during pregnancy.

## CARBOHYDRATE AND LIPID METABOLISM IN PREGNANCY

In pregnancy carbohydrate metabolism is altered with the reduction of carbohydrate tolerance. There is a delay in the exchange of glucose between the blood and the tissues, and higher concentrations of glucose are found in the blood.

The increased blood glucose concentration is due in part to the increased circulating oestrogen and progesterone which may oppose the glucose lowering effect of insulin. In part it is due to the effect of human placental lactogen. HPL mobilizes free fatty acids, in some way increases insulin resistance, and also 'spares' carbohydrate for the glucose-dependent fetus, by enabling the mother to obtain metabolic energy supplies from the fatty acids. Paradoxically, in pregnancy, reduced carbohydrate tolerance is associated with an increased secretion of insulin, and the production of raised levels of circulating glucose, after eating a carbohydrate-rich meal.

A factor, recently postulated, is that the placenta has an active insulin degrading system which increases in activity as pregnancy advances. Since the levels of HPL, oestrogens and progesterone also progressively rise as pregnancy advances, insulin resistance and carbohydrate intolerance increase as term approaches. This can be demonstrated by the fact that as pregnancy advances, a standard dose of insulin causes a smaller fall in the blood glucose level.

Since the fetus largely is a glucose-dependent parasite, the higher levels of maternal blood glucose permit a more ready transfer of glucose to the fetus, provided that placental function is not impaired. The fetus responds to the hyperglycaemia by hypertrophy of the beta-cells of its pancreas which synthesize and release increasing amounts of insulin to maintain glucose–insulin homeostasis. The hyperinsulinaemia has other effects on the fetus, particularly after the 30th week of pregnancy. First, it stimulates adrenocortical activity, which could account for the cushingoid appearance of many infants of diabetic mothers. Secondly, it promotes the growth of fetal organs and the deposition of fat and protein in the tissues. This is the reason for the abnormally large size of many infants. It has been observed that about 20 per cent of infants are either growth-retarded or of normal weight, and such infants are often delivered by mothers who have diabetes with vascular complications. The reason appears to be that although there is maternal hyperglycaemia, there is also defective uterine and placental vascularization, which reduces the quantity of glucose and other nutrients transferred to the fetus.

To summarize: pregnancy acts as a provocative for the appearance of diabetes. The disease may appear for the first time in pregnancy and disappear between pregnancies. Established diabetes is made worse in pregnancy, and there is an increasing incidence of diabetes with increasing parity.

## CLASSIFICATION OF DIABETES

Much confusion has arisen in the classification of diabetes, and a scheme proposed by the British Diabetic Association, and adopted by the World Health Organization, is of value. In this classification, diabetes is divided into several groups:

### POTENTIAL DIABETES

A condition in which there is a normal glucose tolerance test (GTT) but there is an increased risk of developing diabetes because the patient (i) is an identical twin, the other twin being diabetic; (ii) has both parents diabetic; (iii) has one diabetic parent and the other non-diabetic parent; (iv) has either a diabetic parent, sibling or offspring, or a sibling with a diabetic child; (v) has borne a live or stillborn child weighing 4.5kg or more at birth, or a stillborn child showing hyperplasia of the pancreatic islets, not associated with Rhesus incompatibility. Certain other pregnant women should be considered to have potential diabetes and investigations made: these include women who have glycosuria; who have had a previous unexplained intra-uterine fetal death; who are excessively obese, particularly if high multigravidae; or who have delivered a baby considerably overweight for its gestation period. The risk of subsequent development of diabetes in these patients has not yet been fully defined, but available evidence suggests that, particularly if the patient is obese, she has a 10 per cent chance of developing clinical diabetes and a 30 per cent chance of developing latent diabetes 3 to 20 years after a pregnancy in which a baby weighing more than 4.5kg was delivered. This risk is increased if, in addition, a family history of diabetes was noted.

### IMPAIRED GLUCOSE TOLERANCE (GESTATIONAL DIABETES)

The patient has no diabetic symptoms and a normal fasting blood glucose, but the 2-hour GTT reading is between 8 and 11mmol/l. If this is found in pregnancy it is referred to as 'gestational diabetes'.

### CLINICAL DIABETES

The patient has symptoms or complications of diabetes and a GTT shows a diabetic response.

## THE DIAGNOSIS OF DIABETES

The WHO expert committee on diabetes mellitus, the British Diabetic Association and the Working Party on Diabetes in Australia have agreed on criteria to establish whether diabetes is present or not. These are as follows:

1. If diabetes is suspected, measure random or fasting blood glucose concentrations. If diabetic symptoms are present, random venous plasma values of 11mmol/l (198mg/dl) or more, or fasting values of 8mmol/l (144mg/dl) or more are diagnostic of diabetes. Postprandial values below 8mmol/l (144mg/dl) and fasting values

| | *Glucose concentration mmol/l (mg/dl)* | | | |
| | *Whole blood* | | *Plasma* | |
| | *Venous* | *Capillary* | *Venous* | *Capillary* |
|---|---|---|---|---|
| Diabetes mellitus: | | | | |
| Fasting value and/or | $\geqslant 6.7\ (\geqslant 120)$ | $\geqslant 6.7\ (\geqslant 120)$ | $\geqslant 7.8\ (\geqslant 140)$ | $\geqslant 7.8\ (\geqslant 140)$ |
| 2 hours after glucose load | $\geqslant 10.0\ (\geqslant 180)$ | $\geqslant 11.1\ (\geqslant 200)$ | $\geqslant 11.1\ (\geqslant 200)$ | $\geqslant 12.2\ (\geqslant 220)$ |
| Impaired glucose tolerance: | | | | |
| Fasting value and | $< 6.7\ (< 120)$ | $< 6.7\ (< 120)$ | $< 7.8\ (< 140)$ | $< 7.8\ (< 140)$ |
| 2 hours after glucose load | 6.7–10.0 (120–180) | 7.8–11.1 (140–200) | 7.8–11.1 (140–200) | 8.9–12.2 (160–220) |

**Table 30/1** The diagnosis of diabetes: diagnostic values for 75g oral tolerance test. From Diabetes Mellitus. Report of WHO Study Group; WHO 1985. Technical Report Series 727.

below 6mmol/l (108mg/dl) exclude the diagnosis of diabetes.

2. Only if these results are equivocal need an oral glucose tolerance test be performed using a glucose load of 75mg. The 75g is mixed with 200ml of flavoured water and drunk over a 5-minute period. This is counted as zero time.

3. When the diabetic symptoms are present the oral glucose tolerance test 2-hour value alone is sufficient to establish the diagnosis, but if they are not, at least one other abnormal reading in the oral glucose tolerance test or a raised fasting or 2-hour test is required for confirmation (Table **30/1**).

An oral glucose tolerance test is preferable to an intravenous test. In pregnancy, a cortisone stressed test confuses rather than clarifies the diagnosis. In doubtful cases, a standard glucose tolerance test and perhaps a cortisone stressed test should be made about 12 weeks after the pregnancy is over.

Although glucose tolerance tests are made on whole venous blood plasma, the day-to-day control of diabetes is made on capillary blood. The capillary whole blood glucose levels are about 7 to 10 per cent *higher* than venous blood plasma levels.

It is to be hoped that international agreement on criteria for diagnosing true diabetes and gestational diabetes can be established in the near future.

## DETECTION OF DIABETES IN PREGNANCY

Diabetes occurs in about 0.2 per cent of all women in their reproductive years and a further 1.5 to 2.5 per cent develop gestational diabetes. Gestational diabetes in women over the age of 25 causes an increased risk to the fetus. As pregnancy is diabetogenic and renal glycosuria not uncommon, the value of testing the urine of a pregnant women for sugar at each antenatal visit has been questioned. In its place it is suggested that at the first visit and again at about 28 weeks, both of which are times when blood is taken for routine tests, the venous blood glucose level should be measured. If the venous blood glucose level is > 6.1mmol/litre within 2 hours of a meal, or > 5.6mmol/litre more than 2 hours after a meal, a standard GTT should be made. All women, except known diabetics, would be screened in this way. The cost has been calculated to be less than using urine tests, with GTT when glucosuria was found.

The presence of an abnormal glucose tolerance test is an indication for an assessment of renal function and the eye grounds of the patient. The final diagnosis is made on the basis of further testing at least eight weeks after delivery.

## EFFECT OF DIABETES ON PREGNANCY

Except in cases with vascular involvement, there is no increased incidence of abortion in diabetics, and the first and second quarters of pregnancy usually pass without incident apart from the possible development of a monilial vulvo-vaginitis.

In the second half of pregnancy, there is an increased incidence of *pregnancy-induced hypertension* (PIH) and hydramnios, and a higher perinatal mortality rate. The incidence of PIH is 10 to 20 per cent (three times that of non-diabetics), but this varies with the management of the case. Should PIH develop, the fetal mortality increases fourfold. The incidence of *hydramnios* also increases in diabetic women, and the condition is an added complication in 20 to 30 per cent of cases, being highest in the uncontrolled case. *Bacteriuria* occurs twice as frequently in diabetic pregnant women as in non-diabetic parturients, and should therefore be sought at prenatal visits. The *perinatal mortality rate* is increased to between 50 and 100 per 1000, and its reduction depends on the efficiency of the management of the case. Most of the *deaths in utero* occur after the 35th week, some during labour, and in a few cases the baby dies in the neonatal period, usually from the respiratory distress syndrome. The cause of the intra-uterine death is unknown, but it may be due to altered exchange mechanisms in the placenta aggravated by maternal acidoketosis. *Congenital malformations* are found in about 8 per cent of babies of diabetic mothers, and although the malformation is trivial in many infants, the severity of the defect in the others makes this a significant cause of perinatal mortality.

It appears that insulin dependent diabetic women have a higher chance of delivering a baby with congenital defects (about 7 per cent) compared with non-insulin dependent diabetic women, whose chance of a congenitally defective baby is no greater than that of non-diabetic women (about 2 per cent). There is evidence that the incidence of congenital defects may be reduced if a known diabetic woman plans her pregnancy. In the 3 months before conception, her 2-hourly postprandial blood glucose levels should be stabilized (2-hourly postprandial capillary glucose < 7.8mmol/l), so that at conception the glycosylated haemoglobin has a normal value. Following conception the same meticulous control of the diabetes is continued.

Apart from congenital defects, the effect of diabetes on the baby depends largely on the degree with which maternal hyperglycaemia is controlled. It is believed that in poorly controlled diabetes, the transfer of excess glucose across the placenta (which is largely impervious to insulin) stimulates the fetal pancreatic beta-cells to produce insulin. The extra insulin causes fat deposition so that the baby becomes large and fat, but likely to develop hypoglycaemia in its early days of life.

As well, poorly controlled diabetes is associated with ketosis, and a consequent metabolic acidosis in the fetus, which may be sufficient to lead to intra-uterine death.

Good control of diabetes largely prevents these two problems.

## EFFECT OF PREGNANCY ON THE DIABETES

The altered carbohydrate metabolism throughout pregnancy, and the increased secretion of HPL, which antagonizes insulin, particularly in late pregnancy, lead to an increase in the severity of the disease although, unless vascular damage is present, it is only temporary. Insulin requirements increase, particularly after the 30th week of pregnancy and because of the increased loss of sugar due to the increased glomerular filtration rate, control cannot be obtained by urine tests. In pregnancy, blood sugar estimations are essential for good control. Ketosis is common, and unless corrected quickly, and its recurrence avoided, may be followed by intra-uterine fetal death. Immediately after delivery the insulin sensitivity increases, and the insulin dosage must be reduced or hypoglycaemic coma will result.

Vascular changes, particularly retinitis, may be aggravated in pregnancy, but usually revert after delivery.

## MANAGEMENT

When severe renal disease, calcification of pelvic vessels or marked retinopathy are present, therapeutic abortion must be considered. Since the disease is transmitted by a defective gene, it should also be considered if both parents are diabetic.

In most cases of diabetes complicating pregnancy, the disease is less severe, and in many instances is only detected initially during pregnancy (gestational diabetes).

### Pre and peri-conceptional control

Ideally the management of diabetes starts in the preconceptional or peri-conceptional period. A known diabetic woman, or a woman who has impaired glucose tolerance, should avoid becoming pregnant until her glycosylated haemoglobin ($HbA_{1c}$) is within the normal range. This is believed to reduce the chance of fetal congenital defects and to obtain optimal control of the diabetes.

### Diabetic control in pregnancy

1. *To maintain euglycaemia for as much of the day as possible.* It is known that if capillary whole blood glucose is maintained within the normal

physiological range, maternal death is eliminated and perinatal death reduced significantly. As well as this the chance that the baby will be large and fat at birth is reduced.

2. *To avoid or to detect major congenital defects.* An ultrasound examination should be made between gestation weeks 10 and 14. If measurement of the crown-rump length indicates that the fetus is smaller than expected, four out of five infants will be found to have a congenital defect. A serum alphafetoprotein (AFP) measurement should be made between the 12th and 15th week as a marker for possible neural tube defects.

3. *To determine the most appropriate gestational time for childbirth.*

4. *To ensure that the neonate can receive the appropriate intensive care if required.*

These objectives are best met if a pregnant diabetic woman is cared for by a team consisting of a physician, an obstetrician, a neonatologist and a dietician, and if she is a participant in her own care. This implies that she is informed and has medical attendants who are able to communicate.

Many cases of gestational diabetes, particularly if associated with obesity, respond to diet alone as do a few late onset insulin-dependent diabetic women. But if the diet fails to maintain the whole blood glucose within the desired limits, additional treatment will be required.

The *diet* should be adjusted, with regular advice from a dietician. A total daily energy intake of 6500 to 8500kJ is usually required. Weight gain is controlled to less than 12kg in the second half of pregnancy. Obese women should be given a weight reducing diet, but should never receive less than 4500kJ a day, to avoid the danger of acidoketosis to the fetus. The average patient should receive 100–120kJ day/kg 'ideal body-weight'. The food should be divided into three main meals and three snacks, the last being eaten at night before sleep.

The diet should provide a daily intake of about 100g protein and 200g carbohydrate.

*Insulin dependent diabetic* women (and a few gestational diabetic women) require insulin. This is given as a mixture of a pure short-acting insulin (e.g. Actrapid) and an intermediate insulin (e.g. Monotard) twice daily.

*General assessment:* When pregnancy is diagnosed in a patient with IDDM, she should be admitted to hospital for renal function testing, blood lipids, examination of the fundi and stabilization of the diabetes. The patient's fasting capillary blood glucose should be stabilized: the preprandial level at < 5.5mmol/l and the 2-hourly postprandial level at < 4.8mmol/l.

*Follow-up during pregnancy:* The patient measures her preprandial blood glucose daily and attends at weekly intervals when she is examined and her home glucose monitoring is reviewed. (If she uses a glucose meter it is calibrated in the hospital's laboratory.) If control is not maintained, or the glycosylated haemoglobin level (measured every four weeks) exceeds 10 per cent, the patient is readmitted for stabilization. From the 28th week the patient is seen weekly. The well-being of the fetus is assessed (fetal kick counts, and, perhaps, ultrasound to detect retarded fetal growth). This regimen, in which the patient is involved because of self-monitoring her glucose levels and the well-being of her fetus, enables a pregnant woman to be treated outside hospital for longer with a good control of the diabetic state. Hospital admission may be delayed to the 36th week (or later) in most cases.

*Gestational diabetics* can generally be managed as outpatients but require the same care in pregnancy, as a proportion need insulin to control the hyperglycaemia.

If the regimen outlined fails to maintain euglycaemia, as defined earlier; if PIH supervenes; if ketosis occurs frequently, or if the fetus appears growth-retarded, admission to hospital for stabilization and evaluation is needed.

In hospital, the dietary regimen is maintained and the chosen dose of a mixture of short- and intermediate-acting insulin is given. If this dose fails to reduce the fasting or 2-hour postprandial blood glucose levels to the normal range, all insulin doses are increased by 20 per cent. Control is re-evaluated every 2 to 3 days, as at least 2 days of constant diet and insulin dose are needed to establish the hypoglycaemic effect.

Some authorities admit all insulin dependent diabetic women to hospital from about the 35th week; but equally good results have been obtained by selective admission, and patients who are able to co-operate fully in the management of their diabetes, may be managed as outpatients.

## TIME OF DELIVERY

If the diabetic condition remains brittle, and admission is required, or if it is needed because of PIH, the welfare of the fetus should be monitored. This is discussed in Chapter 36.

In some cases, where the maturity of the fetus is in doubt, ultrasound may be used to help in estimating its maturity and to identify the placental site, so that this is avoided should amniocentesis be required to determine the lecithin–sphingomyelin ratio.

The presence of deteriorating PIH, of increasing hydramnios, or of frequent attacks of ketosis may make termination of pregnancy imperative as early as the 32nd or 34th week. However, most diabetics, with good control, may be permitted to continue the pregnancy to about the end of the 38th week or later. The time decided upon for delivery is not immutable. The history of the disease and the development of the fetus must be considered and a separate decision made for each patient. Pregnancy in most gestational diabetics may continue to term, but in some patients premature induction of labour is advisable.

The decision regarding the best way to deliver the baby is controversial, but the trend is increasingly towards vaginal delivery. Several groups recommend that, in the absence of pregnancy-induced hypertension and with good diabetic control, the patient should be permitted to go into labour spontaneously. They claim that this approach is not associated with an increased perinatal loss and has advantages (psychological, social and financial) for the parents. Other groups recommend induction of labour (oxytocin infusion) at about 37-weeks gestation. This regimen enables all hospital facilities to be available for the care of the mother and the neonate. Following induction, if labour is not established within 6 hours, if fetal distress or lack of progress occurs, caesarean section is performed. A few groups perform elective caesarean section at 37 weeks, and caesarean section may be required if complications arise during pregnancy.

*Management of labour:* Control of the patient's blood glucose levels is essential in labour as maternal hyperglycaemia may cause neonatal hypoglycaemia. An intravenous infusion of 5 per cent glucose is run to provide 5 and 7.5g per hour and between 1 and 3 units of insulin per hour, depending on the preceding total daily insulin needs. Blood glucose levels are obtained 1-to 2-hourly and the rate of the infusion adjusted. Following the birth of the baby, the infusion rate is reduced by half and continued for 12 hours or longer.

The alternative regimen is to set up the 5 per cent dextrose infusion and to give subcutaneous or intramuscular injections of insulin at intervals. The first injection is given when the infusion is set up and is half the woman's usual dose, the dose of subsequent injections relate to the woman's blood glucose level.

When the baby is born, the infusion rate is reduced by 50 per cent, and is continued until the next morning, when the woman's pre-pregnancy insulin dose is started (if known). In the case of gestational diabetics who required insulin for control of blood glucose, the intravenous line may be removed.

*Follow-up of women who have gestational diabetes:* Women who have gestational diabetes should be screened for diabetes mellitus each year, as 5 per

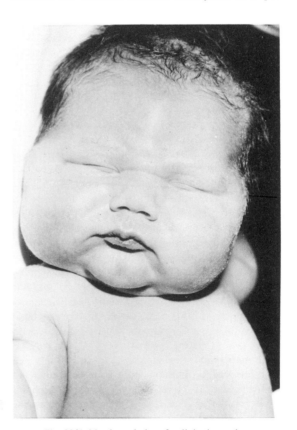

**Fig. 30/1** Newborn baby of a diabetic mother

cent will continue to have impaired glucose tolerance and about 10 per cent of these women will develop diabetes within 10 years.

## THE NEWBORN BABY

The baby born to a diabetic mother is usually larger than a baby of similar gestational age born to a non-diabetic mother. The increased body-weight is mainly due to overnutrition and fat deposition, but physiologically the infant is immature and the weight of the brain is less than in a non-diabetic baby. The heart usually is enlarged due to myocardial hypertrophy, whilst the liver and adrenal glands are occasionally enlarged. Most infants have neuromuscular excitability and a cushingoid appearance (Fig. 30/1), but this has not been correlated with increased adrenal corticosteroid secretion. The thymus is smaller than normal. The total body water is decreased, and the blood volume is increased.

Since 8 per cent of neonates have congenital abnormalities (half of which are cardiac lesions), the child must be examined carefully. This examination includes passing a fine catheter into the stomach with aspiration of the stomach contents.

Although the baby looks mature, it is particularly prone to develop hypoglycaemia ($< 1.7$ mmol/litre), hyperbilirubinaemia ($> 200 \mu$mol/litre), polycythaemia ($> 7.0$ per cent), hypokalaemia ($< 1.8$ mmol/litre) and the respiratory distress syndrome. The last complication usually develops within 24 hours of birth, after which the likelihood decreases. The baby is at 'high risk' and is best cared for in a special unit where blood gases, blood glucose and other biochemical measurements can be made at appropriate intervals.

The cord is clamped early to reduce the chance of polycythaemia. The baby is dried and placed in a warmed cot, or incubator, immediately after birth to prevent heat loss. Vital signs are monitored, and feeding is started early, when the baby shows it is hungry, usually 2 to 6 hours after birth. Oral feeding or intragastric feeding is started, as appropriate. Hypoglycaemia, which may occur within 2 hours of birth, can be prevented by early oral feeding, but if it occurs should be treated by further feeding or by intravenous glucose. The babies of diabetic mothers lose considerable weight and tend to be lethargic for the first week of life, but after this their progress is the same as that of other children. In the first 96 hours of life, sedation may be needed to control the neuromuscular excitability.

# THYROID DISEASE

The thyroid gland enlarges in pregnancy, mainly due to increased deposition of colloid, but there is some epithelial hyperplasia. These changes are due to physiological alterations in pregnancy, including increased secretion of the thyrotrophic hormone.

The common symptoms and physiological changes of normal pregnancy also mimic the clinical signs of hyperthyroidism. Tachycardia, increased cardiac output, heat intolerance and emotional instability are common to both. Because of this, the diagnosis of thyrotoxicosis in pregnancy must be made with care.

In pregnancy an increase in circulating sex hormone-binding globulin occurs, and the levels of thyroxine ($T_4$) and tri-iodothyronine ($T_3$) are raised. However, the level of thyroid stimulating hormone (TSH) is unaltered. This means that the most useful test for thyrotoxicosis is to measure TSH using the immunoradiometric assay (IMRA). If the level of

TSH is low, confirmation may be obtained by measuring $T_3$, $T_4$, and $T_3$ resin uptake. From this the thyroxine index can be calculated. A raised level of $T_3$ is confirmatory of thyrotoxicosis.

### Hyperthyroidism

Auto-immune hyperthyroidism (Graves' disease) which is due to circulating abnormal thyroid stimulating immunoglobulins may impair fertility, or may arise during pregnancy because of the hypermetabolic state. If the condition is not treated, curtailed pregnancy with premature labour may occur. The baby is usually euthyroid, but if the mother has high concentrations of thyroid-stimulating antibodies, these may cross the placenta and cause congenital thyrotoxicosis.

Maternal thyrotoxicosis is treated with the thiourea drugs, carbimazole or propylthiouracil. The latter is to be preferred as it is less readily transferred across the placenta. The objective of treatment is to keep the free $T_4$ index in the normal range. If possible the drug should be discontinued in the last 4 weeks of pregnancy to avoid the chance of fetal goitre.

There is no benefit in giving the mother thyroid medication to 'protect the fetal thyroid' as the drugs do not cross the placenta.

About 10 per cent of babies of hyperthyroid mothers become thyrotoxic in the neonatal period, due to the transplacental passage of thyroid stimulating immunoglobulins (TSIg). These affected babies can be identified during pregnancy if TSIg levels in the maternal blood (measured as long-acting thyroid stimulator protector or LATS-P) exceeds 20U/ml in the last 10 weeks of pregnancy (whether or not the mother is receiving anti-thyroid medication).

Surgery is rarely required, but if the patient has a deteriorating severe thyrotoxicosis in the second quarter of pregnancy thyroidectomy should be considered.

Labour is usually uneventful, but there is a slight danger that heart failure from toxic myocarditis may occur. In the patient who has received adequate antenatal care, this is unlikely.

**Parenchymatous goitre (colloid)**

Despite further enlargement of the goitrous thyroid gland during pregnancy, it is uncommon for any further symptoms to develop. The main risk is that the fetus will also develop colloid goitre and this can be avoided by giving the mother iodized table salt. During labour there is said to be further increase in size of the gland, with pressure on the trachea, due to venous congestion. This is very rare and occurs in the second stage during the expulsive efforts of the mother. The treatment is to give oxygen and to deliver the baby by forceps.

## Chapter 31

# Infectious Disease in Pregnancy

Pregnancy does not alter the susceptibility of the woman to infection by viral or microbial agents. The effect of the infection depends on the virulence of the invaders and the resistance of the patient. In general, pregnancy does not alter resistance, the exception being anterior poliomyelitis. Statistics suggest that a woman in early pregnancy is more likely to develop paralysis following infection with the virus, and it is therefore recommended that if immunization has not been completed before pregnancy, it should be done as early as possible in pregnancy. This is particularly important in the case of unprotected women going to an area, such as the tropics, where poliomyelitis is endemic.

Studies of many viral and microbial infections show that there is a positive correlation between the severity of the mother's infection and the effect it has on the fetus. The more severe the infection, and the earlier it occurs in pregnancy, the greater is the risk of abortion or stillbirth. This applies whether the infection is due to influenza, measles, rubella, poliomyelitis, smallpox or to bacterial infections such as enteric fever, cholera or pneumonia. With potent chemotherapeutic and antibiotic agents available, severe infections due to bacteria are rare, but no decline has occurred in the incidence of viral infections.

## THE EFFECTS OF VIRAL INFECTIONS

Examination of the abortus or stillbirth occurring after an infection does not always produce the recovery of the infective agent, and the abortion in these cases must have been due to *indirect effects* of the organism, perhaps by altering the oxygenation of the placental blood, or by reducing nutrient exchange through the placenta.

The *direct* effects of infection are more important,

and depend on the ability of the agent to cross the placental barrier. Viruses, being smaller than bacteria, are better able to do this. Viral infections occurring during pregnancy may be manifested by clinical signs or may occur without any observable effect. Such infections have two effects on the pregnancy, the indirect effect, which has been mentioned, and the direct effect due to the multiplication of the organism in the maternal system, the development of a viraemia and the subsequent invasion of, and multiplication in, the placental trophoblastic cells. The final stage is the passage of the virus to the fetal circulation and the invasion of fetal organs.

Since the essential prerequisite for invasion of the conceptus is a maternal viraemia, maternal circulating specific immunoglobulins reduce the danger, and infection of the fetus is unlikely except following a primary infection.

### The response of the conceptus to infection

The effect of infection upon the fetus is directly related to the virulence of the organism. Severe infection causes intra-uterine death of the embryo or fetus, which is subsequently expelled as an abortus or as a stillborn infant. Less severe infections do not kill the fetus, and with three exceptions appear to have no harmful effects upon its growth and development. The three exceptions are infection by rubella, cytomegalovirus and toxoplasmosis. Acute herpes simplex infection acquired at the time of delivery is also associated, in some cases, with damage to the neonate. These viral infections are designated TORCH infections, an acronym for Toxoplasmosis, Rubella, Cytomegalovirus and Herpes simplex virus. The clinical effects of TORCH virus infections include abortion, fetal death and growth retardation; while the neonate may show one or other of microcephaly, congenital heart disease, eye damage such as cataract, deafness, hepatosplenomegaly with jaundice, purpura, and later in childhood, mental handicap.

The time in gestation at which the infection occurs also has a bearing upon the degree of damage inflicted upon the fetus. Until the fetus is able to mobilize its own immunocompetent cells, and manufacture its own immunoglobulins any infection is likely to be severe. Fetal immunocompetence first becomes apparent after the 14th week of gestation but remains at a low efficiency until the second half of pregnancy.

The second protective factor is the transplacental transfer of maternal immunoglobulin. The effect of this factor is delayed in primary infections as the mother initially manufactures IgM, which is unable to cross the placenta, and it is only after a period that her immunocompetent cells secrete IgG. IgG can, and does, cross the placenta and affords some degree of passive protection to the fetus, although simultaneously depressing its own immune response.

For these reasons, a maternal infection which becomes established in the fetus in the first trimester is likely to be severe.

# RUBELLA

The virus which causes rubella is widespread, and the disease endemic in most countries. Surveys in Europe, the USA and Australia show that by the age of 19 more than 85 per cent of women have immunological evidence of a previous infection which in many cases was subclinical. Immunity is life-long in 99 per cent of cases.

Should rubella occur during the first 14 weeks of pregnancy in a non-immune woman, viraemia and infection of the fetus is almost certain, and a large proportion will develop congenital malformations or other evidence of congenital rubella. The initial response of an immunocompetent individual to infection is the production of IgM by immunocompetent cells. After a short period of time IgG is produced. The large molecular IgM is unable to traverse the placenta, so the virus is able to thrive in the fetus at a time when its own immunocompetence has not become effective. After the 14th week of gestation, fetal immunocompetence develops and the effects of an invading virus are less evident. The congenital malformations develop because the rubella virus invades actively dividing fetal cells at a period of rapid organogenesis. The virus produces an inflammatory reaction within the cytoplasm of the cell, or alters the genome so that the normal development of the organ is prevented. The organ, or organs, affected are those which are actively forming at the time of the infection. The lens of the eye forms between the 4th and 12th weeks, as does the ear, whilst the chambers of the heart form between the 5th and 7th weeks. In those cases in which congenital malformations have followed rubella, the evidence is

that specific anomalies follow when rubella occurs at a specific time: cataract is found if rubella occurs during the 5th to 7th week, deafness at 8 to 9 weeks and cardiac anomalies between the 5th and 10th weeks. In addition to damage to specific organs, congenital rubella may cause widespread cellular growth retardation, leading to the birth of dysmature infants, and continued cellular cytoplasmic reaction producing thrombocytopenia; hepato-splenomegaly, 'nephritis'; vasculitis, especially renal artery stenosis, and osteitis. In some cases the defects only become apparent in infancy, and it is hypothesized that this is due to a persistent excretion of virus which occurs in some infants. In support of this, live virus was isolated from 60 per cent of 18 cataracts aspirated from 12 infants, the oldest being over 2 years old.

The incidence of major congenital malformations varies in different epidemics, but an average of 40 per cent of women infected in the first 12 weeks of pregnancy will abort or deliver deformed infants. If the infection occurs in the first 6 weeks of pregnancy, the risk of a major congenital anomaly in the infant is 50 per cent, and between weeks 6 and 12 it is 30 per cent. Because of this, therapeutic abortion should be offered to all women who have developed rubella in the first 12 weeks of pregnancy. If the woman decides to continue with the pregnancy, she should be reassured that there is no danger to herself, although the effect of the rubella on the fetus cannot be predicted.

Until recently it was believed that the fetuses of women exposed to rubella, or developing rubella in early pregnancy, could be protected by giving the mother immune human gammaglobulin in a dose of 0.5mg per kg body-weight. It is now known that the protective value of immunoglobulins is minimal, and there is no place for the use of human immunoglobulin for this purpose.

The clinical diagnosis of rubella is difficult, as a rubelliform rash can occur with other diseases. Studies have shown that a serological diagnosis of rubella was obtained in fewer than 50 per cent of patients showing a rubelliform rash. Luckily in non-immune patients infected with rubella, haemag-glutination inhibiting antibodies develop at about the time of the appearance of the rash, and reach a peak 14 days later.

The original haemagglutination-inhibition test (HAI) test, for the presence of anti-rubella anti-bodies, which indicates a previous infection by and immunity to rubella, is being replaced by the more reliable and sensitive single radial haemolysis test (SRH test).

A pregnant woman who has been in close contact with a case of rubella, should have a blood specimen examined as soon as possible, but a specimen collected within 14 days will still give a clear indication of her immunity to rubella at the time of contact. If the SRH test is positive in a titre of $\geqslant 15\,000\mathrm{IU/litre(l)}$ ($>1:10$ in the HAI test) she is immune to rubella and need have no anxiety. A woman who has no antibodies, or a low titre, should be retested three weeks later, when a two-tube rise in titre indicates infection.

A pregnant woman who develops a rubella-like rash should have a blood specimen examined as soon as possible. A value of $\geqslant 15\,000\mathrm{IU/l}$, or more, in a specimen obtained within 4 days of the appearance of the rash indicates that the illness is unlikely to be rubella. A further SRH test is made 21 days later. A static or reduced titre at the time confirms that the illness was not rubella. In the latter case, termination of pregnancy may be properly offered to the patient.

The problem of inadvertent, or suspected rubella in early pregnancy would be avoided if all girls were given an injection of attenuated rubella virus between the ages of 11 and 14, using the RA 27/3 strain. Many women, who intend to become pregnant, will not have received the injection, and should be offered protection at a later date. Two approaches are possible. They may be offered the vaccination at marriage (but should avoid becoming pregnant for 3 months) or in the early puerperium. The alternative is to determine the SRH titre in their blood,

and only offer the injection to those women who have low, or negative titres, either when they are not pregnant, or in the puerperium.

Some concern has been expressed if a pregnant woman is inadvertently given rubella vaccination. Although this should be avoided, collected experience shows that the risk of a rubella-induced severe congenital malformation is low, less than 2 per cent of babies being affected, which is no greater than the rate in non-vaccinated women. However, the mother should be offered the choice of induced abortion or of continuing the pregnancy.

## CYTOMEGALOVIRUS (CMV)

Over half of all pregnant women show evidence of previous CMV infection and about 1 per cent develop CMV infection in pregnancy, all of which are asymptomatic. These infections are associated with an increased perinatal mortality and between 5 and 20 per cent of infected fetuses suffer congenital defects.

Unfortunately antibody screening in early pregnancy has proved of no value, as many infections occur later in pregnancy, and screening will not identify babies with congenital defects.

Until a vaccine is available, prevention of CMV infections is impossible and no treatment is currently available.

## TOXOPLASMOSIS

*Toxoplasma gondii* infections acquired during pregnancy may result in a spontaneous abortion or in congenital infection of the baby. In about 8 per cent of affected babies, the eyes or central nervous system are severely damaged, and more are affected to some degree. Statistics from the USA suggest that the incidence of congenital toxoplasmosis is 2.7 per 1000 live births.

About 3 to 6 pregnant women in every 1000 will acquire the infection during pregnancy and 90 per cent have no clinical illness. This makes prospective testing necessary if a programme to reduce congenital toxoplasmosis is decided upon. One fetus in every 4 is congenitally affected.

Serological screening tests are available. A screening programme would begin ideally before pregnancy so that sero-negative women could be identified. If this cannot be done, pregnant women should be tested in the first 10 weeks of pregnancy. Those who are sero-negative, should be retested at 20 weeks and again in the last quarter of pregnancy. Sero-conversion in the first half of pregnancy should lead to discussions about therapeutic abortion or to treatment with spiromycin which is thought to reduce the risk of congenital toxoplasmosis.

The cost of such a programme is considerable and preventive measures should be taken by pregnant women. They should avoid touching cat faeces; they should wash the hands after handling raw meat and avoid touching the eyes or mouth whilst handling raw meat.

# SEXUALLY TRANSMITTED INFECTIONS

## SYPHILIS

Early syphilitic infection in the female is often less noticeable than in the male, and indeed the primary and secondary phases may pass unnoticed. Untreated syphilis leads to the premature delivery of a stillborn infant or to the birth of a child infected in utero by *Treponema pallidum* in 50 per cent of cases. For this reason all women should have a diagnostic serological test for latent syphilis performed in early pregnancy (although the incidence of syphilis is less than 0.1 per cent in most areas). If the disease is discovered and treated before the end of the 15th week the fetus will not be affected; but if the mother is not treated until later, the infant may have some stigmata of prenatal syphilitic infection.

Two types of serological test are available. The first measures a substance called reagin, which increases considerably when the person has been infected with syphilis, and can be quantified. Following cure the reagin test becomes negative within 12 months. Two reagin tests are available. The VDRL test and the Rapid Plasma Reagin (RPR) test. False-positive reactions may occur in pregnancy, in liver disease, in drug addiction, infectious mononucleosis and autoimmune disease. For this reason a specific test is required if a pregnant woman has a positive reagin test and no clinical signs of syphilis. The specific tests detect anti-treponemal antibodies in the woman's serum. Currently three tests are favoured. These are (1) the TPHA (*Treponema pallidum* haemagglutination assay), (2) the FTA-ABS (fluorescent treponemal antibody test) and (3) the TPI (*Treponema pallidum* immobilization test). Once positive, these tests tend to remain so for life, even after cure. In some centres the VDRL and TPHA are done on the sera of all pregnant women. It is recommended that serological screening tests should be made in early pregnancy and repeated at about the 30th week. In positive cases the husband should also be examined and tested serologically.

The *treatment* of syphilis is by the daily intramuscular injection of 1 000 000 units of penicillin-G for 10 days. Alternatively, a long-acting penicillin, such as procaine penicillin in oil with 2 per cent aluminium monostearate (PAM), may be used. The initial injection of 2.4 mega-units of PAM is followed by nine biweekly injections each of 1.2 mega-units of PAM. If the patient is sensitive to penicillin, erythromycin 20 to 30g over 10 to 15 days may be substituted.

Follow-up serological tests in early syphilis detected in pregnancy are made at monthly intervals for 3 months, every 2 months for 6 months, then every 3 months for a further year. Retreatment is required: (1) if there is evidence of clinical progression; (2) if there is evidence of clinical relapse; (3) if there is evidence of serological 'relapse' shown by the conversion of a non-reactive reagin test to a reactive test or by an increase in a previously declining titre. Retreatment is also required if a titre greater than 1 in 4 persists for more than 6 months, or if re-infection occurs.

### Detection of syphilis in the child of an untreated mother

The signs of syphilis are often equivocal in the newborn and serology inaccurate. For these reasons, the infant of a mother who has contracted syphilis in pregnancy and has received no treatment or who is found to have positive serological tests in pregnancy and does not obtain treatment, should receive a full course of antibiotic treatment in the form of aqueous procaine penicillin 50 000U/kg body-weight daily for a minimum of 10 days. An alternative is to give benzathine penicillin 50 000U/kg body-weight as a single injection. If the mother has been treated adequately it is unlikely that her baby will be infected.

However, the infant must be followed both clinically and by serology.

As there may be a 'transfer' of reagin and treponemal antibody into the baby's blood, the first serological test should be delayed until he is 4 weeks old and repeated when he is 12 weeks old. If the reagin test is positive at 12 weeks, treatment should be given. Clinical signs, especially radiological signs in the long bones, or positive serology are an indication for treatment.

## GONORRHOEA

Studies in Canada and the USA using the Thayer–Martin medium for the culture of gonococci show that between 1 and 6 per cent of prenatal patients have gonorrhoea. Patients with acute gonorrhoea present with urethritis, dysuria, vaginal discharge and occasionally cervicitis within 5 days of the infection. If clinical signs and symptoms are suggestive of gonorrhoea, urethral, vaginal and cervical swabs should be taken and inoculated directly onto preheated plates of culture medium. Swabs should also be taken from all sexual contacts. If the patient is a contact and the initial swabs are negative, they should be repeated after an interval of 7 days.

Treatment in pregnancy must take into consideration the fact that syphilis may have been acquired at the same time as gonorrhoea.

Acute gonorrhoea is treated by a single injection of 4.5 mega-units procaine penicillin-G, preceded by probenecid 1g, and followed by probenecid 0.5mg 6-hourly for 4 doses. Serological tests are made for syphilis at the same time, and if negative these tests are repeated at monthly intervals for 3 months.

Careful follow-up to determine that the gonorrhoea has been cured is essential. Urethral, vaginal and cervical swabs are taken at the completion of treatment and twice more at monthly intervals. Persistence of infection, relapse, or re-infection demands retreatment, whilst laboratory evidence of bacterial resistance indicates that the dose of the antibiotic must be increased or the drug changed. Patients who are sensitive to penicillin should be treated with erythromycin. If bacterial resistance to penicillin is found, spectinomycin in a dose of 2 to 4g may be injected intramuscularly.

## GENITAL HERPES

Herpes simplex virus infections of the genital tract are becoming more common. About 90 per cent are due to HSV type II, and the remainder to HSV Type I, which is the virus usually associated with 'cold sores' on the lips or nose. HSV genital infections show as painful vulvo-vaginal or cervical ulcers, but two-thirds of those whose cervix is infected are asymptomatic. HSV genital infections occur in between 1 and 10 per 1000 sexually active women, and younger age groups appear to be at higher risk. Five per cent of those infected develop recurrent infections.

The risk of fetal infection is greatest if the mother has a primary HSV2 infection in the last quarter of pregnancy and is symptomatic (or is shedding virus from her cervix) at the time of childbirth. HSV infection may lead to intra-uterine growth retardation and 50 per cent of the infants will develop neonatal herpetic infection. A case can therefore be made for giving acyclovir to a pregnant woman who develops primary HSV2 infection in the last 10 weeks of pregnancy. If the woman is asymptomatic and not shedding virus from her cervix at the time of childbirth, the risk that the infant will be infected is less than 1 per thousand.

Recurrent HSV2 infections cause fewer problems to the fetus, the risk that the infant will be infected during childbirth being less than 8 per cent. Three reasons are given: (1) in recurrent infections HSV2 virus is present in the genital tract at a lower titre and for a shorter time, (2) the cervix is less likely to be infected and (3) the fetus is likely to have developed HSV2 antibodies.

These findings suggest that: (1) a woman with a history of genital herpes needs to have no anxiety and may anticipate a vaginal delivery unless a recurrence or a new infection occurs during pregnancy, (2) if genital herpes occurs or recurs in pregnancy, from the 34th week of pregnancy, cultures of material taken from the cervix should be made each week to determine the presence or absence of the HSV2 when the membranes rupture or labour starts, (3) if herpetic lesions are present, or the culture shows HSV2 when the membranes rupture or labour starts, caesarean section should be made within four hours to reduce the risk that the neonate will develop herpes.

## HEPATITIS B VIRUS

Although fewer than 0.5 per cent of women in the developed nations are hepatitis B carriers, up to 30 per cent of migrants from parts of Africa, East and South East Asia have hepatitis B surface antigen (HB$_s$Ag) in their blood and are potentially infectious to health care workers who may be infected by contact with blood and body secretions. For this reason, screening of pregnant migrant women and drug addicts for Hb$_s$Ag is now recommended. Precautions are made when caring for such women in childbirth and most hospitals have developed protocols.

It is also known that the hepatitis B virus is readily transmitted to the baby, probably during the birth. Babies at special risk are those whose mothers have HB$_e$Ag as well as HB$_s$Ag in their blood. If not treated, many of the babies will develop hepatocellular carcinoma when adult. This event can be avoided to a large extent if babies at high risk are given hepatitis B globulin at birth together with hepatitis B vaccine 10$\mu$g, and two further injections of the vaccine at the age of 1 and 6 months.

## HUMAN IMMUNODEFICIENCY VIRUS INFECTION (AIDS)

Although in western countries most cases of HIV infection occur in homosexual or bisexual men, intravenous drug users who share needles are increasingly being infected, as are some heterosexual men and women, who do not abuse drugs. Infected women who become pregnant have a 20 to 40 per cent risk of transmitting the virus to the fetus, all of whom will be antibody positive and will develop AIDS. There is a strong argument that screening for HIV infection should be offered to all pregnant women, particularly as there is evidence that the use of drugs such as zivudine may delay the progression of the disease. HIV infection has no adverse effect on the pregnancy nor has the pregancy any adverse effect on the progress of HIV infection. As the HIV infects the amniotic fluid as well as the women's blood, full infectious control precautions should be taken by attending medical staff during labour and child birth. Vaginal delivery may be anticipated and there is no place for Caesarean section purely because the woman has HIV infection. Because of all the problems involved, women infected with HIV should be given the opportunity to choose to have an abortion rather than giving birth to a baby which may have HIV infection.

# INFECTIONS IN THE TROPICS

## HELMINTH INFESTATIONS– HOOKWORM DISEASE

Endemic infections by helminths are almost universal amongst rural dwellers in the tropics and subtropics, and the most serious of these is hookworm disease. Two types of hookworm are found, *Ancylostoma duodenale* and *Necator americanus*, and their distribution can be seen in Fig. **31/1** (overleaf). In the gut the worms attach to the villi by suckers, and feed on blood obtained from the villi which, after passing through their bodies, is excreted into the lumen of the bowel. In studies in Malaysia, the blood loss due to hookworm related closely to the hookworm load, and varied from 2 to 90ml per day. Hookworm infestation is a cause of iron deficiency anaemia, and this is particularly serious in pregnancy. Treatment is to eliminate the worms by administering bephenium hydroxynapthoate (Alcopar) in a dose of 5g, daily for 3 days, and to treat the anaemia with iron.

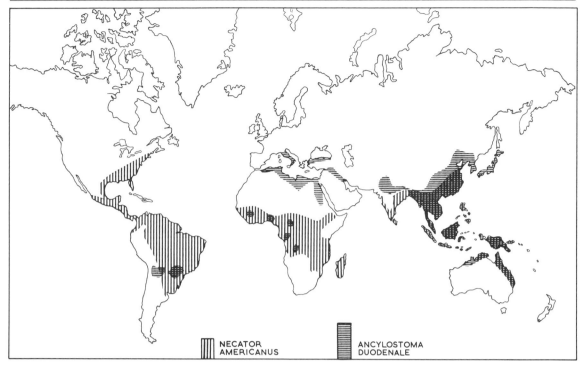

**Fig. 31/1** Distribution of hookworm disease

## MALARIA

Exacerbation or relapse of malaria in a partially immune female is particularly common during pregnancy, and each attack may precipitate abortion or the onset of premature labour. The fetus is protected by the placenta in most cases, although large numbers of immobilized parasites may be found in the placenta, particularly if the infection is by *P. falciparum*. Occasionally in non-immune patients, congenital transmission of malaria occurs.

Pregnant women travelling to an area where malaria is endemic should take prophylactic antimalarial drugs. If the strains of *P. falciparum* in the area are chloroquine resistant problems arise. The alternative drugs, Fansidar and Maloprim, affect folic acid synthesis and may induce a fatal Stevens–Johnson syndrome. They should be avoided. If the risk of chloroquine resistance is low, chloroquine and proguanil should be given. If the risk of chloroquine resistance is high, a pregnant woman should postpone her visit until she has given birth.

Any pregnant woman developing a high fever in a malarial area should be suspected of having the infection, and if this is confirmed by finding parasites in a thick blood film, treatment is given with chloroquine 600mg (base) initially, followed 8 hours later by 300mg, and 300mg daily on the next 3 days.

## Chapter 32

# Iso-immunization in Pregnancy

All humans can be divided into two groups by determining whether or not their erythrocytes contain an antigen found in the erythrocytes of Rhesus monkeys. Studies have shown that the proportion of the population with the factor (Rhesus positive) and without the factor (Rhesus negative) varies from region to region (Table **32/1**), but that the proportion of Rhesus negative people diminishes the nearer one gets to East and South-east Asia.

| | *Rhesus positive* | *Rhesus negative* |
|---|---|---|
| USA, UK | 85 | 15 |
| North India | 90 | 10 |
| South India | 95 | 5 |
| China/South-east Asia | 99 | < 1 |

**Table 32/1** Percentage of population having the Rhesus factor

The Rhesus factor is a complex antigen consisting of three pairs of alleles occupying a specific locus on a chromosome, but only one of the pairs, named D, is likely to cause iso-immunization. Thus if a Rhesus negative individual receives a transfusion of Rhesus positive blood, the immunologically competent cells in the body become sensitized to the Rhesus D antigen, provided the amount is sufficiently large. Following a subsequent exposure to the antigen, the cells are stimulated to produce specific anti-D antibodies which combine with antigen sites on the injected erythrocytes, and lead to their destruction. The Rhesus antigens are quite different from the ABO antigens found in humans but, as they are carried on the erythrocyte plasma membranes, act in a similar way, causing agglutination of the erythrocytes and subsequent haemolysis, provided complement is present.

Since the genotype of the fetus is derived from maternal and paternal genes it is quite possible for a woman to have a fetus with a different ABO and Rhesus group. As far as ABO iso-agglutinins are concerned, there is little problem. If the fetus has a different ABO group from that of the mother and fetal cells cross the placenta into the maternal circulation, normal immunological processes take place so that the cells are coated with antibody and are destroyed in the reticulo-endothelial system. The antibody formed is of large size (a macro immunoglobulin, IgM) and this is unable to pass through the placenta to affect the fetus.

The situation with Rhesus antigens is different. If a mother who is Rhesus negative has a baby which is Rhesus positive, and if sufficient fetal cells from that baby enter the maternal circulation, antibody production is stimulated. The anti-D antibodies include both the IgM and IgG immunoglobulins and the latter are sufficiently small to pass through the placenta and enter the fetal circulation, where they immediately fix onto the antigen sites on the surface of the fetal erythrocytes. In the presence of complement the antigen–antibody complex causes small holes in the cell envelope and lysis of the erythrocyte. This shows clinically as fetal haemolytic disease.

Thus the consequence of maternal iso-immunization may be haemolytic disease in her fetus or newborn baby. The extent of the problem can be gauged by the fact that 1 in 200 pregnancies is complicated by iso-immunization.

### How does iso-immunization occur?

In a few instances the Rhesus negative mother forms antibodies because of a previous injection, or transfusion, of Rhesus positive blood. Since the consequences of such an injection have been realized few cases have been reported but it is essential to remember that no Rhesus negative female should ever receive Rhesus positive blood.

In the majority of cases, the cause of the iso-immunization is due to a previous pregnancy. Usually the pregnancy has continued to viability, but on occasions, a woman may be sensitized by an induced, or a spontaneous abortion.

It is known that, in pregnancy, fetal cells enter the maternal circulation, but the numbers are small and, in general, they are destroyed before they can provoke an allergic response with the production of antibodies. This is especially so if the ABO group of the fetus is incompatible with that of the mother. In such cases any fetal erythrocytes which leak through the placenta are rapidly destroyed, usually before they can provoke an antibody response.

During labour and delivery, a much larger transfusion of fetal blood may occur, and this is more likely to provoke antibody production. Should the woman become pregnant again, the circulating antibodies persist, which may pass through the placenta and cause haemolysis of fetal erythrocytes; or a further feto-maternal transfusion at the time of delivery may lead to a marked allergic response which will affect any subsequent pregnancy.

## THE 'RHESUS' PROBLEM

The chance of a Rhesus negative mother bearing a Rhesus positive child is 75 per cent, but even so she has only a 15 per cent chance of being sensitized at the time of delivery of the first child. Unless she has had a transfusion of Rhesus positive blood, the small amounts of fetal blood which may enter her circulation in pregnancy are usually insufficient to sensitize her, and it is only the larger quantity entering her circulation during labour which causes the hyper-immunity. As well, about one-third of Rhesus negative people are 'non-responders', failing to produce anti-D antibody when injected with Rhesus positive cells. Once the mother is sensitized only small infusions of fetal erythrocytes are needed to stimulate antibody production. The first baby is almost never affected, the second baby has a 15 per cent chance of being affected, but the risk of the fetus developing haemolytic disease increases with each subsequent pregnancy. The first affected baby is usually only affected mildly (although 10 to 20 per cent are severely affected) but subsequent babies have an increased risk of being severely affected.

## CONDUCT OF PREGNANCY

In view of the above it is essential to know whether a mother has developed iso-agglutinins, and whether the agglutinins have passed across the placental barrier and are causing fetal erythrocyte haemolysis. This information can be obtained by two methods and treatment decided upon after scrutinizing the results.

### Routine serum testing

All pregnant women should be tested to determine their Rhesus group at the first prenatal visit. If the woman is Rhesus negative, her husband, or partner, should be asked to have his Rhesus group determined. If he is found to be Rhesus positive, or refuses to be tested, the pregnant woman should have her serum examined for iso-agglutinins during pregnancy. Even with enzyme testing mild iso-immunization may not be detectable in early pregnancy. For this reason, the blood of all Rhesus negative women should be tested at 4-weekly intervals from week 20. If iso-agglutinins are found in a titre of 1 in 8 or higher by the indirect Coombs' method in any test, further assessment should be made by amniocentesis, as the degree of haemolysis of fetal erythrocytes does not correlate with the maternal antibody titre.

### Amniocentesis

The basis for amniocentesis in determining the severity of fetal haemolysis depends on what is known about fetal excretion of bilirubin. Bilirubin circulates bound to serum albumin. Most of this is excreted into the maternal circulation via the placenta, but a small quantity is filtered into the amniotic fluid through the mucosa of the upper respiratory tract. Although the fetal liver is unable to deal with this unconjugated bilirubin, it has a limited capacity to conjugate it with glucuronic acid. This capacity is about 40 per cent of that of the adult liver and is due to enzymatic immaturity. The conjugated bilirubin is water-soluble and is excreted by the fetal kidneys into the amniotic fluid. The level of bilirubin in the amniotic sac correlates fairly well with the amount of erythrocyte destruction, and hence with the degree of fetal anaemia. This is the basis of amniocentesis in the management of Rhesus iso-immunization. The quantity of bilirubin in the liquor amnii can be estimated by spectrophotometry.

In the absence of bilirubin the absorption spectra of amniotic fluid for the range 360 to 630nm in a

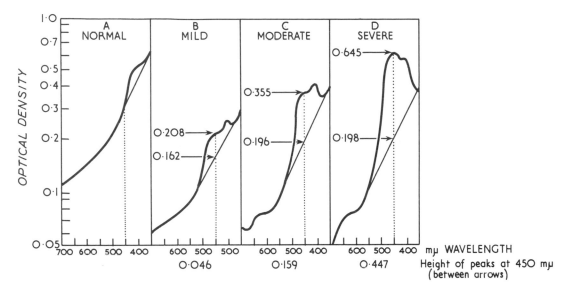

**Fig. 32/1** Spectral absorption curves of amniotic fluid in (from left) normal late pregnancy, mild, moderate and severe haemolytic disease. The method of measurement of the peaks is shown (redrawn from Liley, A. W. *Triangle* 1966, 7, 184, published by Sandoz)

spectrophotometer is expressed as a relatively straight line (Fig. **32/1A**). If albumin-bound bilirubin is present in the liquor, increased absorption is found at a wavelength of 450nm and this shows as a characteristic peak (Fig. **32/1B**). The measurement of the height of the peak above the 'normal' optical density at 450nm gives a fairly close indication of the amount of bilirubin present and of the severity of the haemolytic process. The condition of the fetus in utero can therefore be assessed by estimating the bilirubin content of the liquor obtained at amniocentesis. 2 to 5ml of liquor amnii are removed using a lumbar puncture needle which is inserted into the uterus just below the mother's umbilicus and on the side opposite to that of the fetal spine. The colour of the liquor is inspected and the specimen is subjected to spectrophotometry. When possible the position of the placenta should first be determined using ultrasound.

If the patient develops antibodies during the pregnancy, in a titre of more than 1 in 8, amniocentesis should be performed at discovery provided the pregnancy has advanced to 28 weeks. If there is a history of previous stillbirths, or if antibodies have been present from early pregnancy the first tap is made at the 24th week or even earlier.

The bilirubin peak is entered on to a chart devised by Liley in New Zealand (Fig. **32/2**). If the level lies in the high zone, the baby will certainly be severely

affected and may die in utero. If the pregnancy has advanced to 32 to 34 weeks, labour should be induced; and before that date intra-uterine fetal transfusion offers a 35 per cent salvage rate, unless the fetus is hydropic when the transfusion is of no benefit. If the peak lies in the mid-zone, a further amniocentesis is performed 2 to 3 weeks later and the height of the peak is noted, treatment being planned on this result. Further taps may be required, as the objective is to maintain the pregnancy at least to the 32nd week when delivery may be indicated. If the peak lies in the low zone, a further tap is made at the 34th week. If this tap shows that the peak is now in the mid-zone, treatment is for that condition, but if the peak remains in the low zone pregnancy may continue to 38 weeks, or to term.

If the reading is within the upper part of the mid-zone or is in the high zone, the fetus is likely to be severely affected, occasionally hydropic with a haemoglobin of less than 4g, and at great risk of dying. This event may be reduced by intra-uterine intravascular fetal transfusion. Under ultrasonic guidance a 22-gauge needle is introduced into an umbilical cord vessel. A fetal blood sample is taken to estimate the haemoglobin level and to calculate the amount of Rh negative blood needed for the transfusion. Transfusions are repeated as required. However, the fetal loss exceeds 75 per cent in spite of these techniques, and there is some doubt if they

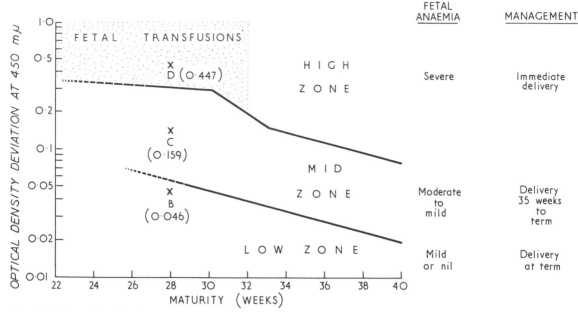

**Fig. 32/2** The relationship between the size of the amniotic fluid pigment peak at different stages of maturity and fetal anaemia and management (redrawn from Liley, A. W. *Triangle* 1966, 7, 184, published by Sandoz). (The peak figures from **32/1** B, C and D are charted in **32/2**)

should be used. A reading in the lower mid-zone is associated with a fetal survival rate of 80 per cent and intra-uterine fetal transfusions are not indicated. Readings remaining in the lower zone are associated with a fetal survival rate of 95 per cent.

**Premature induction of labour**

The decision to deliver the baby prematurely is made on the amniotic fluid findings. Since the patients are multiparous, induction of labour by amniotomy is the usual method. If labour has not started within 6 to 12 hours, an oxytocin infusion may be given to stimulate contractions. Caesarean section has a limited place but should be considered if oxytocin fails to induce labour or if termination of pregnancy is thought advisable before the 34th week, as at this stage induction of labour is often not successful.

The placenta in cases of babies affected by haemolytic disease is usually enlarged, oedematous and friable, and disruption is common during delivery, with possible retention of a cotyledon. On histological study the villi are greatly enlarged with increased density of collagen tissue. The fetal vessels are not enlarged but because of the haemolysis contain few erythrocytes and consequently appear larger. The cytotrophoblast is increased in amount

when compared with a normal placenta at a comparable period of gestation.

**THE PREVENTION OF RHESUS ISO-IMMUNIZATION**

About 98 per cent of cases of Rhesus iso-immunization can be prevented by giving every unsensitized Rhesus-negative woman, who gives birth to a Rhesus-positive baby, an injection of Rhesus anti-D gamma globulin within 72 hours of birth. A similar injection should be given to unsensitized Rhesus-negative women after an abortion, an amniocentesis or an external cephalic version. The Rh-anti-D IgG either occupies D-antigen binding sites on the fetal erythrocytes, which prevent them expressing their antigenicity, or blocks maternal lymphocytes from detecting the fetal cells.

A few Rhesus-negative women (1 to 2 per cent) will develop Rhesus antibodies during late pregnancy. These women will be protected if given anti-D immunoglobulin injections in late pregnancy. The injections are of no value to women already sensitized, so that every Rhesus-negative woman should be screened for Rhesus antibodies from early pregnancy.

The following scheme would solve the 'Rhesus problem'.

1. All Rhesus-negative, unsensitized women who abort spontaneously needing curettage or have an abortion induced are given an injection of 125µg Rh-anti-D IgG within 72 hours of the abortion.
2. All Rhesus-negative, unsensitized women who require amniocentesis, receive a similar injection, unless the father is Rhesus negative.
3. All Rhesus-negative, unsensitized women, whose pregnancy progresses normally receive an injection of 100µg Rh-anti-D IgG at 28 and 34 weeks' gestation, unless the father is Rhesus negative.
4. All Rhesus-negative, unsensitized women, who give birth to a Rhesus-positive baby are given an injection of 250µg (2ml) of Rh-anti-D IgG within 72 hours of birth. As the amount of transplacental haemorrhage is unknown, an indirect Coombs' test is made 24 hours after the injection. If the Coombs' test is negative (indicating no circulating anti-D IgG) a Kleihauer test is made on the mother's blood. The test permits an estimate of the number of fetal cells in her blood to be made. If a transplacental haemorrhage > 5ml of fetal cells is discovered (> 80 fetal blood cells per 50 low-power fields), an additional injection of anti-D gamma globulin is given so that the dose is 20µg per ml of red cells.

The third recommendation, although logical, poses a problem. Only about 1.5 per cent of Rh-negative women will become sensitized during pregnancy, but if all Rh-negative women are given an injection of anti-D IgG at 28 weeks, the quantity of antibody required will be increased fourfold.

Anti-D IgG is prepared from plasma from human donors, who have to be subjected to regular plasmophoresis and who require periodic injections of Rh-positive red cells to maintain a higher titre of antibodies in their plasma. The two procedures are not without risk, but if they are carried out by experienced people the risk is small.

In the next few years this problem may be solved by the production of anti-D Rhesus antibody by tissue culture.

## HAEMOLYTIC DISEASE OF THE FETUS AND NEWBORN

The effect of the transplacental passage of iso-agglutinins depends upon the amount of immunoglobulin and the duration of its action. The infant responds to the haemolysis by hyperplasia of its erythropoietic tissues; the bone marrow becomes hyperactive and later the spleen and liver enlarge and begin erythropoietic activity. The clinical appearance of haemolytic disease depends on the balance of these two factors; and three grades of severity are found.

### 1. HAEMOLYTIC ANAEMIA OF THE NEWBORN

The haemoglobin level is reduced from the normal 18g/dl but is more than 14g/dl. Jaundice is usually absent, or slight, at birth, but may develop during the 2nd week of life when further haemolysis occurs. The prognosis is good, provided that haemoglobin concentration and serum bilirubin levels are kept at reasonable levels.

### 2. ICTERUS GRAVIS NEONATORUM

The baby is anaemic (haemoglobin concentration 10 to 14g/dl) and jaundice usually appears soon after birth and always within 48 hours. The liver and spleen are enlarged and the serum bilirubin level exceeds 210µmol/litre (10mg/dl) in the first 24 hours.

### 3. HYDROPS FETALIS

In this condition the haemolytic process has outstripped the capacity of the erythrocyte-producing organs to correct the anaemia, and intra-uterine death from anaemic heart failure is usual. The fetus is grossly oedematous with ascites, pleural effusion and hepatosplenomegaly.

**Investigation of the infant at birth**

Blood is taken for haemoglobin concentration, ABO and Rhesus grouping, a Coombs' test is performed and a serum bilirubin estimation made. Assessment of these investigations indicates whether exchange transfusion is needed. Because the anaemic babies have a raised venous pressure, exchange transfusion is preferable to simple transfusion so that the blood volume is not increased. The purpose of the exchange of blood is to correct the anaemia, by replacing the sensitized Rhesus positive erythrocytes with compatible Rhesus negative erythrocytes; to remove circulating antibody; and to reduce the circulating bilirubin.

Exchange transfusion is given to all Rhesus positive and Coombs' positive affected babies: (a) when the cord haemoglobin is 14.8g or less; (b) when the cord bilirubin level is 105.5$\mu$mol/litre (5mg/dl) or more at birth; (c) with borderline cord haemoglobin and bilirubin levels if the baby weighs less than 2500g at birth.

The exchange transfusion is carried out within 16 hours of birth, the optimum time being about 10 hours after birth. The blood for exchange transfusion should be Rhesus negative but of the same ABO group as that of the baby and it is concentrated to give a haemoglobin level of 14.8g/dl. Fresh blood should be obtained if possible, as stored blood becomes increasingly acid and can produce a fetal acidosis. If stored blood is used it should be transfused slowly (3ml per minute) and 1mmol of sodium bicarbonate given intravenously for every 100ml of blood exchanged. Transfusion is made into the umbilical vein and blood is exchanged until a total of 80 to 100ml per 0.5kg body-weight has been exchanged. The exchange is stopped at any time if the baby's condition deteriorates.

Further haemoglobin concentration and serum bilirubin studies are made 24 hours after birth, and if the serum bilirubin exceeds 300$\mu$mol/litre (18mg/dl) at this time an exchange transfusion is given or repeated.

The condition of the baby is followed for the first 10 days and should the serum bilirubin level exceed 300$\mu$mol/litre (18mg/dl) or the haemoglobin level fall below 14.8g further transfusion is required.

### Dangers of exchange transfusion

Without premature induction of labour and exchange transfusion of the affected baby the perinatal mortality would be not less than 25 per cent. With exchange transfusion the mortality falls to less than 10 per cent. The more severely affected the baby, the earlier is the transfusion needed; but these babies have a markedly raised venous pressure and cardiac failure is common. To avoid this the blood must be exchanged slowly.

### Prognosis for the baby of the Rhesus negative sensitized mother

The chances of survival of the next Rhesus positive infant can be summarized as follows:

|   |   | % |
|---|---|---|
| a. | If the mother has never been given a Rhesus positive blood transfusion, and it is her first pregnancy | 100 |
| b. | If she has no previous affected children | 95 |
| c. | Previous child affected but did not require treatment | 85 |
| d. | Previous child moderately affected, required treatment | 75 |
| e. | Previous child severely affected, required treatment | 40 |
| f. | Previous child died or was stillborn | 30 |
| g. | More than one child lost from haemolytic disease | 20 |

## OTHER TYPES OF ISO-IMMUNIZATION

Increasingly sophisticated methods of detection of iso-agglutinins in human blood have revealed that about 5 per cent of cases of haemolytic disease of the newborn are due to antibodies other than anti-D. With the increasing protection of Rhesus negative women by an injection of anti-D immunoglobulin after abortion or childbirth, haemolytic disease due to the other 'irregular' antibodies will become relatively more frequent.

This argues that there is a case for screening every pregnant woman, not only for her Rhesus status, and the presence of anti-D iso-agglutinins but also for the presence of the other irregular antibodies.

*Chapter 33*

# Tumours of the Genital Tract Complicating Pregnancy

## MYOMATA

The uterine myoma is the commonest gynaecological tumour and occurs more frequently with advancing age and in infertile patients. Pregnancies in early womanhood appear to protect against the development of the tumour. For this reason myomata are more commonly found complicating the pregnancy of the older primigravida.

### Incidence

The incidence of myoma associated with pregnancy is about 1 in 200 but the majority of the myomata are small and cause no trouble, so that the incidence of myomata potentially capable of complicating pregnancy or labour is 1 in 800. Complications which occur depend on the number, the size and the position of the myomata in the uterus.

### Effect of pregnancy on the myoma

The increased vascularity of the uterus and increased circulating oestrogen and progesterone often lead to an increase in size of the myoma. This is largely due to oedema, but some hypertrophy of the muscle fibres occurs. The growth may reduce the blood supply to the depths of the tumour, with hyaline or cystic degeneration. In a few cases, 'red degeneration', or necrobiosis occurs. The affected myomata are generally at least 3cm in diameter and intramural in position. The cause of necrobiosis is not clear but it is probably due to an aseptic degeneration with haemolysis of cells within the blood vessels supplying the tumour. The cut tumour looks like raw beef. Necrobiosis is a rare complication. The patient complains of pain and low grade fever between the 12th and 22nd week of pregnancy, and on palpation

the uterus has an area of localized tenderness. With rest and sedation the pain and tenderness diminish over a few days and finally cease. The pregnancy continues.

Since myomata increase in size during pregnancy, torsion may occur in a pedunculated myoma, or the tumour may become impacted in the pelvis. These complications are extremely rare.

### Effect of the myoma on pregnancy

This depends mainly upon the size and position of the tumour. Small subserous or intramural myomata have no effect. Tumours involving the uterine cavity, either intramural or submucous, are associated with lowered fertility, twice the risk of abortion and an increased risk of premature labour. Larger tumours in this position can lead to malposition and malpresentation of the fetus. If the tumour is cervical or involves the lower part of the corpus uteri it may obstruct labour, although many tumours are drawn out of the pelvis as the lower uterine segment develops.

Pressure symptoms may occur when the tumour is large and in the posterior uterine wall. The pressure is usually felt on the rectum and pelvic nerves. Myomata in the anterior uterine wall may press upon the bladder, but it must be emphasized that the symptoms are not commonly encountered.

### Effect on labour and puerperium

Once again the position of the myoma is important. Distortion of the uterine cavity may lead to malpresentation or malposition of the fetus and complicated labour, whilst a myoma which remains in the pelvis will cause obstruction to vaginal delivery. However, myomata cause no alteration in the type and quality of uterine contractions until the third stage of labour when the distorted cavity, or altered muscle retraction, can lead to postpartum haemorrhage and retention of the placenta.

In the puerperium infection is said to be more common but there is no real evidence of this. Very rarely, due to the puerperal uterine contractions, an intramural myoma may pedunculate into the uterine cavity. Such an occurrence could lead, in theory, to inversion of the uterus, but this is exceptional.

## DIAGNOSIS

If all the patients, and particularly those with a long history of infertility, are examined vaginally between the 6th and 10th week of pregnancy, patients with myomata will be detected. The pregnancy lies to one side and the irregular firm mass of the myoma to the other. Occasionally a single fundal myoma may cause difficulty in diagnosis but scrutiny of the menstrual history will usually resolve the matter. It is important not to confuse a myoma in a non-pregnant uterus with a normal pregnancy, and if any doubt exists an immunological pregnancy test will resolve the issue, and prevent the embarrassment of operating on a normal pregnancy.

Occasionally the differential diagnosis is important. A single fundal myoma complicating pregnancy may be mistaken for a trophoblastic tumour, or for a uterus containing a multiple pregnancy. More important, ectopic pregnancy, normal pregnancy, or a firm ovarian mass must be eliminated before making a diagnosis. The use of ultrasound helps to establish the diagnosis if doubt persists.

A pelvic myoma may resemble a retroverted gravid uterus or a bicornuate uterus with the rudimentary horn in the pouch of Douglas. The position of the cervix distinguishes the former and the treatment for the latter is the same as that for a myoma complicating pregnancy.

## TREATMENT

In general no treatment is indicated if the myoma is diagnosed before labour. Myomectomy is troublesome to perform, haemostasis is difficult and abortion likely to follow the operation. It is best deferred until after the puerperium.

Threatened abortion is treated in the usual way, and necrobiosis is treated conservatively. Bed rest and analgesics are prescribed and operation avoided.

If the diagnosis is not made until late pregnancy, treatment depends upon the position and size of the myoma and the presence of any other obstetrical complications. The final decision cannot be made until the 37th week. Examination at this time will determine if the myoma is occupying the pelvic cavity and obstructing the engagement of the fetal head. Should this occur an elective caesarean section may be planned for the 39th week. If no myoma is detected in the pelvis and the lie is longitudinal a vaginal delivery can be anticipated, but each labour must be treated as a trial labour. An exception to this rule is if the patient is an infertile older primigravida, when elective caesarean section is preferable in selected cases, particularly if the baby presents as a breech. If no tumour is found in the pelvis and the fetal lie is transverse, the case must be reviewed regularly. Should the lie remain transverse, caesarean section in early labour is the treatment of choice.

### Myomectomy at the time of caesarean section

Unless the myoma is easily accessible, and adequate haemostasis can be assured, myomectomy should be avoided at the time of caesarean section. Bleeding may prove intractable and there may be difficulty in obliterating the myoma cavity so that hysterectomy is unavoidable.

Occasionally multiple myomata complicate the pregnancy of a woman who wants no further children and who has to be delivered per abdomen. Such women are best treated by caesarean hysterectomy.

# OVARIAN TUMOURS

One pregnancy in 1500 is complicated by a clinically detectable ovarian tumour, which usually measures more than 5cm in diameter. Routine ultrasound scanning detects one ovarian tumour in 200 pregnancies. Most of them are cysts, usually an enlarged corpus luteum, and resolve. If the tumour is a neoplasm, serous cystadenomas are more common than mucinous cystadenomas, and these two tumours account for 65 per cent of all ovarian neoplasms found in pregnant women. Teratoma account for 25 per cent. The remaining 10 per cent are made up of a wide and bizarre variety of ovarian neoplasms.

### Effect of the pregnancy on the tumour

The size of the tumour is unaltered in pregnancy, but by displacement it may become more evident to palpation. With the growth and movement of the uterus, torsion may occur if an ovarian cystectomy is not performed. In the past haemorrhage and infection of twisted cysts were reported, but today these complications are rare, as is rupture of a cyst.

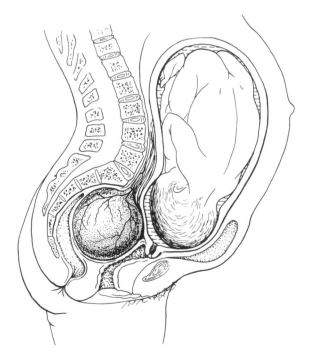

**Fig. 33/1** Ovarian cyst obstructing labour

### Effect of the cyst on pregnancy and labour

In early pregnancy, provided that torsion does not occur, abortion is no more frequent than normal. In late pregnancy incarceration of the cyst in the pouch of Douglas is a possibility and if adherent this would cause an obstruction to vaginal delivery (Fig. **33/1**).

## DIAGNOSIS

In early pregnancy the diagnosis is usually easy as pelvic examination demonstrates two masses. The pregnant uterus has a boggy feeling and moves when the cervix is pushed to one or other side. The ovarian mass tends to be firmer. Occasionally an 8-week pregnant uterus with a positive Hegar sign is mistaken for an ovarian tumour. Other conditions requiring consideration are ectopic gestation, particularly if a peritubal haematoma has formed and a pedunculated uterine myoma in a pregnant uterus. Scrutiny of the menstrual history and an ultrasound examination will resolve the problem.

## TREATMENT

If the clinical examination and the ultrasound scan show an ovarian tumour, treatment depends on the size of the tumour and its acoustic consistency. Ovarian tumours which are less than 8cm and echo free should be observed and repeat scans made to find out if the tumour increases in size or becomes smaller. If the tumour is 8cm or more in size or, if smaller, is multilocular, thick walled or semi-solid, the neoplasm should be removed by surgery after the 12th week of pregnancy.

If the ovarian tumour is detected for the first time after the 30th gestational week, its removal is technically more difficult and premature labour may follow. The decision to operate is made after full consideration of the findings, including the position of the tumour.

An ovarian tumour detected in labour and impacted in the pouch of Douglas makes caesarean section and ovarian cystectomy mandatory. An extrapelvic position of the tumour will permit the patient to deliver vaginally. However, in this case and in those in which the ovarian tumour is detected in the puerperium, surgical intervention is recommended with minimal delay as the risk of torsion of the ovarian tumour is increased considerably. This is because of the laxity of the abdominal wall and the movement and involution of the uterus.

# CARCINOMA OF THE UTERINE CERVIX

This complication is rare, the incidence being about 1:3000. Since the disease is more common in the 4th or subsequent decade it is more common in older pregnant women. With general application of routine cervical smears the incidence of carcinoma should fall considerably. Carcinoma-in-situ of the uterine cervix is rather more common, and in clinics where routine cervical cytology is performed on all pregnant women, about 1 in 200 will show 'abnormal smears'. These may indicate the presence of intra-epithelial carcinoma, but a single smear has limited diagnostic value. A single abnormal smear should be repeated as errors may occur. If the second smear shows abnormal cells, a colposcopic examination is made and punch biopsies are taken of colposcopically suspicious areas. The punch biopsies may show normal epithelium, dysplasia, carcinoma-in-situ or invasive carcinoma. Dysplasia requires follow-up by further smears taken 6 weeks postpartum. Carcinoma-in-situ may require cone biopsy to exclude areas of invasion; however, cone biopsy in pregnancy is attended by a 20 per cent risk of abortion or of preterm birth, and a 15 per cent risk of haemorrhage either immediate or delayed. For this reason, clinical judgement is required and many gynaecologists avoid cone biopsy until after childbirth. Invasive carcinoma, diagnosed by colposcopically directed punch biopsy, or cone biopsy, requires treatment.

Pregnancy does not increase the growth potential of carcinoma-in-situ or invasive carcinoma, although, due to oedema and changes in the stroma, the tumour may appear to grow more rapidly.

Treatment of invasive carcinoma of the cervix is the same in the pregnant and non-pregnant woman, although the complication of the fetus requires consideration. If the disease is detected before the 30th week, hysterectomy, followed 10 to 14 days later by external radiation and radium to the cervical area, is the treatment of choice. If the pregnancy has advanced beyond the 30th week, treatment may be withheld until the 35th week when the baby is delivered by caesarean section. Radiation therapy is again started 10 to 14 days later. The alternative treatment is surgical, and Wertheim hysterectomy with lymphadenectomy is recommended by many gynaecologists.

## Chapter 34

# Abnormalities of the Placenta and Membranes

## THE AMNIOTIC FLUID

The origin of the amniotic fluid is unknown. Early in embryonic life there is active secretion by the amniotic cells, and it is likely that this secretion continues throughout pregnancy. Only those cells overlying the placenta and umbilical cord are thought to be active. The regulation of the secretion of these cells is controlled by endometrial prolactin, and when prolactin receptors are insufficient, polyhydramnios may result. In addition, an ultrafiltrate of maternal plasma passes through the amniotic cells to add to the quantity of liquor. Amniotic fluid is not a stagnant pool, except perhaps in the first few weeks of pregnancy. After this time the fetus begins to swallow the liquor and a 'circulation' of liquor amnii is established. Most of the fluid swallowed is absorbed by the intestinal villi, and enters the fetal circulation. Between the 20th and 30th weeks additional fluid is added to the total by diffusion through the fetal skin, which at this time is poorly developed, and by renal glomerular filtration. The skin diffusion diminishes or ceases by the 30th week, but with increasing kidney function, fetal urine forms the main source of the liquor amnii. Since the fetal kidneys become increasingly active in late pregnancy, urine is constantly secreted and each time micturition occurs additional fluid enters the amniotic cavity. Because of these mechanisms a constant circulation of amniotic fluid occurs, half

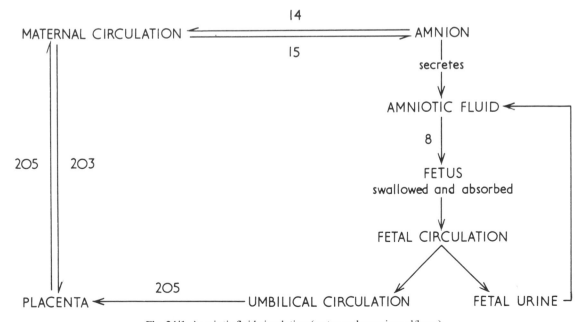

**Fig. 34/1** Amniotic fluid circulation (water exchange in mol/hour)

the volume being exchanged every 90 minutes (Fig. **34/1**).

Amniotic fluid is 99 per cent water, and contains about 0.25 per cent of protein, the pattern suggesting that it is mainly a dialysate of maternal serum protein, at least in early pregnancy. In late pregnancy its osmolarity and sodium content exceed that of maternal plasma, suggesting that fetal urine is added increasingly at this time.

The amount of liquor amnii increases from 30ml at 10 weeks to 300ml at 20 weeks, 600 at 30 weeks, 1000 at 38 weeks, and then drops to 600ml at term.

## POLYHYDRAMNIOS

Hydramnios is defined as the clinical finding of excessive liquor amnii, more than 3000ml being present. It occurs once in every 250 pregnancies.

## AETIOLOGY

Hydramnios is caused by a defect in circulation of the liquor, which may be temporary, in which case the amount of liquor will vary from week to week, or may be permanent. Any condition leading to a greater area of secreting amnion, such as the large placenta associated with diabetes, or chorioangioma, can cause hydramnios. Malformations of the fetus, particularly anencephaly, spina bifida and atresia of the upper gastro-intestinal tract which prevent swallowing, or absorption through the intestinal villi, are commonly associated with hydramnios. The anencephalic baby, in addition to being unable to swallow, is unable to produce any antidiuretic hormone, and consequently hydramnios is found in association in over half the cases. Hydramnios is found in 5 to 15 per cent of multiple pregnancies, being commoner with uniovular twins and usually affecting only one sac.

## CLINICAL VARIETIES

The symptoms of hydramnios depend on the rapidity of accumulation of fluid rather than the total amount, and the slow accumulation (chronic hydramnios) is ten times more common than the rapid increment (acute hydramnios).

### Chronic hydramnios

Although the fluid may accumulate from mid-pregnancy, clinical signs usually do not appear before the 32nd week. Dyspnoea or oedema of the legs may occur, but generally abdominal discomfort is the main complaint. The uterus is larger than normal, tense and a fluid thrill can be obtained. Premature labour may occur, and should the membranes rupture, prolapse of the cord or malpresentation of the fetus may be found. The course of labour is not altered, but postpartum haemorrhage should be anticipated and prevented. Diagnosis is usually easy but ultrasound is necessary to detect multiple pregnancy or fetal malformation. A large ovarian cyst may lead to confusion but ultrasound will resolve the problem.

The patient with minor degrees of hydramnios requires additional rest and sedation at night, but no other treatment is needed, unless a gross fetal malformation is found when labour should be induced, provided conditions are suitable. If the symptoms become severe in mid-pregnancy and the fetus is normal, abdominal amniocentesis using a spinal needle may give relief without bringing on labour, although half of the patients treated in this way will go into labour. Labour is less likely to occur if the amount of fluid removed at any one time is less than 500ml. Aggravation of symptoms in late pregnancy may necessitate induction of labour. The fluid should be released slowly to avoid sudden alteration in the position of the fetus and to prevent prolapse of the cord.

Labour is usually normal, but postpartum haemorrhage is a hazard, and a prophylactic injection of oxytocin is advisable. Since many babies are malformed careful scrutiny must be made, attention being paid to oesophageal and duodenal atresia, which is only amenable to surgery in the early hours of life.

### Acute hydramnios

Rapid abdominal distension occurs at about the 20th to 28th week, with severe abdominal pain, dyspnoea, tachycardia, nausea and vomiting. Oedema of the legs and lower abdominal wall follows and the patient becomes very ill. The abdomen is tense, the skin shiny and stretched, a fluid thrill is present and fetal parts cannot be felt. Ultrasound may show a multiple pregnancy or an abnormal fetus, and because of the excessive liquor the picture is often hazy and hard to read.

Treatment is to remove amniotic fluid by amniocentesis repeated if necessary, but the outlook for the fetus is poor as abortion usually occurs, or labour has to be induced by amniotomy.

## OLIGOHYDRAMNIOS

Oligohydramnios is usually defined as an abnormally small amount of liquor detected before term. It is rare, and probably due to failure of secretion by the cells covering the placenta, or by malformations of the fetal renal tract preventing micturition. If it occurs early in pregnancy abortion is usual, but should pregnancy continue adhesion of fetal skin and amnion, or the formation of amniotic bands are likely. When oligohydramnios occurs later in pregnancy pressure deformities such as alterations of the shape of the skull, wry neck and club foot may be expected. The fetus is cramped, its skin dry and leathery. Labour is often premature and fetal survival low.

## ABNORMALITIES OF THE UMBILICAL CORD

The usual length of the umbilical cord is 45 to 60cm, but extremes of up to 200cm and down to 2cm have been reported. Apart from the greater risk of coiling round the neck, long cords have no clinical significance. A cord may be absolutely short, and shortened relatively by coiling. Such shortening may lead to premature separation of the placenta and malpresentations, but the condition is only diagnosed after delivery. Coiling of the cord around the fetus is only of clinical significance if the coils are tightly pulled by fetal movements or descent, in which case they may lead to fetal death, but this is rare. Knots occur in the cord, and can be true or false. The true knot may lead to diminished fetal circulation in labour. False knots are caused by varicosities of the umbilical vessels and accumulations of Wharton's jelly, and are of no importance.

The cord usually contains one vein and two arteries, but in 1 per cent of cords, only one artery is found. Half the babies supplied by such vessels have congenital malformations.

### Abnormal insertions

In about 15 per cent of cases the cord is inserted at the edge of the placenta (battledore insertion). If the placenta is low lying, the cord may be compressed by the descent of the fetal head, or may prolapse when the membranes rupture.

In 1 per cent of cases the cord originates in membranes some distance from the placental margin, and the vessels then run in the membranes to reach the placenta. The condition is known as velamentous insertion of the cord and is more common in cases of multiple pregnancy. If the vessels happen to run across the cervical os, they may rupture during the second stage of labour leading to fetal blood loss, but this is exceedingly rare.

## TROPHOBLASTIC DISEASE

The abnormalities which may occur in the shape of the placenta are discussed in Chapter 2, whilst the functional disturbances of the placenta are considered in Chapter 3. In this chapter, trophoblastic disease is discussed, although the condition is dealt with in greater detail in Volume 2. Benign trophoblastic disease, or hydatidiform mole, occurs in about 1 in 2000 pregnancies in Western developed nations, and is three times more common in the developing nations of the world. The condition develops when excessively active trophoblast, or reduced maternal resistance, permits the accumulation of nutrients in the villi, which then become distended and swollen resembling a bunch of hydatid cysts, or small grapes (Fig. 34/2). Because there are few, or no, blood vessels within each villus, the fetus is starved, dies and is resorbed. The villi continue to proliferate.

### Clinical features

The first sign of hydatidiform mole is usually uterine bleeding which is no different from that of threatened abortion, but tends to occur in the second quarter of pregnancy and to persist. A few patients start to vomit excessively but this symptom is not diagnostic.

Four main diagnostic criteria are usually described. These are: (1) the size of the uterus is larger

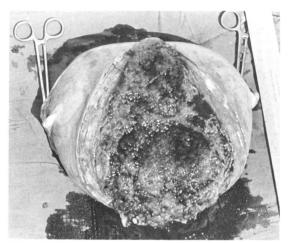

Fig. 34/2 Hydatidiform mole (benign trophoblastic tumour)

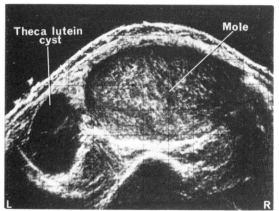

Fig. 34/3 The echogram shows the characteristic vesicular pattern of a hydatidiform mole (by kind permission of Dr W. J. Garrett)

than expected as estimated from the date of the last menstrual period; (2) the excretion of human chorionic gonadotrophin tends to remain markedly elevated after the 16th week; (3) the fetal heart cannot be detected using an ultrasonic fetal heart monitor, and fetal parts cannot be felt after the 18th gestational week; (4) hypertension and proteinuria may be present. One or more of these findings may suggest benign trophoblastic disease, and it can be confirmed by ultrasonic echography when no fetal echoes will be seen. Instead a diffuse vesiculated effect is found in the uterus (Fig. **34/3**).

**Treatment**

In at least half of the cases the diagnosis is only made when the patient begins to expel the hydatidiform mole. Blood loss is frequently heavy but may be reduced by the use of an oxytocic infusion, the expulsion being aided by the suction curette, used carefully. Three to 5 days later a curettage, using a sharp curette, is made to remove residual trophoblast.

If the tumour is diagnosed prior to its expulsion, treatment is either to use the suction curette and oxytocin, or to perform a hysterectomy with the tumour in situ. The choice depends on the desire of the patient for further pregnancies and on her age. This is discussed in greater detail in Volume 2, where details of the meticulous follow-up that is required after a hydatidiform mole has been evacuated are given.

*Chapter 35*

# Variations in the Duration of Pregnancy: Fetal Maturity

The duration of pregnancy in the human female averages 260 days from conception, or 280 days from the first day of the last menstrual period in a woman who has a normal 28 ($\pm 5$) day cycle. Fifty per cent of women deliver within the period of 7 days before, or 7 days after, the estimated date, and 80 per cent deliver between the 266th and 293rd day (38 to 41 weeks inclusive). In about 10 per cent of the population, pregnancy is curtailed and ends before the 266th day, and in a further 10 per cent pregnancy is prolonged beyond the 294th day.

## CURTAILED PREGNANCY

Curtailed pregnancy, that is termination before the 37th week of gestation, is of obstetric significance only in so far as a low birth-weight baby is born which is less able to adapt to extra-uterine life. The incidence of curtailed pregnancy is difficult to compute as in many instances the exact date of the last menstrual period, and the rhythmicity of the menstrual cycle, are not known or have been forgotten. For this reason it has been customary to decide that pregnancy is curtailed when it is known to be less than 36 completed weeks in duration, or if the infant weighs less than 2500g at birth. The latter definition, however, includes not only true preterm babies, but a group of infants whose growth in utero has been retarded. These dysmature infants which are 'small-for-dates' have a gestation period exceeding 36 weeks, but weigh less than 2500g at birth (Table **35/1**). They constitute at least 6 per cent of all low birth-weight babies. The Perinatal Mortality Survey in Britain studied the correlation between birth-weight and period of gestation for the first time in a national sample, and showed that the mortality is more closely related to birth-weight than to period of gestation, but that the combination of curtailment of pregnancy and low birth-weight carries a greater risk of fetal mortality. The problems of low birth-weight are considered further in Chapter 60.

About 6 per cent of all pregnancies are curtailed.

| Period of gestation | Percentage of babies of birth-weight | |
| --- | --- | --- |
| | 2500g or less | More than 2500g |
| Less than 34 weeks | 99.7 | 0.3 |
| 34 and 35 weeks | 49.5 | 50.5 |
| 36 and 37 weeks | 19.0 | 81.0 |
| 38 to 41 weeks | 3.4 | 96.6 |
| 42 weeks or more | 2.8 | 97.2 |

(From the Perinatal Mortality Survey, Britain, 1958)

Table **35/1**  Relationship between the period of gestation and birth-weight

The curtailment is more likely to occur if the mother is aged less than 20 or more than 35, and in women pregnant for the fourth or subsequent time, irrespective of age. The socio-economic status of the parents is also implicated, although poor socio-economic conditions are more likely to lead to the growth retardation of the fetus in utero, and the delivery of a low birth-weight infant after the 37th week (i.e. a 'small-for-dates' baby) than the actual curtailment of pregnancy. Heavy continuous work in the last ten weeks of pregnancy may cause curtailment of pregnancy, but no definite correlation has been obtained and the factor cannot be separated from that of social class. Other factors are low maternal age, low maternal weight at the onset of pregnancy, smoking, threatened abortion and a history of a previous preterm baby (20–35 weeks gestation).

If a patient has one curtailed pregnancy she has an 85 per cent chance that her next pregnancy will be at term. If she has had two preterm births, the chance that the next birth will be at term is 70 per cent.

## AETIOLOGY

The causes of curtailment of pregnancy are shown in Table 35/2, which has been constructed from information obtained in Australia, Britain, Malaysia and the USA. These matters are considered further.

|  | (%) |
|---|---|
| No cause found (including premature rupture of the membranes) | 35 to 45 |
| Hypertensive disorders | 18 to 30 |
| Multiple pregnancy | 12 to 18 |
| Maternal disease | 5 to 15 |
| Abruptio placentae | 5 to 7 |
| Placenta praevia | 3 to 4 |
| Fetal malformations | 1 to 2 |

Table 35/2 Causes of curtailment of pregnancy and prematurity

### Maternal causes

Essential hypertension, chronic nephritis and diabetes are conditions which themselves produce curtailment of pregnancy, or in which pregnancy is terminated prematurely to rescue the baby from a hostile environment. In a like manner, heart disease which is not controlled is likely to be attended by premature labour. If there is a malformation of the uterus, labour is likely to start prematurely, and in many of these cases the baby is also small.

In tropical countries maternal anaemia accounts for curtailment of pregnancy, but is more commonly a cause of a 'small-for-dates' baby being born at term. Acute infectious diseases, particularly malaria and enteric fevers, may also lead to curtailment of pregnancy.

Severe hypertensive disorders are the largest single cause of premature termination of pregnancy, and account for between 18 and 30 per cent of all cases (Table 35/2). In some cases labour starts spontaneously, in others labour is induced in order to obtain fetal salvage. There is no evidence that mild PIH has any marked effect on the duration of pregnancy or on the incidence of prematurity. Placenta praevia may be attended by curtailment of pregnancy, but with 'conservative treatment' the importance of this cause is reduced. Accidental haemorrhage (abruptio placentae) continues to be an important cause of curtailment of pregnancy, and if the haemorrhage is moderate, or severe, pregnancy must be terminated. Rhesus incompatibility may require that pregnancy be curtailed.

### Fetal causes

The most common fetal cause is multiple pregnancy, and this accounts for 12 to 18 per cent of cases of curtailed pregnancy. The factor does not operate alone, for anaemia and PIH are more common in patients with a multiple pregnancy, as is hydramnios. Hydramnios itself frequently leads to curtailment of pregnancy, and the greater the degree of hydramnios, the greater the chance of premature labour. Congenitally malformed fetuses tend to be 'small-for-dates', and to be delivered prematurely.

### PREVENTION

Since in at least half of the cases the cause is unknown, prevention can only be empirical. There is some evidence that increased protein and folic acid (in a dose of 1 to 2mg per day) from conception may reduce the incidence of fetal retardation of growth. Patients who have previously had unsuccessful or curtailed pregnancies should be advised to spend most of the day in bed during the first 12 weeks of pregnancy in order to obtain better placentation, although once again the value of this regimen has not been proved scientifically.

A careful examination of the whole patient (and not just the abdomen) in early pregnancy may detect maternal disease, which may then be treated before it exerts any deleterious effect. Regular antenatal examinations will detect hypertensive disorders which should be treated without delay. Although there is no proof that the regimen is effective, it is generally recommended that patients carrying a multiple pregnancy should rest as much as possible between the 32nd and 36th week of pregnancy, or if the socio-economic conditions are poor, should be admitted to hospital. Supplements of folic acid (1 to 3mg daily) should be given to these patients. Nothing can reduce the incidence of placenta praevia, but conservative treatment in an attempt to prolong the pregnancy to the 37th week will reduce the incidence of prematurity. Diabetes, syphilis and pyelonephritis are relatively uncommon causes of curtailed pregnancy, but should be sought, and if detected, treated vigorously.

No drugs, including tocolytics have proved of any benefit when used prophylactically.

Cervical circlage is of value in treating patients with recurrent abortion whose cervix is shown to be 'incompetent' (see p. 188). This has led a number of obstetricians to insert a 'prophylactic' cervical suture in patients with a history of preterm labour, but no evidence of cervical incompetence. Recent randomized, blind studies have shown that cervical circlage has no benefit in reducing preterm births in these patients, and may have possible hazards (antepartum haemorrhage, increased uterine activity, cervical laceration and infection).

The birth of preterm babies increases the neonatal and the perinatal death rates significantly. Consequently a reduction in the frequency of the onset of labour, prior to the 36th week of pregnancy, would play a significant role in reducing the perinatal mortality. Prevention, in one of the ways suggested, plays a part, but suppression of premature labour would play a much larger part if satisfactory methods were available, particularly in the large group where no reason for the onset of premature labour can be detected.

In the past 5 years the perinatal mortality rate of babies, whose gestation period is 34 to 37 weeks, has fallen and is not significantly greater than that of babies born after the 37th week, at least in hospitals which have intensive neonatal care units (level 3 nurseries). For this reason it is now probable that if labour threatens after the 34th week of pregnancy, no attempt should be made to suppress it, as the danger of intra-uterine infection, usually chorio-amnionitis, is greater than that of preterm birth. The exception to this statement is that drugs may be given to suppress labour for sufficient time to enable the pregnant woman to be transferred to a hospital which has a level 3 nursery.

## PRETERM (PREMATURE) LABOUR

The diagnosis of preterm labour is not easy and the criteria used by different centres demonstrate that it is often arbitrary. Labour only becomes progressive when cervical dilatation is effected by contractions with a pressure of >24mmHg and a frequency >3 per 20 minutes. A useful set of criteria for diagnosing premature labour are (1) the gestational period is less than 37 weeks, (2) uterine contractions (observed in hospital for at least 1 hour) occur every 5 to 10 minutes, last for 30 seconds and persist for the 60 minutes (the frequency and pressure of the contractions should be recorded using a tocograph), and (3) a vaginal examination shows the cervix to be >2.5cm dilated and >75 per cent effaced.

### Suppression of preterm labour with tocolytic drugs

Using these criteria, two-thirds of all patients presenting with presumed preterm labour will be found not to be in labour, and no treatment is required. If preterm labour is diagnosed and the pregnancy is less than 34 weeks gestation (and/or the fetus weighs less than 1500g, as determined by real time ultrasound), the cervix is <5.0cm dilated and the membranes are intact, treatment may be offered. The main modality is bed rest which is thought to improve the uterine blood supply.

If the patient is apprehensive, promazine 50 to 100mg intramuscularly may be of value, but morphine and pethidine are contra-indicated in the absence of severe pain, as the narcotics more frequently enhance than depress uterine activity. Additional measures are available which may delay or suppress the onset of labour. Currently, two methods are advocated. These are to use: (1) the beta sympathomimetic agents, (a) salbutamol infusion, (b) ritodrine infusion, or (2) ethanol infusion.

The beta sympathomimetic agents (beta-agonists) are so called because they mimic certain actions of the sympathetic nervous system. In the uterus, beta-receptors, if stimulated, inhibit uterine contractions, so that the agonists should be useful in treating preterm labour. However, the beta-receptors are also present in smooth muscle and cardiac muscle. Stimulation may lead to vasodilatation, cardiac acceleration, a widening of the pulse pressure, and an increase in cardiac output. Beta-receptor stimulation in the liver and muscle may lead to glyconeogenesis, a rise in blood glucose and an increase in insulin and glycogen secretion. For these reasons, all women given beta-agonists to reduce uterine activity, develop tachycardia, hyperglycaemia and hyperinsulinaemia. Fluid retention occurs in all; pulmonary oedema and myocardial ischaemia occurs in about 5 per cent, usually after 24 to 48 hours treatment. Careful monitoring is essential.

Because of this only certain cases of preterm labour are suitable for receiving the drugs:

1. Pregnancy advanced to less than 34 weeks
2. Contraction pressure > 24mmHg
3. Contraction frequency > 3 per 20 min over 1 hour's observation
4. The cervix < 5cm dilated
5. The patient has no cardiac disease, is not hypertensive, is not a diabetic, has not had abruptio placentae, and has no evidence of infection
6. The fetus is alive and has no evident congenital defect (as determined by ultrasound).

With these exclusions, only 25 per cent of women in threatened premature labour are suitable for drug treatment, using salbutamol or ritodrine.

1. *Salbutamol* is infused at a rate of 4μg/minute increasing by 4μg/minute every 10 minutes until uterine contractions are suppressed. This dose is maintained for 6 hours and then reduced incrementally over the next 6 hours. Oral salbutamol, 8mg every 8 hours is then started and given for 5 to 7 days.
2. *Ritodrine* is infused at a rate of 50μg/minute, increasing by 50μg/minute every 10 minutes to a maximum of 350μg/minute until uterine contractions are suppressed or unacceptable side-effects occur. The infusion is run for 24 hours. Oral ritodrine 10 to 20mg, 2- to 6-hourly is then given.

   The drugs are relatively ineffective when cervical dilatation exceeds 4cm and if the membranes have ruptured.

3. *Ethanol* is infused to provide 1.25g per kg/body-weight per hour for 12 to 24 hours, and is followed by oral cognac 30g every 4 hours

for a further 24 hours. A problem of this regimen is that the high blood alcohol levels may not be desirable either for mother or fetus.

There seems no significant difference in the outcome which of the methods is used: each is as effective or as ineffective as the others.

In fact, the few randomized controlled trials of the beta-agonists show that their only significant effect is to delay childbirth by an average of 24 hours. They do not reduce the frequency of delivery before the 37th week, nor the proportion of infants whose birth weight is less than 2500g, nor the incidence of hyaline membrane disease. Nor do they reduce the perinatal mortality rate. These data suggest that the beta-agonists should only be used during the transfer of a mother to a hospital which has a level 3 nursery.

Curtailed pregnancy implies the birth of a preterm baby, who is at increased risk of developing respiratory distress syndrome (RDS or hyaline membrane disease). The shorter the gestation period, the greater is the risk.

The incidence of severity of RDS is reduced by the administration of betamethasone (Celestone chronodose) 24mg, in two doses preferably 24 hours apart, or of dexamethasone 4mg, 8-hourly until delivery or until six doses have been given. Corticosteroids are believed to increase the secretion of surfactant by the fetal lung thus reducing the development of hyaline membrane. To be effective corticosteroids have to be given more than 24 hours and less than 7 days before birth. They have no value if the pregnancy has advanced to > 34 weeks.

Corticosteroids should be given to all mothers who are in premature labour, or in whom induction of labour is indicated if the gestation period is 34 weeks or less, if the membranes are intact (and if the lecithin : sphingomyelin ratio is less than 2, when the test has been made, see page 276). To enable the corticosteroid to work it may also be necessary to try to suppress labour, using the drugs mentioned in the previous paragraph, for at least 24 hours.

## MANAGEMENT OF PREMATURE LABOUR

If the membranes are intact, they should be kept intact as long as possible, and the patient should therefore remain in bed. When the membranes rupture, a vaginal examination should be performed to exclude a prolapsed cord. Analgesics such as pethidine may be given during the first stage of labour if required, but should be avoided if possible. If pethidine is given, the depressant effect of the drug upon the infant's sensitive respiratory centre can be counteracted by giving the baby naloxone 0.01mg intravenously and intramuscularly. As there is a risk of a haemorrhagic diathesis in the 'premature' fetus, due to a reduced prothrombin level in the fetal blood, vitamin $K_1$ 5mg should be given to the mother, 6-hourly during labour, or as a single injection of 1mg to the infant immediately after delivery.

During the second stage of labour considerable stress is applied to the fetal head, and delivery may be aided by a judiciously made episiotomy or, if the head is delayed on the perineum for more than ½ hour, by applying forceps. The entire second stage should not be allowed to exceed 1 hour.

The place of caesarean section in the management of premature labour is controversial. Many obstetricians believe that for a fetus weighing between 750 and 1499g (i.e. 26–31 weeks gestation) caesarean section should be considered (1) if the fetus does not present as a vertex or a breech with extended legs, (2) if there is associated antepartum haemorrhage, (3) if labour fails to progress or (4) if fetal distress occurs. The increased use of caesarean section has been associated with a lower perinatal and neonatal mortality. Similar recommendations have been made for gestation periods of 32 to <37 weeks (1500g–2499g); but the more advanced the gestation the less is the risk, so that each case needs to be evaluated.

## PREMATURE RUPTURE OF THE MEMBRANES (PROM)

In about 5 per cent of all births (and in 1 per cent of preterm births) the amniotic membranes rupture spontaneously before the onset of labour. This is called 'premature rupture of the membranes'. The cause is unknown. The further from term the membranes rupture, the longer is the interval between rupture and delivery. For example, if the membranes rupture before the 36th week of pregnancy, the latent period exceeds 5 days in 20 per cent of cases, but after the 36th week the percentage falls to less than 5 per cent.

The diagnosis of premature rupture of the membranes is usually obvious but if any doubt exists, a sample of the fluid should be taken from the posterior vaginal fornix. This is tested using a colorimetric monoclonal alphafetoprotein antibody test, which has a sensitivity of 98 per cent. This test replaces the older nitrazine yellow (Amnistix) test.

The management depends on the duration of the pregnancy when the membranes rupture. If the pregnancy has advanced to 34 completed weeks of gestation, uterine activity should be stimulated, if spontaneous labour has not started 24 hours after the membranes have ruptured, provided that the fetal head is engaged in the pelvis, the cervix is favourable and neonatal care facilities are available. If these conditions are not fulfilled, it is better to delay delivery. In this case the patient should be monitored carefully to detect chorio-amnionitis. If found, the patient should be delivered. In all cases of premature rupture of the membranes a decision has to be made whether the potential danger of intra-uterine infection exceeds that of the birth of a small, less mature, baby.

Should the membranes rupture before the 34th week, the risks of preterm birth and immaturity of the baby exceed those of possible intra-uterine infection, and efforts should be made to prevent the onset of labour. The patient is confined to bed, at least initially, and is given sedation if she is apprehensive. Apart from an initial aseptic vaginal examination (with a speculum) to confirm the diagnosis of ruptured membranes and to exclude prolapse of the umbilical cord, vaginal examinations are prohibited in order to minimize the chance of intra-uterine infection.

There is no evidence that tocolytic drugs, given to a woman who has PROM before the 34th week of pregnancy, have any value in delaying delivery or improving fetal outcome. Corticosteroids to reduce the incidence of hyaline membrane disease should be avoided, as their value is dubious and they may increase the risk of infection.

Intra-uterine infection (chorio-amnionitis) complicates about 20 per cent of cases of PROM, and is usually shown clinically as tachycardia, fever (>38°C), leucocytosis and offensive vaginal discharge. These signs are late, and the early diagnosis of chorio-amnionitis using measurement of C-reactive protein is under investigation. Prophylactic antibiotics are not indicated, but antibiotic treatment should be given to a mother who develops clinical chorio-amnionitis. In this event, large doses of piperazine (2g i.v. 4-hourly), ampicillin (750mg 4-hourly), cephaloridine (1g 12-hourly) or tinidazole (2g single dose) may be required.

If labour does not start within 48 hours of rupture of the membranes, the patient may get up, and if in hospital may go home, provided her home conditions permit her to rest for most of the day. Coitus should, of course, be prohibited, and she should be reminded that if she develops a fever she should at once contact her doctor. Apart from these pre-autions, no treatment is required, and it must be emphasized that neither hormones nor pharmaceuticals are of any value in delaying the onset of labour, when the membranes have ruptured spontaneously.

# PROLONGED PREGNANCY

Pregnancy lasts for 42 completed weeks in about 8 per cent of women and is defined as being prolonged. Prolonged pregnancy (also called postdatism) is believed by some obstetricians to pose dangers to fetus and mother; other obstetricians deny that it does.

Assuming that the menstrual dates are known accurately, or that an ultrasound scan has been made in the first half of pregnancy two groups of women who are 'postdate' can be identified. The first group consists of women whose baby matures slowly and only reaches maturity at 42 weeks gestation or more. The second group of women are those whose baby shows evidence of postmaturity and is at potential risk of dying. These fetuses have a hard skull with narrow skull sutures and small fontanelles, well-developed finger and toe nails, and well-developed genitalia. Some of them show signs of intra-uterine malnutrition: they have absent subcutaneous fat and dry skin. These babies account for the observed doubling of perinatal mortality which occurs between the end of the 42nd and 44th weeks of pregnancy.

If the mother has a pregnancy complication, such as PIH, which reduces uteroplacental blood flow, prolonged pregnancy may pose a real hazard to the fetus.

## DIAGNOSIS

If the menstrual history is not accurately known, and an ultrasound scan has not been made in the first half of pregnancy, this should now be made. The abdominal circumference of the fetus and the length of the femur should be measured and related to a nomogram. The length of the longest column of liquor amnii should also be measured. These tests enable the obstetrician to estimate the gestational period plus or minus 10 days. Older methods, such as placental calcification, ossification of the upper tibial epiphysis, and amniotic fluid examination, are obsolete.

## MANAGEMENT

In the absence of PIH, diabetes mellitus or other pregnancy complications, the pregnancy can continue beyond 42 weeks, provided fetal well-being is monitored. This is done by daily fetal movement counts and twice weekly non-stress testing using a cardiotocograph, or fetal blood flow velocity (see p. 278). The volume of amniotic fluid or the length of amniotic fluid columns should also be measured using ultrasound, if this facility is available. The condition of the cervix should be checked each week to find out if labour is imminent. A low fetal movement count (less than 10 per day), a non-reactive non-stress test, or a decrease in amniotic fluid volume (the longest vertical column less than 30mm long) are indications for intervention. In the absence of these findings, there is no indication for intervention to deliver the baby. Routine surgical induction of labour at the end of the 42nd week is followed by a caesarean section rate >25 per cent, and an increase in babies requiring resuscitation. If the clinical and laboratory findings indicate fetal risk, the management of the patient will depend on clinical examination, particularly the state of the cervix and the position of the fetal head. The choices are induction of labour, by amniotomy and oxytocin, if the cervix is 'favourable', and prostaglandin $E_2$ pessaries if it is not, or elective caesarean section. The patient is examined to determine whether there is cephalopelvic disproportion, and to what extent the head is engaged in the pelvis. This should be followed by a vaginal examination to assess the pelvic size, feto-pelvic relations, and the state of the cervix.

Certain primigravidae, particularly if over the age of 30 and with a history of previous infertility, or women who have had PIH and whose cervix is unripe, are best treated by caesarean section, but labour should be induced in all other cases. The use of vaginal $E_2$ prostaglandin pessaries are usually sufficient to start labour. Alternatively amniotomy (surgical rupture of the forewaters) may be chosen (see Chapter 49). If amniotomy is chosen and the liquor is found to be scanty or meconium-stained, the patient is prepared for immediate caesarean section should fetal distress supervene.

Following amniotomy an oxytocic infusion may be started at once, or the obstetrician may prefer to wait for 6 to 12 hours for spontaneous labour to start. Should the infusion fail to produce effective uterine contractions within a period of 6 hours, caesarean section may be indicated. All women who have a prolonged pregnancy require fetal monitoring during labour. (See Chapter 36.)

# FETAL MATURITY

The discussion in this chapter has stressed the relationship of fetal maturity to fetal and neonatal survival: the less mature the fetus, or the more the fetus is postmature, the higher is the perinatal mortality.

Unfortunately curtailed and prolonged pregnancy can only be diagnosed when the patient has an accurate recollection of her last menstrual period, and a knowledge of the rhythmicity of her menstrual cycle. If the patient has forgotten the date of her last menstrual period or has a completely irregular menstrual cycle, it is impossible to estimate the duration of her pregnancy with any exactitude, unless she has been seen by a doctor in the first quarter of her pregnancy. In all other cases, an exact determination of the duration of the pregnancy and the degree of fetal maturity is difficult to establish.

As mentioned earlier in this chapter and in Chapter 6, many of the problems associated with variations in the duration of pregnancy would be reduced considerably if all patients who had the possibility of being pregnant saw a doctor within 10 weeks of the onset of amenorrhoea. Scrutiny of the menstrual history, together with a careful bimanual vaginal examination at this stage of pregnancy goes a long way to calculating estimated date of delivery.

However, in a number of cases, the patient does not attend for prenatal care until the 3rd, or even the 4th, quarter of pregnancy. In these cases the determination of fetal maturity may be important, so that an unnecessary premature induction of labour and the hazards of prolonged pregnancy are avoided. The problem is compounded if the patient develops pregnancy-induced hypertension or some other condition which is hazardous to the fetus. In these cases the decision which has to be made is at what stage of pregnancy the hazard to the fetus in utero exceeds the hazard to the prematurely born neonate.

The clinical estimates of fetal maturity are not very accurate, and are based on fundal height, and a 'guesstimate' of fetal size. Until recently, radiological estimation of fetal maturity was utilized to supplement the clinical assessment, but it is not very accurate.

Fetal maturity may be determined by biophysical or biochemical methods.

## Biophysical: ultrasound

If the gestation period is known from clinical observations, the measurement of the biparietal diameter of the fetal skull confirms fetal maturity. Because some women are uncertain of the date of their last menstrual period, some obstetricians recommend that all women have an ultrasound examination between the 12th and the 20th week (determined by clinical examination) to establish the period of gestation and fetal maturity.

In the last quarter of pregnancy, the calculation of crown-rump length times the area of the fetal trunk compared with a nomogram gives a reasonable indication of fetal maturity, in cases where clinical methods fail to provide an estimate.

## Biochemical measures

In the past several methods of estimating fetal maturity from a sample of amniotic fluid have been popular. The concentration of amniotic creatinine, for example, increases as kidney function becomes more mature in late pregnancy. A level of 2.0mg/dl or more suggested that the fetus was more than 36 weeks mature, but the converse was not true. Another method was to estimate the proportion of anucleate fetal fat-filled cells by mixing a drop of amniotic fluid with a drop of 0.1 per cent aqueous Nile blue and counting the orange coloured cells. If more than 20 per cent of the cells were orange, the fetus was probably 36 weeks mature, but the converse was not true. These tests have been largely superseded by the measurement of the lecithin–sphingo-myelin ratio.

### FETAL LUNG MATURITY

To enable the lung to expand properly and to func-

tion as an organ of respiratory exchange, two surface-acting phospholipids, lecithin and sphingo-myelin, are formed. As pregnancy advances, and as the lung matures, increasing amounts of the phospholipids appear in the amniotic fluid (Fig. **35/1**). In normal pregnancies the ratio between lecithin and sphingomyelin (the L/S ratio) correlates fairly closely with gestational age, and with fetal lung maturity (Fig. **35/2**). If the baby's lungs are immature, the respiratory distress syndrome (hyaline membrane disease) is likely to occur. If the lungs are mature it is likely that the baby's liver function and neurological maturity is adequate for extra-uterine life.

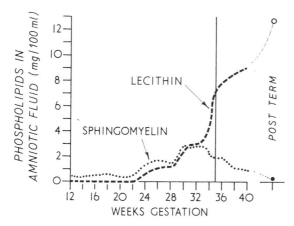

Fig. **35/1** Changes in the concentration of lecithin and sphingomyelin in amniotic fluid

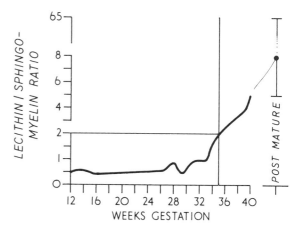

Fig. **35/2** Mean L/S ratios during normal gestation

## Chapter 36

# The At-risk Fetus in Pregnancy and Labour

PLACENTAL DYSFUNCTION OR RETARDED FETAL GROWTH

The birth-weight of the infant depends upon its ability to achieve its growth potential in utero, and this in turn depends on the growth support obtained from the mother. Within genetically set limits, the actual fetal growth will depend on: (1) an adequate supply of nutrients (especially of glucose) and of oxygen from the maternal circulation; (2) an adequate placental transfer of nutrients; (3) an adequate fetal circulation; and (4) an adequate release of insulin by the fetal pancreatic beta-cells, as insulin is the main regulator of fetal growth, provided adequate supplies of glucose and free fatty acids are transferred across the placenta. So long as the maternal growth support exceeds the fetal growth potential, the fetus will thrive, but should the support be inadequate, or the placenta be unable to transfer the available nutrients to the fetus, its growth will become retarded.

Fetal growth will also be retarded when its growth potential is reduced as in malformed and chromosomally abnormal fetuses (e.g. anencephaly and Down's syndrome) but these conditions are relatively uncommon.

It is obvious that the uteroplacental environment, and in particular the uteroplacental blood supply, is crucial in regard to fetal growth, and indeed to fetal survival. For example, if gross placental dysfunction occurs, as in severe abruptio placentae, fetal death in utero is usual, whilst if the dysfunction is less, fetal growth retardation may occur.

In most cases where retarded fetal growth is detected by ultrasound or suspected clinically, the cause is an inadequate blood supply to the placental bed. It will be recalled that in the first half of pregnancy trophoblastic cells invade the lumen and then the wall of the uterine spiral arteries, first in their endometrial portion and later in their myometrial portion. The effect of the trophoblastic invasion is to convert relatively rigid vessels into flaccid dilat-able arteries which supply additional blood to the placental bed. If the trophoblast fails to invade the arteries or its action is insufficient, the blood supply to the placental bed is reduced and the fetus is denied the supplies of oxygen and nutrients it needs for adequate growth. In other words it is chronically undernourished in utero, and becomes growth retarded. The placenta responds to the reduced blood flow by cytotrophoblastic hyperplasia in an attempt to improve fetal nutrition.

Until these facts were discovered, fetal growth retardation leading to a small-for-dates or dysmature baby was thought to be due to placental dysfunction. However, this term failed to emphasize that the primary problem is a reduction in maternal blood flow to the placental bed.

Several medical complications of pregnancy aggravate the reduced blood flow (Table **36/1**). Not all women who have these conditions have a growth-retarded fetus. This may be explained by postulating that if a pre-existing inadequate blood supply to the placenta is present it is made worse by the conditions, but if the placental-bed blood supply is adequate, the decrease caused by the conditions may

| *Maternal causes* | *per cent* |
|---|---|
| Hypertensive disorders | 60 |
| Prolonged pregnancy | 5 |
| Maternal diseases (esp. renal disease and severe anaemia) | 5 |
| *Fetal causes* | 10 |
| Malformations, transplacental infections | |
| Multiple pregnancy | |
| Unknown | 20 |

**Table 36/1** Aetiological factors in fetal growth retardation (placental dysfunction)

not be so great as to impair transfer of nutrients to the fetus, and growth retardation.

A growth-retarded fetus may develop metabolic disturbances. These include acidosis, hyperlactaemia, hypercapnia, hypoglycaemia and erythroblastosis. If the disturbances are severe the fetus may die in the uterus. Less severe metabolic disturbances tend to worsen in labour, and may cause clinical or monitor-detected fetal distress, or the infant may be born with signs of severe hypoxia.

The fetus in affected pregnancies is at greater risk of dying or, if born alive, needing resuscitation, and the pregnancy is said to be 'high risk'.

## HIGH-RISK PREGNANCY

Women with a high-risk pregnancy require greater attention during pregnancy and, if these women could be identified early, the fetal loss might be reduced. No reliable tests have been devised, but a Swedish study helps to identify such women, at least at the known 32nd week of pregnancy. The Swedish obstetricians looked at eight variables, and gave them weighted values (Table 36/2). They showed that if the score was 3 or less no baby was born small-for-dates. If the score was 4 or more, all small-for-dates babies were identified, but 66 per cent of babies in this group were not growth retarded (sensitivity 100 per cent; specificity 95 per cent; positive predictive value 34 per cent).

Another method is to measure the symphysis-fundal height and relate this to the period of gestation. The method depends on the patient's knowing accurately the date of her last menstrual period, or on an ultrasound examination made in the first half of pregnancy. The technique of symphysis-fundal height measurement is simple. The height of the fundus is determined by gentle palpation with the ulnar border of the hand and is marked. The distance between the upper border of the symphysis pubis and the mark is measured using a length of taut string or a measuring tape. The result is related to the expected measurement on a chart (Fig 36/1). If the measured distance falls below the 10th centile, fetal growth retardation is likely, although the false positive rate is greater than 70 per cent. Thus the finding is an indication for further, more accurate investigations. Some obstetricians use ultrasound to detect the presence of fetal growth retardation by examining all women, or women suspected of having a growth-retarded fetus, at the 32nd week of pregnancy. The biparietal diameter, the length of the femur and the abdominal circumference are measured. The last of these has the highest positive predictive value.

## TESTS FOR EVALUATING FETAL CONDITION IN HIGH-RISK PREGNANCIES

Tests for determining the degree to which the fetus is compromised, in other words to determine fetal

| Variable | Weighted value |
|---|---|
| 1. Previous birth of baby weighing ≤ 2500g, stillbirth or first week neonatal death | 1 |
| 2. Blood pressure ≥ 140/90 | 1 |
| 3. History of renal disease, repeated urinary tract infection (UTI) or UTI in present pregnancy | 1 |
| 4. Bleeding in current pregnancy | 1 |
| 5. Weight gain > 0.5kg in any week after 20 weeks | 1 |
| 6. Decrease or no increase in girth | 1 |
| 7. Smoking | 2 |
| 8. Decrease or no increase in fundal height | 3 |

**Table 36/2** 'At-risk fetus' scoring system

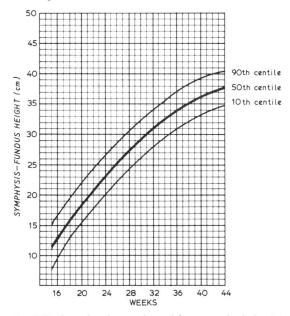

**Fig. 36/1** Gestational age estimated from symphysis-fundal height

well-being, may use biophysical or biochemical methods. In vogue in the 1960s and 1970s, the biochemical methods of serial astral measurement and human placental lactogen (hPL) measurement have been superseded by more accurate biophysical methods. One biochemical method continues to be used. This is the measurement of the ratio between lecithin and sphingomyelin in the amniotic fluid as an indication of fetal-lung maturity (see p. 276).

The biophysical methods currently used include (1) recording fetal movements, (2) cardiotocography, (3) serial ultrasound examinations, (4) Doppler flow-velocity waveforms in the umbilical artery or fetal aorta. None of these tests has a high positive predictive value, but each has a high negative predictive value.

## Fetal movements (kick counts)

Several ways of counting fetal movements have been reported, none being superior. A mother whose baby is at 'higher risk' should count the number of fetal movements from 9 a.m. or from 9 p.m. whichever is more convenient, until she has counted 10 movements in a 1- to 3-hour period. If she feels fewer than 10 movements in the time period, she should report to the attending doctor or nurse midwife. The fetal movement count is performed 3 or more times a week.

## Cardiotocography (CTG)

Cardiotocography, using a fetal heart monitor, is proving to be an efficient method of monitoring the well-being of the fetus in utero. The tests depend on the assumption that a healthy fetus, which is receiving adequate supplies of oxygen and nutrients will normally be more active than a malnourished or hypoxic fetus, and its heart rate will respond to 'stress' more effectively.

To determine the fetal response to activity or to the 'stress' of a uterine contraction, or to manipulation, an external cardiotocograph is applied to the woman's abdomen and a recording of the fetal heart is made for a 30-minute period. If spontaneous uterine contractions do not occur during a 30-minute period, they may be obtained by nipple stimulation. During the test the woman should not lie on her back as false non-reactive results may occur in this position. During this time, the variations in the fetal heart rate are observed in response to observed fetal movements (as reported by the mother) or in relation to Braxton Hicks contractions. The latter procedure is referred to as the *non-stress test*.

A '*reactive*' fetus is one in which an acceleration of the fetal heart of at least 15 beats per minute, lasting for at least 15 seconds occurs at least twice in the 30-minute test period in response to fetal movements. A reactive fetus is not at risk. If this pattern of fetal heart acceleration is not observed over a period of 60 minutes it is classified as '*non-reactive*' and this indicates some degree of fetal hazard. If the fetus does not show spontaneous movements, it may be stimulated into activity by external manipulation of the uterus; failure to induce fetal movements by this technique suggests that the fetus is at risk. A positive non-stress test (i.e. a 'reactive' test) gives reasonable reassurance that the fetus is well, but there are a proportion of false positive tests. For this reason, the prognostic value of the test may be enhanced if the relationship of the fetal heart-rate pattern to 2 to 4 Braxton Hicks contractions is evaluated by non-stress cardiotocography.

Four cardiotocographic patterns have been described (Table **36/3**). These are: (1) normal, (2) suboptimal, (3) decelerative and (4) preterminal. The *suboptimal* pattern suggests that the fetus is at minor risk, and that the test should be repeated in three or four days. The *decelerative* pattern indicates that the fetus is at greater risk, and the test should be repeated the next day, unless conditions for delivery are suitable, when labour should be induced. The *preterminal* pattern indicates that the fetus is at considerable risk of dying in utero and delivery should be effected quickly.

Some obstetricians add an intravenous infusion of oxytocin to the above method – the oxytocin challenge test (OCT). A baseline reading is obtained and oxytocin is infused incrementally until three uterine contractions lasting 30–90 seconds are obtained in a 10-minute period. The infusion is maintained at this rate for 30 minutes. If a fetal heart deceleration pattern is observed the oxytocin challenge test is positive, and the fetus is at risk.

The OCT has the disadvantage that the patient has to be monitored carefully for up to 2 hours, which is time consuming and expensive. As well, fewer than 7 per cent of OCTs are positive. The evidence currently available is that the non-stress test is less dangerous, requires less supervision, is cheaper and is as effective a method as the OCT for detecting fetal hazard.

## Serial ultrasound examinations

Fetal growth retardation can be monitored by serial

| | *Normal* | *Suboptimal* | *Pattern* *Decelerative* | *Preterminal* |
|---|---|---|---|---|
| Variation in baseline FHR beats per min | > 10 | > 10 | < 10   > 5 | > 5 |
| Acceleration on fetal movement (over a 30–45 min period) | At least 2 of 15 bpm | At least 2 of 10 bpm | At least 1 episode of acceleration (10 bpm) every 20 min | None |
| Deceleration (in relation to Braxton Hicks contractions) | None | None | Variable | Late |

**Table 36/3** Patterns found on antepartum cardiotocography

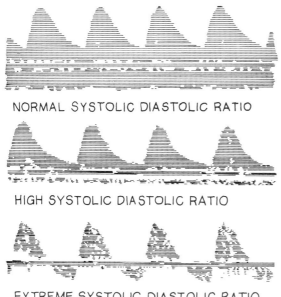

NORMAL SYSTOLIC DIASTOLIC RATIO

HIGH SYSTOLIC DIASTOLIC RATIO

EXTREME SYSTOLIC DIASTOLIC RATIO

**Fig. 36/2** Blood flow in pregnancy

ultrasound examinations. Usually the biparietal diameter, the length of the femur, the abdominal circumference and the volume of the liquor amnii are measured and related to normograms. The examination is made each week.

### Fetal blood flow velocity

Doppler ultrasound, either as a continuous wave system or a pulsed wave system, is used to study fetal well-being. Uteroplacental and fetoplacental circulations are low resistance systems in which flow towards the placenta continues throughout the cardiac cycle. When fetal vascular resistance increases due to acute atherosis consequent on maternal disease, fetal disease or unknown causes the wave forms are altered. The difference between the peak systolic flow and the least diastolic flow in the umbilical artery produces a ratio (the A/B ratio). The greater the ratio the more likely is the fetus to be compromised (Fig. **36/2**). At present, fetal blood flow measurements should be considered experimental and not introduced into general clinical practice until a proper assessment has been made. It is not yet clear whether a single test (for example, the non-stress test), or a battery of tests provide the best predictive values. A reasonable compromise would be to do a non-stress test and an ultrasound measure of abdominal area and amniotic volume (a column of > 20mm is normal).

## BIOCHEMICAL TESTS

As the quantities of plasma and urinary oestriol and of hPL increase during pregnancy, estimations have to be related to the normal range for each week of gestation. This means that unless the period of gestation is known, with some accuracy, the interpretation of the test is difficult. A knowledge of the history of the pregnancy and a clinical examination may establish the gestation period. In cases of doubt an ultrasound examination may help.

### Estimation of plasma or urinary oestriol

It will be recalled that the placenta lacks certain

enzymes needed for the synthesis of oestriol, and that these are available in the fetal adrenals and liver.

If placental dysfunction is present, causing fetal malnutrition, oestriol synthesis may be affected with resultant lower plasma oestriol levels, and a reduced urinary oestriol excretion. The measurement of unconjugated oestriol provides some indication of fetal well-being, but a single reading is of limited prognostic value and serial readings are required. Further, the correlation between persistently low plasma oestriol levels and fetal well-being is poor.

### Estimation of human placental lactogen (hPL)

Human placental lactogen (hPL) is a protein synthesized exclusively in the placental syncytiotrophoblast. hPL has a half-life of only 20 minutes. The blood levels rise from early pregnancy reaching a level of $5\mu g/ml$ at 32 weeks and $7\mu g/ml$ at 40 weeks. As maternal blood levels correlate with placental and fetal weight, a small placenta (and fetal growth retardation) may be associated with low levels of hPL in the maternal scrum. Clinical experience has shown that an hPL level in the maternal serum of less than $4\mu g/ml$ from the 30th week indicates some degree of fetal hazard. A low hPL level also indicates the need for more precise biochemical or biophysical estimates of fetal well-being.

### Lecithin/sphingomyelin ratio in amniotic fluid

If the tests mentioned indicate that the fetus is 'at risk' in utero, and that the placental dysfunction is becoming increasingly severe, the obstetrician may decide that premature induction of labour, or delivery by elective caesarean section is in the best interests of the baby.

A problem of premature delivery is that 'at-risk' babies are at especial risk in the early neonatal period of developing the respiratory distress syndrome (hyaline membrane disease), due to insufficient phospholipid surfactant in their lungs. The affected babies require intensive care if they are to survive.

It would clearly be an advantage to know if a particular baby was likely to be affected. This information can be obtained by taking a sample of amniotic fluid by amniocentesis, and by measuring the lecithin/sphingomyelin ratio (the L/S ratio) using thin layer chromatography and densitometry. An L/S ratio of 2:1 or more indicates that the respiratory distress syndrome is unlikely to arise; whilst if the L/S ratio is less than 2:1, it may be advisable if possible to delay inducing labour or performing an elective caesarean section until the fetal respiratory system is more mature.

A second test is to determine if phosphatidylglycerol is present in the amniotic fluid. Although phosphatidylglycerol appears earlier than the change in the L/S ratio, the false positive rate is higher.

Recently, two relatively simple tests have been proposed. Both appear to correlate reliably with the L/S ratio or phosphatidylglycerol level. In the 'shake test', 5 dilutions of amniotic fluid are made by adding normal saline. An equal volume of 95 per cent ethanol is added to each tube, which are shaken vigorously for 15 seconds, and allowed to stand for 15 seconds. If a complete ring of stable bubbles is present, the fetal lungs are considered mature.

The alternative is the 'tap' test. In this test 1ml of amniotic fluid is added to 1 drop of 6N hydrochloric acid and 1.5ml of diethyl ether is added to make a superficial layer in the tube. The test tube is tapped 4 times and after 5 minutes the number of bubbles in the ether layer is observed. If no more than 5 bubbles persist in the ether layer, the test indicates mature lungs. In general the shake or the tap test should be done as a first step, care being taken to ensure that contamination is not introduced into any tube. If the shake test is positive the baby's lungs are mature. If the test is negative, the L/S ratio should be evaluated in an experienced laboratory, as a negative shake test has > 60 per cent false positive rate.

# MANAGEMENT OF HIGHER-RISK PREGNANCIES

Primary placental dysfunction leads to retarded fetal growth at all stages of pregnancy. Secondary placental dysfunction is not usually observed until about the 30th week of fetal growth, and retardation is unusual before this time. The effects of placental dysfunction usually become manifest some time

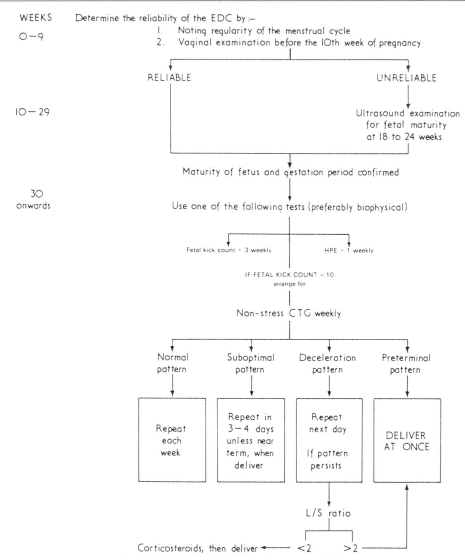

WEEKS    Determine the reliability of the EDC by :—
0—9                1.    Noting regularity of the menstrual cycle
                   2.    Vaginal examination before the 10th week of pregnancy

RELIABLE                                      UNRELIABLE

10—29                                         Ultrasound examination
                                              for fetal maturity
                                              at 18 to 24 weeks

Maturity of fetus and gestation period confirmed

30
onwards        Use one of the following tests (preferably biophysical)

Fetal kick count · 3 weekly        HPE · 1 weekly

IF FETAL KICK COUNT < 10
arrange for

Non-stress CTG weekly

Normal          Suboptimal        Deceleration      Preterminal
pattern         pattern           pattern           pattern

Repeat          Repeat in         Repeat
each            3—4 days          next day          DELIVER
week            unless near                         AT ONCE
                term, when        If pattern
                deliver           persists

L/S ratio

Corticosteroids, then deliver ◄——— <2        >2 ———

**Fig. 36/3** A scheme for monitoring the 'at risk' fetus

between the 30th and 35th weeks, and are most marked after the 35th week. As 70 per cent of cases of placental dysfunction are associated with a clinically identifiable disease pattern, and as the clinical observation of growth retardation can be made, these cases require additional care in pregnancy.

Whilst little can be done to alter placental function, placental efficiency is increased if the supply of nutrients and oxygen available to it is high. The conditions which lead to secondary placental dysfunction are associated with a reduced uteroplacental blood flow. Although some studies have shown that

bed rest improves uteroplacental blood flow, there is no evidence that it improves fetal growth, at least when pregnancy complications such as PIH are absent.

Recent evidence, which requires confirmation, suggests that if fetal growth retardation is detected aspirin in a dose of 60–150mg a day may improve fetal growth. In addition, the maternal diet should be rich in protein; and anaemia, if present, should be corrected. Beyond this, little can be done to improve fetal growth.

Higher-risk pregnancies should be monitored from about the 28th week, in an attempt to detect when the risk to the fetus becomes critical, so that the baby may be rescued by immediate delivery. It is recommended that biophysical rather than biochemical tests are used, for several reasons. First, biophysical tests reflect fetal well-being more accurately than biochemical tests. Second, if fetal kick counts are used as a screening procedure, the patient is involved in her own care. Third, non-stress cardiotography can be performed quickly on outpatients, and collecting blood or urinary samples is avoided.

It must be stated that antenatal fetal monitoring, using biophysical or biochemical methods, will not prevent every antepartum fetal death, but the tests enable the obstetrician to decide with greater accuracy if termination of the pregnancy is indicated to remove the fetus from a potentially lethal environment, or so it is hoped. However, a controlled study of the value of weekly non-stress cardiotocography in high-risk patients admitted to a Melbourne hospital found that weekly CTG made no difference in perinatal morbidity or mortality. It is possible that the problem lay in the criteria adopted for admission.

A scheme for monitoring the 'at-risk' fetus is shown in Fig. **36/3**.

# MONITORING THE 'AT-RISK' FETUS IN LABOUR ('FETAL DISTRESS')

The growth-retarded fetus is at greater risk during labour than the normal fetus, as it has few reserves on which it may draw for energy should placental gas and nutrient exchange be diminished still further at this time. This means that the progress of labour and the condition of the fetus in cases of placental dysfunction must be monitored with care. The principal clinical signs of fetal danger are an alteration in the fetal heart rate and the passage of meconium. Infants showing these signs are said to have developed fetal distress although the clinical diagnosis often is inexact and confusing and the term inaccurate.

Fetal distress may also affect infants whose progress in pregnancy has been normal, and these constitute the majority of cases of fetal distress encountered in labour (Table **36/4**). The aetiological factors leading to fetal distress in labour are considered later in this chapter, but since modern methods of monitoring the condition of the fetus in labour require some knowledge of the physiological changes which occur when the fetus is challenged by hypoxia, this is discussed first.

## PHYSIOLOGICAL CONSIDERATIONS

The fetus depends for its energy requirements on the transfer from the mother of adequate supplies of glucose and oxygen. Part of the glucose is used for immediate metabolic needs; the rest is converted into glycogen or fat. The glycogen is stored in the liver, in skeletal and in cardiac muscle, whilst the fat is deposited around the heart and behind the scapulae. These stores can be drawn upon for anaerobic respiration if the maternal supplies of glucose and the oxygen needed for aerobic respiration are temporarily diminished.

Normally the fetus converts the glucose by anaerobic pathways into ketopyruvic and pyruvic acids, and then in the presence of oxygen via the Krebs cycle into carbon dioxide and water, a method which

|  | Per cent |
|---|---|
| *Complications of labour* | 55 |
| Cord complications | |
| Abruptio placentae | |
| Fetal malpresentation | |
| Fetal distress* | |
| *Complications of pregnancy* | 41 |
| Hypertension in pregnancy (usually severe) | |
| Prolonged pregnancy | |
| Retarded fetal growth | |
| Diabetes mellitus | |
| Preterm birth | |
| *Neither of the above* | 8 |

*Fetal heart rate >160 or <110bpm; meconium stained liquor

**Table 36/4** Aetiological factors in intrapartum fetal death from hypoxia

provides 30 'high energy bonds' per molecule of glucose, and is highly efficient. When the supply of oxygen is limited, the conversion cycle stops before the Krebs cycle is initiated, and only the anaerobic cycle operates. Anaerobic glycolysis releases 8 'high energy bonds' and leads to the accumulation of lactic acid (derived from ketopyruvic acid) and of pyruvic acid in the fetal blood, which consequently becomes acidotic. The degree of acidosis can be assessed with fair accuracy by determining the pH of a fetal blood sample.

Because of the glycogen stores and relatively limited metabolic requirements, the fetus can sustain life in hypoxic states for much longer than the infant. But the progressive accumulation of lactic acid leads to increasingly severe acidosis. In lambs, glycolysis ceases when the blood pH falls below 6.7, and a similar pattern of events is probable in the human fetus. The cardiac muscle component is especially important, and an adequate circulation is essential for survival in the presence of hypoxia. Since glycogen stores are laid down progressively during pregnancy, a premature infant, and more particularly a dysmature or growth-retarded infant, has smaller glycogen stores, and is at greater risk from the effects of hypoxia than is the mature infant. These infants react less well to intra-uterine hypoxia, and intra-uterine death may occur in the presence of only mild hypoxic episodes. Labour is a particularly dangerous time, as the transfer of maternal oxygen may be interrupted either because of uteroplacental dysfunction, or because of compression of the umbilical cord.

A further danger of persisting hypoxia or repeated episodes of hypoxia is that the accumulation of lactate in the blood may lead to its accumulation in fetal brain tissue. This may cause brain swelling and damage, although this may be reversible in babies who survive.

A sensitive measure of the degree of fetal hypoxia and consequent acidosis is an alteration in the fetal heart rate. The fetal heart rate is the result of a balance between the opposing effects of vagal nerve stimulation which tends to produce bradycardia, and the sympathetic nerve stimulation which tends to produce tachycardia.

Since the heart rate is influenced by several physiological factors which are themselves immature and continually adjusting, it is to be expected that wide variations in the rate will occur, and marked variations in the rate over a short period may mean no more than a temporary adjustment to new condi-

tions. Studies using continuous monitoring of the fetal heart rate by electrocardiography or instantaneous rate metering during late pregnancy and early labour, indicate that the rate normally varies considerably, ranging from 100 to 170 beats a minute, with a mode of from 120 to 140.

The fetal heart rate also varies depending on whether the fetus is in an 'active' phase or is sleeping. The duration of these two phases is similar during labour to the activity–sleeping patterns adopted by the fetus in pregnancy and in the early neonatal period.

When fetal hypoxia occurs, the altered composition of the blood leads to a rise in the vagal and sympathetic tone, which are different in character and effect. The sympathetic response occurs in mild hypoxia, its onset is delayed, after which it develops progressively and persists for from 10 to 30 minutes after the cause has ceased to operate. The vagal response is stimulated by moderate or severe hypoxia, is rapid in onset, lasts as long as the cause operates, and then disappears rapidly.

From this it will be evident that mild fetal hypoxia results in tachycardia, but severe episodes of fetal hypoxia will result in bradycardia, which may only be intermittent, at least in the early stages.

## THE CAUSES OF FETAL HYPOXIA

The causes of fetal hypoxia may be maternal, fetal or iatrogenic. Any *maternal condition* which reduces the amount of oxygen available to the villi may cause fetal hypoxia, and the effects of this will be more severe if placental dysfunction has existed for some time. The conditions associated with placental dysfunction – severe hypertension disorders, chronic nephritis, prolonged pregnancy, untreated maternal anaemia, and severe cardiac disease – may cause 'fetal distress' in labour. Similarly, episodes of acute placental dysfunction such as abruptio placentae may lead to fetal distress. Maternal pyrexia or acute infections, by diverting the supply of oxygen from the placenta, or by increasing the oxygen requirements of the fetus, may also be a cause. On the *fetal side*, entanglement of the cord round a limb or round the neck with reduced or obliterated circulation, or prolapse of the cord with reflex spasm of the umbilical vessels, are causes. Reflex bradycardia, with consequently reduced placental circulation, may result from stress upon the fetal skull in cases of disproportion and prolonged labour, particularly if hypertonic uterine action reduces the inter-villous blood flow. *Iatrogenic causes* include the abuse of oxytocin injections, hypotension following epidural anaesthesia, and the misuse of inhaled anaesthetics.

## THE DIAGNOSIS OF FETAL DISTRESS

Traditionally, fetal distress is diagnosed by: (1) a fetal heart rate of more than 160; (2) a fetal heart rate of less than 110; (3) the passage of meconium. The condition is more likely if alterations of the heart rate are associated with the passage of meconium. Unfortunately, because of the normal variation of the fetal heart rate, the diagnosis of fetal distress is not exact. In studies in which fetal heart variations have been related to depressed Apgar scores taken immediately after birth, the only significant correlation was a fetal bradycardia of less than 100 beats a minute which occurred during a contraction and persisted for a minute or more after the contraction. Meconium staining of the liquor was not a reliable sign, as depressed Apgar scores (less than 6) were only found in 2 to 10 per cent of cases, and in 75 per cent of stillborn babies no meconium was found in the liquor amnii.

The clinical detection of signs indicating fetal distress can be made more exact if the fetal heart is auscultated during and for 2 minutes after a contraction, rather than the current method of auscultating the fetal heart *between* contractions. The heart should be auscultated for periods of 15 seconds, with 10 second intervals, from the time the contraction starts to 2 minutes after it ceases, and a mean rate computed from the several observations. In this way bradycardia related to a contraction may be detected. This is a significant sign of fetal distress in labour and indicates inadequate transfer of oxygen across the placenta. Unless more sophisticated methods of monitoring the fetal condition are available, it is usually an indication for urgent delivery – in the first stage of labour by caesarean section, and in the second stage by the application of obstetric forceps or the vacuum extractor.

Two complementary methods are available which will enable obstetricians to monitor the 'at-risk' fetus and to detect evidence of severe fetal hypoxia early. The methods are: (1) continuous fetal heart monitoring by a fetal heart machine; and (2) sampling the fetal scalp blood to determine its acidity.

### The fetal heart monitor

The fetal heart monitor is now established as a useful method of continuously monitoring the fetal heart rate during labour. Experience has shown that certain patterns of fetal heart rate, shown on the tracing, indicate fetal risk as judged by an increased chance of fetal death in labour and low Apgar scores at 1 and 5 minutes. The studies have shown three predominant patterns, although the interpretation of the tracings is not always easy. The patterns are shown in Fig. **36/4**.

*Early deceleration* (also called Type I Dips) are probably due to pressure on the fetal head during uterine contractions and are without prognostic significance. *Variable decelerations* (Type IIa Dips) may be due to compression of the umbilical cord, and, if severe are of significance. *Late decelerations* (Type IIb Dips) indicate impairment of uteroplacental blood flow and consequent fetal hypoxia, and indicate that the fetus is at risk of dying. Without further investigation the risk is impossible to quantify precisely, but it is generally accepted that marked variable decelerations and *all* late decelerations indicate fetal hazard in labour.

In addition to evaluating changes in fetal heart rate, variations in the beat-to-beat tracing give additional information. When beat to beat variation is less than 5 bpm, in other words when the tracing shows a nearly straight line, fetal hazard is increased.

However, as this may indicate only that the fetus is sleeping, the lack of variability should be observed for 45 minutes before considering other tests, for example, fetal blood scalp sampling, or intervening to deliver the baby.

The development of sophisticated electronic fetal monitors has led to their widespread use. In some centres, all women in labour are monitored in this way. The argument is that by this technique, intrapartum deaths of the fetus will be eliminated. Against this are the facts that fetal heart monitoring is invasive (in one technique an electrode has to be inserted into the baby's scalp); intervention by forceps or caesarean section is higher; the mobility of the patient is reduced, and the psychological effects of making labour a pathological process are increased.

Most proponents of routine electronic fetal heart monitoring would agree that only 1 to 2 babies would be 'saved' per 1000 births.

Five prospective trials have been conducted to

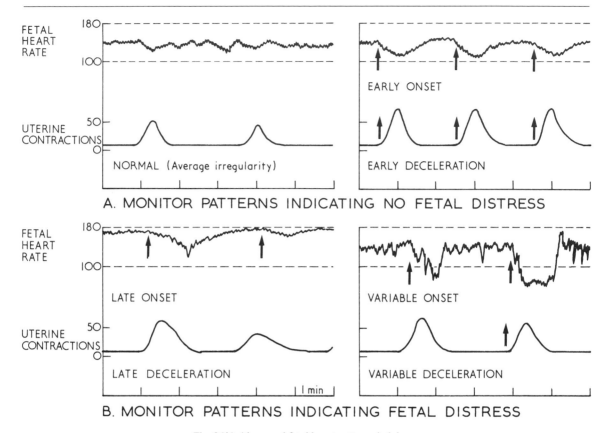

**Fig. 36/4** Abnormal fetal heart patterns in labour

determine if *routine* electronic fetal heart monitoring should be introduced. Three indicated that routine monitoring failed to reduce the perinatal morbidity or mortality. Two showed a significant reduction when monitoring (combined with biochemical assessment of fetal acidaemia) was used *selectively* for high risk cases.

It appears from this evidence that *routine* electronic fetal heart monitoring is inappropriate, but the method is of value in the management of the 'at risk' fetus in labour although its ability to predict severe neonatal hypoxia is limited.

**Biochemical assessment of fetal acidaemia**

It will be recalled that fetal hypoxia results, after a period, in fetal acidaemia, and the more severe the acidaemia, the greater the chance of fetal death. From this it follows that a better assessment of fetal health can be obtained if electronic fetal heart monitoring is supplemented by measurements of the pH

of the fetal scalp blood. Fetal scalp blood sampling is recommended if the fetal heart monitor shows abnormal patterns which persist, and the patient is not ready for delivery. The membranes are ruptured artificially, if they have not already broken spontaneously, and a tubular speculum is introduced through the cervix, capillary hyperaemia of the scalp vessels is obtained by spraying the scalp with ethyl chloride, a small incision is made into the scalp, and the blood is drawn by capillary action into a specially prepared tube. The pH of this blood is then estimated on a pH meter. A pH of < 7.20 is indicative of fetal hypoxia. The method has limitations in that the membranes must have ruptured, and its accuracy is only high in the late first stage and second stage of labour. In addition, serial estimations (which may lead to damage to the scalp and to haematoma) are more accurate than single readings.

The method is not in competition with electronic fetal heart monitoring, but complementary to it. The fetus at 'high risk' in labour is monitored by the fetal heart monitor. If patterns of monitor fetal distress are found, which do not disappear on repositioning the patient, fetal scalp blood is sampled, unless it is feasible to deliver the patient without undue trauma. A pH of less than 7.20 is an indication for urgent delivery, but levels of 7.20 or more indicate that labour may proceed, further blood samples being taken. As the equipment is expensive and a high degree of 'quality control' is needed, 'fetal intensive care' units should be established in large regional hospitals which would care for patients at high risk of fetal distress from peripheral hospitals.

Immediately following birth, blood should be taken from the umbilical artery to determine its pH and base deficit.

## MANAGEMENT OF FETAL DISTRESS

The management of fetal distress will depend on whether the patient is in the first or the second stage of labour. If the patient is in the second stage, delivery of the baby by forceps or caesarean section is urgently required. In the first stage of labour, problems are greater. The degree of maternal acidoketosis should be checked. In the past, maternal acidoketosis was assumed to lead to fetal acidoketosis and, if found, an infusion of 1 litre of 10 per cent dextrose given over a 60-minute period was recommended. Recent studies question the value of this therapy. Although this treatment corrects maternal acidoketosis, fetal blood shows a significant fall in the pH and a rise of lactate, which may precipitate brain oedema. Maternal acidoketosis seems to have no clinical significance on the progress of labour, and the infusion of glucose-saline as recommended on page 122 is all that is required.

Uterine activity is monitored, and if excessive due to oxytocic infusion, this is stopped. The position of the patient should be changed, and she should not lie supine because of the possible pressure of the uterus upon the inferior vena cava reducing the venous return to the heart. It is traditional to give oxygen via a face mask, but it is doubtful whether this improves fetal oxygenation. Often these techniques are sufficient to alter the pattern of the fetal heart to normal, in which case labour may continue in the hope that vaginal delivery will occur. The obstetrician's confidence is enhanced if facilities for fetal scalp blood sampling are available. If they are, a sample of blood is taken and its pH measured. A level of 7.20 or more indicates that labour may proceed; a level of less than 7.20 suggests that delivery should be effected urgently. Where facilities for scalp blood monitoring are not available, caesarean section is generally indicated, particularly if thick green meconium and fetal bradycardia are found. If there is any doubt about the condition of the fetus, a caesarean section is performed.

## Chapter 37

# Occipito-posterior Position

In about 10 per cent of all pregnancies the occiput lies in the posterior segment of the pelvis at the onset of labour. In over half of the cases the position is due to an abnormal shape of the pelvis, particularly the long oval (anthropoid) pelvis in which the forepelvis is narrow so that the head has to adjust to fit into the pelvic brim. In the remainder the pelvis is normal and the position arises because the head is deflexed at the onset of labour, which results in a longer diameter presenting at the brim.

## DIAGNOSIS

In pregnancy, the fetal back is felt away from the midline, and may be difficult to outline clearly, and the fetal limbs are easily felt anteriorly. The head is usually high, and since the narrow forehead is palpated in the midline, it may give the erroneous impression of being small. On using the pelvic grip the occiput and brow are found at the same level, and on suprapubic palpation, the fingers on the side of the occiput sink more deeply than the fingers on the side of the sinciput. The fetal heart is loudest far out in the flank. During labour the same abnormal findings are present on abdominal examination (Fig. **37/1**); and on vaginal examination the posterior fontanelle is found in a posterior quadrant of the pelvis. This clinches the diagnosis.

## MECHANISM OF LABOUR

In 65 per cent of cases, descent of the head with some degree of flexion occurs and the occiput rotates in the midpelvis through 135° to lie behind the symphysis pubis (Fig. **37/2**), after which delivery is as for the normal vertex (Fig. **37/3**). In 20 per cent

of cases, rotation of the occiput occurs to the transverse position, after which movement ceases despite uterine contractions – the transverse arrest of the head. Arrest in this position is favoured by a diminished sacral curve. In 15 per cent of cases, rotation of the occiput occurs through 45° into the hollow of the sacrum, and the head descends into the lower pelvis in this position. Delivery from this position is by further flexion, to allow the occiput to escape over the perineum, and this is followed by extension of the head so that the forehead, eyes, nose, mouth

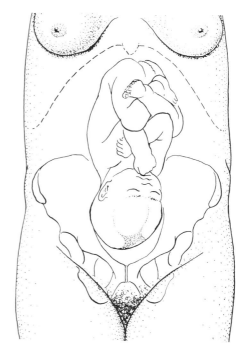

**Fig. 37/1** Occipito-posterior position – abdominal findings

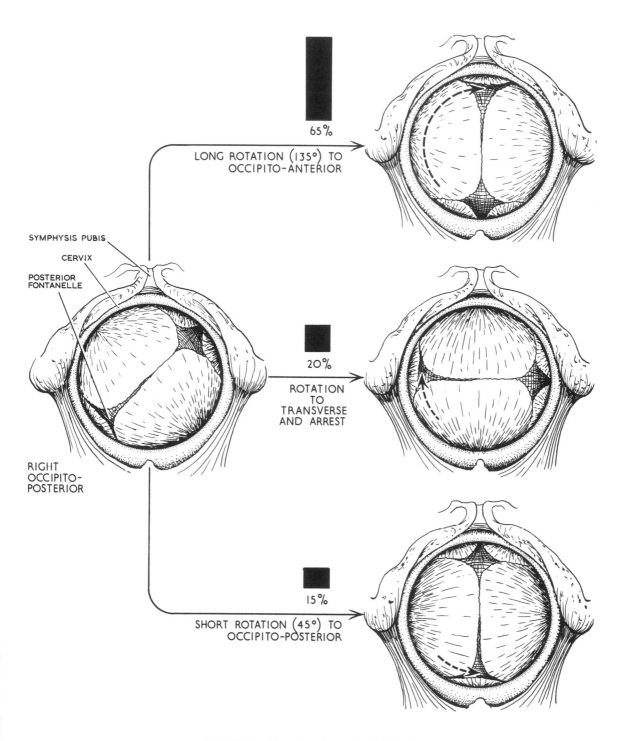

**Fig. 37/2** Possible modes of rotation of the head

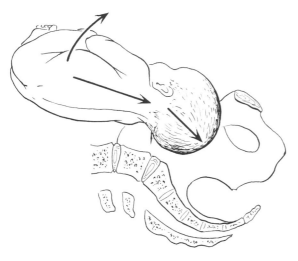

(A) The uterus and fetal axis move forward, and the head flexes as it is forced down into the pelvis

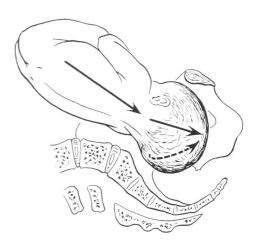

(B) Early second stage. The occiput has reached the pelvic floor. Anterior rotation now begins and the head flexes still more

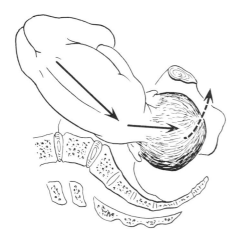

(C) Anterior rotation is occurring through 135°

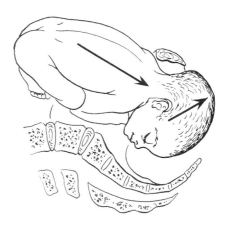

(D) Anterior rotation is complete and the remainder of the delivery is as for an occipito-anterior position

**Fig. 37/3** Occipito-posterior. Long rotation

and chin are successively born (Fig. **37/4**). This type of rotation is often found in association with the long oval (anthropoid) types of pelvis. Whatever the mechanism, labour is likely to last longer than usual because: (1) the pelvis may have an abnormal shape; (2) if the head is deflexed, a larger diameter presents (the suboccipito-frontal, 10.5cm or the occipito-frontal, 11.5cm) and flexion and moulding take

longer; (3) abnormal uterine contraction patterns are common, particularly inco-ordinate uterine action.

**TREATMENT**

There is no effective treatment of the position prior to labour, and pads and binders are of no value.

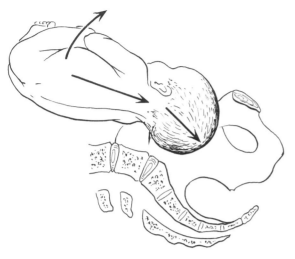

(A) The uterus and fetal axis move forward, and the head enters the pelvis

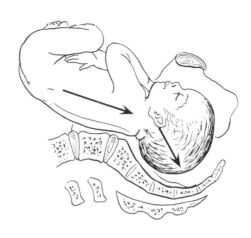

(B) The head fails to flex and descends into the pelvis in the posterior position

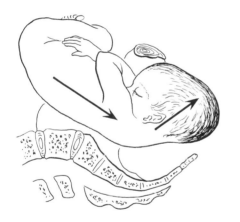

(C) The occiput rotating backwards through 45° when it reaches the pelvic floor to lie in the hollow of the sacrum

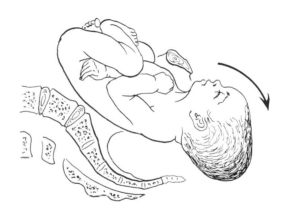

(D) Birth of the head occurs by further flexion to permit the occiput to crown and escape over the perineum. Then by extension, the brow, nose, face and chin appear from behind the symphysis

**Fig. 37/4** Occipito-posterior. Short rotation

When the position persists to term, pelvic assessment, and if necessary, radiological pelvimetry must be made, and prolongation of labour anticipated. If an occipito-posterior position is diagnosed in early labour, treatment should be instituted early. This consists of: (1) giving adequate sedation; (2) ensuring that dehydration and ketosis do not arise; (3) seeing that the patient has no food by mouth. The progress of labour is judged by descent of the head, by the movement of the anterior shoulder inward to the midline and, on vaginal examination, by the progressive dilatation of the cervix and further flexion of the fetal head. In a few cases (about 7 per cent) labour has to be terminated before full dilatation of the cervix because of maternal exhaustion and fetal distress, but the majority of patients continue labour until the second stage. Rotation usually does not occur until this time. If it does, delivery will be spontaneous, or if there is any delay, can be aided by forceps. When transverse arrest of the occiput occurs despite good contractions, delivery is effected by Kielland's forceps rotation and extraction, or by manual rotation of the occiput to the anterior position and the application of forceps.

If delivery has not occurred after $1\frac{1}{2}$ hours in the second stage of labour and the occiput is persistently posterior, treatment depends on the level of the occiput. If this is in the mid-pelvis, rotation anteriorly and forceps extraction is the correct method of management, but if the occiput has rotated posteriorly and advanced to below the ischial spines, forceps delivery without rotation, but with a wide episiotomy, is to be preferred.

## PROGNOSIS

What is the outcome in cases of occipito-posterior position? The following statistics give some indication:

|  | *Per cent* |
|---|---|
| Spontaneous rotation and delivery | 65 |
| Manual, or forceps, rotation and forceps delivery | 15 |
| Spontaneous delivery as occipito-posterior | 8 |
| Forceps delivery in posterior position | 7 |
| Caesarean section | 5 |

It can be seen that there is a 1 in 4 chance that operative interference will be required. This, together with the longer labour commonly encountered, increases both fetal and maternal mortality. But it is to be remembered that occipito-posterior positions are only found in 10 per cent of women and that three-quarters of them cause no trouble and the baby is delivered spontaneously. Early unnecessary interference can cause as much damage as undue delay.

## Chapter 38

# Breech Presentation

In early pregnancy breech presentation is common. At the 20th week, over 40 per cent of babies present by the breech, by the 28th week the incidence has fallen to 15 per cent, by the 34th week to 6 per cent, and by 40 weeks only about 3 per cent of babies present as a breech. To put it in another way: by the 34th week of pregnancy, over three-quarters of those babies who previously presented by the breech have undergone spontaneous cephalic version.

## CLASSIFICATION

The babies which remain in the breech presentation may be classified in three groups (Fig. **38/1**).

1. *Breech with extended legs*. The breech presents with the thighs flexed and the legs extended along the fetal abdomen. Amongst primigravidae, 70 per cent, and in multigravidae, 50 per cent of breech presentations are of this type.

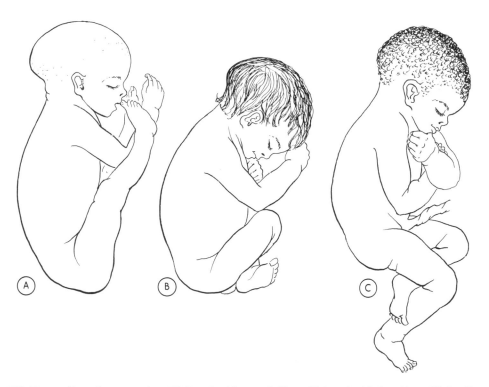

**Fig. 38/1** Types of breech presentation. (A) Breech with extended legs; (B) breech with flexed legs; (C) footling

2. *Breech with flexed legs.* In this variety the fetus lies in a flexed attitude, and the legs are flexed on the abdomen. The presenting part is therefore bulky, and consists of the buttocks, the external genitalia and both feet.

3. *Footling and knee presentations.* These are uncommon, and the name describes the condition.

For the purposes of determining the dangers in delivery in these groups due to the presentation alone, two groups of breech presentation have been described; the uncomplicated and the complicated breech presentation.

Uncomplicated breech presentation is defined as any baby presenting by the breech which weighs more than 2000g and where no other obstetric complication is present. Twin pregnancies fulfilling the above are included in this category. Complicated breech presentation comprises all the others.

## CAUSE OF BREECH PRESENTATION

It would appear that the main reason for the reduction of breech presentation as pregnancy advances is that the large pole of the fetus seeks room by entering the large pole of the uterus. The buttocks and feet require more room than the head, and consequently try to occupy the fundal area, particularly after the 34th week of pregnancy, when the size of the fetus relative to the available space in the uterus is increasing rapidly. The spontaneous version is aided by the flexed attitude of most fetuses; if the attitude is one of deflexion as in the case of a breech with extended legs, whose back is 'splinted' by the legs, version may not occur. Deflexion attitudes are the main cause for breech presentation in late pregnancy, and account for the preponderance of breech with extended legs. In a few cases, not more than 10 per cent, the cavity of the uterus is mis-shaped either because of a septum or a myoma, or the fetus is abnormal (particularly hydrocephalic), which hinders spontaneous version. Placenta praevia is often stated to be a cause, but this is doubtful, and the association is casual rather than causal.

## DANGERS OF BREECH PRESENTATION

Since breech delivery frequently requires operative intervention, there is a slightly greater risk to the mother. The risk to the fetus is considerable, and depends mainly on (1) the skill of the attendant obstetrician and his team, and (2) the weight of the baby. The fetal loss in cases of uncomplicated breech delivery varies from 3 to 12 per cent. If the baby weighs less than 2250g the mortality is 12 per cent, prematurity being the main cause of death. Between 2250g and 3500g the fetal mortality is 5 per cent; above 3500g it rises steeply to 10 per cent. The principal causes of death of babies weighing more than 2250g are intracranial haemorrhage, tentorial tears from traumatic delivery, or asphyxia from prolapsed cord. As well, 6 per cent of babies presenting as a breech have congenital abnormalities (compared with 2 per cent of babies presenting as vertex). In the larger babies, fracture of femur, humerus or clavicle may occur. These dangers can be reduced by skilled obstetrics, particularly by teamwork, by the use of caesarean section in selected cases, and by slow, gentle delivery in all other cases.

## DIAGNOSIS OF BREECH PRESENTATION

Since the mortality of breech presentation is at least double that of vertex presentations, it is important that the presentation should be detected by the 34th week of pregnancy, so that version may be attempted. Not infrequently a pregnant woman whose fetus presents by the breech complains of discomfort under the ribs, especially when the fetus moves. In about 25 per cent of cases, the breech presentation is not suspected until a vaginal examination early in labour shows that the buttocks have entered the pelvis.

The diagnosis may be made by palpation, auscultation and, if in doubt, by medical imaging, using ultrasound or radiography.

### Palpation

The fundus contains a firm, smooth, rounded mass, which 'ballotts', or bounces, between the two examining hands if flicked with the fingers. On lateral palpation, the lie is noted to be longitudinal, and on pelvic palpation, no head can be detected. The pelvic area is occupied by an irregular soft mass. This is often better detected by Pawlik's grip than the ordinary bimanual one.

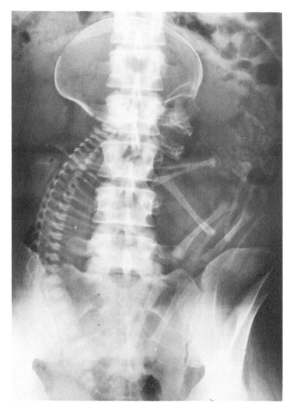

**Fig. 38/2** Radiograph of breech with extended legs

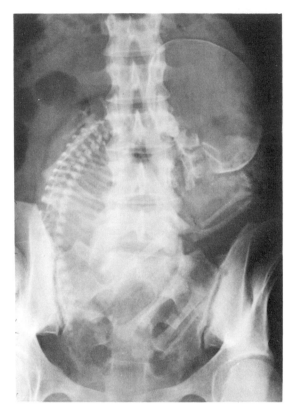

**Fig. 38/3** Radiograph of breech with flexed legs

### Vaginal examination

In cases of breech with extended legs, the diagnosis can be missed, particularly when the breech is engaged in the pelvis. Routine vaginal examination of all patients at the 37th week will detect these cases before the onset of labour. The breech is soft, irregular in shape, and not smooth and round, with palpable sutures, as is the head.

### Auscultation

In most cases of breech presentation, the fetal heart is heard with greater clarity above the umbilicus, but if the breech has extended legs and the buttocks are engaged in the pelvis, this sign may be equivocal.

### Medical imaging

In 10 per cent of primigravidae, tense muscles of the abdominal wall, or uterine irritability, hinder diagnosis by palpation. In these cases, and in other cases where there is uncertainty after clinical examination, a radiograph should be taken (Figs **38/2** and **38/3**), or ultrasound may be used. Many obstetricians prefer radiography, taking a lateral film, which includes the pelvis, so that pelvimetry can be made at the same time.

### MANAGEMENT IN PREGNANCY
(see Table **38/1**)

Because of the increased fetal loss associated with breech delivery, external cephalic version should be tried between the 34th and 37th week. Version before the 34th week is pointless, as many babies immediately revert to breech, and spontaneous version to vertex is usual. After the 37th week, the manipulation is difficult to accomplish. The dangers of version are separation of the placenta, rupture of the membranes, the onset of premature labour, and possible knotting of the umbilical cord. The first three can be avoided if the version is done without undue force, and without anaesthesia. Patients who are frightened, or find relaxation difficult, can be given an analgesic (such as pethidine 100mg intravenously), or a tocolytic agent, but anaesthesia should be avoided except in very exceptional circumstances, and then only if the version is being attempted by an experienced obstetrician (see Chapter 52 for further details).

## CAESAREAN SECTION IN BREECH DELIVERY

If the pelvic measurements are small, as determined by x-ray pelvimetry, or a maternal or fetal condition exists, caesarean section is the method of choice for the delivery of a baby presenting as a breech. In recent years, even in the absence of these unfavourable criteria, an increased trend has occurred to use caesarean section to deliver a baby presenting by the breech. In some institutions the caesarean section rate in breech presentation has risen to 60 per cent, although the mean is about 25 per cent.

The change has occurred because of several factors: (1) if the baby weighs less than 2500g the trauma of vaginal delivery to the relatively soft fetal head is believed to be greater than that of caesarean delivery, and (2) if the baby weighs more than 4000g vaginal delivery is often difficult, and the baby has to be extracted forcibly. In both situations the baby may sustain intracranial damage, fractures of clavicle or limbs, or, more seriously, may suffer severe hypoxia during birth, resulting in cerebral palsy.

Additional arguments are: (1) demographic changes to smaller families which have reduced the incidence of breech delivery, so that obstetricians are unable to obtain the needed skills for vaginal delivery; (2) caesarean section is now a safe operation; (3) the perinatal mortality is less, if the breech baby is delivered by caesarean section.

Counter arguments are: (1) caesarean section is an invasive procedure and early 'bonding' between mother and baby is hindered; (2) the morbidity to the mother is greater after caesarean section than after vaginal delivery; (3) if the baby is preterm, the incidence of congenital defects is at least 15 per cent; and (4) the long-term morbidity, especially neurological handicap, of low birth-weight babies delivered by caesarean section is 3 times that of those surviving vaginal delivery, and affects at least 25 per cent of babies. The reason may be that many preterm breech babies have pre-existing brain damage, and

the method of delivery does not affect the outcome. If these findings are confirmed, delivery by caesarean section should be reserved for low birth-weight babies (<1500g) presenting as footling breeches, as cord prolapse is a real risk during labour in these cases.

If vaginal delivery is decided upon the labour must be treated as a 'trial', and the attendants be aware that the possibility of caesarean section is increased. Such evidence as there is suggests that preterm babies presenting as breeches with extended or flexed legs may be delivered vaginally with no increased mortality; but that footling breech presentations are best delivered by caesarean section. All large (>4000g) breech presentations are best treated by caesarean section.

## MECHANISM OF BREECH DELIVERY

Part of the increased fetal loss in breech delivery is due to the fact that three deliveries take place: that of the buttocks, that of the shoulder girdle, and that of the head. The buttocks and body, unless excessively large, and firmly splinted by extended legs, rarely cause any difficulty, as they are compressible. Difficulty in delivery of the shoulder girdle only arises if the baby's arms are displaced from their normal position of flexion across the thorax. Various degrees of extension of the arms may occur, which by increasing the volume of tissue at the pelvic brim, cause delay in descent and delivery of the shoulder girdle. The delivery of the head is generally the most difficult, and critical, part of the confinement. This is particularly so if the cervix is not completely dilated, and the head is large and firm. Each of the three components go through the normal mechanism of engagement, descent, internal rotation, birth and external rotation, and whilst one part is at one phase of the process, another part is at an earlier phase.

### 1. The breech

Engagement usually occurs before labour, with the bitrochanteric diameter of the buttocks in the transverse diameter of the pelvic brim (Fig. **38/4**). With full dilatation of the cervix, the buttocks *descend* to the pelvic floor and, guided by the gutter formed by the levator ani muscles, undergo *internal rotation* through 90°, so that the bitrochanteric diameter now lies in the antero-posterior diameter of the pelvic outlet (Fig. **38/5**). With the further contractions lateral flexion of the trunk takes place so that the trunk may be accommodated to the curve of the birth canal, and the buttocks distend the perineum, the anus 'winking' between the labia minora (Fig. 38/6). The anterior buttock then passes the pubis and is born, followed by further lateral trunk flexion and the birth of the posterior buttock. If the feet are flexed they now drop out of the vulva; if extended, they are born later. The delivered breech finally undergoes external rotation through 90° to lie in the transverse diameter of the pelvic outlet.

## 2. The shoulder girdle

External rotation of the buttocks is caused by the shoulders entering the pelvis with the bis-achromial diameter in the transverse diameter of the pelvic brim (Fig. 38/7). Descent takes place and as the pelvic floor is reached, *internal rotation* occurs through 90° so that the bis-achromial diameter is now in the antero-posterior diameter of the outlet. (At this time, the head is entering the pelvis, the sagittal suture lying in the transverse diameter of the brim (Fig. 38/8).) The delivered body flexes posteriorly, so that the anterior shoulder stems from behind the symphysis pubis and is born (Fig. 38/9). The posterior shoulder than appears over the perineum, by anterior flexion of the delivered trunk.

## 3. The head

The head *engages* in the brim as the shoulders rotate anteriorly in the mid-pelvis. Descent occurs with further flexion of the head, so that the sub-occipitobregmatic circumference is applied to the birth canal. On reaching the pelvic floor, *internal rotation* through 90° occurs, the occiput entering the anterior pelvic quadrant. Further descent with further flexion occurs, and the occiput comes to lie directly behind the symphysis. The head pivots under the symphysis and is born in flexion, the chin, mouth, nose, forehead and occiput appearing over the perineum. If the delivery of the head is assisted, as is usual, the mechanism does not take place as described.

The course of the mechanism may be altered at any stage, particularly if the patient pushes the buttocks and trunk through a cervix which is not dilated fully, or if the size of the baby has been misjudged. Extended legs are considered to interfere with the mechanism of lateral flexion, but since a breech with extended legs is the usual form, this must be considered normal. The point is that the perineum in a primigravida is subjected to much stress and may tear. A prophylactic episiotomy is therefore desirable. Delay may be occasioned by extended arms, or by a large fetal head, particularly if it is hydrocephalic, or by imperfect flexion which places the larger occipito-frontal circumference in contact with the birth canal. If this occurs the head may become impacted at the brim or at the pelvic floor.

## MANAGEMENT OF BREECH DELIVERY

If version fails or is not attempted, a pelvic assessment must be made in all primigravidae, and in multigravidae when the history of previous deliveries is not explicit. If any doubt exists after the pelvic assessment, a radiological pelvimetry should be made. The choice of method of delivery will depend on: (1) the age of the mother, if she is primigravid; (2) the size of the baby; and (3) the presence of other obstetrical complications. Three methods are available: (1) to allow labour to start naturally; (2) to induce labour at or before the expected date of delivery; (3) to perform an elective caesarean section.

Most patients should be permitted to come into labour spontaneously, and this includes each young primigravida who has a normal pelvis.

Labour in cases of breech presentation must be considered a 'trial', and if any delay occurs the case must be reviewed carefully. Delay in the descent of the fetal buttocks through the maternal pelvis after full dilatation of the cervix is a particularly worrying finding, and if this is detected, the method of delivery must be reassessed. Caesarean section may well be chosen, but the choice will depend on the clinical experience of the obstetrician.

Induction of labour has a very limited place, because of the risk of miscalculation of the duration of the pregnancy and the danger of prolapse of the cord. It is of value if the patient is multigravid, the pregnancy advanced to 37 weeks and the baby big, and in cases when pregnancy is prolonged beyond 42 weeks and the baby is of normal size.

Elective caesarean section is the method of choice in primigravidae over the age of 35; if the baby is estimated to be more than 4000g in weight or less than 1500g; or if other obstetric complications for which caesarean section is required are present.

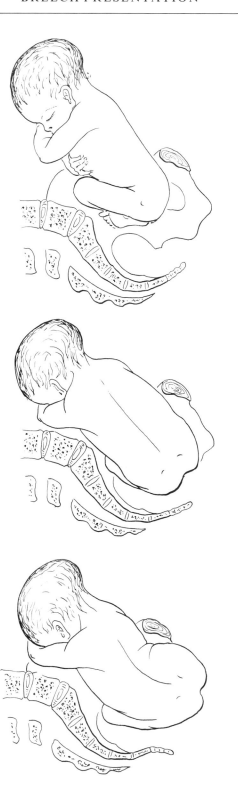

**Fig. 38/4** Mechanism of breech delivery. RST at the onset of labour, engagement of the buttocks usually occurs in the oblique or transverse diameter of the pelvic brim

**Fig. 38/5** Early second stage. The buttocks have reached the pelvic floor and internal rotation has occurred so that the bitrochanteric diameter lies in the antero-posterior diameter of the pelvic outlet

**Fig. 38/6** Late second stage. The anterior buttock appears at the vulva by lateral flexion of the trunk around the symphysis pubis. The shoulders have not yet engaged in the pelvis

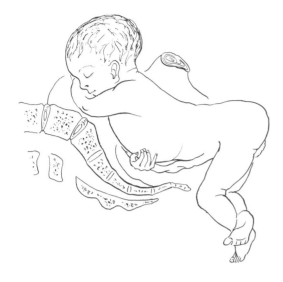

**Fig. 38/7** The buttocks have been born, and the shoulders are adjusting to engage in the transverse diameter of the brim. This movement causes external rotation of the delivered buttocks so that the fetal back becomes uppermost

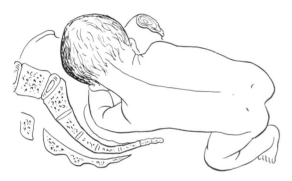

**Fig. 38/8** The shoulders have reached the pelvic floor and have undergone internal rotation so that the bis-achromial diameter lies in the antero-posterior diameter of the pelvic outlet. Simultaneously the buttocks rotate anteriorly through 90°. This is called *restitution*. The head is engaging in the pelvic brim, and the sagittal suture lying in the transverse diameter of the brim

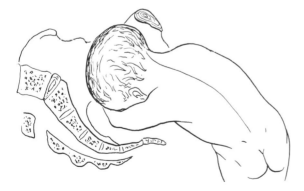

**Fig. 38/9** The anterior shoulder is born from behind the symphysis pubis by lateral flexion of the delivered trunk

## MANAGEMENT OF LABOUR

### First stage

A vaginal examination should be made in early labour to confirm the presentation is a breech, and that the pelvis is adequate in size. A second vaginal examination is mandatory when the membranes rupture to exclude prolapse of the cord. Apart from this the management is identical with that described for normal labour.

### Second stage

Contrary to general belief, the second stage is not usually prolonged, and if the breech has not reached the lower pelvis and distended the perineum within 1½ hours of full dilatation of the cervix, the case must be reassessed. With the appearance of the anterior buttock at the vulva, the patient is placed in the lithotomy position, the vulval skin is cleansed and sterile drapes are put on. In a short time the anus appears to 'wink' between the labia minora. This is a crucial time, for from now on the breech delivery is assisted.

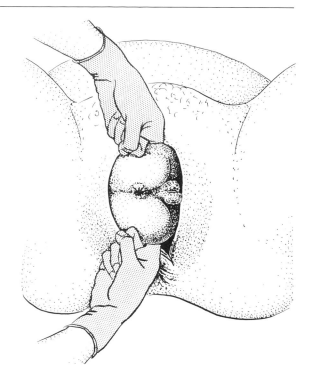

**Fig. 38/10** Groin traction

## DELIVERY OF THE BUTTOCKS

The obstetrician, gloved and gowned, performs a mediolateral episiotomy extending backwards from the posterior commissure at 35° from the midline. During the next two contractions, in cases of flexed breech, the buttocks are expelled from the vulva followed by the feet. If the buttocks are not expelled, the obstetrician's finger is inserted in the fold of the anterior groin, or of both groins, and slight traction is applied during uterine contractions (Fig. **38/10**). This expels the buttocks, which usually rotate through 90° on delivery, and the baby slips out to the level of the umbilicus, the back uppermost. If the legs are extended, the popliteal fossae can now be seen and the legs are released by pressure outwards behind the knees to abduct and flex the thighs (Fig. **38/11**). From this point on the delivery is in the hands of the obstetrician, and, if an epidural has not been established, anaesthesia is induced, using thiopentone, in all primigravidae and in a tense and nervous multigravida. This prevents the patient struggling and straining at the wrong time, and eliminates the pain of delivery. A loop of cord is brought down, merely to see that it is of sufficient length, but pulsations in the cord are not determined

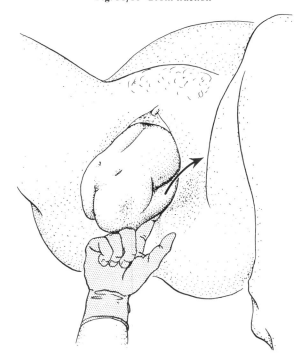

**Fig. 38/11** Flexion and abduction to deliver the anterior extended leg

as they have no prognostic value. The time is also checked, and the rest of the delivery must be carried out slowly and deliberately over a 5-minute period. Each minute should be called out by a nurse.

## DELIVERY OF THE THORAX AND SHOULDER GIRDLE

The baby is held by the feet, or by the flat hands placed along the sides of the pelvic girdle, with a sterile towel between the hands and the baby, to prevent slipping. The thorax is rotated back through 90°, if this has not occurred spontaneously, so that the shoulders lie in the antero-posterior diameter of the outlet, and traction is made downwards and backwards until the lower border of the scapula appears (Fig. **38/12**).

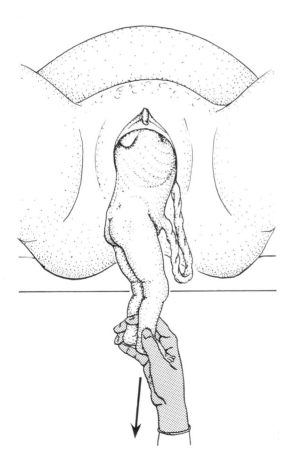

**Fig. 38/12** Delivery of the thorax – traction is made downwards and backwards

Two methods are commonly used for the delivery of the shoulder girdle; these are: (1) Lövset's rotation; and (2) hooking down the arm. Both are effective, but Lövset's rotation has the advantage that it can be used in dealing with complicated as well as normal deliveries, whilst hooking down the anterior arm can only be used safely when the arms are flexed across the child's chest.

### Lövset's manoeuvre

The manoeuvre is based on the fact that owing to the inclination of the pelvic inlet, the posterior shoulder enters the pelvic cavity before the anterior. The fetal body is lifted slightly and supported by the obstetrician's hands, and is rotated with slight traction through 180°, the back passing anteriorly, so that the posterior shoulder comes to lie in front. Since it is on a lower level than the anterior shoulder, it either delivers spontaneously, or can be lifted out by one finger placed in the bend of the elbow. The body of the child is now rotated through 180° in the opposite direction, so that the other arm is brought into the anterior position again, but at a much lower level, and the arm and shoulder are born spontaneously, or can be hooked out. The back then rotates to lie uppermost (Fig. **38/13**).

### Hooking down the arm

When the lower border of the anterior scapula is visible and the back is in the antero-posterior diameter of the pelvis, the arms are felt for on the front of the chest, by lifting the trunk, and if found, are delivered by placing a finger on the tip of the acromion. The finger is then run along the humerus to the elbow, and the arm is dislodged downwards and delivered by pressure of the finger. Once the anterior arm is delivered the body rotates slightly, the back upwards, and the posterior arm is freed in a similar manner.

## DELIVERY OF THE HEAD

### Liverpool technique

This is the crucial stage of the delivery, and the stage in which most babies are damaged, or die. The aim in delivering the head is to maintain full flexion, so that the most favourable diameter is presented to the pelvic cavity. Once the shoulders are born, the baby is allowed to hang unsupported, and slight

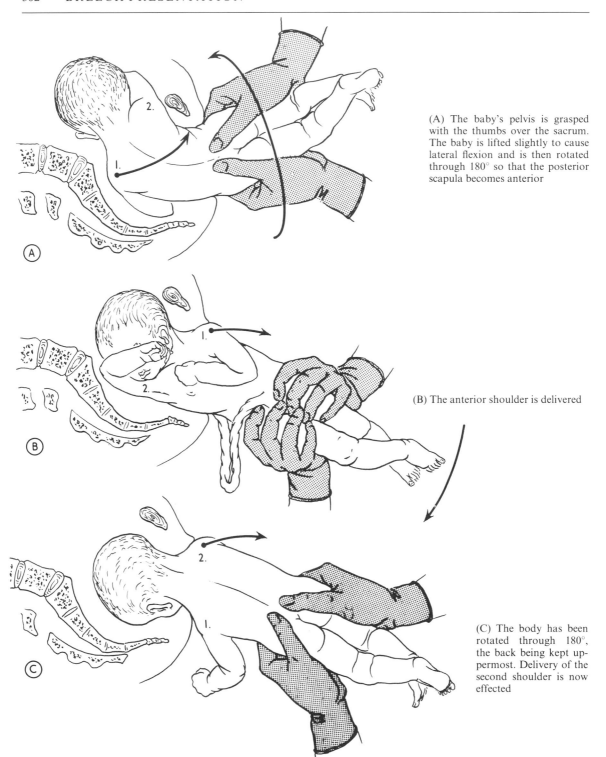

(A) The baby's pelvis is grasped with the thumbs over the sacrum. The baby is lifted slightly to cause lateral flexion and is then rotated through 180° so that the posterior scapula becomes anterior

(B) The anterior shoulder is delivered

(C) The body has been rotated through 180°, the back being kept uppermost. Delivery of the second shoulder is now effected

**Fig. 38/13** Lövset's manoeuvre in breech with extended arm

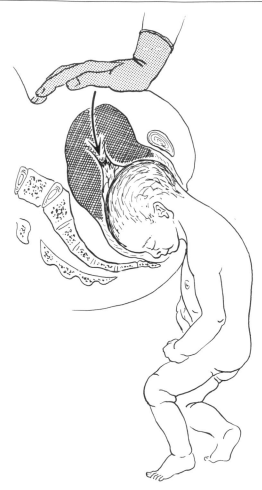

Fig. **38/14** The baby hangs from the vulva. This increases flexion of the head

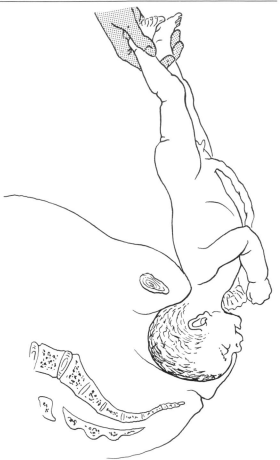

Fig. **38/15** Traction is applied to the legs and the body swung in an arc

suprapubic pressure encourages flexion and further descent (Fig. **38/14**). Within 1 minute the nape of the neck appears in the subpubic angle. If it does not, the operator applies suprapubic pressure using the flat of his hand, in a downward and backward direction. When the nape of the neck has appeared the baby is grasped by the ankles, or pelvic girdle, and maintaining traction, is swung through a wide arc over the vulva. This movement, by using the lower border of the symphysis as a fulcrum, pulls the head down and rotates it through the outlet so that the chin and mouth appear at the vulva (Fig. **38/15**). Mucus is extracted from the mouth and pharynx. In primigravidae the delivery of the head is completed slowly by forceps, the long-shanked Neville-Barnes or Piper forceps being used, and

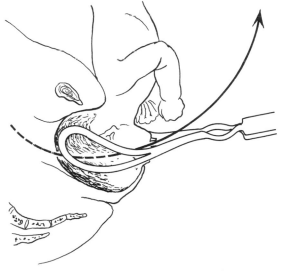

Fig. **38/16** Delivery of the head is completed using forceps

traction applied in an arc which follows the axis of the birth canal (Fig. **38/16**). In multigravidae slight suprapubic pressure will normally complete the delivery without difficulty.

### Mauriceau–Smellie–Veit technique

An alternative method for the delivery of the head is to use a 'grip' described by three pioneer obstetricians independently, the Mauriceau–Smellie–Veit grip. The middle finger of the fully pronated left hand is placed on the baby's suboccipital region, the ring and index fingers placed over the shoulders. The supinated right hand is placed below the baby, which lies astride the arm. One finger of the right hand is placed in the mouth and one on each malar bone. This hand maintains flexion of the head whilst two hands apply traction to the baby smoothly and steadily in the axis of the pelvis – first downwards and backwards, then downwards, then downwards and forwards, in an arc (Fig. **38/17**). Once the baby is born, the vagina is examined for

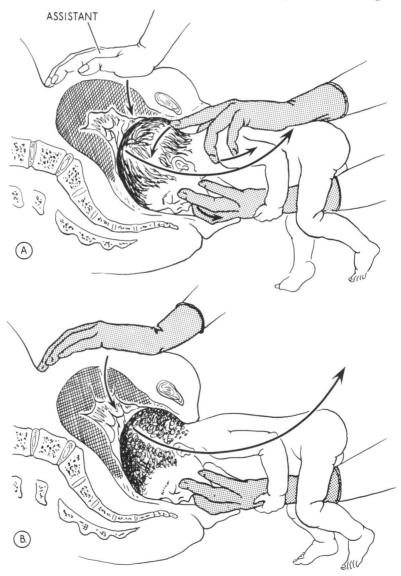

**Fig. 38/17** Methods of delivering the head. (A) Mauriceau–Smellie–Veit manoeuvre; (B) Wigand–Martin manoeuvre. The methods are basically similar but in the first the help of an assistant is required

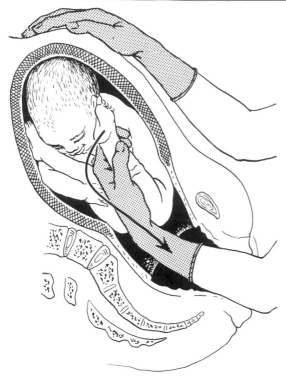

**Fig. 38/18** Method of bringing down a leg after the breech has been dislodged from the pelvis

lacerations and the third stage is conducted in the usual way.

## UNEXPECTED COMPLICATIONS OF BREECH DELIVERY

### 1. Delay in the descent of the buttocks

If the buttocks do not reach the ischial spines within $1\frac{1}{2}$ hours of the start of the second stage, either the baby is larger than had been anticipated, or the pelvis is contracted. The feto-pelvic relations should be reassessed and in most cases delivery should be by caesarean section. In a few cases the arrest may be resolved by dislodging the breech from the pelvis and bringing down a leg. Deep anaesthesia is required. The fetal mortality from this procedure is high so that great care must be taken to select the patient in which this method is appropriate. The operator introduces his left hand along the curve of the sacrum, and between uterine contractions reaches inside the uterine cavity until he finds a leg which he traces to the foot. For preference the anterior leg is sought, but this is not essential (Fig. **38/18**). The foot is grasped between fingers and thumb and is delivered. The rest of the delivery is effected by

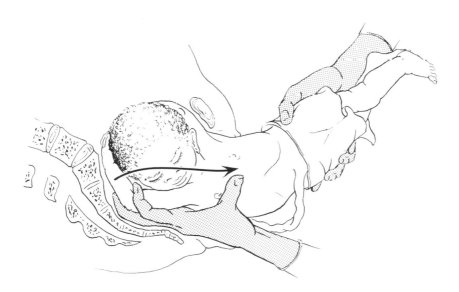

**Fig. 38/19** Method of bringing down an arm when the baby's back is to the mother's left side

traction from below and pressure from above, Lövset's technique being used for the shoulders, and forceps applied to the aftercoming head. The whole procedure is termed *breech extraction*. Delay of the buttocks in the lower pelvis, or on the perineum, is treated by groin traction, but again an estimate of the feto-pelvic sizes must be made.

## 2. Extension of the arms

Full extension of the arms so that they stretch above the head, or even lie behind the neck (in the 'nuchal' position) is uncommon unless traction or other manipulations have been used in attempting delivery. The first sign of the complication is that the trunk of the child is expelled as far as the costal margin

and is there arrested. A finger should be introduced along the baby's thorax and the elbow sought. If it cannot be found the arms are probably extended. The arms may be disimpacted by using Lövset's manoeuvre, or by the following method: the baby is grasped by the pelvic girdle and traction is made to bring the anterior scapula into view. The body of the baby is now swung forward and two fingers of the left hand are introduced along the curve of the sacrum until the elbow of the posterior arm is reached. The fingers seek the antecubital fossa and with firm pressure on the humerus, efforts are made to swing the arm towards the midline of the child's body and downwards over the thorax (Fig. **38/19**). The manoeuvre requires great skill, or fracture of the humerus will result. Once the posterior arm is

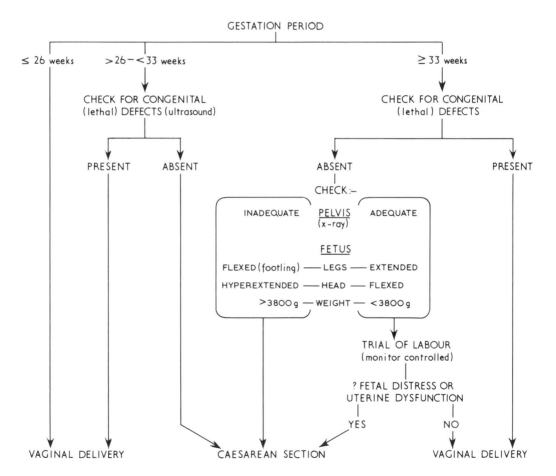

**Table 38/1** Management of breech presentation. If detected at 33–35 weeks confirm gestation period by checking date of LMP, visits during pregnancy, ultrasound examination. Attempt external cephalic version (ECV) without anaesthesia, ? using tocolytics and real-time ultrasound. If failure of ECV wait for labour

delivered, the body of the baby is swung backwards and the anterior arm is disengaged in a similar manner.

### 3. The arrest of the aftercoming head

The arrest may occur at the pelvic brim, in the cavity or at the outlet. Arrest at the brim may be due to pelvic contraction or to hydrocephalus, but is most commonly due to a deflexed head, or an incompletely dilated cervix. Both are more likely when the baby is large. Any manipulation requires deep anaesthesia for success, and it must be remembered that the head enters the pelvic cavity with its long axis in the transverse diameter of the brim. The usual manipulations tried are jaw and shoulder traction, with suprapubic pressure from an assistant or attempted application of Kielland's forceps. If the baby dies during the procedures craniotomy should be performed, after which delivery will be easy. If the delay is due to an *incompletely dilated cervix*, this may grasp the fetal neck, causing a partial vacuum. A finger should be introduced between the cervix and the head and cervical incisions made. If the baby dies, craniotomy is preferable to awaiting spontaneous delivery. Arrest at the mid-cavity or outlet may indicate mid-pelvic contraction and is best treated by application of forceps, or by craniotomy if the baby dies during attempts at extraction.

### 4. Prolapse of the cord

This complication is more common in footling or flexed breech presentations, than if the breech has extended legs. If the cervix is not fully dilated caesarean section gives the best fetal results; whilst if it is, the choice lies between caesarean section and breech extraction.

### BREECH EXTRACTION

The most frequent, and safest, indication is for the delivery of a second twin. Less commonly, and less safely, breech extraction may be required for (1) prolapse of the cord; (2) fetal distress; (3) impaction of the breech in the mid-cavity or lower pelvis; (4) following internal version for oblique or transverse lie. The operation should only be performed (1) if there is no cephalopelvic disproportion; (2) if the cervix is fully dilated; (3) if the patient is adequately anaesthetized; (4) if the operation can be performed with full asepsis by a skilled obstetrician.

## Chapter 39

# Other Malpositions and Malpresentations

## FACE PRESENTATION

Face presentation occurs in about 1 in 500 births, and in 70 per cent of cases it occurs by chance, the head undergoing a change in attitude from incomplete flexion to extension at the moment of engagement in the maternal pelvis. In these cases the head and spine are extended and the legs flexed. In 15 per cent of cases a congenital malformation, usually anencephaly, a tumour of the fetal neck, or shortening of the fetal neck muscles is the cause of the presentation. In the few remaining cases, a primary brow presentation undergoes further extension to become a face presentation during labour.

### DIAGNOSIS

Rarely, face presentation may be present and be diagnosed before labour, but in most instances the diagnosis is only made in labour, and even then the presentation may be missed until the swollen distorted lips appear at the vulva in the second stage.

On abdominal palpation the shape of the fetal spine is that of an S, and the uterus a long ovoid with no bulges in the flanks. On using the 'pelvic grip', the round occiput is very prominent, may be 'ballottable', and a deep groove can be felt between it and the back. The feet are felt on the opposite side to the occipital prominence, and the fetal heart is loudest on the same side as the feet (Fig. **39/1**). In many cases the diagnosis is not clear on abdominal palpation, and provided the cervix is sufficiently dilated, vaginal examination is helpful. The orbital ridges and eyes, the irregular nose, and the mouth, can be recognized (Fig. **39/2**). But in late labour, when much oedema has occurred, it may be difficult to differentiate the face from the breech.

### MECHANISM OF LABOUR

The majority of face presentations engage in the transverse diameter of the pelvis, and a right mento-transverse position is more common than a left one.

The diameter applied to the pelvis is the submento-

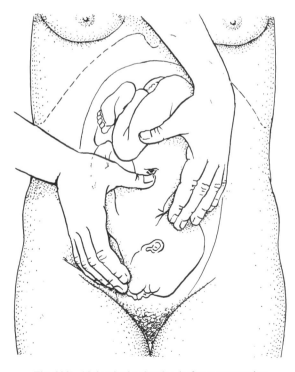

**Fig. 39/1** Abdominal palpation in face presentation

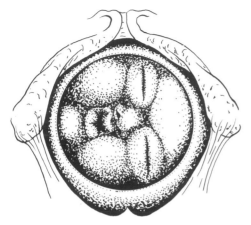

**Fig. 39/2** Touch picture of the face (RMT)

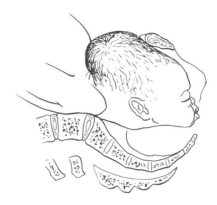

**Fig. 39/4** Impacted mento-posterior position. Birth of the head by flexion is impossible

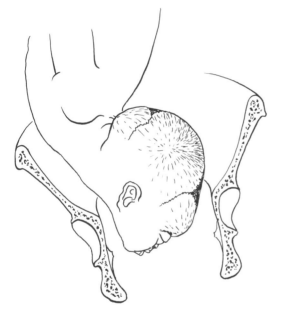

**Fig. 39/3** Diagram of engagement. In face presentation engagement occurs late as the parietal prominences do not enter the brim until the face has reached the pelvic floor

bregmatic which measures 9.5cm. Descent to the mid-pelvis occurs with further extension of the head, but it must be remembered that even when the face has reached the ischial spines, full engagement of the head has not occurred (Fig. **39/3**). Rotation occurs at, or below, the level of the ischial spines, the chin turning anteriorly through 90° to lie behind the symphysis in the antero-posterior diameter of the outlet. Anterior rotation of the chin occurs in 90 per

cent of cases, but in 10 per cent the rotation is posterior, the chin coming to lie in the hollow of the sacrum, from which position spontaneous delivery is impossible (Fig. **39/4**). Mento-anterior positions are favourable and further descent occurs, the chin escaping from the vulva and the head being born by flexion. The remainder of the birth does not differ from that of vertex presentations. Since the facial bones are less flexible than the bones of the vault, moulding is less and consequently minor degrees of pelvic contraction more serious than in vertex presentations. Owing to poor venous return, marked caput formation distorts the entire face, often to a pulpy diffuse mass, from which distended lips and swollen eyelids emerge (Fig. **39/5**). The head is elongated, and after birth the baby lies on one side with its back straight and its head extended. In a few days the oedema and distortion disappear. The mother must be reassured that this will occur, as soon as possible after the delivery. Anencephalic babies should be removed from the labour room immediately, as they may make feeble cries within the mother's hearing, unless the diagnosis has been made before the onset of labour and the problem has been discussed with the parents who have received counselling. In such cases, the parents may wish to see the child.

## PROGNOSIS

Although labour is only prolonged when there is the added complication of cephalopelvic disproportion,

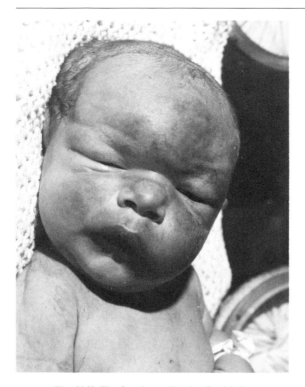

**Fig. 39/5** The face immediately after birth

operative interference may be necessary in up to 20 per cent of cases, and the maternal morbidity is raised. Face presentation offers a considerable risk to the fetus, even when malformed babies are excluded, and amongst normal babies the mortality is about 10 per cent. This is due to a higher incidence of operative procedures, to cerebral congestion, and to hypoxia in labour due to the poor venous return from the head and neck.

## MANAGEMENT

If the presentation is diagnosed before labour, pelvic contraction must be excluded, and the size of the fetus estimated. A large baby, or a reduction in pelvic measurements is an indication that labour should be a 'trial'. Caesarean section may be required if progress is not rapid. A radiological examination is usually necessary to detect fetal malformations, and to give some indication of the size of the baby.

In most cases the diagnosis is not made until labour has started, and in half, not until delivery. It must be remembered that the majority of face presentations deliver spontaneously. However, in a few cases of mento-anterior position, low forceps may be required. In some cases rotation from the transverse does not occur and rotation with Kielland's forceps is indicated to avoid a prolonged second stage of labour. Should the chin rotate posteriorly in the mid-pelvis, spontaneous delivery cannot occur, and a decision will have to be made whether to deliver by caesarean section before the head is impacted further into the pelvis, or whether to attempt rotation of the head by Kielland's forceps. This manoeuvre requires considerable skill, and should only be performed in an operating theatre, with preparations made for caesarean section. If the patient is admitted in late labour with a dead baby impacted in the mento-posterior position, craniotomy and forceps extraction is required to effect delivery.

Two intra-uterine manipulations used in the past should be avoided. Conversion of the face to a vertex by internal manipulation in labour is not easy, and usually fails; and disengagement of the head, followed by internal version, is lethal to mother and fetus, and is condemned.

# BROW PRESENTATION

Brow presentation is the most unfavourable of all cranial presentations, as the mento-vertical diameter (13cm) presents. It occurs when a vertex extending to become a face is interrupted by engaging in the pelvis. When the brow becomes engaged in the pelvic brim, further progress is halted unless the baby is very small. However, brow presentation is uncommon, the incidence being 1 in 1500 deliveries.

## DIAGNOSIS

As the position is transient until the head is fixed in labour, it is rarely diagnosed before this. In labour the finding of a large unengaged head, with a sulcus between occiput and back, should make the physician suspicious that a brow presents. The diagnosis can be confirmed on vaginal examination by palpating the anterior fontanelle and supra-orbital ridges, or by radiology.

## TREATMENT

In pregnancy no treatment is required as conversion to vertex or face is usual. The patient should be instructed to come into hospital immediately labour starts, or if the membranes rupture. Although 10 per cent of brow presentations encountered in labour will convert spontaneously into face or vertex, or can be converted by manipulation, this only occurs when the fetus is small, and should not be anticipated. The proper treatment of a brow presentation diagnosed in labour is caesarean section, unless the baby is dead or gross fetal abnormality (such as hydrocephaly) exists. In these cases, craniotomy and vaginal delivery is to be preferred.

# TRANSVERSE LIE AND OBLIQUE LIE (SHOULDER PRESENTATION) AND UNSTABLE LIE

Transverse and oblique lie are the most dangerous of all fetal malpresentations. The presenting part is the shoulder, and the back may be anterior (in 60 per cent of cases) or posterior (in 40 per cent of cases). An oblique lie tends to be unstable and to become longitudinal or transverse when labour starts. The incidence of the presentation is 1 in 200, but it is not commonly found in primigravidae.

## AETIOLOGY

Transverse lie is favoured if the uterus is large and of poor tone (as in many high multigravidae), or over-distended by excessive liquor amnii, or by a multiple pregnancy. In 10 per cent of cases a placenta praevia is present. Amongst primigravidae the finding of the presentation is more sinister, and may indicate an arcuate, or subseptate, uterus, a contracted pelvis, or rarely, placenta praevia.

## DIAGNOSIS

Inspection of the abdomen will show that the uterus is enlarged transversely and has the shape of a transverse oval (Fig. **39/6**). On abdominal palpation, no head can be found in the pelvis or in the uterine fundus, and the fetus lies 'cross-wise'. On one side of the uterus the hard head is felt and on the other the softer indefinite breech. Vaginal examination confirms the absence of the fetal head, or breech, in the lower uterine pole and if labour has been in progress the shoulder may be identified (Figs **39/7** and **39/8**). If the presentation is not detected until labour is in progress, prolapse of one or more limbs, or of the umbilical cord, may draw attention to its presence.

## TRANSVERSE LIE IN PREGNANCY

The diagnosis is usually easy, but before any treatment is attempted it must be ascertained that there is no contracted pelvis or placenta praevia. Once these conditions, and multiple pregnancy, have been excluded, a gentle external cephalic version should be attempted if the pregnancy has advanced to 36 weeks' gestation. In many cases, because of uterine laxity, the fetus will return to the transverse position, but this is not an argument for failing to do the version. Because of this risk the patient must be instructed to report to hospital immediately labour starts, or if the membranes rupture. The alternative is to admit the patient to hospital to await the onset of labour if the abnormal lie persists or recurs after the 38th week of pregnancy.

Another alternative, which is probably preferable provided the cervix is ripe and suitable for amniotomy, is to induce labour at about the 38th week. The transverse lie is corrected by external cephalic version, and with an assistant maintaining the fetal head over the pelvic brim, a high amniotomy is performed. As the liquor escapes through the Drew–

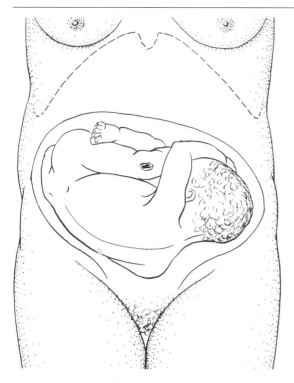

**Fig. 39/6** Transverse lie

Smythe catheter, the head is led into the pelvis, a low amniotomy is performed, and a dilute oxytocin infusion set up. The presentation of the fetus is checked periodically and the labour carefully monitored, as in about 15 per cent of cases caesarean section becomes necessary. Another approach is to perform an elective caesarean section.

## COURSE OF LABOUR IN TRANSVERSE LIE

If labour starts with the shoulder presenting, the effect of the uterine contractions is to push the shoulder deeper and deeper into the pelvis. Should premature rupture of the membranes occur, either before the onset of labour or in early labour, a prolapsed arm or cord, or both, may further complicate the progress of labour. In very rare instances spontaneous expulsion of the baby occurs, particularly if the child is small. It should not be anticipated and if treatment is not undertaken the shoulder will so obstruct labour that uterine rupture is inevitable (Fig. **39/9**).

## MANAGEMENT OF THE MALPRESENTATION RECOGNIZED IN LABOUR

Transverse lie may be detected at different times during labour: (1) early in labour, the membranes being intact or recently ruptured; (2) late in labour, the fetus being alive; and (3) late in labour, the fetus being dead.

### Early in labour

If the membranes are intact, or recently ruptured, and the fetus of normal size, external, or bipolar cephalic version should be attempted. Once the fetus is in a longitudinal lie, amniotomy is performed and most of the liquor is allowed to drain away. In cases where the fetus is large or the patient primigravid, and gentle version fails, caesarean section is indicated. Podalic version in these cases is contra-indicated as the fetal loss is high.

### Late labour: live fetus

Unless the membranes are still intact, the baby of normal size, and a practised obstetrician is prepared to sit by the patient and perform an internal podalic version and breech extraction at full dilatation of the cervix, the treatment of choice is caesarean section. Indeed, caesarean section is a superior method in all but a small minority of cases as it is attended by a much lower fetal loss. The opportunity can also be taken to ligate the Fallopian tubes of high multigravidae who have no wish for further children. If the membranes have been ruptured for some time, the shoulder is impacted in the pelvis and the fetus alive, caesarean section is mandatory, as internal podalic version is hazardous and traumatic uterine rupture probable. Internal version in these cases is to be condemned.

### Late labour: dead fetus

If the uterus is tightly wrapped around the fetus and the lower segment so distended that it is paper-thin, caesarean section is the safest line of treatment. If the danger of rupture of the uterus is less, and the baby small, decapitation of the fetus, using a decapitating wire, or a long scissors, followed by vaginal extraction of the body and later the head, will avoid the need for abdominal operation. The decision of what to do can only be made after assess-

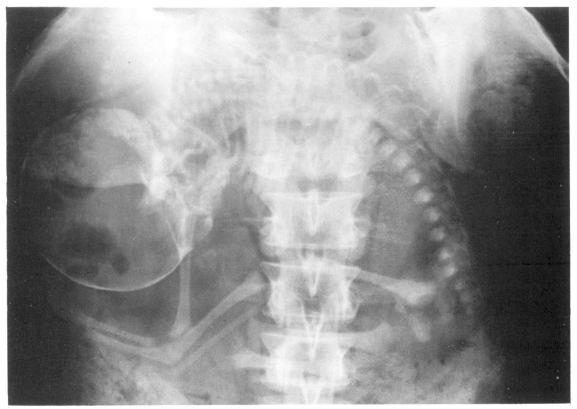

Fig. 39/7 Transverse lie, radiological findings

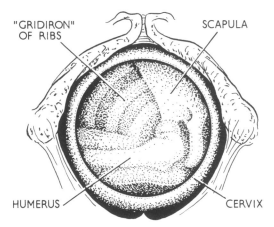

"GRIDIRON" OF RIBS

SCAPULA

HUMERUS

CERVIX

Fig. 39/8 The vaginal findings in shoulder presentation

ment of each case, and if the obstetrician has limited experience, caesarean section is safest. It must be stressed once again that in this situation there is no place for internal version.

Following delivery after any intra-uterine manipu-lation, the cavity of the uterus must be palpated carefully over all its contours to determine if a rupture has occurred. This examination can be combined with a prophylactic manual removal of the placenta.

### The second twin as a transverse lie

In 5 per cent of all cases of multiple pregnancy, examination immediately after delivery of the first twin will reveal that the second twin lies transversely, or obliquely. This is much less hazardous to the mother than in the case of a single baby and can generally be treated by obstetric manipulations. If the membranes are intact an external cephalic (or podalic) version should be performed. If this should fail or if the membranes rupture, an internal podalic version and breech extraction can be performed safely, provided the baby is not too large. Only if the baby is big, or if considerable time has elapsed since the birth of the first baby and the uterus is

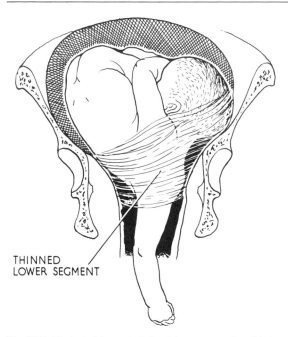

THINNED
LOWER SEGMENT

**Fig. 39/9** Neglected impacted shoulder presentation. Note the thinned lower uterine segment

consequently tightly wrapped round the baby, need caesarean section be considered.

## PROGNOSIS FOR MOTHER AND CHILD

### Maternal

Unless the condition is detected early in labour and treated skilfully the maternal mortality is increased. This is because the undetected case may lead to uterine rupture, and treatment demands either intra-uterine manipulation or abdominal operation.

### Fetal

The overall fetal loss is high, varying between 25 and 60 per cent, depending on the time of detection of the malpresentation in labour and on the treatment adopted. In many instances the baby is premature, or has died in utero, or the mother is admitted late in labour, and this influences the overall mortality. It has been shown that the prognosis for the fetus is best following caesarean section, and worst after internal version.

# PROLAPSE OF THE HAND IN A VERTEX PRESENTATION (COMPOUND PRESENTATION)

Compound presentation is rare, but may occur in any condition interfering with the proper engagement of the head such as hydramnios or contracted pelvis or when the baby is premature. The condition is unimportant both before labour, and in labour before rupture of the membranes, as the arm usually floats away from the head. When encountered in late labour after rupture of the membranes, full cervical dilatation should be awaited when disimpaction of the arm is easy to perform under anaesthesia, after which the baby is delivered by forceps or with a vacuum extractor.

## Chapter 40

# Multiple Pregnancy

Multiple pregnancy can occur from the simultaneous release and fertilization of two or more ova (dizygotic multiple pregnancy), or from the early division of a fertilized single ovum (monozygotic twins). The incidence of twins is 1 in 90 pregnancies, of triplets 1 in 90 × 90 pregnancies, and of quadruplets 1 in 90 × 90 × 90 pregnancies in Western countries, but twins are more frequent in Africa and Asia. This increased frequency is due to a higher population of dizygotic twins amongst the women, as the incidence of monozygotic twins is not affected by heredity, race or age. On the other hand, dizygotic twins are proportionally more common amongst families with a history of twins, in older women, and women of high gravidity.

The incidence reported relates to twins diagnosed by clinical methods. The routine use of ultrasound in the first quarter of pregnancy has revealed that the real incidence is twice that reported by clinical methods. In half of all twin pregnancies one twin disappears – the 'vanishing twin syndrome'.

## TWINS

Binovular twins arise from the chance fertilization of two ova released at the same time. These ova may come from the same or from different ovaries. Each fetus is a separate individual (fraternal twin) and has its own placenta, amnion and chorion. The placentae are distinct, and although they may be close together and apparently joined, no connecting circulation exists. The sex of the children may be the same or different.

Uni-ovular twins arise from the complete and equal division of the ovum at the inner cell mass stage, or earlier. Later division is rare and leads to conjoined twins of various forms. The fetuses have a single placenta, and one chorion, but each fetus has its own amniotic sac. There is usually a communication between the vessels in the placenta and one fetus may receive a reduced supply of nutrients and grow more slowly than the other. Occasionally one fetus dies early in pregnancy and becomes dehydrated and mummified (fetus papyraceous).

### GENERAL CHARACTERISTICS

Twins usually differ considerably in size from each other, and the difference is greater amongst monozygotic twins. Each twin is smaller and lighter at birth than a singleton birth, but their combined weight is greater.

In utero the frequency of presentation varies from week to week, but in the last month of pregnancy the order of frequency is approximately: both cephalic 45 per cent; cephalic and breech 25 per cent; breech and cephalic 10 per cent; both breech 10 per cent; cephalic and transverse, breech and transverse, or both transverse, in the remainder.

### DIAGNOSIS OF MULTIPLE PREGNANCY

1. The girth of the abdomen and size of the uterus is greater than expected from the period of amenorrhoea, and hydramnios is common.
2. Palpation shows an excess of fetal parts and two fetal heads can often be detected. The finding of a small fetal head in a large uterus is suggestive of twins.

3. If a doubt exists, confirmation of a multiple pregnancy can be made by ultrasound (Figs **40/1** and **40/2**). Because about 20 per cent of multiple births are undiagnosed at the onset of labour, some obstetricians recommend routine ultrasound examination of all women between the 18th and 24th weeks of pregnancy. Although such an examination would identify all multiple pregnancies earlier, it is uncertain that this would reduce the morbidity or mortality associated with the condition.

At present more errors are made in diagnosing multiple pregnancy, on clinical grounds, than in missing the condition.

Errors in the period of gestation, a large single baby, a pregnancy complicated by myomata or an ovarian tumour, and a benign trophoblastic tumour may cause confusion.

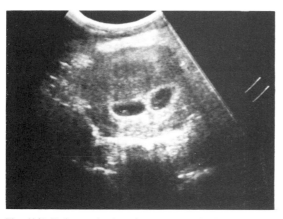

**Fig. 40/1** Twin sacs in 6-week pregnancy. Scale caliper 1cm on right. Real-time ultrasound showed fetal heart movement in each sac (transverse scan)

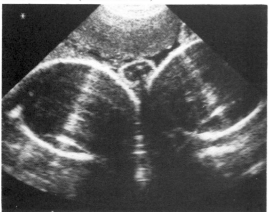

## COMPLICATIONS IN MULTIPLE PREGNANCY

### Pregnancy

*Pregnancy-induced hypertension.* The incidence of PIH is about 15 to 20 per cent and is frequently severe in type.

*Anaemia* is more common than in a single pregnancy, and megaloblastic anaemia is a particular hazard because of the requirements of the two babies for folic acid. There is good evidence that all women carrying a multiple pregnancy should routinely receive folic acid 1mg daily from the 28th week.

*Hydramnios* complicates about 5 per cent of multiple pregnancies. Not only does it cause maternal discomfort, it also leads to difficulty in diagnosis.

*Premature labour* is more common, 10 per cent of pregnancies terminating before the 34th week and 25 per cent before the 36th week. Moreover the weight of each twin is less than that of a singleton of the same maturity (Fig. **40/3**) so that the frequency with which babies of low birth-weight (less than 2500g) are born is increased. The frequency ranges from 35 to 60 per cent of all twin births in the different nations. The cause of the lower mean birth-weight of a child of a multiple pregnancy compared with a singleton is due mainly to growth retardation, rather than to curtailed pregnancy. It is not due to placental dysfunction, for the placenta of a multiple is often larger than that of a singleton. It is probably due to the fact that the maternal organism can only support 3000 to 3600g of total fetal weight without the onset of fetal growth retardation.

Neither placenta praevia nor abruptio placentae are more frequent in multiple than in singleton pregnancy.

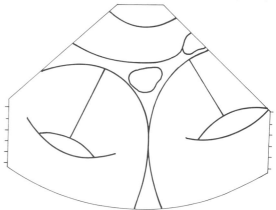

**Fig. 40/2** Multiple pregnancy. Transverse scan at 32 weeks – two heads visible.

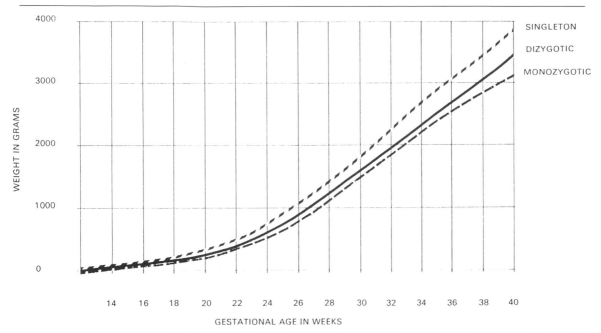

**Fig. 40/3** The intrauterine growth of multiple and single pregnancies as assessed by ultrasound fetometry (**Source**: G. Geuser and P. H. Persson. *Clinics in Obstetrics and Gynaecology*, 1986, 533)

### Labour

Since the lie of the babies is longitudinal in over 90 per cent of cases and uterine activity is not altered, the length of labour is not increased beyond that of a single pregnancy. However, because of the larger placental bed the incidence of postpartum haemorrhage is double (7 to 9 per cent) that which follows the birth of a single fetus.

### MANAGEMENT OF PREGNANCY

The patient is advised to rest more in early pregnancy to improve placental blood flow, and should increase her protein intake. Iron and folic acid should be given to prevent or treat anaemia. She should be seen at fortnightly intervals from the 24th week. It is usually recommended that women carrying a multiple pregnancy should rest, either in bed or in a chair, for at least 4 hours a day from about the 30th to the 36th week. The belief is that additional rest during these weeks will reduce the risk of premature labour, and to increase the number of babies of 'normal' birth-weight (greater than 2500g) although recent studies cast doubt on these findings. There is no place for the prophylactic use of beta-mimetic drugs, such as ritodrine; or for prophylactic cervical circlage.

Some obstetricians monitor the growth of each fetus at two-week intervals from about the 30th week using serial ultrasound. Should either fetus show evidence of no growth, intervention to deliver the twins is considered.

### LABOUR

Apart from checking that no maternal anaemia exists, labour may be allowed to proceed normally. The delivery of the first fetus usually causes no difficulty. Following its birth the lie of the second twin must be determined by abdominal palpation, and if it is transverse, an external cephalic, or podalic, version attempted. A vaginal examination is then made, and the bulging bag of membranes of the second twin ruptured artifically and the liquor allowed to drain slowly, the presenting part being led into the pelvis, if it has not already engaged. If the second twin is a breech or a transverse lie and its weight is estimated at <1500g or >4000g caesarean section is probably advisable rather than attempted vaginal delivery.

If the mother has not been anaesthetized she should be encouraged to push with the contractions, but if there is no progress, forceps delivery or breech extraction should be employed. Should the lie of the second twin be transverse, and external version a failure, internal version and extraction should be performed under anaesthesia.

If the mother has been anaesthetized for the birth of the first baby she should be delivered of the second infant by forceps or breech extraction. Since the babies are frequently premature, all manipulations must be performed gently.

In the past ten years, increasing proportions of twins are being delivered by caesarean section in an attempt to reduce respiratory difficulties and neonatal mortality. Careful studies indicate that caesarean section does not produce the desired results, and a high rate of caesarean section is not justified. Nor does caesarean section to deliver the second twin improve the outcome for that twin.

The third stage of labour is managed actively to prevent postpartum haemorrhage, intravenous ergometrine 0.25mg or intramuscular Syntometrine, 1 ampoule being given with the birth of the second baby and controlled cord traction practised.

### Locked twins

This abnormality occurs once in 100 000 deliveries and is very dangerous. Treatment depends on the conditions encountered in each patient, but caesarean section gives the best fetal results.

## TRIPLETS

Triplets usually arise from two ova – as twins from one, and a single baby from the other. The complications and management of pregnancy and labour are as described for twins. The perinatal loss is double that of twins.

## PROGNOSIS IN MULTIPLE PREGNANCY

### Maternal

The risk to the mother is slightly highly than in singleton pregnancies because of the increased incidence of pregnancy-induced hypertension, anaemia and postpartum haemorrhage.

### Fetal and neonatal

The risk to the infant is much higher than in singletons, preterm birth being the commonest cause of perinatal loss, which is increased fourfold to 50 to 75 per 1000. The risk to the second twin is greater than that to the first because of its lower birth-weight and of the added complication of intra-uterine anoxia and operative delivery. Provided the twin survives the neonatal period he has no greater chance of physical or mental defects compared with a singleton child of similar birth-weight.

The death in utero or in the neonatal period of one or more of the infants presents parents with particular problems. They have to adjust to the joy of having a living baby and the grief of having a dead baby. The issues are discussed on p. 135. Because the parents have a surviving baby, the birthday of that child may be attended by memories of and sadness about the dead sibling. Counselling may be needed at that time.

## Chapter 41

# Prolapse of the Cord

Prolapse of the cord occurs about once in 200 deliveries. The cord may lie enclosed in the intact bag of forewaters (often called presentation of the cord), or may have prolapsed into the vagina after rupture of the membranes (Fig. **41/1**).

## AETIOLOGY

Anything which interferes with the snug application of the presenting part in the lower uterine segment or its engagement in the pelvis, or which offers space between fetus and pelvis may be a predisposing cause.

Malpresentation (which is sometimes associated with contracted pelvis) is the most common cause, and the more marked the malpresentation the greater is the risk of cord prolapse. In a personal series of

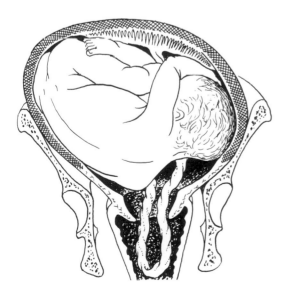

**Fig. 41/1** Prolapse of the cord

400 cases, the incidence in various presentations was: vertex, no other complication, 1 in 1300; vertex, unengaged or with minor disproportion, 1 in 800; breech, 1 in 22; shoulder (transverse lie) 1 in 5. The prolapse usually occurred when the membranes ruptured, especially when the presenting part was not engaged in the pelvis. Prematurity, by offering space between the fetus and the pelvis, is often associated with the condition, and in the series referred to, the baby weighed less than 2000g in 20 per cent of cases, Prolapse of the cord may also occur at amniotomy, during version of the fetus, and in other obstetric manipulations.

## DIAGNOSIS

The complication must be kept in mind when any of the foregoing predisposing factors are present. Since the condition is more serious after the membranes have ruptured, a vaginal examination is mandatory immediately they rupture in all cases of unengaged fetal head, abnormal presentation and when labour is premature.

## TREATMENT

The method to be employed depends on: (1) the condition, maturity and lie of the fetus; and (2) the degree of cervical dilatation. As a principle, the longer the delay between detection and delivery, the higher is the fetal mortality.

### 1. The condition of the fetus

Absence of pulsations in the cord indicates fetal death, but this must be confirmed by careful auscultation of the fetal heart before the diagnosis is confirmed. If the fetus is dead and the lie longitudinal no treatment is required and spontaneous delivery can be anticipated, but if the lie is transverse, further action is required. (See Chapter 39.) If the fetus is alive and sufficiently mature to survive, treatment depends on the degree of cervical dilatation.

### 2. The degree of cervical dilatation

Unless the cervix is fully dilated, the safest treatment is immediate caesarean section. Whilst preparations for operation are being made, the patient is put in the knee-chest position and immediately before operation the condition of the fetus and degree of cervical dilatation is reassessed.

If the cervix is fully dilated, when the prolapsed cord is detected, and the vertex, or breech is engaged, a forceps delivery or breech extraction may be performed. If the lie is tranverse and the shoulder presents, caesarean section has replaced the older method of internal version and breech extraction except in rare circumstances.

### PROGNOSIS

There is an increased maternal risk, particularly if traumatic obstetric manipulations are attempted. Unless delivery is prompt, there is a considerable risk to the fetus and the perinatal mortality ranges from 20 to 60 per cent, being lowest where prompt delivery is effected.

# Part Four

# ABNORMALITIES OF LABOUR AND THE PUERPERIUM

*Difficult labour arises either from the woman who bears the child, or from the child itself, or from the secundines, or from some external circumstances. From the woman in labour, either because she is gross and fat, or because her whole womb is small, or because she has no pains, or is affected with fear. . . . From the child, either because it is too large or because the position is preternatural. Or from the secundines, either because the membranes cannot be torn, owing to their thickness; or because they have been torn prematurely, owing to their thinness; for when the waters are evacuated unseasonably, the fetus gets out with difficulty, from the dryness of the parts. From external circumstances, either from cold contracting or immoderate heat dissipating the powers, or from some accidental occurrence.*

Paulus Aegineta (AD 607)

*Chapter 42*

# Dystocia: Faults in the Passenger

It was noted earlier that difficulty in labour, or dystocia, may arise because of 'faults' in the powers, the passages or the passenger. In this and in the following two chapters, these faults and their rela-

tionship to prolonged labour are considered. Because malpresentation and malposition of the fetus have just been discussed, the faults in the passenger which may cause dystocia are dealt with first.

## DYSTOCIA

Dystocia may result from a fault in: (1) the presentation of the fetus; (2) the position of the presenting part; (3) the size of the fetus; or because of (4) gross congenital malformation of the fetus.

### PRESENTATION OF THE FETUS

The mechanism of labour in the various abnormal presentations has been discussed, and it will be recalled that in most cases labour proceeds normally and no dystocia results. Exceptions occur when the fetus is big and particularly if the baby presents by the face (in the mento-posterior position) or by the shoulder.

### POSITION OF THE PRESENTING PART

This factor cannot be dissociated from that of presentation, but is of greatest significance in face and vertex presentations. If the vertex fails to flex during descent and retains a 'military attitude' a greater area of the head fills the narrow straight of the pelvis and rotation may fail to occur, the head becoming arrested. Similarly the occipito-posterior position of the head may be associated with prolonged labour.

### THE SIZE OF THE FETUS

The larger the baby the greater is the chance of dystocia, particularly as both the position of the presenting part and the presentation itself may be unfavourable for vaginal delivery in these cases. It is almost impossible to define, in absolute terms, what constitutes an excessively large baby but dystocia, in a normal-sized pelvis, is unusual if the baby weighs less than 3500g.

#### Aetiology

The aetiology of excessively large babies is obscure. Some women habitually produce large babies, and in many women there is a tendency for a large baby to be produced with each successive gestation. This is of importance in high multigravidae, particularly in the developing countries. The first four or five pregnancies end with a spontaneous delivery, and the mother does not seek antenatal care in subsequent pregnancies because the previous deliveries have been easy. Unfortunately, the subsequent baby, being bigger, causes dystocia and the labour is often neglected, the patient being brought to hospital in obstructed labour. Diabetic mothers are liable to have excessively large babies (the biggest recorded weighed 11kg) and certain women who subsequently develop diabetes tend to have large babies in the few years before the diabetes becomes apparent. Excessive eating in pregnancy has no effect on the birth-weight and dietary restriction will not reduce the birth-weight of the baby, although the child of the mother undernourished from birth tends to be small. Postmaturity may be complicated by an excessively large baby, but not all large babies are postmature.

### Diagnosis

The condition may be suspected if: (1) the abdomen is excessively enlarged; (2) the fetus seems larger than normal and distends the uterus, little or no liquor being present; and (3) the fetal head is not well engaged in the pelvis at term or in early labour.

### Management

The course of labour may be normal or delayed, particularly by transverse arrest of the head in the mid-pelvis. Even if delivery of the head is normal, difficulty may occur in delivering the shoulders (shoulder dystocia). If the patient habitually has excessively large babies, induction of labour prematurely, by amniotomy, some time after the 36th week is justifiable, but in most cases the onset of spontaneous labour is awaited, although disproportion at the pelvic brim may lead to caesarean section, either electively at term, or after a trial of labour. The majority of patients deliver vaginally, but forceps may be required to deliver the baby from the mid-cavity of the pelvis because the head fails to rotate.

### SHOULDER DYSTOCIA

If, after delivery of the head, the shoulders are impacted at the brim, delivery must be performed expeditiously, or the baby will die. The delay occurs because the bis-acromial diameter fails to rotate to enter the transverse diameter of the brim. The condition can be diagnosed if there is difficulty in delivering the face and chin, and the face is seen to be fat.

The patient is put in the lithotomy position and her thighs are flexed on to her abdomen. After inducing anaesthesia the following manoeuvres are attempted:

a. The head is grasped on each side with both hands, and without rotation, traction is made downwards and backwards in the axis of the pelvic brim (Fig. 42/1A). At the same time the patient bears down strongly, or controlled fundal pressure is applied by an assistant. Traction should be intermittent and made carefully as the brachial plexus is put under tension and may be damaged. Once the anterior shoulder is dislodged it descends rapidly and the posterior shoulder is brought into the pelvic cavity by traction forwards and upwards (Fig. 42/1B).

b. If the disproportion is greater, the shoulders may only be made to enter the pelvis by introducing one or two fingers into the posterior axilla of the child. The posterior shoulder is then pressed anteriorly whilst the other hand attempts to manipulate the anterior shoulder in the opposite direction. Once movement has been obtained traction of the head is attempted again. If this manoeuvre fails, all that can be done is to attempt to bring down the posterior arm, which is a traumatic procedure to mother and baby. Vaginal lacerations are usual, and fracture of the clavicle or humerus frequent.

At present no clinical or technological methods are sufficiently accurate to predict shoulder dystocia. However, women weighing more than 82kg, diabetic women and women who have previously delivered a baby weighing more than 4000g should alert the obstetrician to the possibility of shoulder dystocia.

## GROSS CONGENITAL MALFORMATIONS OF THE FETUS

### Hydrocephaly

The most common cause of dystocia due to a fetal malformation is hydrocephaly, the incidence of which is about 1 in 1000 deliveries, being half this in Asian countries, and almost twice the mean in Australia. The malformation is often associated with a meningocele or a spina bifida (Fig. 42/2). Gross enlargement of the head should be diagnosed clinically in pregnancy and confirmed by ultrasound or radiology, but lesser enlargement may be missed until labour is established, particularly as the baby presents as a breech in 25 per cent of cases.

Although treatment is possible for cases of minor hydrocephaly, in 80 per cent of infants the distended ventricles have caused severe cortical damage, and the prognosis for the child is bad. If diagnosed in pregnancy and the fetus presents as a vertex, labour should be induced by amniotomy at the 37th week,

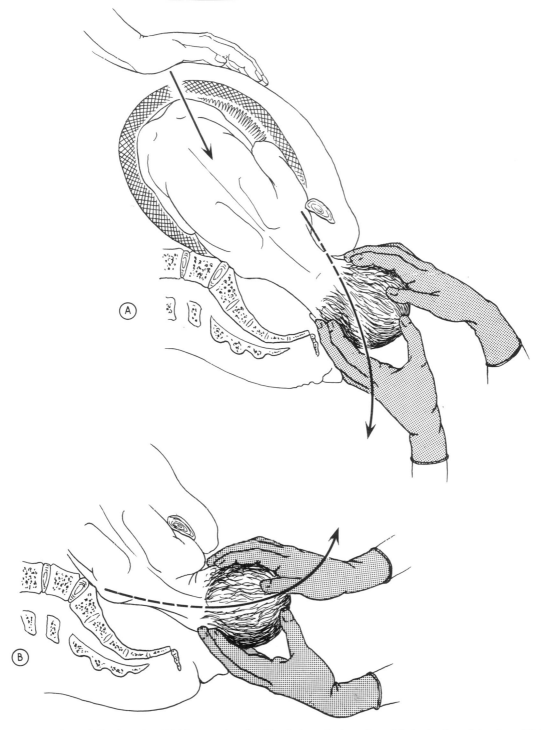

**Fig. 42/1** Shoulder girdle dystocia. (A) The anterior shoulder is brought into the pelvis by backward traction; (B) the posterior shoulder is brought lower in the pelvis by anterior traction

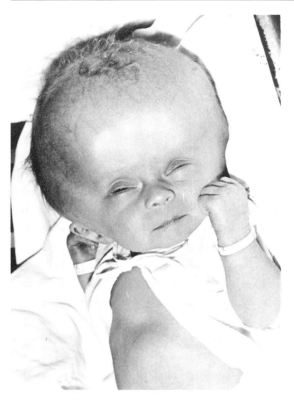

**Fig. 42/2** Hydrocephaly, associated with spina bifida

and fluid withdrawn from the skull by perforating through one of the gaping sutures. If the condition is detected early in labour similar treatment is adopted.

When the baby presents as a breech the condition is frequently not noticed until the body of the baby has been delivered, and delay occurs with the head. If a spina bifida is also present hydrocephaly should be suspected. Treatment is to introduce a catheter (either a gum-elastic or a Drew–Smythe metal instru-

ment) into the cranium via the spinal canal or directly through the foramen magnum.

**Anencephaly**

In this malformation the bony vault of the skull and scalp are absent, the facial portion being normal. It may be due to a recessive gene but environmental factors have been incriminated. Two-thirds of the cases are in females and it is commonly associated with other abnormalities. The mean birth-weight of an anencephalic fetus is about 850g less than that of a normal infant of similar maturity. Clinically, hydramnios is usually present (in 60 per cent of cases), the excess liquor being due to transudation through the exposed choroid plexus and meninges, and to the inability of the fetus to swallow liquor.

Screening in the first half of pregnancy to detect anencephaly and other neural tube defects is now practised (see p. 56) and fewer cases of anencephaly should reach term in the future. For those which do labour is usually premature because of the hydramnios, but occasionally postmaturity occurs and shoulder dystocia results. If diagnosed in late pregnancy, surgical induction of labour should be performed during the last 3 weeks to avoid this complication.

**Other malformations**

Swelling of the neck, or of the abdomen due to a renal tumour, an enlarged liver or spleen or to a distended bladder, occasionally occur, and may cause dystocia. In these conditions delay arises after delivery of the head, and stillbirth is usual.

Double monsters of varying types cause severe dystocia but as the incidence is less than 1 in 50 000 deliveries are not likely to be encountered.

## Chapter 43

# Dystocia: Faults in the Passages

## ABNORMALITIES OF THE SIZE AND SHAPE OF THE PELVIS

The size and shape of the pelvic cavity is a function of the size and shape of the surrounding bones which make up the pelvic girdle.

Alterations in the size of the cavity can be judged by observing alterations in the size of the pelvic brim, and generally speaking, a satisfactory brim area and shape indicates that the rest of the pelvic cavity is also satisfactory. The size of the 'normal' female pelvic brim varies from race to race, and is influenced by the social status of the woman within that race. Caucasian (European) women, from the Atlantic seaboard countries and Australia, tend to have bigger pelves than women from South-east Asia, although the incidence of difficult labour is less in the latter area. Within each race women who have had good nutrition prenatally and during infancy and childhood are more likely to have normal pelves than women from the deprived sections of the community. Genetic influences also play a part and big parents tend to have big children with big pelves, although this is not always so.

The shape of the female pelvis is subject to many influences which operate during infancy and puberty before the bony ring of the pelvis is fully ossified. In the past, poor socio-economic conditions, shortage of protein and calcium in the diet, and lack of sunshine produced rickets in many cities of the Northern Atlantic countries, and with the increased malleability of the bones due to the disease, gross distortion of the pelvic cavity resulted.

In certain parts of Central Asia calcium deficiency in adult life gives rise to osteomalacia and similar softening and distortion of the pelvic bones. Such gross deficiencies are now rare, but minor degrees of malnutrition in childhood may affect the shape of the pelvis. The African pelvis tends to resemble a transverse oval at the brim, but is of adequate size. This has the effect of delaying the engagement of the head until labour is well established, after which delivery is rapid.

### THE IDEAL OBSTETRIC PELVIS

Because of the many variations in the 'normal', the ideal obstetric pelvis is an abstraction rather than a reality, but it does have importance for it is against this that abnormalities in pelvic shape and size are judged. The ideal obstetric pelvis was described on page 79, and the description is summarized here:

The *brim* should be round or slightly oval transversely, with no undue projection of the sacral promontory. The measurements of the brim should be as follows:

| | |
|---|---|
| Antero-posterior diameter | 12cm |
| Widest transverse diameter | 13cm |
| Mid-transverse diameter | 12.5cm |
| Brim index (which is: | |

$$\frac{\text{antero-posterior diameter}}{\text{widest transverse diameter}} \times 100) \quad 85 \text{ to } 100$$

The *cavity* should be shallow with straight side walls, from which the ischial spines do not project unduly. The sacrospinous ligament should measure at least 3.5cm (2 finger-breadths). The distance between the ischial spines should measure at least 10.5cm.

The *pelvic arch of the outlet* should be rounded and subpubic angle 85°. The intertuberous diameter should measure 10cm.

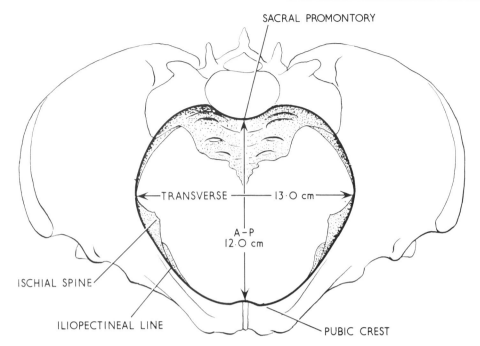

**Fig. 43/1** The ideal obstetric pelvis: the pelvic inlet or brim

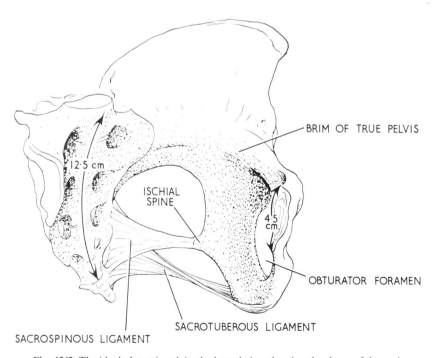

**Fig. 43/2** The ideal obstetric pelvis: the lateral view showing the shape of the cavity

# CONTRACTED PELVIS AND CEPHALOPELVIC DISPROPORTION

Any pelvis in which one or more of the important diameters is reduced by 2cm is considered contracted. Since the brim is usually affected, a reduction in the antero-posterior diameter or transverse diameter of the brim by 2cm is the usual criterion. The definition is not completely satisfactory as the shape of the pelvis may be abnormal and difficult labour may arise even when there is no marked shortening of the main diameters. To meet this objection the pelvic brim index is often used as a measure: a pelvic brim index of less than 85 indicating a contracted pelvis.

In cephalopelvic disproportion the size of the fetus relative to the size of the pelvis is assessed. The term will therefore include cases of contracted pelvis with normal-sized babies, and cases of normal pelvis with excessively large babies. In many cases of disproportion the head negotiates the brim, but difficulty arises in the mid-pelvis. The large head does not flex so well and consequently presents a larger diameter than usual to the mid-pelvis, and arrest occurs.

The incidence of disproportion and contracted pelvis varies, being influenced by selection of cases for hospital care. In most hospitals in Western European countries 1 to 2 per cent of cases fall into this category, whilst in Asia and Australia the incidence is less than 0.5 per cent of all admissions.

## DETECTION OF CONTRACTED PELVIS

If the patient is Caucasian, a height of less than 150cm may indicate pelvic contraction, although of course many small women have a normally shaped pelvis and are able to deliver a small baby with ease. The patient's appearance and her gait may also indicate the possibility of pelvic abnormality. If the patient is multigravid, the history of previous labours, the duration of the labour, the type of delivery and the weight of the child is informative. A patient who has had a labour of 10 hours and delivered a 4000g baby is unlikely to have a pelvic abnormality! 

Pelvic examination at the first visit will enable the obstetrician to determine if bony tumours, or other space-occupying lesions, are present.

The most important pointer in a primigravida is the non-engagement of the fetal head in the pelvis by the 37th week of pregnancy. Whilst the cause may not be pelvic contraction, this must be excluded first. It has been recommended earlier in this book that all patients should be examined vaginally at the 37th week of pregnancy. In the case of patients who are less than 150cm tall, or who have a history of previous difficulty in labour, or who are primigravid and are found to have a fetus with an 'unengaged' head, a careful pelvic assessment is mandatory.

### Pelvic assessment

The questions the obstetrician should ask when performing a pelvic examination are:

1. Can the sacral promontory be reached?
2. Is the sacrum flat or curved?
3. Are the side walls of the pelvis convergent?
4. Are the ischial spines prominent?
5. Will the sacrospinous ligaments accommodate two fingers?
6. Will the head enter the pelvis?
7. Will the tuberosities accommodate the clenched fist?
8. What is the shape of the pubic arch?

In most cases the pelvic assessment will indicate whether or not the fetal head will engage in the pelvis. When any doubt exists, particularly if the fetus presents by the breech, a radiological pelvimetry should be arranged.

### Prognosis for vaginal delivery

The final arbiter of vaginal delivery is the quality of the uterine contractions, but the outcome is influenced, in addition, by the size of the fetal head and its ability to mould. For these reasons clinical or radiological pelvimetry can only give a guide to prognosis. In this, two mathematical calculations are helpful. These are the measurement of the antero-posterior diameter of the brim, and the calculation of the brim area:

*The antero-posterior diameter*

| Less than 9cm | Vaginal delivery improbable. |
| 9 to 10.5cm | Vaginal delivery possible. |
| 10.5 to 11.5cm | Vaginal delivery probable. |

*The brim area*

| Less than 85cm² | Vaginal delivery unlikely, elective caesarean section at term justified. |
| 85 to 100cm² | Vaginal delivery possible; trial of labour in most cases; elective caesarean section occasionally. |
| 105 to 130cm² | Vaginal delivery probable, forceps may be required. |

## MECHANISM OF LABOUR IN CASES OF PELVIC ABNORMALITY

The long axis of the fetal head adapts itself to the long axis of the pelvic brim in all cases. Thus with a normally shaped brim the head descends through an axis which bisects the pelvis, and engages in the occipito-lateral position with its longest diameter in the transverse diameter of the brim. Often the head is slightly tilted laterally and forwards so that the posterior parietal bone leads, and this tilt is corrected as the head descends into the cavity (Fig. **43/3**). In the long oval pelvis, the head engages with its longest diameter in the antero-posterior diameter of the brim, the occiput either lying directly anterior or directly posterior. If the pelvic brim is triangular or flat, and the head enters the pelvis in the occipito-lateral position, its engagement may be delayed.

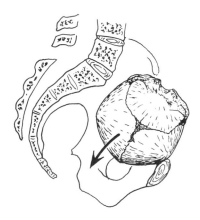

**Fig. 43/3** Posterior parietal presentation

Once the head has negotiated the brim, the next narrow zone is at the level of the ischial spines. If the cavity is round, the head descends to this level in the occipito-lateral position when the occiput rotates forwards. If the head has engaged in the occipito-posterior position and the brim is a long oval the cavity is usually roomy and rotation through 180° may, or may not, occur. The shape of the sacrum has considerable influence on the rotation. When the brim is triangular the sacrum is likely to lack concavity and the descending head is pushed forwards. The mid-pelvis is frequently reduced in size and consequently rotation may be hindered and the head arrested at the mid-pelvic level.

### Arrest of the head in the pelvis

The effect of a triangular brim and a flat sacrum is to prevent rotation occurring, since the flat side of the head is applied to the flat sacrum. In extreme cases, marked pelvic funnelling may cause the arrest above the spines but below the brim. Even if the pelvis is normal, arrest at the mid-pelvic level may occur, particularly if the baby is large and the uterine contractions poor.

The arrest usually occurs with the head lying in an occipito-lateral position ('*deep transverse arrest of the head*') but occasionally the occiput is posterior ('*posterior arrest of the head*').

In both situations the condition is diagnosed when the head fails to descend below the spines after full dilatation of the cervix and despite strong contractions. If no descent or rotation has occurred within 1½ hours of full dilatation, operative delivery must be effected. It is cruel to the mother, and dangerous to the baby, to persist beyond this time.

Delivery of a 'deep transverse arrest' or a 'posterior arrest' is by forceps rotation and extraction using Keilland's forceps, by manual rotation and forceps extraction, by the use of the ventouse or, increasingly, by caesarean section. The attempts at vaginal delivery should be treated as trials of delivery and skill, not strength, used. Should rotation, or descent, not occur despite moderate force, skilfully applied, the attempt should be abandoned and caesarean section carried out. It is no mark of obstetric prowess to deliver a baby which dies from the injuries received during a traumatic delivery, and leaves a mother scarred vaginally and mentally. Mid-forceps delivery should not be attempted except by trained obstetricians in the operation room of a well-equipped maternity hospital.

## DANGERS TO THE MOTHER

In any case of contracted pelvis or disproportion, labour should be conducted as a trial – the object being to see 'what the patient can accomplish, not what she can endure'. Provided that an adequate assessment of cephalopelvic relationships and of maternal attitudes has been made, the dangers of labour in cases of disproportion are small, and many will end with a vaginal delivery. Careful attention to determine progress during labour, and the experience to know when to interfere, further reduce the risk to mother and child. In inexperienced hands, or in those of the doctor who is unwilling to seek advice, the risks increase considerably, the main hazards being trauma and infection.

### Uterine damage

Although in most cases of disproportion labour progresses normally, abnormalities of uterine action may arise at any time. Whether these are caused by the disproportion or are the cause of the perpetuation of an unfavourable position of the fetal head, is disputed. The association of an abnormality of uterine action with disproportion frequently leads to prolonged labour with an increased risk of intra-uterine infection. Moreover if the degree of pelvic contraction, or the size of the fetus, has been miscalculated, labour may become obstructed. Should this happen two patterns of uterine activity result: in the primigravida uterine inertia occurs; but in the multigravida the uterus continues to contract more and more forcibly until uterine rupture threatens. A patient who reaches this stage has been grossly neglected.

### Damage to the bladder

If the fit of the head into the pelvis is tight, once full dilatation of the cervix has occurred marked pressure is exerted on the bladder base which is pressed between the head and the posterior surface of the symphysis pubis (Fig. **43/4**). In such cases, a second stage prolonged beyond 2 hours may lead to devitalization to the tissues of the bladder base from pressure and its sloughing 5 to 7 days after delivery. Alternatively, attempts by an inexperienced obstetrician to deliver the baby by forceps and force may damage the bladder directly. In either case a vesicovaginal fistula will result. Such fistulae occur rarely in developed countries, but in countries where obstetric services are not yet fully developed, and where many women are attended in labour by unqualified helpers, fistulae continue to occur. They are all preventable.

### Vaginal and cervical damage

Vaginal delivery in cases of contracted pelvis requires experience, and attempts to deliver before full cervical dilatation has been reached, or with undue force in the second stage, will result in cervical or vaginal lacerations.

## DANGERS TO THE FETUS

Until the membranes rupture the fetus is at little risk; after this time increasing danger is present. Moulding of the head may be marked, and caput formation excessive, caput being seen at the vulva whilst the greatest diameter of the head is still above the brim. If a rough forceps delivery is attempted, the extra compression may be sufficient to cause

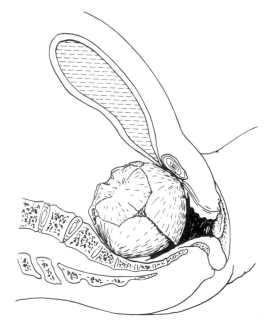

**Fig. 43/4** The bladder in mid-pelvic contraction. The patient had been in labour for 41 hours, the cervix was fully dilated and the head arrested in the transverse position at the level of the ischial spines. Delivery was by forceps. The bladder base has risen in the pelvis and is being compressed between the symphysis pubis and the fetal head (redrawn from Malpas, P., Jeffcoate, T. N. A. and Lister, U. M. *J. Obstet. Gynaecol. Brit. Emp.* 1949, **56**, 944)

intracranial damage to the child whose tentorium is already markedly stretched. Intra-uterine infection may occur with prolonged labour and may infect the baby; and stress asphyxia due to excessive uterine contractions, which cause interference with the placental circulation, may be a factor in the aetiology of cerebral palsy.

Obviously the prognosis for the child depends on the degree of pelvic contraction, the length of labour, and the skill of the obstetrician should operative delivery be required. Above all it depends upon judgement after careful analysis of the case.

## CONDUCT OF LABOUR IN CONTRACTED PELVIS OR DISPROPORTION

In all such cases labour should be conducted by an experienced obstetrician in a well-equipped hospital. There are two methods of treatment: (1) elective caesarean section at term; and (2) trial of labour.

### Elective caesarean section at term

If the antero-posterior diameter of the pelvic brim is less than 9cm in length and the baby of average size, elective caesarean section is probably unavoidable. If, however, the baby is small, trial of labour may be permitted in selected cases. If the degree of pelvic contraction is less marked, but some other obstetrical complication is present, such as postmaturity or PIH, which are known to increase the risk to the fetus; or if the patient has a history of a long period of infertility, the decision may be that caesarean section is the best treatment. Similarly when caesarean section has been performed because of a contracted pelvis, a repeat section is probably unavoidable.

The timing of the caesarean section is important, and the nearer it is done to term, the better is the fetal prognosis. If the patient has been seen from the first quarter of pregnancy, the expected date of confinement will have been established either clinically or by the use of ultrasound. In such cases the date of the operation can be decided in advance. The advantage is that the operation can be done deliberately and slowly; the patient and her relatives are prepared, and nursing staff is available. When the date of delivery cannot be estimated there is much to be said for waiting until the onset of labour and performing the caesarean section within a few hours of this time.

### Trial of labour

If the cephalopelvic disproportion is not of major degree, the outcome of the trial, that is vaginal delivery or operative delivery, will depend to a large extent on the quality of the uterine contractions. Strong, well co-ordinated uterine contractions may permit the vaginal delivery of the infant. The quality of the uterine contractions can only be assessed in labour and for this reason a trial of labour is carried out. The implication of the term is that should no progress be evident after a reasonable time, labour is terminated by operation. It is the decision of what constitutes 'reasonable time' which causes most of the difficulty.

#### CONDITIONS TO BE FULFILLED BEFORE CONDUCTING A TRIAL OF LABOUR

(1) Gross pelvic contraction must be excluded; (2) the head must be the presenting part; and (3) unless the pregnancy is prolonged, labour must start spontaneously. Very occasionally it is permissible to induce labour prematurely in a patient who previously has had difficulty in delivering at term. The danger of this method is that the duration of the pregnancy may be miscalculated, the size of the baby estimated wrongly, and induction is not always successful. If labour is induced prematurely the course of labour must be treated as a trial.

The attendants (but not the patient) must be fully aware that operative delivery, either by forceps or caesarean section, is a possible outcome, and must pay careful attention to avoid introducing infection and to maintaining the patient's hydration.

#### CONTRA-INDICATIONS TO A TRIAL OF LABOUR

Trial of labour is contra-indicated: (1) if pelvic contraction is gross; (2) if the patient has some other medical or obstetrical complication, e.g. severe cardiac disease or severe pre-eclampsia as well as disproportion; and (3) if the fetus presents by the breech, particularly if its weight is estimated to be more than 3500g.

#### CONDUCT OF THE TRIAL

1. Once labour is established the patient is given no solid food by mouth, hydration and electrolyte balance being maintained by intravenous fluid therapy.

The pulse rate, temperature, fluid intake and urinary output are recorded at 4-hourly intervals, and the urine tested for the presence of acidoketones.

2. The character and frequency of the uterine contractions are recorded regularly: if the contractions are inco-ordinate or infrequent, treatment is given as appropriate (see Chapter 44). In some cases the trial has to be abandoned because of poor contractions, rather than because the head has failed to negotiate the pelvic brim.

3. The station of the fetal head is noted regularly. The crux of a successful trial is that the head enters the brim. If it can do this in most cases it will pass through the mid-cavity with little difficulty.

4. The time the membranes rupture and the character of the liquor are noted. If the head is not deeply engaged in the pelvis a vaginal examination must be done to determine the dilatation of the cervix and to exclude a prolapsed cord.

5. Sterile vaginal examinations are performed at defined intervals. At each vaginal examination the questions asked when the pelvic assessment was made are asked again. In addition answers to the following are sought:

a. What is the degree of effacement and dilatation of the cervix, and is it well applied to the head?

A cervix which dilates slowly and is not well applied to the head, or is markedly oedematous, indicates that the disproportion is more marked than had been expected and vaginal delivery improbable.

b. How much has the head descended since the previous examination?

In this respect it must be remembered that only slight descent of the head occurs before full dilatation of the cervix.

The findings are recorded on a partograph and are assessed at intervals so that an analysis of the progress of the trial is made. Each case must be considered individually, for the personality of the patient (and of the doctor) will often influence the outcome. Occasionally a radiograph of the lateral view of the pelvis is helpful in formulating a decision. On the film the position and degree of engagement of the fetal head can be seen, and the shape and capacity of the pelvis can be estimated accurately. The investigation is especially helpful when oedema of the bladder tissues, or tenseness of the patient prevents adequate clinical assessment.

### DURATION OF THE TRIAL

The trial should be abandoned: (1) if no increase in cervical dilatation occurs over a period of 4 hours despite co-ordinated well-sustained contractions; (2) if, after rupture of the membranes, the cervix fails to dilate demonstrably within 2 hours despite co-ordinated contractions; (3) if, after rupture of the membranes, the uterine contractions do not improve in quality and frequency over a 4-hour period; (4) if, after full dilatation of the cervix the head does not engage within 1 hour or the baby has not been delivered within $1\frac{1}{2}$ hours; (5) if there is any deterioration in the general condition of the mother or signs of the development of fetal distress; and (6) if no significant progress has been made and labour has lasted 18 hours.

In assessing the prognosis of a trial of labour a humane attitude must be adopted: after all it is the patient who is undergoing the pain and discomfort, not the doctor, although he may be mentally disquiet.

An indication of the value of trial labour can be gauged from hospital statistics: about 50 per cent of patients deliver spontaneously, 30 per cent require forceps to complete the delivery, and in 20 per cent the trial is abandoned, and delivery effected by caesarean section.

# APPENDIX: A CLASSIFICATION OF PELVIC ABNORMALITIES

In the developed nations of the world, contracted pelvis has diminished as a cause of dystocia. However, amongst the less privileged groups in the rich nations and amongst the urban poor in the developing nations, contracted pelvis still occurs and may lead to a difficult labour. Of the many classifications of pelvic abnormalities available, that suggested by Baird is one of the most helpful. Studies by his

ROUND                    LONG OVAL

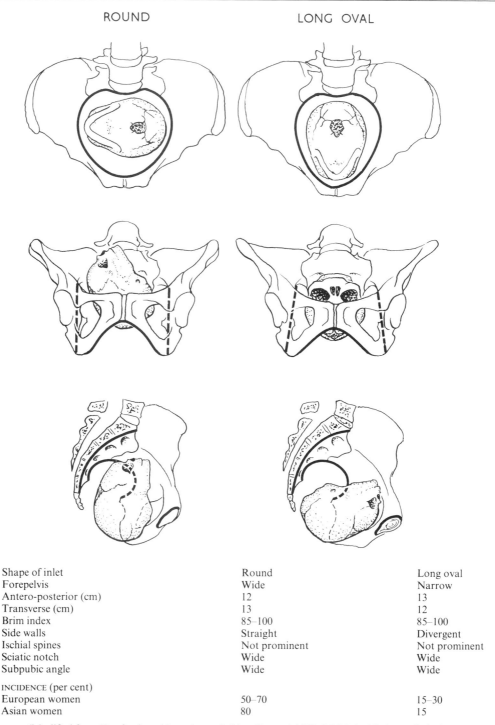

| Shape of inlet | Round | Long oval |
|---|---|---|
| Forepelvis | Wide | Narrow |
| Antero-posterior (cm) | 12 | 13 |
| Transverse (cm) | 13 | 12 |
| Brim index | 85–100 | 85–100 |
| Side walls | Straight | Divergent |
| Ischial spines | Not prominent | Not prominent |
| Sciatic notch | Wide | Wide |
| Subpubic angle | Wide | Wide |
| INCIDENCE (per cent) | | |
| European women | 50–70 | 15–30 |
| Asian women | 80 | 15 |

(Modified from Danforth and Ivy. *Amer. J. Obst. Gynecol.* 1963, **86**, 29, by kind permission)

**Figs 43/5 and 43/6** Pelves with normal shape and bone development

TRIANGULAR                    FLAT

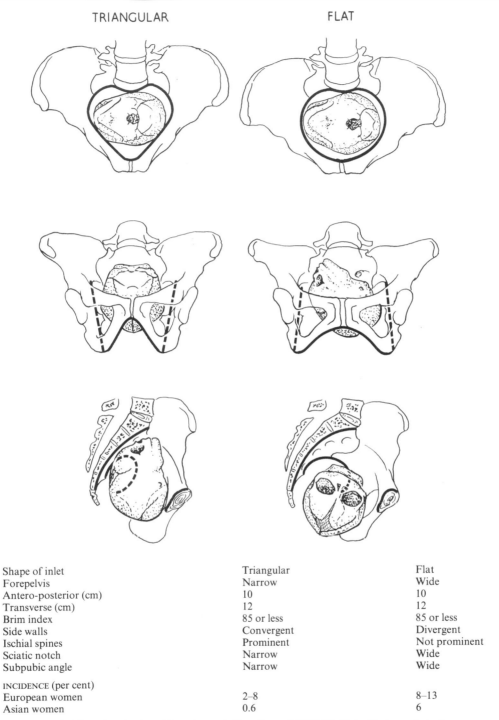

| Shape of inlet | Triangular | Flat |
|---|---|---|
| Forepelvis | Narrow | Wide |
| Antero-posterior (cm) | 10 | 10 |
| Transverse (cm) | 12 | 12 |
| Brim index | 85 or less | 85 or less |
| Side walls | Convergent | Divergent |
| Ischial spines | Prominent | Not prominent |
| Sciatic notch | Narrow | Wide |
| Subpubic angle | Narrow | Wide |
| INCIDENCE (per cent) | | |
| European women | 2–8 | 8–13 |
| Asian women | 0.6 | 6 |

(Modified from Danforth and Ivy. *Amer. J. Obst. Gynecol.* 1963, **86**, 29, by kind permission)

**Figs 43/7 and 43/8**  Pelves with abnormal shape and bone development

group in Aberdeen found that nutritional influences in infancy and childhood were the major factors in causing minor alterations from the normal, whilst gross alterations were due to disease or injury. The classification is based on brim size and shape, as it has been found that mid-pelvic or outlet contraction is rare if the brim shape and size are normal. There is one exception to this: tall thin girls, whose growth has spurted during puberty, may have mid-pelvic narrowing with no brim contraction (Table **43/1**).

### Peives with normal shape and bone development

The *round* brim is obstetrically ideal (Fig. **43/5**) and in the developed countries is found in 70 per cent of women whose height exceeds 163cm, the percentage dropping to 55 in women less than 153cm tall. The factor of height does not apply in Asian countries, where the overall incidence of the round pelvis is more than 80 per cent.

The *long oval* brim (Fig. **43/6**) is relatively uncommon and is found in about 15 per cent of women; in Asia the incidence is similar.

1. *Pelves with normal shape and bone development*
   (Measurements usually normal, may be small)
      Round ('gynaecoid')
      Long oval ('anthropoid')
2. *Pelves with abnormality of shape and bone development*
   (Measurements usually decreased)
   a. Defects of nutrition and environment
      1. Minor defects—Triangular brim
                                    (android)
                              Flat brim (platypelloid)
      2. Major defects—Rachitic
                                Osteomalacic
   b. Disease or injury
      1. Spinal (kyphosis, scoliosis, spondylolisthesis)
      2. Pelvic (tumours, fractures, caries)
      3. Limbs (poliomyelitis in childhood, congenital dislocation of the hip)
   c. Congenital malformations
      1. Naegele's pelvis and Robert's pelvis
      2. High assimilation pelvis
3. *Mid-pelvic contraction*

   **Table 43/1** Pelvic classification (after Baird)

### Pelves with abnormality of shape and bone development

#### MINOR DEFECTS OF NUTRITION OR ENVIRONMENT

The *triangular* brim, with some degree of funnelling of the pelvis, is relatively uncommon, and in a British study was found in only 2 per cent of women. It appears to have a higher incidence amongst women from Southern Europe, but is not particularly common in Asia. The mid-pelvis is also likely to be narrowed (Fig. **43/7**).

The *flat* brim is the commonest minor abnormality of pelvic shape and the incidence increases from less than 5 per cent in tall European women to more than 30 per cent in Europeans whose height is less than 150cm. It is even more common amongst Africans (Fig. **43/8**).

#### MAJOR DEFECTS OF NUTRITION OR ENVIRONMENT

*Rickets and osteomalacia*
In the past 20 years most developed countries have paid increasing attention to social and preventive medicine, and rickets, a disease of poor nutrition, particularly a lack of vitamin D and calcium, has largely disappeared. Since the developing countries have an abundance of sunshine (which converts ergosterol in the skin into vitamin D), and in most the drinking water is rich in calcium, rickets is not common amongst the children, although protein deficiency is usual.

In a young child suffering from rickets the weight of the upper body presses down through the spine on to the softened pelvic bones. The sacral promontory is pushed forwards and downwards, whilst the sacrum itself pivots backwards. At the same time the ligaments of the back draw the spinous process medially so that the ilia flare outwards, as do the ischial tuberosities. In extreme cases the softened acetabulae may be forced inwards. The main altera-tion in pelvic shape is a marked reduction of the antero-posterior measurement of the brim, with some irregular widening of the cavity (Fig. **43/9**).

Osteomalacia, due to an acquired deficiency of calcium and encountered in adult life, causes the same deformities as rickets but is rare, except in certain inland parts of Northern India and in China (Fig. **43/10**).

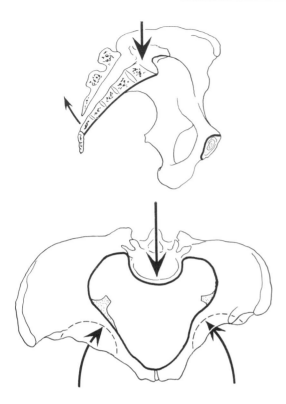

Fig. 43/9 The rachitic pelvis. Tracing from a radiograph showing the antero-posterior diameter of 8cm, the widest transverse diameter of 11.7 and a brim index of 69. The arrows show how pressure of the softened bones alters the shape of the pelvis

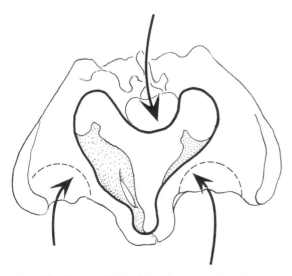

**Fig. 43/10** Osteomalacic pelvis. The arrows show how pressure deforms the softened bones

### DISEASE OR INJURY

*Spinal*

Kyphosis of the lower dorsal or lumbar region which started in childhood may alter the shape of the brim of the pelvis, as the weight of the body pushes the upper part of the sacrum backward and the lower part forward. The side walls of the pelvis converge forming a funnel. In scoliosis the altered pressure distribution on the soft bones may cause bays on each side of the sacral promontory, so that the shape of the brim is asymmetrical (Fig. **43/11**). Spondylolisthesis, which means slipping forward of the fifth lumbar vertebra so that it projects beyond the sacral promontory, is rare (Fig. **43/12**).

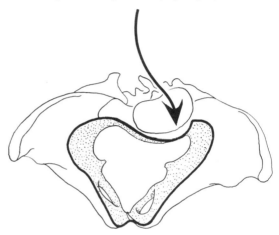

**Fig. 43/11** Scoliosis and kyphosis

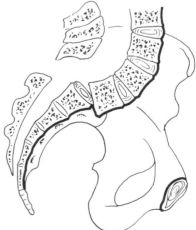

**Fig. 43/12** Spondylolisthesis; tracing from the radiograph showing the subluxation of the fifth lumbar vertebra upon the sacrum. The diagnosis can only be made by radiography

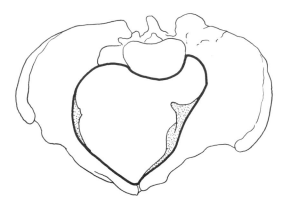

**Fig. 43/13** Naegele's pelvis. Note the absence of the sacral ala

*Pelvic*
Osteomata may develop, or an injury may lead to excessive bone formation over the site of the fracture. If all patients are examined vaginally at the first visit these abnormalities will be detected.

*Limbs*
Poliomyelitis in childhood, or congenital dislocation of the hip, may cause pelvic deformity. The child puts most of its weight on the stronger leg, and on this side the pelvis is pressed in, with flattening of the brim on the same side.

CONGENITAL MALFORMATIONS

*Naegele's pelvis* and *Robert's pelvis*
These are due to the defective development of one or both sacral lateral masses so that the sacrum fuses with the ilium on one or both sides (Fig. **43/13**). The *high assimilation pelvis* occurs when the fifth lumbar vertebra is fused to the sacrum, thus increasing the inclination of the pelvic brim. This hinders engagement of the fetal head.

*Mid-pelvic contraction*
The incidence of this condition in the absence of brim abnormality is difficult to estimate. As has been mentioned the condition is found in certain women over 163cm in height, who have had a sudden 'spurt' of growth at about the time of puberty. Another type of woman in whom the abnormality is found, often in association with some degree of triangular brim, is the short, squat, hirsute woman who is frequently obese and occasionally of reduced fertility. These women have heavy bones and the pelvic cavity and outlet resembles that of the male.

*Chapter 44*

# Dystocia: Faults in the Powers

The normal contractile wave which is propagated over the entire uterus in labour is characterized by a triple descending gradient of activity.

The characteristics of the triple descending gradient are that: (1) the intensity of the contraction is stronger in the upper muscular part of the uterus than in the lower, less muscular, part; (2) the duration of the contraction is longer in the upper part of the uterus; (3) the propagation of the wave is downwards towards the cervix from the pacemakers; and (4) the peak of the contraction occurs in all parts of the uterus simultaneously. These components cause fundal dominance, and the progressive dilatation of the cervix, but occasionally a disorder of uterine activity occurs, and has the effect of prolonging labour.

Two types of abnormal uterine activity may be distinguished: (1) the over-efficient uterus; and (2) the inefficient uterus (Table **44/1**).

## UTERINE OVER-EFFICIENCY

### Precipitate labour

This term is self-explanatory and indicates that the course of labour has been rapid with intense and

*Over-efficient uterine activity*
1. Precipitate labour
2. Tetanic uterine activity
*Inefficient uterine activity*
1. Hypoactive states
2. Hyperactive, inco-ordinate states
   (a) hyperactive lower uterine segment
   (b) colicky uterus
   (c) constriction ring dystocia
3. Cervical dystocia

**Table 44/1** Classification of abnormal uterine activity

frequent contractions, and delivery has occurred within 1 hour.

The condition is not frequent and recurs in the same woman who often has a developmental weakness of the pelvic musculature. The danger to the mother is in the first delivery when lacerations of cervix or vagina may occur, but in fact are infrequent. A greater danger exists for the baby which may become anoxic in utero due to the intense and frequent contractions causing a hypertonic state; or may suffer intracranial haemorrhage during its rapid descent through the birth canal; or may be injured by being delivered in an unsuitable place and falling on the floor.

### MANAGEMENT

If the baby has been born before the attendant arrives, the mother is examined for bleeding, the uterus palpated and the lower genital tract inspected for injury. If the baby has not yet been born, labour may be slowed by giving a general anaesthetic, but under no circumstances should the head be held back during delivery. To do this is to risk rupture of the uterus and intracranial damage to the fetus.

Since precipitate labour tends to recur, a woman who has had a labour lasting 2 hours or less should be admitted to hospital before term, and labour may be induced in special cases.

### Tetanic uterine action

The main cause of temporary uterine overactivity is the misuse of oxytocin, particularly when this is given intramuscularly. Marked uterine spasm prevents placental circulation and, unless relieved, may lead to fetal death. The treatment, if the oxytocin is being given intravenously, is to stop the infusion.

## INEFFICIENT UTERINE ACTION

It is difficult to determine with accuracy how many women have labours which are complicated by inefficient uterine action, but the most reliable estimates puts between 1 and 2 per cent of all labours, and between 4 and 6 per cent of first labours into this category.

Two main types of inefficient uterine activity are described: (1) hypo-active states (erroneously referred to as uterine inertia) and (2) hyperactive, inco-ordinate states (which includes inco-ordinate uterine action, 'colicky' uterus, and its end result, constriction ring dystocia).

Disorders of uterine activity seem predominantly a disease of primigravidae, and over 85 per cent of cases occur amongst them. The effect of age is less marked, but amongst primigravidae uterine dysfunction is more common after the age of 30, particularly if the patient has a squat, thickset, obese physique and is relatively infertile, and if the pregnancy is prolonged beyond term.

The aetiology of inefficient uterine action is unclear. In some cases a minor degree of cephalo-pelvic disproportion is present, in others the fetal head is not well-engaged in the pelvis, although no disproportion can be detected. In the former case a proposed explanation is that the poor application of the fetal head to the uterine cervix fails to initiate the cervical or 'Ferguson' reflex, which is believed to cause the release of oxytocin from the posterior pituitary gland. In the latter it is postulated that the lower uterine segment fails to dilate, or that fundal 'dominance' fails to become established.

Psychological factors have been postulated. Since the emotions are known to affect hypothalamic activity it is not unreasonable to postulate that the releasing factor required to liberate oxytocin from the posterior pituitary gland is inhibited. Alternatively emotional factors may affect cervical dilatation by altering the ratio of adrenaline, which is inhibitory, and noradrenaline, which is stimulatory at nerve endings. It must be confessed that although it is agreed that emotions may affect uterine activity, the mechanism of their effect is not known.

The role of psychological factors is further obscured by the fact that no matter how inefficient uterine action is during a first labour, whether the labour ends by caesarean section or by forceps extraction, the uterus tends to function better in the next labour. To the surprise of the patient, who was apprehensive of the outcome, the second confinement is generally unlike the first and is easy and rapid. It is for this reason that uterine dysfunction is predominantly a disorder of primigravidae.

## TYPES OF ABNORMAL ACTION

**Hypoactive states** (so-called uterine inertia) (Fig. **44/1**)

In this pattern of abnormal uterine activity, the resting tone of the uterus is usually lowered and the intensity of the contractions reduced, so that only a feeble contractile wave is propagated towards the lower segment which is scarcely affected. Fundal dominance is present but is not marked. The frequency of the contractions may be normal or reduced, so that they only occur at long intervals. The commonly used term 'inertia' is really a misnomer for there is always some evidence of uterine activity.

Clinically the patient is not distressed by the contractions, and any pain which is felt is abdominal in distribution with little or no backache. If the fundus is lightly palpated with the tips of the fingers during a contraction, the contraction is palpable before the patient complains of pain. At its peak the muscle of the fundus can be indented, and the pain is of shorter duration than the palpable contraction.

This pattern may be primary or may arise at any time during labour, and may occur intermittently. It must not be confused with a similar pattern which occurs in primigravidae when labour is obstructed, and in which the uterus, having failed to overcome the obstruction, becomes inert.

**Hyperactive, inco-ordinate states** (inco-ordinate uterine action)

In the varieties of this pattern of uterine activity there is usually some increase of uterine resting tone. This is most marked in the colicky types of uterus, but may occur in the hyperactive lower uterine segment pattern.

The perception of pain in labour is only reached when the uterine tone exceeds about 25mmHg. Since the resting tone of the muscle is often raised in inco-ordinate uterine action, the pain threshold is reached earlier in the contraction and the pain is felt for a longer time (Fig. **44/2**).

Despite strong contractions, cervical dilatation occurs slowly, if at all, and since energy is constantly

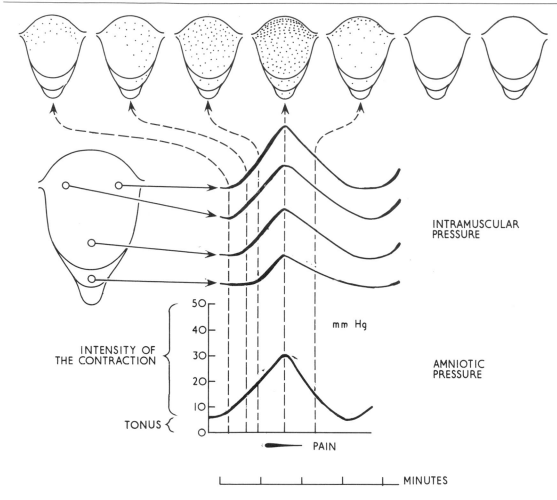

INTRAMUSCULAR
PRESSURE

INTENSITY OF
THE CONTRACTION

mm Hg

AMNIOTIC
PRESSURE

TONUS

PAIN

MINUTES

**Fig. 44/1** Hypoactive uterus. Note that the intensity of the contraction is diminished and the tone lowered slightly (drawn from information from the writings of R. Caldeyro-Barcia)

expended in maintaining uterine tone as well as during uterine contractions, ketosis may occur.

The most common type of uterine dysfunction is the *hyperactive lower uterine segment*, which often occurs in association with minor degrees of disproportion or malposition of the fetal head. In this pattern the normal triple descending gradient of activity does not occur, and fundal dominance is lost, a 'reversed' gradient of activity occurring. The abnormal contractile wave starts in the lower uterine segment and passes upwards towards the fundus, and downwards towards the cervix (Fig. **44/3**). The contraction is more intense and lasts longer in the lower portion of the uterus, and as a consequence the cervix fails to dilate despite strong uterine activity. This is the most common type of uterine dysfunction encountered, and is often associated with minor degrees of disproportion or malposition of the fetal head.

Clinically the patient is distressed and complains constantly of backache, which increases during each contraction when the pain radiates into the lower abdomen. The pain, and particularly the backache, is complained about before the contraction can be felt on fundal palpation; the peak of the contraction is extremely painful; and the pain is of longer duration than the palpable contraction. Often the patient has a desire to 'bear down' during the contraction,

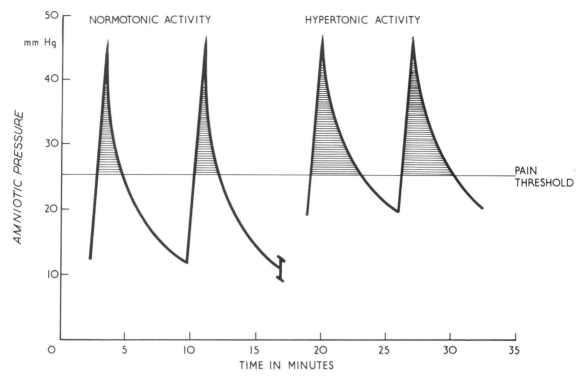

**Fig. 44/2** Pain in inco-ordinate uterine action. Because the resting tone is raised, the pain threshold is reached earlier in the contraction, and remains above the threshold for longer (redrawn from Caldeyro-Barcia, R. *Trans. Conf. Int. Gynecol. et Obstet., 1958.* Librairie Beauchemin, Montreal, 1959)

although examination shows the cervix to be thick and not to have reached full dilatation. The fetal head frequently is not well applied to the cervix and caput formation may be minimal.

The remaining two patterns are uncommon. In the first, or *colicky uterus,* various parts of the uterus contract independently. The contractions may be most intense in the lower segment (when backache and lower abdominal pain are the main complaints) or in the fundal area (when intense colicky cramps are complained of) (Fig. **44/4**). The second pattern, that of *constriction ring dystocia,* is rarely encountered (incidence less than 1:10 000 confinements). An annular spasm occurs in the myometrium, usually at the junction of the upper and lower uterine segment, but occasionally at the level of the internal os (Fig. **44/5**). In primigravidae, constriction ring dystocia may be the end result of a colicky uterus; but in multigravidae constriction rings are caused by interference, particularly the use of intramuscular oxytocin injections, or manipulations under light

anaesthesia, neither of which is often used today.

The ring tends to form around the neck of the fetus, and thus prevents its descent. The uterus above the ring continues to contract; that below is usually quiescent, as the normal propagation of the contractile wave is prevented.

The diagnosis is rarely made in the first stage of labour. In the second stage failure of the fetal head to descend during a contraction may make the obstetrician suspect the condition. It may also be suspected if the fetal head fails to descend during an attempted forceps delivery, although the forceps have been properly applied and there is no obvious disproportion. A definite diagnosis can only be established if the constriction ring is felt on intra-uterine palpation.

Treatment is to anaesthetize the patient deeply before attempting delivery; no drug has any effect on a constriction ring.

In the past a further abnormality of uterine action was included. This was diagnosed as *cervical dys-*

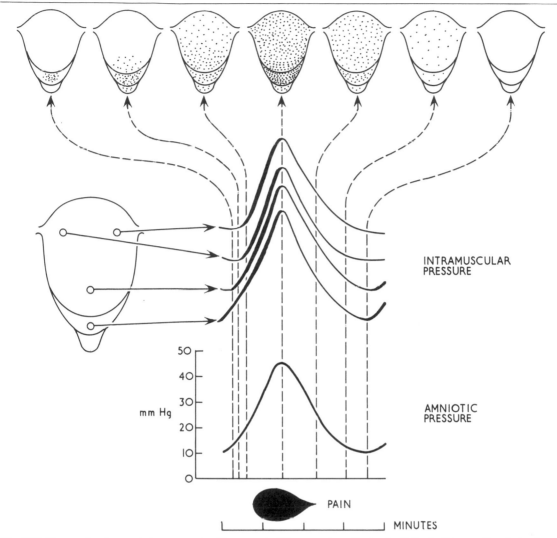

**Fig. 44/3** Hyperactive lower uterine segment, with reversal of the normal gradients of activity. In this case the uterine tone is still normal but the cervix fails to dilate (redrawn from Caldeyro-Barcia)

*tocia.* Clinically, in spite of strong co-ordinated uterine contractions, the cervix failed to dilate becoming stretched paper-thin in late labour over the fetal head which had descended to lie in the zone of the fetal outlet (Fig. **44/6**). Labour tended to be prolonged and the patient to complain of severe backache. Cervical dystocia is very rare and its physiopathology unclear. Treatment is to make small (2cm) incisions in the cervix at the 10 o'clock position, and to deliver the baby with forceps. If treatment is delayed too long, the cervix may undergo pressure necrosis and become detached.

## PROBLEMS OF CLASSIFICATION IN MODERN OBSTETRIC PRACTICE

The differentiation between the two most common varieties of inefficient uterine action – hypertonic lower uterine segment (or reversed gradient of uterine activity) and hypoactive uterine activity, depends on the patient's perception of pain and on the clinical findings. With the increasing use of epidural ananalgesia the patient no longer has pain. However, delay in cervical dilatation due to inefficient uterine activity continues to occur. If the partographic

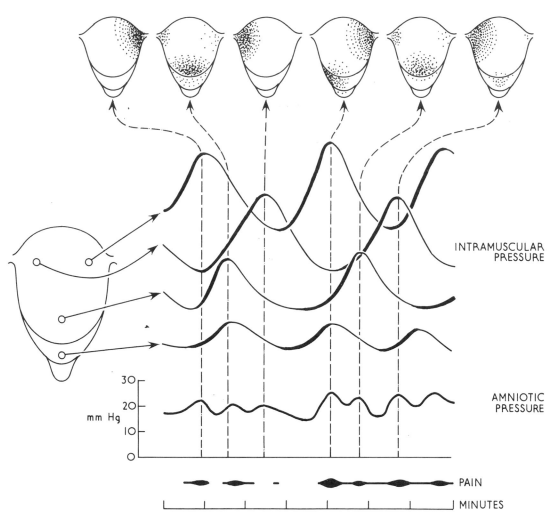

**Fig. 44/4** Colicky uterus. Isolated segments of the uterus contract independently, and without any pattern, in a completely inco-ordinated way. The tonus is raised because at no time are all the parts of the uterus relaxed, and the amniotic pressure is unable to fall (redrawn from Caldeyro-Barcia)

method of recording the progress of labour is utilized, abnormal patterns of cervical dilatation can be observed (Fig. **44/7**).

A *prolonged quiet (or latent) phase* may be due to the use of excessive sedation, or the institution of the epidural nerve block too early in labour. In most cases the pattern of uterine activity is hypoactive. If the cervix fails to dilate after 2 to 4 hours, the membranes should be ruptured and uterine activity stimulated with a dilute incremental infusion of oxytocin.

A *protracted active phase* is more likely to be due to the hyperactive lower uterine segment pattern of

uterine dysfunction. Cephalopelvic relationships should be reassessed and in the absence of fetal malposition or disproportion, a dilute oxytocin infusion may be tried. *Secondary arrest of cervical dilatation* probably equates to inco-ordinate uterine action.

## THE MANAGEMENT OF INEFFICIENT UTERINE ACTION

Ninety per cent of cases of inefficient uterine action are due either to hypoactive states or to inco-ordin-

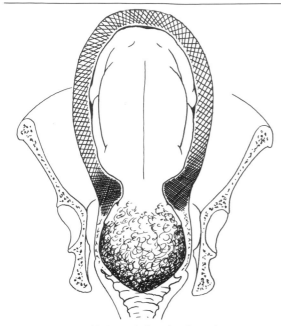

**Fig. 44/5** Constriction ring dystocia

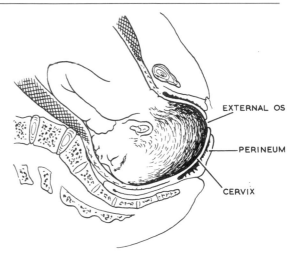

**Fig. 44/6** Cervical dystocia

ate uterine action. The treatment of constriction ring dystocia (which is rare) has been discussed, and in this section only the management of cases of hypo-activity and of inco-ordinate uterine action will be considered.

**General**

Before any specific therapy is introduced, a review of the course of labour must be made, and the physical condition of the patient reassessed. Dehydration and acidoketosis should be sought and if present, an intravenous infusion of Hartmann's solu-tion, alternating with 5 per cent glucose set up. The first 500ml may be infused quickly, but after this, a rate of 50 to 100ml per hour is sufficient. No further fluids should be given by mouth as an operative delivery is likely.

Abdominal palpation is made to confirm the presentation of the fetus, the position of the fetal head and the degree of its 'engagement' in the pelvis (see p. 66). An attempt is made to determine, clinically, the type of abnormal uterine activity but if the patient has an epidural analgesic this may be diffi-cult. Consideration should be made whether or not to apply a cardiotocograph to record the uterine activity and the fetal heart rate.

A vaginal examination is made to determine the condition and the degree of dilatation of the cervix and the level of the fetal biparietal diameter in rela-tion to the ischial spines.

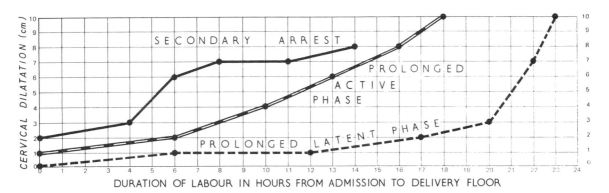

**Fig. 44/7** Abnormal patterns of cervical dilatation

**Specific**

### HYPOACTIVE UTERINE STATES

This pattern of uterine activity, as recorded by the partogram, may be associated with a prolonged latent phase or with a prolonged active phase. In the former condition two approaches may be adopted. Either no treatment is given and the onset of the active phase awaited, or the membranes are ruptured and a dilute oxytocin infusion set up. In each case a vaginal examination should be performed to determine the dilatation of the cervix and the presence or absence of cephalopelvic disproportion. If the active approach is chosen, the oxytocin infusion should be increased incrementally (pp. 416–17) and vaginal examinations made at 2-hourly intervals. The aim is to obtain cervical dilatation in excess of 1cm/hour. If this rate of cervical dilatation does not occur in spite of the oxytocin infusion, the case should be reviewed and caesarean section considered. (In the future the use of monitor computer controlled evaluation of the area under the contraction may give the obstetrician more information on which to base the management of the problem.)

If the hypoactive state is identified in the active stage of labour, treatment is to rupture the membranes and to set up an incremental oxytocin infusion.

Using this regimen over 85 per cent of patients will deliver vaginally, either spontaneously or by forceps and 10 per cent will require caesarean section.

### HYPERACTIVE UTERINE STATES

These patterns are usually associated either with a prolonged active phase or with secondary arrest in the active phase of labour. As has been mentioned, the increased use of epidural analgesia has limited the ability of the clinician to make a clinical diagnosis of the uterine dysfunction. If a hyperactive uterine state is diagnosed in a woman who does not have epidural analgesia, either an epidural is established or the patient is sedated with an intravenous infusion of pethidine 300mg, together with diazepam 10mg, in 5 per cent glucose. The rate of the infusion is adjusted so that the woman sleeps between contractions. Vaginal examinations are made every 2 hours, and if the cervix fails to dilate over a 4-hour period the case is reviewed, and, if possible, epidural analgesic initiated.

Patients who have an epidural analgesic, and whose cervix fails to dilate at a rate exceeding 1cm/hour in the active stage, require to be re-evaluated. Provided major cephalopelvic disproportion is excluded, an incremental oxytocin infusion may be set up. If no cervical dilation has occurred after 2 to 4 hours labour is terminated by caesarean section.

*Outcome*: The type of uterine pattern as judged by the partogram and the outcome for a series of 684 British primigravidae is shown in Table **44/2**.

| | Per cent of all cases | Outcome | | |
| | | Spontaneous per cent | Forceps per cent | Caesarean per cent |
|---|---|---|---|---|
| *Pattern* | | | | |
| Normal pattern | 65–70 | 80 | 18 | 2 |
| Prolonged latent phase | 2–5 | 75 | 10 | 15 |
| Prolonged active phase | 20–30 | 55 | 30 | 15 |
| Secondary arrest | 5–10 | 40 | 35 | 25 |

**Table 44/2** Type of uterine activity and method of delivery in 684 British primigravidae (Cardozo, L. D. et al. *Brit. J. Obstet. Gynecol.*, 1982: **89**, 33–8)

## Chapter 45

# Prolonged Labour and Obstructed Labour

The concept of prolonged labour, which is a retrospective diagnosis, poses two problems. The first is that the time of onset of labour is imprecise and often difficult to establish. The second problem is to decide after what time labour should be considered prolonged. The time of onset of labour depends on the opinion of the patient together with objective data once she has reached hospital and has been examined. Confirmation that the patient is in labour will be obtained if the uterine contractions are regular and increasing in duration and severity and if vaginal examination shows that the cervix is dilating progressively. With this information an estimate can be made of when labour started.

The definition of when labour should be considered prolonged adds to the confusion. As was noted in Chapter 12 a first labour lasts about 13 hours, and subsequent labours average 8 hours' duration. By the time 18 hours have passed between 85 and 95 per cent of primigravidae will have delivered (unless the philosophy of the obstetrician is to manage the labour actively). By the time 18 hours have passed between 95 and 98 per cent of multigravidae will have given birth.

For these reasons it is customary to define labour as being prolonged if its duration has exceeded 18 hours, which is a much more humane concept than that of a decade ago when the definition included only those labours which had lasted for more than 48 hours.

A further refinement is to classify the onset of labour as the time the woman seeks admission to hospital (irrespective of the duration of painful contractions prior to admission), and to designate labour as prolonged if delivery has not occurred within 12 hours of admission.

It does not matter whether the definition of prolonged labour is one in which regular uterine contractions, with a dilating cervix have been present

for 18 hours or more, or for 12 hours since admission, provided the medical attendants are aware of the definition which has been adopted by the institution.

In several studies it has been found that prolonged labour is four times as common in primigravidae as in multigravidae, and the incidence rises with increasing age, particularly amongst primigravidae over the age of 30. In Europe, the incidence is doubled if the woman is less than 153cm tall, but the influence of height is not found amongst Asian women.

## CAUSES OF PROLONGED LABOUR

In considering the cause of prolonged labour, four different factors should be taken into account, although in most cases more than one factor plays a part. The factors are the four 'Ps': (1) faults in the powers; (2) faults in the passenger; (3) faults in the passages, and (4) faults in the patient's psychology. The importance given to each factor depends on the doctor's analysis of the case, and interpretations may vary. For example, in many cases it is difficult to decide if the malposition of the fetal head, or a minor degree of disproportion is the cause of the disordered uterine action, or if the abnormal uterine action is preventing the proper rotation or flexion of the fetal head.

In most series collected from hospital reports about 55 per cent of cases of prolonged labour are due to faults of the powers; about 30 per cent due to faults in the passenger, usually malposition, and about 20 per cent are due to cephalopelvic disproportion.

In a few cases no definite cause is found. There is no cephalopelvic disproportion, no fetal malpresentation and uterine activity appears normal. The only significant finding is an anxious, apprehensive patient. It can be speculated that the anxiety and apprehension may be interfering with the neuro-hormonal and muscular events which maintain the progressive dilation of the cervix. In other words, the fault lies in the patient's psychology.

## HAZARDS OF PROLONGED LABOUR

### Maternal

In past years, when prolonged labour was defined as a labour which had lasted for 48 hours or more, both the maternal mortality and morbidity, and the perinatal mortality were increased; and the longer the duration of labour the higher was the mortality. Most of the maternal deaths were due to infection, to trauma during delivery and to shock, particularly from a ruptured uterus. In the developed countries such deaths are rare, but in the developing nations a significant proportion of the deaths occur in women whose labour is prolonged.

Maternal morbidity is increased. Dehydration and ketoacidosis cause alterations in cellular chemistry, as potassium is mobilized leaving the cell relatively depleted which, in muscle cells, leads to hypotonia and the potential occurrence of postpartum haemorrhage. Myohypotonia may also account for the dilatation of the colon which frequently accompanies prolonged labour. Puerperal infection is increased five-fold, the infection being that of the urinary tract or of the uterine cavity, and the latter is of greater danger to the fetus.

### Fetal

The longer the duration of labour the higher is the perinatal mortality, particularly if pregnancy is also prolonged. For example, when gestation periods of 38 weeks or more are considered, the perinatal mortality doubles if labour lasts for more than 24 hours.

The main causes of the perinatal death are pneumonia following intra-uterine infection; hypoxia and stress from a reduced placental circulation, which increases fetal acidaemia, and trauma from a difficult delivery.

## INVESTIGATION OF A CASE OF PROLONGED LABOUR

When labour has lasted 18 hours (or 12 hours since admission to hospital) the antenatal history and the

details of previous deliveries (if any) are reviewed and the following questions are asked and answered:

1. Is the mother dehydrated or acidotic?
2. Is she infected or anaemic?
3. Is she mentally distressed? (The personality)
4. Is there evidence of contracted pelvis or tumour? (The passages)
5. Is there evidence of disproportion or malposition? (The passenger)
6. Is there evidence of disordered uterine action? (The powers)
7. Is the cervix effaced and dilating?
8. Are the membranes ruptured?
9. Is the bowel or bladder distended?

In order to answer the questions a careful general physical, abdominal and vaginal examination has to be made, laboratory investigations have to be evaluated, and the pattern of uterine action assessed. When the process is complete the observer should have a fairly clear indication of the main reason for the prolongation of labour and rational treatment can be adopted.

## TREATMENT

### General

If the patient is dehydrated or ketoacidotic, hydration and normal metabolic pathways should be restored by giving 500 to 1000ml of 5 per cent glucose intravenously, fairly rapidly. If the patient has been permitted oral feeding this must cease, as over 50 per cent of patients will require operative delivery. If anaemia is detected, this should be corrected by a blood transfusion and even if no anaemia is present two units of cross-matched blood should be made available on the delivery floor. If there is evidence of infection, it should be treated by intramuscular injections of ampicillin, or cephaloridine. A distressed nervous patient must be reassured and sedated: she should be treated as a person and not as a 'case of prolonged labour'.

### Specific

The specific treatment is directed to what is considered the main cause, and the appropriate treatment for faults in the powers, the passenger and the passages has been discussed in the previous chapters. As has been noted, primigravidae account for 75 per cent of cases, and in first labours minor degrees of disproportion and abnormal uterine action are often associated, the value given to each factor being determined by experience. But in all cases a further review should be made 4 to 6 hours after instituting treatment, and if no further cervical dilatation has occurred, labour should be terminated by caesarean section. As an axiom the obstetrician should 'seek to determine what the woman can accomplish, not what she can endure'.

## THE NEXT LABOUR

The memory of a prolonged labour, harshly handled by unsympathetic attendants and terminated by a difficult operative delivery, can leave a deeper scar on the patient's mind than the operative scar on her abdomen or perineum. So much so that between 25 and 35 per cent of couples deliberately avoid a further pregnancy.

Should the couple decide on a further pregnancy, both partners will require reassurance that the next delivery will be less traumatic. This reassurance can only be given after studying the details of the first confinement and assessing the progress of the present pregnancy. Since over half the cases of prolonged labour are due to disordered uterine activity, and since the uterus functions better with each confinement, spontaneous vaginal delivery or a low forceps delivery, may be anticipated. A low forceps delivery cannot be considered abnormal as the instruments are used merely to help the baby over a perineum damaged in the previous confinement.

A rather higher proportion of women whose first labour was prolonged are delivered by caesarean section in a subsequent labour. Some have a caesarean section because this method of delivery was used to terminate the previous pregnancy, others fail to progress in labour, and caesarean section is required. About 10 to 20 per cent of women whose previous labour was prolonged will need to be delivered by caesarean section once again.

# OBSTRUCTED LABOUR: RETRACTION RING DYSTOCIA

Obstructed labour is the end result of a badly managed, or neglected, labour, when cephalo-pelvic disproportion or a pelvic tumour have prevented the birth of the baby.

The uterus, by contracting, attempts to overcome the obstruction in two ways. In first labours, in other words in primigravid labours, the uterus contracts strongly for a while and then, on failing to effect delivery, the pattern of uterine activity changes to one of hypotonic inertia. If such a patient is given an oxytocin, the uterine activity will be enhanced and death of the fetus and, probably, rupture of the uterus will result.

The multigravid uterus meets obstruction in a different way. The uterus continues to show the normal pattern of activity with fundal dominance. The upper muscular segment contracts excessively and the muscle fibres retract (or shorten) slightly with each contraction, and consequently the lower uterine segment is increasingly distended as the fetus is forced into it, and at the same time drawn up over the fetus, becoming elongated and thinned (Fig. **45/1**).

The junction between the thick upper segment and the thin lower segment becomes increasingly marked and obvious, and rises in the abdomen. This pathological retraction ring is known as Bandl's ring. Ultimately the lower uterine segment will rupture, either spontaneously, or following interference.

### Aetiology

Obstructed labour is an indictment of the inadequate care a patient has received in labour, and should not occur. In countries where obstetric services are well developed, cases are rare, but in the developing countries where obstetric services are not yet fully established, and where many women are still attended by unqualified midwives, the accident is more common. The cause in many cases is the lack of recognition that with succeeding pregnancies there is a tendency for the baby to get progressively bigger. The fact that a woman has delivered spontaneously her fifth child, does not mean that the sixth will not be slightly larger and cause obstruction. Other causes

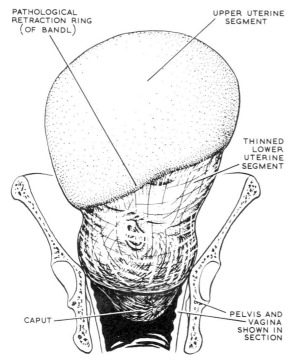

PATHOLOGICAL
RETRACTION RING
(OF BANDL)

UPPER UTERINE
SEGMENT

THINNED
LOWER
UTERINE
SEGMENT

CAPUT

PELVIS AND
VAGINA
SHOWN IN
SECTION

**Fig. 45/1** Threatened rupture of the uterus in a case of cephalopelvic disproportion and obstructed labour

are brow presentation, hydrocephaly, impacted breech and shoulder presentation. Rarely the obstruction may be due to an ovarian tumour occupying the pelvis, or a tumour of the bony pelvis.

### Clinical features

These can be deduced from the description of the pattern of uterine activity. The uterus meets the obstruction and tries to overcome it by contracting with increasing force and frequency, but as the contractions are co-ordinate, the pain distribution is normal. Because of the increased uterine activity, dehydration and ketosis develop early, and the patient becomes anxious, flushed and obviously in pain. Her temperature and pulse begin to rise.

With increasing activity the lower uterine segment becomes thinner and the ring marking the junction between the upper and lower segments begins to rise in the abdomen. Soon the contractions are almost continuous, the patient's pulse rate more than 120 beats a minute and Bandl's ring is seen as an oblique ridge two or more finger-breadths below the umbilicus. It may be confused with a full bladder, but the obliquity of the line is diagnostic and the bladder contains little urine as catheterization shows. The patient is now markedly dehydrated with a coated tongue and dry mouth and a rapid pulse and has concentrated urine, which is often bloodstained and contains acetone. The fetus is certainly in danger of death and may be dead, either from intra-uterine infection or from the stress caused by the overactive uterus. The patient herself is in danger of death from rupture of the uterus, internal haemorrhage and infection.

## MANAGEMENT

### Prevention

Prenatal care of all pregnant women and reference for special attention of those who show signs of disproportion either before, or in labour, or in whom labour is prolonged beyond 18 hours, would eliminate obstructed labour.

### Treatment

The dehydration and infection are treated by giving intravenous fluids and antibiotics whilst preparations are made for operation. In most cases caesarean section is to be preferred, even if the baby is dead and infection has occurred. It is less traumatic than a difficult vaginal delivery, particularly an intra-uterine manipulation or complicated embryotomy, which may cause the thinned uterus to rupture. In a few cases, and depending on the experience of the obstetrician, vaginal delivery is possible, particularly if the obstruction is due to a hydrocephalic child.

## Chapter 46

# Postpartum Haemorrhage

*Primary postpartum haemorrhage* is defined as blood loss per vaginam in excess of 500ml occurring in the first 24 hours after delivery. It is sometimes divided into third stage haemorrhage, which occurs before the expulsion of the placenta, and true postpartum haemorrhage which occurs after placental expulsion.

*Secondary postpartum haemorrhage* is defined as undue bleeding occurring more than 24 hours after delivery, usually between the 5th and 15th day postpartum.

## PRIMARY POSTPARTUM HAEMORRHAGE

Better obstetric care and the use of oxytocic drugs has reduced the incidence of primary postpartum haemorrhage from over 15 per cent to under 4 per cent of all deliveries in the developed countries, but it is still a real hazard to the mother in the developing countries, where it is the commonest cause of maternal death.

### AETIOLOGY

With the complete separation of the placenta, strong myometrial retraction causes shortening and kinking of the stretched uterine vessels as they pass along the side of the uterus. Further kinking of the vessels occurs as they pass through the retracted and contracted lattice of uterine muscle fibres. This effectively prevents blood flow and encourages thrombosis of the vessels (Fig. **46/1**). However, if placental remnants remain in the uterus, or if muscle retraction is poor, the constriction of the vessels is not so efficient and bleeding occurs. 'The empty contracted uninjured uterus does not bleed,' is a useful axiom to remember.

Primary postpartum haemorrhage is caused by: (1) inefficient retraction of the uterine muscle leading to bleeding from the placental site; (2) lacerations of the genital tract; or rarely (3) by blood dyscrasias which, by preventing clotting, lead to the condition.

In Table **46/1** it can be seen that in 80 per cent of cases of postpartum haemorrhage the bleeding is from the placental site. Most frequently this is due to inadequacy of myometrial activity (uterine atony) but in a few cases retention of placental tissue occurs despite normal or exaggerated myometrial action.

1. Bleeding from the placental site (80 per cent of cases)
   a. Inadequacy of uterine activity ('uterine atony')
   b. Retention of placental tissue
2. Bleeding from lacerations of the genital tract (20 per cent of cases)
   a. Lacerations of the vagina
   b. Ruptured uterus, or torn cervix

**Table 46/1** Classification of postpartum haemorrhage

Occasionally postpartum uterine atony is unexpected but in most cases the presence of predisposing factors serves to alert the obstetrician that haemorrhage may occur. The predisposing factors are as follows:

1. A history of previous postpartum haemorrhage.

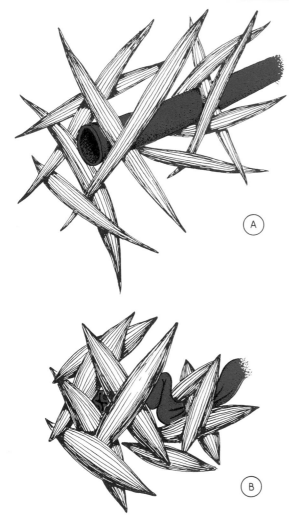

Fig. 46/1 Diagram of 'living tourniquet' of contracted uterine muscle

2. Overdistension of the uterus by hydramnios, multiple pregnancy, or myomata. The overstretched uterus responds less efficiently to endogenous oxytocin. In multiple pregnancy the blood vessels supplying the larger placental site are less efficiently controlled, whilst myomata may interfere with proper myometrial retraction.
3. Prolonged labour.
4. Deep general anaesthesia.
5. Antepartum haemorrhage. Postpartum haemorrhage may follow both abruptio placentae and placenta praevia. In abruptio placentae haemorrhage can be brisk after delivery: some of this blood is due to the release of the retroplacental clots, some is due to inadequate retraction of muscle and some to associated hypofibrinogenaemia. In placenta praevia, the placental site is mainly in the less thickly muscled lower uterine segment and retraction is less efficient.
6. Induction of labour, especially if amniotomy and oxytocin infusion is the method used.

Less frequently, postpartum haemorrhage occurs following the partial separation of the placenta, or the retention of a cotyledon, or fragment of placental tissue. In both cases the blood vessels supplying the placental site are inadequately compressed by the myometrial lattice and bleeding may result. The most frequent cause of retention of placental tissue is mismanagement of the third stage. Kneading of the fundus before the placenta has separated may cause partial retention above a localized (hour glass) constriction of the uterus (Fig. 46/2), with bleeding from the inadequately controlled placental site.

**Hazards of postpartum haemorrhage**

In all countries where surveys have been made it has been observed that more women die of complications of the third stage than of those of the pregnancy, the puerperium and the first and second stages of labour combined. That is the measure of the importance of the condition.

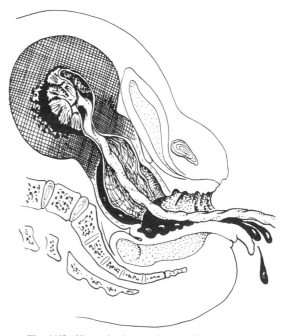

Fig. 46/2 'Hour glass' constriction of the uterus

Pre-existing maternal anaemia, although not a cause of postpartum haemorrhage, is a considerable hazard, as the anaemic mother is unable to adjust to the blood loss, and shock develops more rapidly and with greater severity. In about 1 per cent of cases of severe postpartum haemorrhage, hypofibrinogenaemia arises during the episode of bleeding, and leads to further bleeding. This must be anticipated and investigations made to detect its presence.

Patients who have a severe haemorrhage with associated shock lasting for more than half an hour, and who survive, may develop partial or complete hypopanpituitarism, and when the haemorrhage and shock are severe, 40 per cent will do so.

## DIAGNOSIS

The diagnosis is usually obvious, but occasionally blood collects in, and distends, the uterine cavity with little external loss. The fundus rises in the abdomen, and if a contraction is obtained, blood clots are expelled. The blood loss is usually discontinuous, as the uterus contracts periodically. When this occurs bleeding ceases, but recurs in between contractions because of the inadequate retraction of the myometrial fibres.

For rational treatment it is important to distinguish between placental site and traumatic bleeding, particularly after the placenta has been expelled. In placental site bleeding, if a contraction is 'rubbed up', the blood loss will diminish and cease when the contraction is at its maximum, recurring with uterine relaxation. Traumatic bleeding is not affected by uterine contractions, and is the likely cause if bleeding continues despite a firmly contracted uterus. But in many instances the distinction between the two types cannot be clearly made.

## MANAGEMENT OF POSTPARTUM HAEMORRHAGE

### Prevention

In the antenatal period anaemia must be detected and, if present, treated. During labour, the possibility of postpartum haemorrhage must be considered in the vulnerable groups already discussed. An important cause of postpartum haemorrhage, unless prophylactic oxytocics have been given towards the end of the second stage, is interference with the normal process of placental descent by unnecessary manipu-

lation of the fundus. The modern methods of active management of the third stage of labour have been a major factor in reducing the incidence and severity of postpartum haemorrhage.

### Third stage bleeding

1. If bleeding occurs before expulsion of the placenta, a contraction should be 'rubbed up', and with fundal pressure or with controlled cord traction an attempt should be made to expel the placenta. If bleeding continues despite a contracted uterus, the vagina and cervix should be inspected to discover if there is any damage.

2. If the methods outlined fail to deliver the placenta, treatment will depend on the place of confinement. If this is in the home, or if an anaesthetic cannot be readily given, an injection of ergometrine 0.25mg intravenously, oxytocin 10 units, or Syntometrine 1ml intramuscularly will control the bleeding and enable the attendant to seek further help. In hospital, continued bleeding should be treated by manual removal of the placenta, preceded if one wishes by Credé's method (Fig. **46/3**).

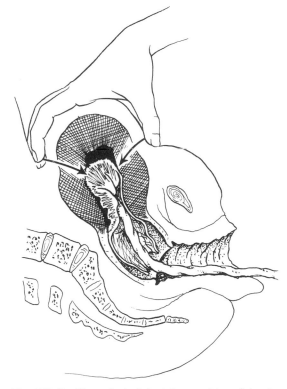

**Fig. 46/3** Credé's method of obtaining expulsion of the placenta

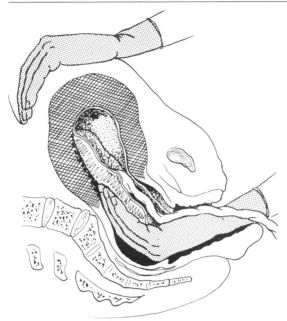

**Fig. 46/4** Manual removal of the placenta

## CREDÉ'S METHOD

A firm uterine contraction is obtained by fundal massage, and at its height the uterus is compressed firmly with the fingers reaching far down behind the fundus and the thumb in front. In some cases this leads to placental separation and descent which can be felt as the uterus appears to empty between the fingers. Further descent is helped by fundal pressure during the next uterine contraction or by controlled cord traction. Credé's method is painful and should be performed once only if at all.

## MANUAL REMOVAL OF THE PLACENTA

Under light general anaesthesia, the vulval area is cleansed and well lubricated with chlorhexidine cream. The gloved hand is also lubricated and is introduced into the uterine cavity, the other hand controlling the fundus per abdomen. If a constriction ring is present this is slowly dilated with the intra-uterine fingers shaped into a cone. The cord, if present, is followed to the placenta and the placental edge identified. With the palm of the hand facing the cavity, the placenta is sheared from its attachments by a sawing motion, mainly using the ulnar border of the hand. In some cases the attachment is too firm and the fingers must be used. The external hand keeps constant control of the fundus during

the manipulation. When the placenta lies freely within the uterine cavity, the cavity is once again gently palpated to ensure that the entire placenta and membranes have been separated. The hand grasps the placenta, and hand and placenta are withdrawn together. The external hand massages the uterus to obtain a contraction during this time, and ergometrine 0.25mg intravenously or 0.5mg intramuscularly is given. The placenta is inspected after withdrawal, and if any doubt about its completeness exists, the hand is reintroduced and placental remnants, chorionic membranes and clots removed (Fig. **46/4**).

### True postpartum haemorrhage

In these cases the placenta has already been delivered but bleeding persists. The placenta should be inspected to see if it is complete, and steps should be taken to control the bleeding and to treat the patient if she is shocked.

### STEP 1

Massage the uterus with a slow firm rotary movement with fingers behind the fundus and the thumbs in front.

### STEP 2

Give an injection of ergometrine 0.25mg intravenously, or Syntometrine 1ml intramuscularly, or an infusion of 30U oxytocin in 1 litre of Hartmann's solution at 200 ml/hour (74mU/minute).

### STEP 3

If the bleeding continues despite this treatment put on a sterile gown and gloves and explore the cavity of the uterus, clearing it of placental tissue, clots and debris, and at the same time palpating the genital tract to detect injury. If cervical, uterine or vaginal damage is suspected after palpation, the genital tract must be inspected under a good light and the damage repaired. Although these procedures can be done without anaesthesia in an emergency, they are potentially shocking, and anaesthesia is advisable.

### STEP 4

Some obstetricians recommend that if Step 3 fails to control the bleeding, an intramuscular or an intra-

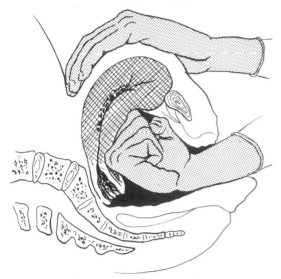

**Fig. 46/5** Bimanual compression of the uterus

myometrial injection of 15-methyl $PGF_{2\alpha}$ 0.5mg (in 1ml of saline) should be given over a 60-second period. Other obstetricians proceed to Step 5 at once.

STEP 5

If Step 3 is not possible, or if it fails to control the bleeding, the uterus should be compressed by lifting the uterus out of the pelvis and compressing it between the hands and the spine. An alternative method is bimanual compression, when one clenched fist placed in the anterior fornix and the other placed abdominally behind the fundus squeeze the uterus between them and compress the placental site (Fig. **46/5**). Both these methods are painful to the patient and tiring to the obstetrician.

STEP 6

If bleeding persists internal iliac artery ligation or

hysterectomy should be done. Hot intra-uterine douches and uterine packing should not be used, as the former is dangerous and the latter ineffective.

**Restoration of the patient's blood volume**

If the blood loss exceeds 1000ml, if the patient is anaemic or if she has signs of shock (tachycardia, a pulse rate raised above 100, or a systolic blood pressure below 100) blood should be transfused in adequate quantities. Blood loss is usually underestimated and at least 1000ml should be given, the first 500ml being given rapidly. Whilst waiting for blood an intravenous infusion of saline, or occasionally a plasma volume expander such as soluble plasma protein solution, or dextran, should be set up. Until the shock has been overcome, intra-uterine manipulations should be avoided. If the patient is apprehensive, morphine 15mg or pethidine 100mg may be injected. Traditionally the foot of the bed is raised in cases of shock. In the puerperal woman this causes the uterus to fall away from the pelvis and the normal stimuli of diaphragmatic movement which induce uterine contractions are lost. For this reason the patient's legs should be raised, but not her body.

If the haemorrhage is severe and the patient shows signs of shock and hypovolaemia, it is wise to monitor biophysical and biochemical indices. An indwelling catheter is inserted to monitor urine flow, a flow of 30ml/hour or more indicating adequate renal perfusion. Central venous pressure is a reliable measure of right atrial pressure and aids in avoiding overtransfusion. Arterial blood gases (PaO, $PaCO_2$, pH) measured serially, enables the medical attendant to correct metabolic acidosis and respiratory alkalosis, both of which increase pH and may lead to a decrease in cardiac output and cardiac arrhythmias. It may also be advisable to give transfusions of reconstituted packed red cells, if large amounts are needed, to avoid the introduction of white cell and plasma antigens.

# SECONDARY POSTPARTUM HAEMORRHAGE

The most common causes of delayed uterine haemorrhage are poor epitheliazation of the placental site or a retained piece of the placenta. In rare instances myometritis may lead to haemorrhage in the absence

of retained products. Even more rarely, recurrent episodes of postpartum haemorrhage, especially more than 4 weeks after delivery, may signify the development of a choriocarcinoma.

The uterus is empty in 75 per cent of patients and, in the remainder, portions of placenta and blood clots are present. An ultrasound scan of the uterus is helpful to exclude retained tissue. In all cases the initial treatment is to control the bleeding with ergometrine 0.5mg intramuscularly, repeated if needed, and to control infection if present with anti-biotics. Curettage is only needed if portions of placental tissue or blood clots are seen in the scan, or if bleeding persists or recurs in spite of oxytocics. An oxytocic must be injected prior to operation and care and skill is essential as the uterine wall is soft and easily perforated.

# RETAINED PLACENTA

A placenta which has remained in the uterus for 1 hour is said to be retained, and action should be taken to remove it. It has been shown that the longer the placenta remains in utero after this time, the greater is the risk to the mother of haemorrhage, shock (particularly if the placenta distends the cervix) and infection.

### Aetiology

*Incarceration of a separated or partially separated placenta* above a constriction ring may occur following meddlesome manipulation of the fundus in an attempt to hurry the third stage, or following the use of an oxytocic agent at the end of the second, or in the early third stage. In the latter case if the placenta has not been expelled within 15 minutes after the injection it is usual to remove it manually.

*Uterine atony* may lead to placental retention and this has been discussed when associated with postpartum haemorrhage. Even in the absence of haemorrhage, the placenta should be removed manually after 1 hour.

A *morbidly adherent placenta* may be the cause of its retention. In such cases the trophoblast has penetrated through the decidua and is attached to the myometrium (placenta accreta), or has penetrated the muscle fibres to a varying degree (placenta increta and placenta percreta). As no plane of easy separation exists, the placenta is retained in utero. Since the abnormality is usually only partial, the placenta separates in some areas, and as muscle retraction is impaired, in these areas the vessels are not constricted and bleeding results. The condition is not common, occurring once in every 1500 deliveries.

### Treatment

In the presence of bleeding the placenta must be delivered at once; in other cases its delivery should be effected within an hour of the birth of the child.

First, it should be determined if the placenta has separated, and if it has it should be expelled as described on page 128. If it has not separated, it should be removed manually. However, if a placenta increta is present, manual removal will be difficult, or impossible, and attended by marked bleeding as the placenta is gouged out of the muscle. As well as this there is a risk of uterine damage or perforation, and in general, the attempt should be abandoned and hysterectomy performed.

# INVERSION OF THE UTERUS

This is an exceedingly rare complication (1 in 20 000 deliveries) and is classified as partial when the inverted fundus appears at the cervix, and complete when the whole uterus is inverted and appears outside the vulva, usually with the placenta attached (Fig. **46/6**).

### Aetiology

If the cervix is dilated, and a strong contraction occurs following a period of uterine flaccidity in a uterus with a fundal implantation of the placenta inversion may occur. More commonly inversion fol-

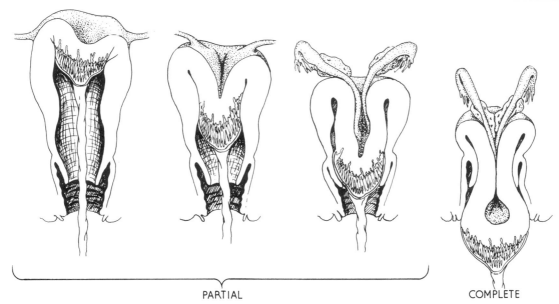

PARTIAL                                                COMPLETE

**Fig. 46/6** Inversion of the uterus – diagrammatic

lows cord traction in a patient whose uterus is atonic and in whom the fundus has not been controlled. It can also be produced by using Credé's method of placental expulsion in a relaxed uterus.

### Symptoms and signs

The patient complains of severe pain, of a dull deep aching nature which is probably due to tension on the ovaries. Shock follows soon, especially if the inversion is complete, and bleeding may be marked, but does not necessarily occur if the placenta is still attached. On abdominal examination the uterus can no longer be palpated, and pelvic examination makes the diagnosis clear.

### Treatment

If the condition is diagnosed early before severe shock has occurred, the placenta should be removed and replacement of the uterus attempted. Without anaesthesia the uterus is pushed back into its normal position with the fingers pressing the fundus upwards.

If shock is severe, it should be treated first, but a completely inverted uterus should be replaced in the vagina if this can be done easily. Once the shock has been treated, replacement of the uterus should be done either manually or by the hydrostatic method. In this the placenta is removed, the inverted uterus replaced in the vagina and the vulval orifice blocked with the forearm, the hand being in the vagina. Up to 5 litres of warm sterile water are run into the vagina through a douche nozzle. The water distends the vagina and, by pressure, leads to replacement of the uterus. Rarely an abdominal operation may be required to deal with the condition.

## Chapter 47

# Damage to the Genital Tract

The assumption of the erect position by mankind, and amongst Western peoples the preference for sitting upon a chair to squatting on the heels, has considerably altered the stresses placed upon the muscles of the pelvic floor and perineum. The evolutionary changes which have expanded the cranium of mankind, and converted it into a sphere, mean that a large non-streamlined object must be propelled into the world along an angled birth canal. In normal childbirth most strain is placed upon the pelvic floor, but in cases of cephalopelvic disproportion, or of difficult forceps delivery, the vagina and cervix may be subjected to damage, and in obstructed labour uterine rupture can occur.

## PERINEAL AND VAGINAL TEARS

The perineal floor and vagina are muscular structures of considerable importance for they act as a barrier to herniation of the uterus and gut. In the past it was customary for birth attendants to 'preserve the perineum' at all costs and a perineal tear was considered due to bad obstetric care. Although in many cases no visible tear occurred, the levator muscles were separated and a uterovaginal prolapse occurred subsequently; and in other cases a perineal tear occurred which was allowed to heal inadequately by granulation.

It is now realized that a damaged perineum, unless treated, predisposes to prolapse, particularly when the hormonal and vascular support of the pelvic tissues is withdrawn after the menopause. It has also come to be understood that a deliberate incision into the perineum to permit the safe delivery of the fetal head is preferable to the occurrence of a ragged tear. Today, between 40 and 80 per cent of primigravidae have an episiotomy (a deliberate perineal incision) performed and between 20 and 25 per cent sustain a perineal tear. The operation of repair of perineal wounds is therefore one of the commonest surgical procedures, but one which is too often performed perfunctorily, inadequately and improperly, so that it is one of the least considered and most painful of all operations performed on the human female. Far too many women leave hospital with the memory of perineal pain, which they say was far worse than the pain of parturition.

**Types of perineal tears**

Four degrees of perineal laceration are generally recognized. In the *first degree* there is damage to the skin of the fourchette and the underlying muscle is exposed. In the *second degree*, the posterior vaginal wall and the perineal muscles are torn to a varying extent, but the anal sphincter is not damaged. In the *third degree* the anal sphincter is torn but the rectal mucosa is intact. In the *fourth degree*, the anal canal is opened and the tear may spread up into the rectum.

Perineal tears may be produced: (1) by rapid delivery of the fetal head and during extraction of the posterior shoulder; (2) when the baby is large; (3) if the pubic arch is narrow so that the head is forced posteriorly to find space; (4) in persistent, occipito-posterior positions; (5) in breech delivery, since there is little opportunity for a slow stretching of the

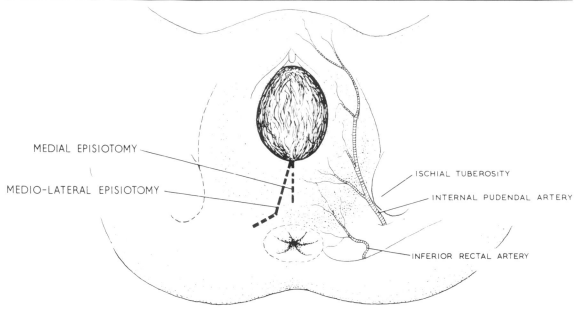

MEDIAL EPISIOTOMY

MEDIO-LATERAL EPISIOTOMY

ISCHIAL TUBEROSITY

INTERNAL PUDENDAL ARTERY

INFERIOR RECTAL ARTERY

**Fig. 47/1** Types of episiotomy

perineal tissues to occur; and (6) in forceps deliveries, since the instruments occupy additional space.

These conditions also favour tears of the labia, which are of little consequence and, unless bleeding, require no suturing. Breech delivery and forceps delivery – especially mid-forceps delivery, may also cause vaginal tears.

### Prevention of perineal and vaginal tears

The slow delivery of the fetal head, preferably between uterine contractions, and the careful delivery of the shoulders will reduce the incidence of perineal tears. However, the best method of avoiding a tear is the judicious use of a deliberate episiotomy.

# EPISIOTOMY

The operation of episiotomy was suggested 200 years ago, but only became commonplace when local anaesthesia and catgut for suture material were introduced. An episiotomy should be performed when the conditions likely to cause a perineal tear are present and in addition it should be made if there is fetal distress; if the head of the premature baby is delayed upon the perineum; if the perineum is 'rigid'; when the patient has had a previous vaginal repair;

or if the perineal skin is obviously about to split at delivery.

In cases where the operation is likely to be required, infiltration of the perineum with 1 per cent lignocaine should be performed as the fetal head begins to distend the pelvic floor.

### Types of episiotomy

The episiotomy may be midline or mediolateral (Fig. **47/1**). The midline incision has the advantage that no large blood vessels are encountered, and it is easy to repair; but it may extend into the rectum. The danger of this has been exaggerated and repair of the rectum is rarely complicated. If a large episiotomy is required (for example, in difficult mid-forceps delivery) the medio-lateral incision is to be preferred. The incision starts at the posterior fourchette and curves at a distance of 2cm to one or other side of the anal sphincter. The incision can be made with scissors or a scalpel, but should be made boldly and not in repeated ineffectual nibbles. If a large vessel is cut, which bleeds, it can be secured with a haemostat.

### Cause of perineal wound pain

Any injury to tissues is followed by a reactionary

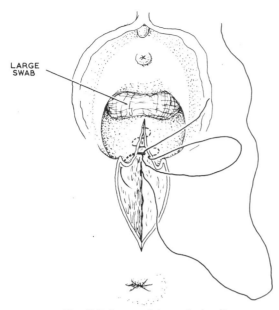

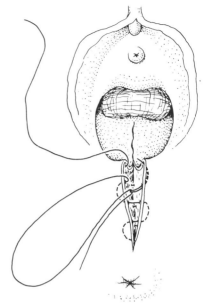

**Fig. 47/2** Suture of the vaginal wall

**Fig. 47/3** The suture of the vaginal wall has been completed and the perineal muscles are being sutured

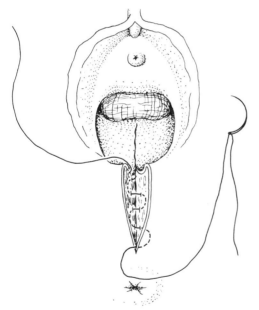

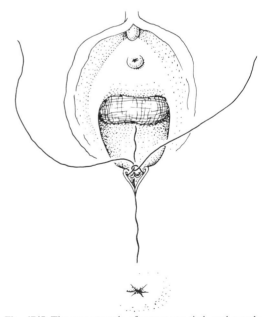

**Fig. 47/4** The subcuticular suture of the perineal skin starting posteriorly and finishing deep to the hymen

**Fig. 47/5** The two strands of catgut are tied, and cut short. The knot disappears beneath the vaginal mucosa

**CONTINUOUS CATGUT SUTURE**

oedema and this is aggravated if a foreign body is inserted into the area. If dead spaces are left in a vascular area, small collections of blood clot occur and increase the irritation of the nerves supplying the area. In puerperal perineal wounds, in addition, irritant lochia may seep into the wound and cause further irritation, whilst sutures involving the skin are disturbed every time the patient moves. It follows from this that the pain of a perineal repair can be minimized if: (1) the wound is clean and the edges are easily defined; (2) accurate approximation of the various tissues is made; (3) the least amount of suture material possible is used; (4) knots are avoided, as they encourage accumulations of blood clot; (5) skin-penetrating sutures are omitted.

## Method of repair

The repair of a perineal tear of second degree and an episiotomy are identical and the latter will be dealt with first. Before starting the repair it is essential to inspect the vagina in a good light to ensure that the apex of the vaginal wound can be seen and that no other vaginal damage has occurred. If local infiltration with anaesthetic has not already been made, 1 per cent lignocaine is injected into the tissues through the wound. So that uterine blood does not obscure the wound a large swab (half of a sanitary pad is useful) is inserted high into the vagina. It must be removed at the end of the operation. The repair is done with the patient in the lithotomy position, the legs and perineum draped with sterile drapes, the operator gowned and gloved.

Two methods are available: (1) using continuous No. 2/0 polyglycolic acid suture material; and (2) using interrupted sutures and fine nylon in the skin. The former is slightly more complex but is much more comfortable for the patient, and 24 hours after operation 65 per cent of women will have no discomfort, 28 per cent will have slight discomfort and only 7 per cent will have pain. This compares with a complaint of pain, or severe pain, in 40 per cent of women using the other method.

## Continuous polyglycolic acid suture

A half circle trochar pointed or cutting needle is threaded with a 2/0 or 3/0 suture so that one-third of the strand is through the eye of the needle. The needle is passed submucosally at the apex of the vaginal wound and a half knot is tied. It is essential to close the apex of the wound. The long portion of

the suture is allowed to fall into the wound, and the short portion is used to close the vagina by a submucosal continuous suture. This ends just below the hymen (Fig. **47/2**).

The needle is now removed and placed on the other strand and the levator ani and perineal muscles are approximated with two or three continuous sutures starting anteriorly and ending just anterior to the anus (Fig. **47/3**). The perineal skin edges are approximated with a subcuticular suture which takes a 0.5 to 1cm bite of the tissues. The suture which approximated the skin edges is drawn tight and tied to the vaginal strand. The knot disappears below the hymenal remnants (Figs **47/4**; **47/5**).

## Standard repair

This method is preferable if the obstetrician is inexperienced, if the wound is ragged, or if infection is present. The steps are as follows:

1. The vagina is closed with a continuous catgut suture of 2/0 polyglycolic acid suture. This suture must include the apex of the tear and seal it. The suture is tied at the level of the fourchette (Fig. **47/6**).

2. The perineal muscles are united with three or more interrupted sutures of 1/0 material, the deep muscles first and then the superficial muscles. A finger in the wound protects the rectum and makes the identification of the muscle more easy.

3. Fine braided nylon is used to co-apt the skin edges in interrupted sutures, or alternatively a subcuticular suture can be used, the initial and final knots being buried inwards.

## Aftercare

The patient with a continuous suture requires no special aftercare. Occasionally analgesics are needed, but most often none are required. The woman may walk as soon as she wishes and can shower twice a day, which obviates the need for swabbing rounds. The patient who has had the traditional type of suturing is rather less mobile for the first 2 or 3 days and during this time analgesics and swabbing may be necessary.

The bowels are not confined, but if the patient wishes to defaecate and the stool is hard, a bisacodyl suppository is inserted into the rectum half an hour before defaecation is attempted.

Twelve weeks after birth 5 per cent of women who have had an episiotomy or a perineal tear repaired still experience some degree of perineal pain,

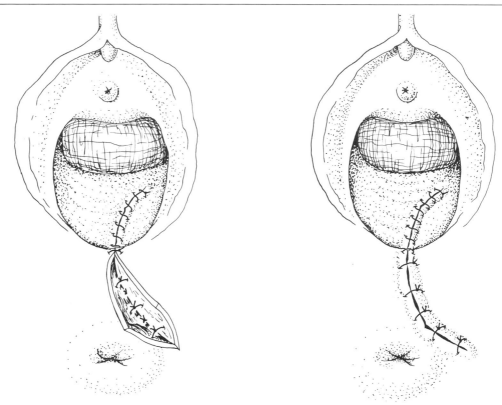

**Figs 47/6** and **47/7** Standard method of repair of an episiotomy or perineal tear

15 per cent have perineal discomfort and 15 per cent find that intercourse is painful.

### Fourth degree tear

If the rectum is involved, the rectal mucosa is first sutured using a submucosal continuous suture of 2/0. It is essential to close the apex of the mucosal tear. The anal sphincter, which always retracts, is sought and identified and is united with two interrupted sutures (Fig. **47/8**). The remainder of the repair is as for an episiotomy.

The aftercare of a fourth degree tear is to give a low residue diet, but if the patient feels a desire to defaecate, a bisacodyl suppository should be inserted into the rectum to soften the stool.

## VAGINAL LACERATIONS

These are fairly common after a difficult mid-forceps delivery, especially if manual or forceps rotation of the fetal head was necessary. The apex of the tear must be identified and is repaired under good light using a continuous 2/0 suture.

## VULVAL LACERATIONS

These are obvious on inspection and the ones which cause the most severe haemorrhage are those which involve the clitoral area. Treatment is to undersew the tear with a continuous catgut suture.

## CERVICAL TEARS

Normally the cervix is sufficiently softened and dilatable to permit the passage of the fetus without incurring damage, and the cervical lacerations commonly reported as indicative of parity are probably more apparent than real. There is no evidence that the cervical epithelium is damaged during a normal delivery although the collagen fibres of the cervical matrix may be separated more widely, so that an apparent 'laceration' occurs.

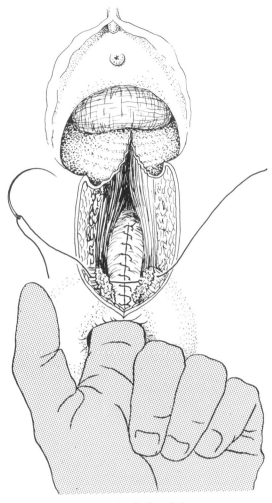

**Fig. 47/8** Repair of a fourth degree tear

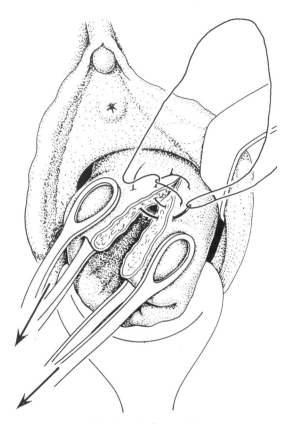

**Fig. 47/9** Repair of a cervical tear

In a few cases tears of the cervix occur during delivery. The commonest cause is surgical interference, particularly attempted delivery by forceps, or the ventouse, before full dilatation of the cervix, or following breech extraction. Less commonly tears may result from the forcible expulsive efforts of the mother pushing the baby through the incompletely dilated cervix, or from the injudicious use of intramuscular oxytocin. Cervical tears only assume importance when they cause postpartum haemorrhage. The bleeding is bright red, variable in amount and can be severe. It is distinguished from placental site bleeding by the fact that it continues even when the uterus is well contracted.

Should haemorrhage continue although the uterus is contracted, the vagina and cervix must be inspected in a good light, and the cavity of the uterus palpated in case a uterine rupture has occurred.

**Technique of repair**

The patient is anaesthetized and put in the lithotomy position. A large Sims speculum is put in the vagina, and the anterior and posterior cervical lips are grasped by one or more sponge forceps. Gauze swabs wipe away the blood. The cervix is usually oedematous, bruised and distorted and the extent of the tear may be difficult to determine. The entire tear and the bleeding points must be brought into view by applying a second sponge forceps nearer to the tear, and pulling the speculum laterally. The first suture may be placed at any convenient level and can be used for traction to make the apex of the tear more accessible. The tear is then sutured with a continuous locking suture, starting above the apex of the tear and continuing to the external os (Fig. **47/9**).

# RUPTURE OF THE UTERUS

Rupture of the uterus constitutes a grave hazard to the mother, and the fetus almost always dies. With the advances of obstetric care in the developed countries, the incidence of the condition is diminishing, and may be expected to occur only once in 4000 births. In the developing countries the incidence is higher and in hospital practice may be as high as 1 in 300 deliveries.

## CLASSIFICATION

Comprehensive classification of uterine rupture is not easy to make, and none is completely satisfactory, but the following has proved useful. The causes are given in order of frequency.
1. Rupture of the uterus in pregnancy
   a. Caesarean section scar
   b. Spontaneous
   c. Traumatic
2. Rupture of the uterus in labour
   a. Spontaneous following obstructed labour
   b. Traumatic (iatrogenic)
   c. Caesarean section scar.

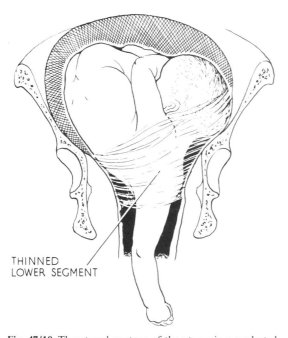

THINNED
LOWER SEGMENT

Fig. 47/10 Threatened rupture of the uterus in a neglected shoulder presentation

### Rupture of the uterus in pregnancy

*Spontaneous rupture of the uterus* is not common in pregnancy but may occur in a patient who has previously had a placenta increta, angular pregnancy, or a pregnancy in a rudimentary horn of the uterus. The most common cause of uterine rupture in pregnancy is *rupture of a caesarean section scar*, particularly of the classical scar. This scar is particularly vulnerable as healing is impaired during the puerperium because of the constant contractions and the involution of the muscle fibres, and because the placenta may be implanted over the scar in a subsequent pregnancy. Three per cent of classical scars rupture, and a half of these give way in the last weeks of pregnancy. The lower uterine scar is much less likely to rupture (0.25 per cent) and if rupture occurs, it usually does so during labour.

### Rupture of the uterus in labour

Most ruptures of the uterus occur during labour, and it is rare for a primigravida's uterus to rupture, almost all cases occurring in multigravidae, particularly high multigravidae.

#### SPONTANEOUS RUPTURE

The response of the multigravid uterus to obstructed labour is spontaneous uterine rupture. Whereas the primigravid uterus meets obstruction to delivery by becoming inert, the multigravid uterus continues to contract. The obstruction may be due to disproportion, as the later the birth order the larger the baby tends to be; to undiagnosed hydrocephaly; to shoulder presentation; and to malposition of the fetal head, such as brow, or to pelvic tumours. In normal labour the lower uterine segment is stretched circumferentially to accommodate the fetal head and there is little increase in its length. However, if labour becomes obstructed, the continued contractions of the fundus increasingly elongate and thin the lower segment. If the condition is not treated, the upper segment becomes thick whilst the lower segment is stretched over the fetus and is paper-thin (Fig. **47/10**). The junction between the two segments forms an oblique line running across the uterus just below the umbilicus, the pathological retraction ring

(Bandl's ring). Pain is constant, the bladder oedematous and the patient in marked distress. Rupture of the uterus is imminent. In a few high multiparae, spontaneous rupture occurs with no evidence of dystocia.

## TRAUMATIC RUPTURE

If the uterus in obstructed labour does not rupture spontaneously, injudicious attempts at vaginal delivery, and particularly attempts at internal podalic version of the impacted shoulder presentation, are liable to be followed by uterine rupture. The lower segment is already overdistended and the additional strain produced by the forceps or by the introduction of a hand into the uterus is sufficient for rupture to occur (Fig. **47/11**). The improper use of oxytocin, generally by intramuscular injection, is another cause of traumatic rupture. Forceps delivery before full cervical dilatation may cause a cervical tear which extends into the lower uterine segment.

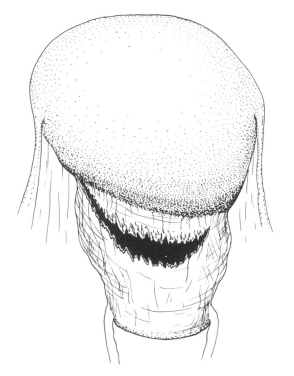

**Fig. 47/11** Ruptured uterus, from a case of obstructed labour (redrawn from Martin, *Atlas of Obstetrics and Gynaecology*. Lewis, London, 1881)

## RUPTURE OF A CAESAREAN SECTION SCAR

The replacement of the classical operation by section through the lower uterine segment has reduced the number of uterine ruptures in labour from this cause.

## SITE OF THE RUPTURE

In most cases of spontaneous or traumatic rupture occurring in labour the tear involves one or other lateral wall usually extending into the upper segment. Anterior and posterior wall tears are less common and the bladder is involved in fewer than 6 per cent of cases. The rupture may be incomplete, in which case the peritoneal cavity is not involved, although haemorrhage occurs into the broad ligament; or complete, in which case haemorrhage involves the peritoneal cavity. This classification is of no particular value. In both instances the edges of the tear are ragged and not easy to define, and uterine vessels and the ureters may course through blood clot and debris.

## DIAGNOSIS

### Rupture in pregnancy

The rupture is in the upper uterine segment and the lower segment is rarely involved. The patient complains of pain and tenderness over the uterus and this is followed sooner or later by signs of intraperitoneal bleeding, with increasing tenderness and progressive collapse. The diagnosis is often not clear until laparotomy is performed because of internal haemorrhage. Treatment is either hysterectomy or, in cases when one wishes to preserve the uterus, by resection of the edges of the tear and its suture.

### Rupture in normal labour, or rupture of a caesarean section scar

In these cases the rupture is usually quiet, and diagnosis may be difficult. Slight vaginal bleeding may occur, and the patient complains of pain which is constant. The pulse rate begins to rise, the contractions usually cease but may continue, and the cervix fails to dilate. Over a period signs of shock increase and laparotomy reveals the rupture. In cases of rupture of a scar of the lower uterine segment, no symptoms may occur and the condition may only be diagnosed by routine intra-uterine palpation after delivery, or because of continued bleeding despite a contracted uterus.

In a few cases the rupture occurs suddenly at the height of one of a sequence of forcible contractions. The patient complains of a feeling of bursting followed by sudden relief, when all pains cease and shock supervenes.

**Rupture in late, obstructed labour**

During the premonitory phase of spontaneous rupture, the lower uterine segment becomes increasingly distended. The patient is in constant pain, mainly in the suprapubic region, with exacerbation each time a contraction occurs. The pulse rate and temperature rise and dehydration is usual. On inspection, the retraction ring is seen, the bladder is oedematous and haematuria may occur. On vaginal examination the presenting part is high and the vagina oedematous.

The rupture usually occurs at the height of a contraction. Suddenly the pattern of constant pain changes to one of a dull ache, and the uterine contractions cease. Vaginal bleeding may occur, but is often not heavy. In some cases the fetus cannot be felt per vaginam, as it has escaped into the peritoneal cavity through the rent in the uterus. If this occurs the shape of the uterus alters, and the fetal parts are easily palpable on abdominal examination. The pulse rate rises, the blood pressure falls and signs of shock supervene. The whole abdomen is very tender when palpated.

## PROPHYLAXIS

In the developed countries, where obstetric care is available to, and accepted by, most of the women, uterine rupture is uncommon and due in most cases to inadequate obstetric care. Either oxytocin is given improperly, obstructed labour is not diagnosed, or improper forceps deliveries, or intra-uterine manipulations, are attempted when the uterus is threatening to rupture. In the developing countries high multiparity is common and most women are at-tended in labour by unqualified attendants. As the previous pregnancies ended with spontaneous deliveries, no reason for anxiety is felt when labour begins. The woman labours for hours without progress; she is given food to strengthen her for the ordeal, prayers are offered or the witch doctor is called in, but to no avail. The pains increase in frequency and severity but the baby remains stubbornly in utero. Finally rupture occurs and a collapsed patient is brought to hospital. If she reaches hospital just before the rupture has occurred, an inexperienced physician may attempt intra-uterine manipulations and cause a rupture in the distended lower segment.

When trained midwives, who have a clear knowledge of when they must send patients to hospital, are placed in every village; when postgraduate experience in obstetrics is given to all doctors who are likely to care for pregnant women, and when each region has a highly efficient well-staffed central hospital, deaths from uterine rupture will cease.

## TREATMENT

If threatened rupture of the uterus is diagnosed, immediate caesarean section should be performed, except in rare cases where an impacted shoulder presentation permits easy decapitation. Should the rupture have occurred, resuscitation by blood transfusion should be followed by immediate laparotomy. On opening the abdomen the operation which can be performed quickest and with least shock should be chosen. If the edges of the rupture can be defined easily, they are freshened and the wound repaired. In most cases a total hysterectomy is performed. Provided the bladder is displaced downwards, the ureters identified and the uterus firmly pulled cephalically during the dissection, the operation can be performed much more easily than would appear when the haemorrhagic torn uterus is first seen. When the patient has no wish for further children, hysterectomy is to be preferred to repair of the rupture.

# SHOCK IN OBSTETRICS

Two types of shock occur in pregnancy or, more commonly, following delivery. In the first, haemorrhage is the predominant feature, although tissue trauma may have occurred; in the second, haemorrhage is minimal and the shock is due to the absorption of bacterial endotoxins.

## HAEMORRHAGIC SHOCK

Haemorrhagic shock may be: (1) *antepartum* (from abruptio placentae or placenta praevia); (2) *intrapartum* (from a ruptured uterus); or (3) *postpartum* (either from an atonic uterus, or due to trauma in the genital tract).

### Physiological considerations

Blood loss leads to a fall in blood volume, a reduced venous filling pressure in the heart, and a lowered cardiac output. This reflexly invokes neurogenically controlled catecholamine production with vasoconstriction of peripheral and visceral arterioles, so that the systemic arterial pressure is maintained and the cerebral and cardiac circulations are unaffected. Simultaneously the blood volume is augmented by fluids passing into the vascular system from the tissues.

However, if the haemorrhage is severe, and not treated, a relative hypoxia and metabolic acidosis results, and should this persist for longer than 3 hours, cellular damage and selective vasodilatation is caused. In the early stages of this phase the vasodilatation is thought to be confined to the precapillary arterioles, the postcapillary venules remaining in spasm, so that more and more blood fills the capillary bed, where it stagnates, and the venous return is reduced. The stagnant blood also exerts a hydrostatic pressure on the hypoxic capillary walls and forces plasma into the tissues, increasing the tissue pressure and causing further tissue damage. Shock is now irreversible, for extensive tissue damage has occurred, and although massive transfusion may temporarily maintain life, death is inevitable.

### Clinical picture

The amount of blood lost is usually underestimated, and the findings of a rising pulse rate, a falling blood pressure, increasing pallor and air hunger are well known. As has been indicated no single sign is diagnostic, and blood volume studies are inaccurate. If facilities are available, a more reliable assessment of the severity of the shock and the adequacy of treatment can be obtained from a catheter introduced into the superior vena cava, or threaded up from the antecubital fossa vein. The aim is to maintain the central venous pressure at 5 to 15mm water. The patient should be nursed with her legs raised and because of possible pressure by the uterus on the inferior vena cava, she should be turned on to one side and not lie in the supine position.

### Treatment

Clinical monitoring (the patient's colour, mental state, pulse pressure and blood pressure and the peripheral circulation) is an important guide to treatment. In most cases restoration of the blood volume is needed. A plasma substitute (such as stable plasma protein solution) or polygeline (Haemaccel) should be given initially whilst waiting for blood. The quantity of blood needed can be determined by the improvement in the patient's clinical condition, but is estimated with greater accuracy by measuring the central venous pressure or preferably by using a flow-directed pulmonary artery catheter, such as a Swan-Ganz catheter. The arterial systolic blood pressure is not a reliable guide, and undertransfusion is a greater danger than overtransfusion. The effective blood volume should be restored by transfusing the estimated blood loss and by giving an additional 500 to 1000ml. If the patient is in pain, morphine 5mg is given intravenously, otherwise it should be withheld. An additional method is to insert a catheter into the bladder and measure the hourly urine volume.

If the patient's condition does not improve rapidly following adequate transfusion, and haemorrhage has been marked and shock is considerable, additional measures are required. Since the main defect is a reduced cardiac output and a diminished venous return, optimal cardiovascular function needs to be restored. The preferred method is to infuse dopamine hydrochloride starting at 2–5 $\mu$g/kg/minute, titrated against the clinical and haemodynamic response. Dopamine increases myocardial output without increasing oxygen consumption and at doses of less than 15 $\mu$g/kg/minute increases renal and mesenteric blood flow. However, the drug must only be given after restoration of the blood volume. Occasionally, corticosteroids are required to combat the shock. If dexamethasone is chosen, it should be given slowly over 30 minutes in a dose of 50mg per kg body-weight intravenously, or half that dose in to the aorta.

Infection should be looked for and if suspected, large doses of antibiotics given.

## BACTERIAL (ENDOTOXIN) SHOCK

The pregnant woman seems especially susceptible to the development of non-haemorrhagic shock caused by the liberation of endotoxins from Gram-negative organisms, particularly *E. coli*. The place of entry of the bacteria is usually the placental bed, particularly after abortion or in puerperal infection, but infection may occur following instrumentation of patients who have chronic pyelonephritis. The shock is usually preceded by rigors, but may occur without marked clinical signs. Despite a rapid thready pulse and hypotension, the skin may be warm and dry, but apart from this the signs are those of shock following haemorrhage.

The aims of treatment are to restore the intravascular volume, to improve cardiac output, to provide antibiotic cover for a wide variety of aerobic and anaerobic bacteria and, when appropriate, to remove infected tissue surgically.

## Chapter 48

# The Complicated Puerperium

## PUERPERAL INFECTION

In the past 25 years there has been a dramatic fall in the incidence and severity of puerperal infection. In part this has been due to better obstetric care and an understanding of the part which maternal resistance plays in combating infection; but most of the fall has been due to the ready availability of potent antibiotics and of blood.

### DEFINITION AND INCIDENCE

A rise in temperature to 38°C (100.4°F) or over, maintained for 24 hours or recurring during that period, from the end of the 1st to the end of the 10th day after confinement or abortion is generally considered indicative of puerperal infection. The definition is not entirely satisfactory, as patients may become infected without being pyrexial, and it fails to distinguish between infection of the genital tract and other forms of infection which may occur in the puerperium, as at other times.

With these reservations, the incidence of infection in the puerperium is 1 to 3 per cent and is dropping; but any patient showing pyrexia must be investigated to determine whether the cause of the fever is (1) genital or (2) non-genital. Although statistics vary between hospitals, it has been found that the proportional frequency of the various types of puerperal infection is

Genital tract in 25 to 55 per cent of infected cases
Urinary tract in 30 to 60 per cent of infected cases
Breast        in  5 to 10 per cent of infected cases
Intercurrent  in  2 to  5 per cent of infected cases

### INVESTIGATION

#### History

Interrogation of the patient and a study of her antenatal record will show whether the infection was present before labour; whether she had a vaginal infection, or was anaemic, in the antenatal period; or if she had a urinary infection. The obstetric record will reveal the duration and character of the labour, if the birth was spontaneous or required forceps and if there were extensive, or minimal, vaginal lacerations.

#### Examination

A general examination of the patient is made, paying special attention to the throat, lungs, heart, breasts and abdomen, and the legs (to exclude venous thrombosis) before special investigations are performed.

#### Special investigations

These include a vaginal speculum examination, the taking of a high vaginal smear, a bimanual examination to detect tenderness and swelling of the uterus or tubes, a midstream specimen of urine, which is sent for microscopic examination and culture, and haemoglobin and leucocyte examinations of the blood.

These investigations should enable the physician to localize the site of the infection, but the bacterial cause of the infection must await the laboratory findings.

## BACTERIOLOGY

The incidence of the causal bacteria varies between hospitals but in recent years the anaerobic streptococcus and *Staphylococcus pyogenes* have become the two forms most often found on puerperal infection, whilst the previously important cause, the *Haemolytic streptococcus (Group A)*, is less frequently encountered (Table **48/1**). In most cases there is a mixed growth, and sensitivity tests are necessary.

Occasionally, particularly after prolonged ruptured membranes, the anaerobic *Bacteroides fragilis* is the causative agent. In such cases the patient has a foul faecal-smelling vaginal discharge, and abscess formation is common.

## PUERPERAL INFECTION

The non-genital causes of infection in the puerperium have been described elsewhere, but puerperal infection requires further consideration.

### Mode of infection

In 60 per cent of cases the infection is caused by bacteria, particularly anaerobes, which normally inhabit the vagina. They only become pathogenic when reduced maternal resistance, or damaged vaginal tissues, permit the anaerobes to grow by virtue of their proteolytic action on devitalized tissue. Should the uterus contain placental remnants, as is frequent after abortion, their growth is enhanced.

In the remaining 40 per cent of cases the infection, usually staphylococcal, is introduced into the genital tract by the patient or her attendants. If the bacteria are introduced by the patient, the mode of transmission is called autogenous; if introduced by the attendants, or the environment, it is exogenous. Autogenous infection arises from organisms introduced into the genital tract from infection in some other part of the patient's body, either carried by the bloodstream, or introduced directly by droplets, or by the patient's fingers. If a patient has a septic spot on her head, and after scratching this, fingers her vulva, the same bacteria can be cultured from pustule and vagina.

Exogenous infection is caused by bacteria introduced from some source other than the patient. This is of importance because it is entirely preventable. In 60 per cent of cases the infection is introduced by the patient's attendants, usually from the upper respiratory tract of doctor or nurses. Infected secretions from the nasopharynx are also readily transferred to handkerchiefs, fingers, and thence to the door knobs and dust of the hospital. In 40 per cent of cases the infection is introduced to the patient's genital tract by infected dust from bed clothes and floors. In closed wards, dust may harbour viable bacteria for many months and these are stirred up during sweeping and bed-making.

| | Per cent |
|---|---|
| GENITAL INFECTION | |
| 1. Potential pathogens which normally inhabit the vagina | |
| Anaerobic streptococci | 65 to 85 |
| Anaerobic Gram-negative bacilli | 5 |
| Haemolytic streptococci (other than Group A, Lancefield) | 1 |
| 2. Bacterial introduced from adjacent viscera | |
| *E. coli* | 5 to 15 |
| *Cl. welchii* | Rare |
| 3. Bacteria introduced from distant organs or from outside | |
| Staphylococci | 5 to 15 |
| *Streptococcus haemolyticus* (Group A) | 3 |
| 4. *Mycoplasma hominis* | Rare |
| NON-GENITAL INFECTION | |
| 1. Urinary tract infection | |
| *E. coli* | 90 |
| 2. Breast infection | |
| Staphylococci (mainly from the baby) | 90 |

**Table 48/1** The main bacterial causes of infection in the puerperium

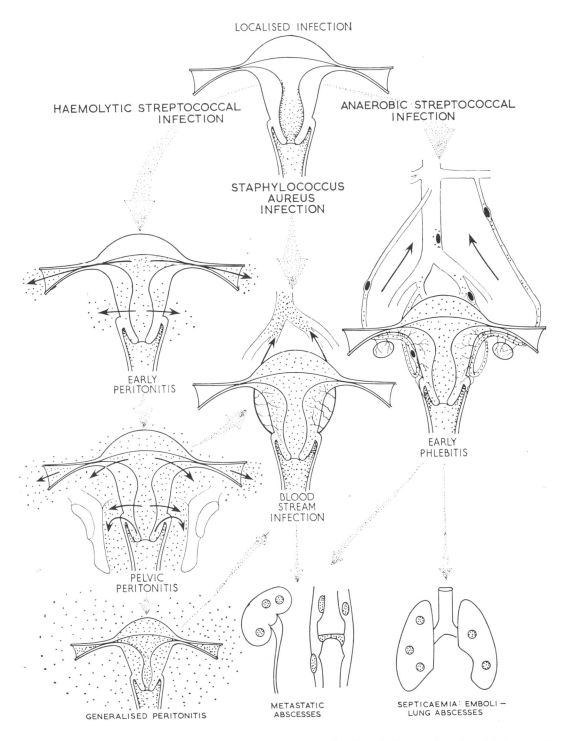

LOCALISED INFECTION

HAEMOLYTIC STREPTOCOCCAL
INFECTION

ANAEROBIC STREPTOCOCCAL
INFECTION

STAPHYLOCOCCUS
AUREUS
INFECTION

EARLY
PERITONITIS

EARLY
PHLEBITIS

PELVIC
PERITONITIS

BLOOD
STREAM
INFECTION

GENERALISED PERITONITIS

METASTATIC
ABSCESSES

SEPTICAEMIA: EMBOLI –
LUNG ABSCESSES

**Fig. 48/1** Pathways of infection showing the routes with various bacteria. Since the introduction of antibiotics spreading infection is not seen frequently (modified from Gibberd, G. F. *J. Obstet. Gynaecol. Brit. Cwlth.* 1966, **73**, 1, by kind permission)

### Site and spread of infection

The ability of the vaginal pathogens, or the introduced bacteria, to invade will depend upon their virulence and the resistance of the patient to invasion. Although the bacterial virulence increases in an epidemic, maternal resistance is much more likely to alter in sporadic infections. Patients who in pregnancy are anaemic, have PIH, are diabetic, or malnourished; patients who in labour become dehydrated, exhausted, or shocked; patients whose labour is prolonged, or have instrumental or operative deliveries, or who have postpartum haemorrhage, are liable to have a reduced resistance to bacteria. Labour is traumatizing to the tissues of the vagina and cervix, and devitalized tissues offer the opportunity for bacterial growth. The placental site in the uterus must be considered a large wound with much dead tissue attached to it, and although a barrier to infection is created behind the placental site, infection can be introduced easily through it.

## TYPES AND CLINICAL FEATURES OF PUERPERAL INFECTION

### Localized infection

#### INFECTION OF VULVA AND VAGINA

Apart from infection of the episiotomy wound, infections of the lower genital tract are uncommon, which is surprising because of the frequency of trauma to the tissues during childbirth, and the proximity of the rectum. Occasionally a cotton wool or gauze sponge may be left in the vagina at delivery. This can cause an offensive discharge and lead to low grade infection. Infection of an episiotomy wound may be suspected if the patient complains of unusual perineal pain or a discharge. The wound edges are swollen and red. Treatment consists of local heat, and, if necessary, antibiotics are given. In a few cases the sutures have to be removed and a secondary repair made when the infection has cleared. A cause of infection is inadequate repair of the wound, particularly omitting to close the apex of the vaginal tear.

#### CERVICITIS

The cervix is often traumatized during childbirth and may readily become infected. However, such infection is usually associated with uterine infection and rarely causes any specific symptoms.

#### ENDOMETRITIS AND MYOMETRITIS

Because of the vulnerable placental site, infection of the endometrium, with spread into the myometrium, is the most frequent cause of puerperal infection. In most cases the infection is limited to the endometrium because of the complex and efficient protective mechanisms of the puerperal woman, but spread throughout the endometrium is usual. The infection usually starts between the 3rd and 6th day after delivery and the clinical picture depends upon the virulence of the invading organisms. In all cases the lochia becomes darker in colour and offensive. This is accompanied by pyrexia, the degree depending on the virulence of the bacteria. Associated with the infection are headaches, malaise and often increased 'afterpains'. Examination shows a tender uterus.

Treatment is to ensure that good drainage from the uterus can occur and to administer antibiotics.

### Spreading infection

#### SALPINGITIS

Infection from the uterine cavity may spread upwards to involve the uterine tubes, which become swollen and tender.

#### PELVIC CELLULITIS

Spread from the lower uterine cavity or the cervix may be laterally through the uterine wall to involve the connective tissues of the cardinal ligaments, leading to pelvic cellulitis. The infection starts quietly but once established, usually in the 2nd week of the puerperium, causes lower abdominal pain. On examination the abdomen is tender, and vaginal examination shows tenderness in the vaginal fornices with relative fixation of the cervix. In many cases the condition is indistinguishable from pelvic peritonitis.

#### PELVIC PERITONITIS

This occurs by spread of infection from the tubes, the uterus or the cervix. The symptoms and signs are similar to those of pelvic cellulitis but occasionally paralytic ileus may occur.

## SEPTICAEMIA

Septicaemia may occur in women infected with virulent organisms (particularly of group A haemolytic streptococci) or whose resistance is low. The patient becomes acutely ill with swinging pyrexia, a rapid pulse and mental confusion. Thrombophlebitis of the uterine veins may arise, and showers of infected clots may be carried to distant organs, particularly the lungs, to produce further symptoms.

### Clinical pattern related to probable organism

To some extent the clinical pattern of the illness indicates the type of infecting organism. If the patient develops early septic shock, *E. coli*, *Streptococcus pyogenes* or *Cl. welchii* are likely. If the fever has an insidious onset, starting 2 to 8 days after childbirth, with swinging fever, gradual development of toxicity and late localizing signs, mixed anaerobic infection is likely. The rare infection with *Mycoplasma hominis*, is associated with a swinging fever, no localizing signs and little toxicity. The treatment of *Mycoplasma hominis* is to prescribe tetracycline.

### Changing patterns

It can be seen from the foregoing that pelvic infection may remain localized to the primary site, or may spread beyond that site to involve adjacent tissues, or even spread in the bloodstream. Spread beyond the primary site is uncommon today, as infection is usually treated early and adequately. With early treatment the exact anatomical delineation of the infection is not so necessary, and indeed may be impossible. For purposes of treatment three conditions can be described: (1) local infection of the lower genital tract; (2) uterine infection; and (3) spreading pelvic infection.

## PROPHYLAXIS

The incidence of puerperal infection can be reduced if certain general measures are undertaken. These are:

1. The provision of properly designed and equipped maternity hospitals. Each ward should be so arranged that potentially infected, or pyrexial, patients can be treated in side rooms, but isolation units are not necessary.

2. All staff attending obstetric patients should have nose and throat swabs taken before starting duty. Any of the staff developing a sore throat should be kept off duty. If haemolytic streptococci or staphylococci are found in nasal swabs, the nose should be treated with antiseptic creams.

3. In the antenatal period septic foci should be treated and the patient should be seen on admission by a doctor, and septic areas sought. She should also have a shower on admission.

4. Labour should be conducted with surgical asepsis, but it is unnecessary to shave the mons veneris or the vulva. The pubic hair should be trimmed with scissors and the area smeared with chlorhexidine cream. Vaginal examinations in labour must only be performed after the hands have been scrubbed, and sterile gloves worn. Repair of cervical, vaginal or episiotomy tears must be performed meticulously and with surgical asepsis.

5. With early ambulation many problems of the lying-in wards are reduced. Wards should be arranged in bays of one, two or four beds, and the baby should remain with the mother unless it is fractious. Because of the danger of bacteria lurking in the dust, sweeping and dusting should be done at a time different from that allocated to bedpan or swabbing rounds, should these still be required.

## TREATMENT

An infected patient should be nursed in a well-ventilated room. Anaemia must be treated and all infected patients require additional fluids. If there is excessive uterine bleeding, due to retained products of conception, digital evacuation of the uterus should be performed.

### Antibiotic therapy

No area of medicine is in a greater state of change than that of the use of anti-infective agents for the treatment of infection. Not only is the pattern of bacterial resistance to drugs changing, but newer, more effective drugs are being developed. What was written only 5 years ago is now largely outdated, and readers must evaluate the opinion expressed here with current opinion in their own hospitals.

The problem of bacterial resistance to drugs continues to cause concern and because of the great variability between hospitals, high vaginal, and cervical, swabs must be taken from all infected patients. The swab is then examined to determine the predominant bacteria present, and sensitivity studies are carried out. As this procedure takes time, the treatment originally prescribed may require to be altered later.

The type of antibiotic, or combination of antibiotics, chosen depends on the severity of the infection, particularly as therapy usually is started before the microbiology of the swab has been reported.

Amoxycillin (250–500mg) 8-hourly is effective against *E. coli* infections, streptococcal infections and anaerobic streptococcal infections. Penicillin has no biological effect against anaerobic Gram-negative (*Bacteroides*) infections. For such infections, clindamycin (150mg) 8-hourly or metronidazole (1g loading dose, and 200mg 8-hourly) should be chosen. If the infection is thought to be penicillinase-producing *Staphylococcus aureus*, intravenous methicillin, cloxacillin or cephalothin (6 to 8g a day in divided doses every 4 to 6 hours is chosen).

Suggested treatment falls into three categories:

1. *Early severe sepsis* (*often with associated shock*)
Intravenous administration of penicillin G (2 to 4 mega units) every 4 hours, *plus* intravenous or intramuscular kanamycin (500mg) or cefoxitin (2g) every 12 hours, *plus* metronidazole (1g loading dose, 400mg every 8 hours).

2. *Predominantly anaerobic infection*
Severe   Regimen as in (1) except that gentamicin (3mg/kg per day in 3 divided doses) is substituted for kanamycin.

Mild     Oral amoxycillin (500mg) every 8 hours, plus clindamycin (150mg) every 6 hours or metronidazole.

3. *Staphylococcus aureus infection*
Methicillin, cloxacillin or cephalothin.

It is frequently forgotten that optimal serum levels of oral penicillin are only obtained if the drug is given at least 3 hours after a meal, and more than 1 hour prior to taking food. This is because food interferes with the absorption of orally administered penicillin. In arranging a regimen of therapy, the patient must be given exact instructions as to when to take the penicillin and when she may eat food. In the absence of these instructions, apparent bacterial resistance to penicillin may be considered present, when the expected response fails to occur. Higher serum levels can be maintained by giving probenecid 0.5 to 1g twice or thrice daily for 2 to 3 days concurrently with the antibiotic.

If the infection is particularly severe, there is considerable merit as noted in giving ampicillin, or cloxacillin, intravenously by intermittent infusion, each infusion of the appropriate dose being given over a period of about 20 to 30 minutes at 4-hourly intervals.

Recently increasing numbers of postpartum genital tract infections have been found to be due to anaerobes (including *peptococci, Bacteroides fragilis* and *Bacteroides* species). This suggests that metronidazole or tinidazole may be the most appropriate drugs to be given initially, usually with a broad spectrum antibiotic. (This is because neither metronidazole nor tinidazole have any activity against aerobic pathogens in soft tissue pelvic infections.)

The precise regimen of medication adopted can only be determined after discussion with the hospital's microbiologist as bacterial resistance varies considerably between institutions. However, the principles of chemotherapy apply in obstetrics as in other branches of medicine. These are:

1. Take high vaginal and cervical swabs to determine the bacteria present and their sensitivity to the available antibiotics.
2. If treatment is considered necessary before this information is available, use the drug most likely to be effective. This demands a knowledge of bacterial resistance in the particular area.
3. Give adequate doses of the chosen drug, and treat for at least 5 days, or until 2 days after the infection is controlled.
4. If no improvement occurs within 72 hours, examine the patient again and consider if the drug or the dosage has been correctly chosen.
5. In general, do not indulge in polytherapy.

# VENOUS COMPLICATIONS IN PREGNANCY AND THE PUERPERIUM

In pregnancy there is a 50 per cent increase in the serum fibrinogen level, a 30 per cent increase in platelets, a rise in the levels of factors VII, VIII and X, and a reduction in fibrinolytic activity. Although the fibrinolytic activity returns abruptly to normal at delivery, the other changes persist into the late puerperium, and additionally there is an increase in platelet adhesiveness.

These chemical alterations in the blood of a pregnant and puerperal woman disturb the coagulation:lysis balance in the direction of hypercoagulation. This, together with the slowing of venous return from the legs in late pregnancy and the puerperium, increases the likelihood of venous thrombosis.

Between 0.1 and 1.5 per cent* of puerperal women may be expected to develop venous thrombosis, which may occur in the superficial or deep veins of the legs. It is usual to distinguish two types, thrombophlebitis in which a primary infective process is present, and phlebothrombosis in which the thrombus formation is due initially to minor damage of the vessel wall, and which is aggravated by circulatory stasis and sepsis. The distinction is of doubtful validity, and venous thrombosis considered here will include both types (Fig. **48/2**).

### Superficial venous thrombosis

This is the commonest form of venous thrombosis complicating pregnancy or the puerperium. It occurs in about 1 per cent of patients and nearly always arises in existing varicose veins. The cause is the altered coagulability of the blood and the marked venous stasis occurring in pregnancy and labour. Extension of the thrombus to involve the deep veins rarely occurs. Treatment is to apply a compression bandage to the elevated leg, to encourage activity and to withhold anticoagulants unless extension to deep veins is diagnosed.

### Deep venous thrombosis and pulmonary embolism

Deep venous thrombosis (DVT) occurs in 0.1 per cent of European patients, and in 0.02 per cent of

* The incidence in the USA and UK is said to be about 1.3 per cent, in Australia 1.0 per cent, and in the developing countries of Asia and Africa about 0.1 per cent.

Asian pregnant or puerperal women. In 20 per cent of cases the disorder appears in pregnancy, and in the rest usually becomes evident between the 5th and 15th days of the puerperium. Women who are over the age of 35, overweight, and who have been delivered by caesarean section, are especially at risk. The thrombotic process may involve deep veins in the calf, or may extend from the calf into the femoral or pelvic veins. Only when the latter occurs is there any great risk of pulmonary embolism. In the United Kingdom, pulmonary embolism is now the second commonest cause of maternal death, and an embolus is likely to occur once in every 4000 deliveries of women of European stock. One patient in four developing an embolus will die. In 75 per cent of cases the embolus occurs without any warning, and in only 25 per cent is there clinical evidence of venous thrombosis.

In Australia, pulmonary embolism is a significant cause of maternal death, but the incidence is lower than in Britain, one case occurring in every 6000 deliveries.

Clinical signs are a poor guide to the diagnosis of deep venous thrombosis, and do not give any indication whether the thrombus is stationary, lysing or progressing. The diagnosis is suggested by the presence of low-grade pyrexia, a raised pulse rate and the appearance of a feeling of uneasiness. Examination of the leg is the most accurate clinical diagnostic method and deep thrombosis is probable when pain and tenderness on firm palpation of the calf muscles are detected. However, these signs may be absent. Pain in the calf on dorsiflexion of the foot (Homan's sign) is misleading.

Because of the inadequacy of the clinical signs, and their diagnostic inaccuracy, deep venous thrombosis should not be diagnosed until further investigations have been made. The most accurate method is radiographic phlebography. This is expensive, invasive, may be painful and may induce venous thrombosis. A non-invasive technique, impedance plethysmography, is nearly as accurate. Impedance plethysmography relies on measuring the electrical impedance between two electrodes wrapped round the patient's calf, while venous blood flow is obstructed and then released by means of an inflatable cuff wrapped round the thigh.

DIRECTION OF
BLOODFLOW →

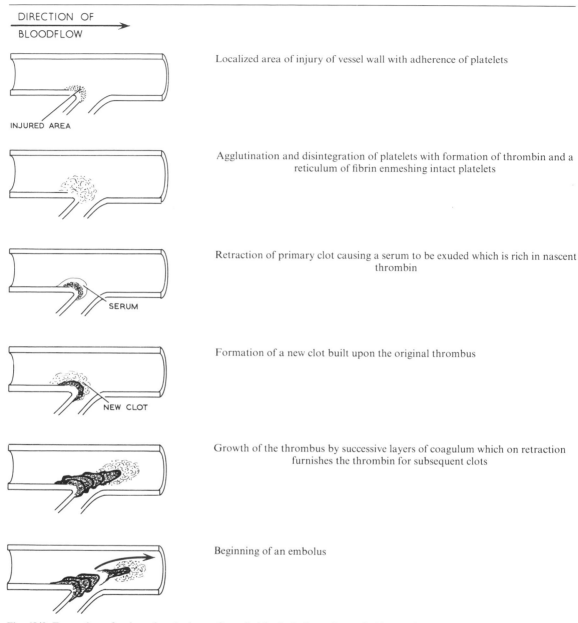

INJURED AREA

Localized area of injury of vessel wall with adherence of platelets

Agglutination and disintegration of platelets with formation of thrombin and a reticulum of fibrin enmeshing intact platelets

SERUM

Retraction of primary clot causing a serum to be exuded which is rich in nascent thrombin

NEW CLOT

Formation of a new clot built upon the original thrombus

Growth of the thrombus by successive layers of coagulum which on retraction furnishes the thrombin for subsequent clots

Beginning of an embolus

**Fig. 48/2** Formation of a thrombus (redrawn from Quick, A. J. *Surg. Gynecol. Obstet.* 1950, **91**, 296, by kind permission of the author and publishers)

Impedance plethysmography detects nearly all thrombi in or proximal to the popliteal vein, but may miss calf-vein thrombi. However, emboli from the calf veins are uncommon and usually of little clinical consequence. The method should be performed on days 3, 5 and 10 to detect the possible development of new thrombi. If normal readings are found, anticoagulants are not required.

If impedance plethysmography is used on all patients suspected of having venous thrombosis on clinical grounds, only one in four will be found to have DVT.

If the clinical signs and the diagnostic tests suggest venous thrombosis in pregnancy, anticoagulant treatment is needed throughout the remainder of the antenatal period and for 6 weeks after delivery.

If pulmonary embolism is suspected on clinical grounds (pleural pain, friction rub or haemoptysis) a chest radiograph, an electrocardiogram (to detect changes indicating right ventricular strain) and pulmonary venography or isotope perfusion lung scan (if available) should be ordered.

## TREATMENT

### Prophylaxis

There is no real evidence that anaemia or dehydration are predisposing causes, but on general principles these should be prevented in pregnancy and labour. The main cause is stasis of blood induced by immobility. Patients must be allowed full mobility as soon after vaginal delivery as possible, and the immobile patient must be forced into activity. Since venous thrombosis is more common after caesarean section, patients must be encouraged into movement. Complaints of leg pain and tenderness must be treated seriously, and further investigations made.

Only patients who have had more than one episode of DVT in the past should be considered for prophylactic heparin treatment because of the risk of demineralization of bone. If the woman is obese, over the age of 35 and has had several episodes of DVT, prophylactic heparin should be recommended because the risk of recurrence of DVT in pregnancy is about 10 per cent.

Women who have had a previous episode of confirmed DVT should be given 1 litre of dextran-70 over a period of 6 hours in early labour, and after delivery should be given prophylactic anticoagulants, as described in the next section.

### Curative

In pregnancy, heparin is usually started by adding 20 000U to 500ml of 5 per cent dextrose, infused intravenously at 25ml per hour. This provides 25 000U of heparin in 24 hours. The rate is adjusted to provide a blood heparin concentration of 0.6–1.0U per ml, as assessed by the protamine neutralization test. An alternative is to measure the activated partial prothrombin time (APPT) maintaining it at 1.5 to 2.0 times the control value.

Recent studies suggest the intravenous heparin may be replaced by subcutaneous injections of calcium heparin, which are as effective and cause fewer problems. The dose of calcium heparin needed is that which maintains the kaolin cephalin clotting time at 1.5 to 2.0 times its normal value.

If DVT is diagnosed after delivery, warfarin is started at the same time as heparin. The heparin is continued until warfarin has prolonged the international normalized ratio into the therapeutic range (> 2.5 to 2.6). Heparin is then stopped and warfarin is continued for 6 to 12 weeks in cases of proven DVT and for 12 to 24 weeks in cases of proven pulmonary embolism.

If the venous thrombosis is found to be iliofemoral in site, and fails to respond to heparin, or if pulmonary embolism occurs, expert advice should be obtained. The choice lies between the use of streptokinase and surgery. Streptokinase converts plasminogen into plasmin, which then attacks the fibrin clot, splitting it into soluble fibrin degradation products. Since these are potent disturbers of the coagulation : lysis balance, haemorrhagic states may occur with possible torrential uterine haemorrhage in the puerperium.

The place for surgery is very limited in uncomplicated deep venous thrombosis, although pulmonary embolectomy may be life-saving in certain cases of pulmonary embolism.

### Other measures

The patient should remain in bed until fully heparinized and until tenderness has gone from the limb. The limb should be supported by a firm crêpe bandage or a properly fitted elastic stocking. During her stay in bed, the limb should be elevated and analgesics given to counter the pain.

# PSYCHIATRIC DISORDERS

In the months after childbirth three psychiatric conditions may occur which seem to be related to pregnancy and childbirth. They are 'third day blues', postpartum depression and postpartum psychosis.

### Third day blues

Between 50 and 70 per cent of mothers become emotionally labile between the third and the fifth day after the birth of the baby. The emotional lability usually lasts for less than a week but may persist for a month. It is discussed under the heading of 'adjustment to childbirth' on p. 135.

### Postpartum depression

From 5 to 10 per cent of women develop clinically diagnosed depression in the first 3 months after childbirth; and twice that proportion have psychometric evidence of depression. Postpartum depression may be a manifestation of persistent maladjustment to parenting. Certain factors are associated with an increased risk that postpartum depression will occur. These are:

* lack of experience of parenting when a child or an adolescent (for example caring for a younger sibling);
* an unstable family during childhood and adolescence;
* lack of positive support from husband or partner during and after pregnancy;
* inaccessibility of a near relative or friend who can care for the baby from time to time.

Postpartum depression must be distinguished from postpartum emotional lability. Women suffering from postpartum depression show the symptoms of ordinary depressive illness. Management requires support and encouragement. The doctor should *listen* to the woman, help her resolve her anxieties and conflicts about her ability to be a parent, and arrange for assistance in caring for the baby from time to time. In some cases (provided that the woman is not profoundly depressed) one of the tricyclic drugs or the newer antidepressants may be needed. In severe depression psychiatric consultation should be obtained.

### Postpartum psychosis

Between one and three women per 1000 develop postpartum psychosis. This is usually an affective psychosis, but may present as schizophrenia. The woman requires admission to hospital and drug treatment. Most patients respond well and make a full recovery within a few months. About 15 per cent will again develop the illness after another pregnancy; and 30 per cent will develop a non-puerperal psychosis.

# Part Five

# OBSTETRIC OPERATIONS

*Those who intend to practise Midwifery, ought first of
all, to make themselves masters of anatomy, and
acquire a competent knowledge in surgery and physic;
but, over and above the advantages of education, the
accoucheur ought to be embued with a natural sagacity,
resolution, and prudence; together with that humanity
which adorns the owner, and never fails of being
agreeable to the distressed patient: in consequence of
this virtue, he will assist the poor as well as the rich,
behaving always with charity and compassion.*

W. Smellie (1756)

## Chapter 49

# Termination of Pregnancy and Induction of Labour

In the first 19 weeks of pregnancy, intervention to terminate pregnancy is synonymous with procuring an abortion. The recent, more rational, liberal attitude to induced abortion has reduced the danger of legal action by the State and, in many nations the anti-abortion laws have been altered to permit abortion with certain safeguards. As has been discussed in Chapter 22, legally induced abortion is now relatively safe, particularly if the abortion is performed before the end of the 10th gestational week,

by a skilled obstetrician, in appropriate surroundings.

In the second half of pregnancy, termination of pregnancy is a proper procedure if it is done to rescue the fetus from a hostile intra-uterine environment, or in a few cases, to save the life of the mother. In the third quarter of pregnancy, termination is occasionally performed when the child is grossly defective, or has inherited some genetic disorder.

## INDUCTION OF ABORTION

**Weeks 2 to 11**

Induced abortion is four times as safe if the procedure is done before the end of the 10th gestational week. In this quarter of pregnancy the mortality is less than 2 per 100 000 abortions. Consequently, all delays which prevent a woman obtaining an abortion must be eliminated.

Abortion in weeks 2 to 11 may be effected by the use of prostaglandin analogues, by suction curette or by using standard curettage. The last is the least suitable as it is followed by more complications.

Between weeks 5 and 7, the conceptus may be removed by using a narrow plastic tube attached to a 50ml syringe (menstrual regulation). Another method used, if the pregnancy is less than 8 weeks, is to give an oral tablet of mifepristone (150mg) daily for 4 days and 48 hours after the first tablet insert a vaginal pessary of gemeprost (prostaglandin $E_1$ analogue) 1.0mg. Bleeding usually starts 36 hours after the first tablet of mifepristone, and uterine contractions follow the gemeprost pessary;

95 per cent of women abort completely, bleeding lasting up to 12 days; the remaining 5 per cent require curettage to remove retained products of conception. After insertion of the vaginal pessary of gemeprost, one-third of women experience nausea or vomiting, and half need an analgesic.

Alternatively, the termination of pregnancy may be delayed until the 7th week, when suction curettage is used. The instrument is a hollow glass, plastic or metal tube, made in various sizes, which relate to the sizes of Hegar's dilators. The curette is connected by heavy transparent tubing to a vacuum pump which can produce a negative pressure (Fig. **49/1**). The patient is anaesthetized, either by intravenous thiopentone, or paracervical nerve block, a bimanual examination is performed, and the cervix is dilated to the appropriate size (Table **49/1**). The corresponding suction curette is introduced and a negative pressure is obtained. An intravenous injection of Syntometrine or of ergometrine 0.25mg is given. The walls of the uterus are stroked firmly from the fundus to the cervix, and the conceptus sac is drawn through

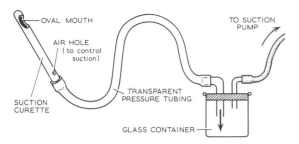

**Fig. 49/1** The suction-curette apparatus. (Source: Kerslake, D. and Casey, D. *Obstet Gynecol.* 1967, **30**, 35)

| Week of pregnancy | Dilatation of cervix (Hegar) mm | Negative pressure kg/cm² |
|---|---|---|
| <8 | 8 | 6.0 |
| 8 to 9 | 10 | 7.0 |
| 10 to 12 | 12 | 8.0 |

**Table 49/1** The suction curette. The degree to which the cervix must be dilated, and the negative pressure required, related to the duration of pregnancy

the curette and the tube. When the cavity is empty, an intramuscular injection of ergometrine 0.25mg is given.

Experience in many countries has shown that the suction curette causes less trauma, and is attended by less haemorrhage than the older method of dilatation and curettage.

If the metal curette is preferred, the vulva and vagina are prepared and draped. A vaginal examination defines the size, the position and the shape of the uterus. An Auvard speculum exposes the cervix which is grasped with a tenaculum. The direction of the cervical canal and length of the uterus is determined by a uterine sound. An injection of pituitrin 10 units intramuscularly, or ergometrine 0.25mg intravenously, is given. The cervix is dilated slowly until it will admit a sponge forceps. The contents of the uterus are evacuated piece by piece with the sponge-holding forceps, in the following manner. The forceps is introduced to the fundus, the jaws are opened and closed whilst being turned through 90°. This grasps fetal tissue without damaging the uterine wall. There is usually a fairly heavy loss of blood, and the procedure takes time. When most of the contents have been removed the uterus is curetted using a large curette. The sponge-holder is re-introduced and the procedure repeated until the uterus is empty. An injection of ergometrine 0.5mg is given intramuscularly at the conclusion of the operation.

## Weeks 12 to 19

Two methods, the use of 20% saline, and that of prostaglandins, have completely altered the management of induced abortion in the second quarter of pregnancy. They have almost replaced the older method of hysterotomy (Fig. 49/2).

The two methods were investigated by a Task Force of the World Health Organization which reported in 1976, and 1977. Their conclusions were as follows:

1. The use of prostaglandins is significantly more effective than hypertonic saline in inducing abortion between the 12th and 19th week of pregnancy. The injection-delivery interval is shorter (18 hours compared with 30 hours), but the problems of haemorrhage, cervical damage, or the need for blood transfusion no greater when prostaglandin is used in preference to hypertonic saline.

2. Following the abortion about 40 per cent of women will require a curettage, performed gently, to remove residual placental tissue.

3. For pregnancies of 12 to 15 weeks' gestation, 15-methyl prostaglandin $F_{2\alpha}$, 2.5mg in viscous dextran-70 (1ml) is introduced into the extra-ovular space. If the pregnancy has advanced to 16 or more weeks, 15-methyl prostaglandin $F_{2\alpha}$ 2.5mg introduced into the amniotic sac is more effective. In each case more than 90 per cent of women abort in 24 hours.

Other methods are to insert a laminaria tent into the cervix 12 hours before giving intramuscular injections of $PGF_{2\alpha}$ alpha (0.25mg every 2 hours); or placing tablets of 15-methyl $PGF_{2\alpha}$ methyl ether (1.5mg) high in the vagina every 3 hours until the abortion occurs.

The abortion rate following any of these regimens is similar, and the interval between starting treatment with prostaglandin and aborting averages 14 hours.

4. The main side-effects of prostaglandins are nausea, vomiting and diarrhoea. Significantly more women have the gastro-intestinal effects when prostaglandins are used (averaging between 2 and 5 episodes per patient) than when hypertonic saline is used (less than 0.5 episode per patient). Vaginal tablets of prostaglandin are associated with more gastro-intestinal side-effects than intra-amniotic or extra-ovular (extra-amniotic) routes of injection.

Abortion, using prostaglandins or hypertonic saline should be delayed until the 15th or 16th week of pregnancy, as both methods are more effective at this time.

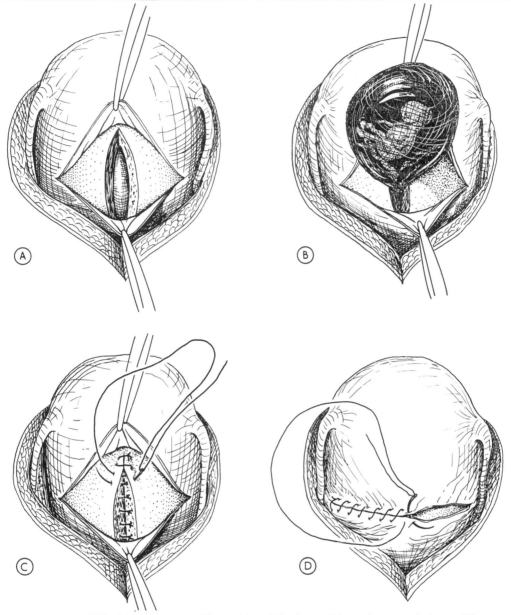

**Fig. 49/2** Hysterotomy. (A) Incision into uterus; (B) expulsion of the fetus within the intact amniotic sac; (C) suture of the wound; (D) the flap of peritoneum is sutured over the wound

A number of gynaecologists believe that vaginal evacuation of the fetus by ovum forceps, curettage and crushing of the fetal head is associated with a morbidity or mortality no greater than that when prostaglandins are used. However, they stress that these results are only obtained when the operation is performed by experienced surgeons.

Termination in the second quarter of pregnancy

should, in general, only be performed in hospitals or clinics where full biochemical and resuscitation services are available.

### Weeks 20 to 29

When termination is required in the third quarter of pregnancy, the chances of survival of the fetus are less than 25 per cent, and the choice of hypertonic saline, prostaglandins or planned hysterotomy depends on the condition of the mother, the maturity of the fetus, and the inclination of the obstetrician.

# INDUCTION OF LABOUR

Termination of pregnancy may be required pre-term (i.e. <37 weeks), at term (i.e. 37 to 41 weeks), or post-term (i.e. 42 completed weeks or more) when: (1) fetal survival is jeopardized if it remains in the uterus; or (2) if the mother's life, or health, is in danger.

The method adopted will depend on: (1) the duration of the pregnancy; (2) the urgency for the delivery; (3) the condition of the cervix; and (4) the degree of engagement of the presenting part in the mother's pelvis. For example, if the patient is primigravid, has severe deteriorating hypertension and proteinuria at 34 weeks' gestation, with the fetal head unengaged in the pelvis, and the cervix unfavourable for induction of labour, caesarean section is the method of choice. In general, however, the aim is to deliver the patient vaginally provided this can be performed without risk to mother or child.

The methods available for induction of labour will be described, but first, it is important to understand the concept of a 'favourable' and 'unfavourable' cervix. A 'favourable' or 'ripe' cervix is soft in texture, usually partly effaced and 2 or more centimetres dilated. An 'unfavourable' or 'unripe' cervix is firm in texture and usually not effaced or dilated (Fig. 49/3).

A more accurate assessment of the probable success rate of induction of labour (in terms of the induction–delivery interval) can be made by taking a cervical score. The higher the score the more favourable is the cervix and the shorter the induction to delivery interval (Table 49/2).

The principal indications for termination of pregnancy after the 28th week vary somewhat in different countries, but in all, hypertensive disease in pregnancy and postmaturity are the most common indications (Table 49/3).

**Hypertensive disease in pregnancy**

PIH is the principal reason for termination of pregnancy, and induction of labour should be carried out when there is an inadequate response to medical treatment, or if there is deterioration in the disease process. Since the decision is made on all the available evidence in each individual case, no precise time for induction can be stated. Clinical experience and judgment remain the principal guides supplemented by the use of biophysical tests for fetal well being. Pregnancy in patients with essential hypertension may continue to between the 38th week and term, when induction should be carried out; but if PIH

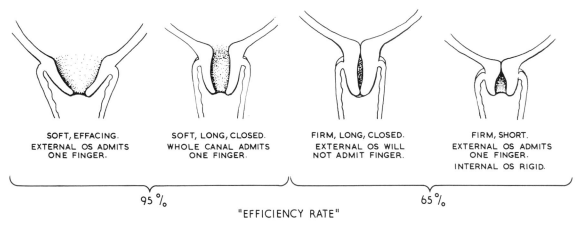

| SOFT, EFFACING. EXTERNAL OS ADMITS ONE FINGER. | SOFT, LONG, CLOSED. WHOLE CANAL ADMITS ONE FINGER. | FIRM, LONG, CLOSED. EXTERNAL OS WILL NOT ADMIT FINGER. | FIRM, SHORT. EXTERNAL OS ADMITS ONE FINGER. INTERNAL OS RIGID. |

95%                                    65%

"EFFICIENCY RATE"

**Fig. 49/3** The relationship between the condition of the cervix and success rate of surgical induction (redrawn from Cocks, D. P. *Brit. Med. J.* 1955, **1**, 327, by permission of the author, editor and publisher)

| Factor | Score rating | | | |
|---|---|---|---|---|
| | 0 | 1 | 2 | 3 |
| *Cervix* | | | | |
| Length (cm) | >4 | >2 | 1–2 | <1 |
| Dilatation (cm) | <1 | <2 | 2–3 | >4 |
| Consistency | Firm | 'Average' | Soft | — |
| Position | Posterior | Other (mid, anterior) | | — |
| *Fetal head* | | | | |
| Position relative to ischial spines (cm) | −3 | −2 | −1 or 0 | +1 or more |

**Table 49/2** A method of cervical 'Scoring'. *Score*: unfavourable 0–4; favourable 5+

| | *Percentage of all inductions* |
|---|---|
| PIH or eclampsia ⎫ | |
| Chronic hypertension ⎬ | 20 to 50 |
| Chronic nephritis ⎭ | |
| Postmaturity | 35 to 60 |
| Placenta praevia ⎫ | |
| Accidental haemorrhage ⎬ | 4 to 12 |
| Fetal abnormality ⎫ | |
| Intra-uterine death ⎬ | 5 |
| Hydramnios ⎭ | |
| Rhesus iso-immunization | 5 to 15 |
| Contracted pelvis, disproportion ⎫ | |
| Unstable lie ⎬ | 1 to 5 |
| Maternal disease or distress ⎫ | |
|   Diabetes | |
|   Cardiac disease ⎬ | 5 to 10 |
|   Tuberculosis | |
|   Obstetric history ⎭ | |

**Table 49/3** Indications for induction of labour. From studies in Australia, Britain and Malaysia

is superimposed upon the essential hypertension, earlier induction is usually required. If the hypertension is labile, pregnancy should in general not continue beyond term, but each case must be assessed individually. In chronic nephritis, placental dysfunction is common, and induction of premature labour should be considered if clinical deterioration of the patient's condition occurs, or if the fetus is considered to be at risk as judged by biophysical or biochemical tests.

**Postmaturity** (prolonged pregnancy)

There is increasing evidence that prolongation of

pregnancy, in a woman with a normal menstrual cycle, beyond 294 days (42 completed weeks), adds a significant hazard to the fetus. Not only is the baby larger, its skull more ossified, and the risk of unexplained death in utero increased, but there is a higher incidence of mental damage amongst surviving children. Increasing numbers of obstetricians feel that pregnancy should be terminated between 10 and 14 days after the estimated date of delivery. No patient with PIH or essential hypertension should be allowed to continue the pregnancy more than 7 days beyond term.

**Antepartum haemorrhage**

Induction of labour, by amniotomy, may be appropriate in cases of moderate or severe abruptio placentae, once blood has been replaced adequately by transfusion. Patients with a minor degree of placenta praevia (anterior wall implantation) should have labour induced by amniotomy at the 37th or 38th week.

**Fetal malformation and fetal intra-uterine death**

In most cases induction of labour is carried out once a gross fetal abnormality incompatible with life (mainly anencephaly) is detected, provided that conditions are suitable. Anencephalic babies may grow to a large size and the malformation is usually accompanied by hydramnios which can distress the mother considerably. Cases of intra-uterine death, once diagnosed, are best treated by induction of labour because of the distress caused to the mother by the knowledge of the condition, and of the danger of hypofibrinogenaemia.

### Rhesus iso-immunization

Premature induction of labour is made when amniocentesis reveals an increasingly severe haemolytic process in the baby provided it is sufficiently mature to survive. Other maternal diseases, or cases where unexplained death of the fetus occurs in the later weeks of pregnancy, may require premature induction. Each case must be assessed on the available evidence before a decision is made.

### Contracted pelvis and unstable lie

A multigravida with a contracted pelvis of minor degree may be treated by premature induction of labour, but the case must be selected carefully, and the method should only be used by experienced obstetricians. If the lie of the baby is unstable, particularly if oblique or transverse, detected after the 37th week and recurring despite correction, labour should be induced by amniotomy after correction, the presenting part being led into the pelvis at the same time.

### Diabetes

In some cases of diabetes the pregnancy should be terminated by the end of the 38th week, but earlier termination may be required if hypertension supervenes. In multigravidae who have previously delivered vaginally and in selected primigravidae, amniotomy is preferred to caesarean section.

### Elective (social) induction

During the late 1960s and early 1970s, increasing numbers of patients were induced electively at or near term. The reasons given were that the mother could more conveniently arrange her house and family if she knew when she was to give birth; the husband could plan for leave of absence from work; and it was more convenient for the doctor and the hospital.

In many hospitals in the USA over 50 per cent of labours were induced electively, whilst in Britain and Australia, the proportion was between 30 and 45 per cent.

Elective induction of labour was associated with a higher forceps and caesarean section rate, a higher incidence of neonatal jaundice and no reduction in the perinatal mortality rate.

Since 1977, the fashion has changed and in most hospitals fewer than 20 per cent of labours are induced electively.

### Fetal intra-uterine growth retardation

In some cases of diagnosed fetal intra-uterine growth retardation, labour may be induced to avoid possible intra-uterine death of the fetus.

## TECHNIQUES OF INDUCTION

If the obstetrician, after analysing the case, determines that induction of labour is necessary, he has the choice of several methods. These fall into two main groups, (1) medicinal and (2) surgical, although in many instances both may be used for the same patient.

### Medicinal

There are two main methods of medicinal induction of labour. These are (1) prostaglandins, $F_{2\alpha}$ and $E_2$ infusion and (2) physiological oxytocin infusion.

#### PROSTAGLANDINS

In recent years prostaglandins (PGs) are being used increasingly to induce labour. The two commonly used PGs are $PGE_2$ and $PGF_{2\alpha}$. The substance may be given as vaginal pessaries, or gels; intracervically as a gel; into the extra-ovular space (between the decidua and the amniotic sac) as a gel; intra-amniotically as a solution; or intravenously.

$PGE_2$ vaginal pessaries, placed high in the vagina at intervals, are the most effective and least invasive way of decreasing cervical resistance. $PGE_2$ acts on the cervical connective tissue and relaxes cervical muscle fibres, thus 'ripening and opening the cervix'. It also increases the contractions of the uterine muscle (i.e. induces labour). The dose of $PGE_2$ varies depending on the duration of the pregnancy and the condition of the cervix. In mid-pregnancy $PGE_2$ 5mg (in triacetin gel) is used; in late pregnancy ($>35$ weeks) the dose is reduced to 2mg. The pessaries are placed in the posterior vaginal fornix. The patient's condition and uterine contractions are monitored for 1 hour, after which she may walk about if she wishes, and the pregnancy is not at 'high risk'. If labour has not become established after 4 to 6 hours, or there is no change in the state of the cervix, a further 2mg pessary is introduced. If the condition of the cervix is suitable, amniotomy is performed. This method and the more invasive intracervical or extra-amniotic installations have a similar success rate to vaginal $PGE_2$ tablets.

Side-effects, usually nausea, vomiting or diarrhoea are unusual, when this dose is used.

The methods may also be used to decrease cervical resistance, before attempting the vaginal evacuation of the fetus in late abortions.

Vaginal, intracervical and extra-ovular prostaglandins in general have superseded the intra-amniotic and intravenous routes, although in some cases the last may be preferred. Intravenous $PGE_2$ in a concentration of $2.5\mu g/ml$ or $PGF_2$ in a concentration of $0.5\mu g/ml$ are equally effective in inducing labour. The drugs are given in an incremental manner.

The appropriate concentration of $PGE_2$ is obtained by mixing stock $PGE_2$ with 0.9 per cent saline to give the concentration of $2.5\mu g/ml$. The infusion is then run initially to supply $10\mu g/kg/ml$, the rate being doubled hourly if required to a maximum of $50\mu g/kg/ml$. Over 95 per cent of the patients studied delivered within 24 hours. If labour does not progress smoothly following prostaglandin induction, an intravenous oxytocin infusion may be set up. In most series, between 20 and 40 per cent of PG inductions require this additional therapy.

If prostaglandins are used carefully, uterine contractions being monitored, the risk of hypertonic uterine activity or of uterine rupture is very small, although both have been reported.

## OXYTOCIN (SYNTOCINON)

Oxytocin should be given by intravenous infusion, preferably using an infusion pump. There is no place for intramuscular injections of oxytocin either in the induction or stimulation of labour, as they have been followed by fetal death, and ruptured uterus. Similarly, oxytocin delivered by nasal spray is to be condemned as inefficient and potentially dangerous. Oxytocin infusion will induce labour in 50 to 60 per cent of patients but is more efficient if used following PG vaginal pessaries or after amniotomy. Its main place, until recently, was to soften the 'unripe' cervix prior to amniotomy in cases of intra-uterine death of the fetus. Prostaglandins have superseded it for this purpose.

## PHYSIOLOGICAL OXYTOCIN INFUSION

Oxytocin is a potent stimulant of uterine activity and for this reason should only be used with due care, and in physiological doses. In general, the infusion should provide no more than 5mU/minute of oxytocin. A convenient regimen described on p. 416 is summarized here: an intravenous infusion of 15U (or 7.5U) of Syntocinon in a litre of normal saline is given via an infusion pump. The rate is increased by 5mU a minute at 20-minute intervals until contractions are obtained which last about 60 seconds and recur at 3–5-minute intervals. Usually the maximum concentration given is 60mU per minute. Because of the risk of water intoxication, the quantity of fluid infused should not exceed 1500ml in a 10-hour period, and no infusion should run for longer than this time (Table **49/4**).

| Rate | Concentration of solution | | |
|---|---|---|---|
| (drops per minute) | 2U/litre | 7.5U/litre | 15U/litre |
| 5 | 0.7 | 2.5 | 5 |
| 10 | 2 | 5.0 | 10 |
| 20 | | 10 | 20 |
| 30 | 4 | 15 | 30 |
| 40 | | 20 | 40 |
| 45 | 6 | | 45 |
| 50 | | 25 | 50 |
| 60 | 8 | 30 | 60 |

**Table 49/4** Oxytocin infusion, relationship between concentration of the solution, the rate of the infusion and the millilitres of oxytocin per minute

### Surgical methods

Artificial rupture of the membranes (amniotomy) is the method of choice when induction of labour is required. Two complementary methods are available: (1) rupture of the forewaters, and (2) rupture of the hindwaters. Originally, it was believed that amniotomy induced uterine contractions by decreasing the uterine volume. This belief is no longer tenable, but it is not clear how amniotomy works.

A possible explanation is that the concomitant stretching the cervix (and stripping the membranes) alters the relationship between the fetal membranes and the decidua with a resulting prompt and substantial release of prostaglandins. These in turn cause cervical 'ripening' and initiate uterine contractions. At the same time oxytocin is released from the pituitary gland because of cervical manipulation (the

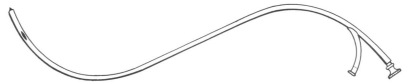

**Fig. 49/4** The Drew-Smythe catheter

Ferguson reflex) and co-ordinates the uterine contractions, so that the triple descending gradient of uterine activity is established.

### THE FOREWATERS

The patient is placed in the lithotomy position and the vulva is swabbed with chlorhexidine solution and the vagina filled with chlorhexidine cream. The operation can usually be performed without anaesthesia, although pethidine 100mg may be given to an apprehensive patient. Two fingers of the right hand are introduced into the vagina and the index finger passes through the cervix and strips the membranes from the lower segment. The membranes are ruptured with a Kocher forceps or some other instrument such as an 'amnihook'. The hole made in the membranes is enlarged with the index finger. About 500ml of liquor is allowed to drain, if necessary by displacing the head of the fetus slightly upwards. Before withdrawing the finger the position of the presenting part is checked and the absence of a prolapsed cord noted. The fetal heart is monitored for 30 minutes after amniotomy to detect irregularities.

### THE HINDWATERS

When the cervix will not readily admit a finger and when induction of labour is essential either the use of vaginal PGE$_2$ pessaries are used or rupture of the hindwaters is performed. The method is identical with that of low amniotomy except that a curved Drew-Smythe catheter (Fig. **49/4**), with the stylette withdrawn, is passed through the cervix between the amniotic membranes and the uterine wall until the hindwaters are reached. The stylette is pushed in and penetrates the membranes. If blood is obtained, the catheter is withdrawn and replaced in another direction. About 200 to 500ml of liquor is allowed to drain away and the remainder of the operation is the same as that of low amniotomy. The method is rarely used today.

### Reducing the induction/delivery interval

Three approaches are possible.
(1) to insert a PGE$_2$ vaginal pessary the evening before amniotomy or 3 hours before the procedure.
(2) to set up an intravenous oxytocin infusion at the time of amniotomy
(3) to delay 6 to 12 hours before setting up the oxytocin infusion as about 50 per cent of women are in labour by this time.

The advantages of using a PGE$_2$ vaginal pessary pre-amniotomy are that the woman can continue to be mobile, about two-thirds of the patients will be in labour within 6 hours of amniotomy (thus avoiding an oxytocin infusion) and the procedure is non-invasive. If an oxytocin infusion is set up at the time of amniotomy, or 6 to 12 hours later, it is given preferably by an automatic infusion pump, in incremental doses (see p. 416–17). Labour should be monitored and large doses (more than 40mU per minute) should not be infused until cephalopelvic disproportion has been excluded.

### Efficiency of surgical induction

Surgical induction is more efficient the nearer the patient is to term. To some extent the duration of the induction–delivery interval is related to the condition of the cervix. If the cervix is favourable (soft as the lips and admitting at least one finger), between 70 and 80 per cent of patients will have delivered with 24 hours and 90 to 95 per cent within 48 hours, particularly if an oxytocin infusion is used in selected cases. If the cervix is unfavourable (firm as the tip of the nose) the 'efficiency rate' falls to about 65 per cent (see Fig. **49/3**). Between 5 and 15 per cent of all inductions 'fail' and the patient has to be delivered by caesarean section.

### Risks of surgical induction

#### PROLAPSE OF THE CORD

This occurs in about 0.5 per cent of cases of amniotomy, more commonly when low amniotomy has been performed, because the head has to be displaced to release the liquor.

### INFECTION

The incidence of this complication is low, but the longer the induction–delivery interval, the greater is the risk. The infection begins as an amnionitis which may spread to the fetus causing pneumonia, or to the mother causing endometritis. Prophylactic antibiotics should not be given at the time of induction because of the danger of development of resistant strains of bacteria. If the induction–delivery interval exceeds 24 hours, the infection rate increases and many obstetricians recommend antibiotics after this time.

### ANTEPARTUM HAEMORRHAGE

Slight but significant bleeding may follow high amniotomy in less than 1 per cent of cases. If this occurs and is accompanied by fetal distress, caesarean section should be performed.

### POSTPARTUM HAEMORRHAGE

The risk of postpartum haemorrhage is doubled amongst women who have labour induced compared with women whose labour starts spontaneously.

### NEONATAL HYPERBILIRUBINAEMIA

Hyperbilirubinaemia (bilirubin concentration greater than $250 \mu mol/litre$ ($15mg/dl$)) appears more commonly in infants of women who have received an oxytocin infusion, especially if the total oxytocin administered exceeds 20 units. The degree of jaundice is usually without harm to the neonate but causes concern.

The degree of hyperbilirubinaemia is related to the total dose of oxytocin administered. There is evidence that it may be due to the antidiuretic effects of oxytocin (especially if diluted with 5 per cent dextrose) which lead to transplacental hyponatraemia, hypo-osmolarity and enhanced osmotic fragility of erythrocytes after birth. Hyperbilirubinaemia is usually without consequence, except when the baby is pre-term or affected by haemolytic disease or if additional risk factors for hyperbilirubinaemia are present.

### A suggested method of induction of labour

The state of the cervix is a major factor in choosing the appropriate method of induction. If the cervix is

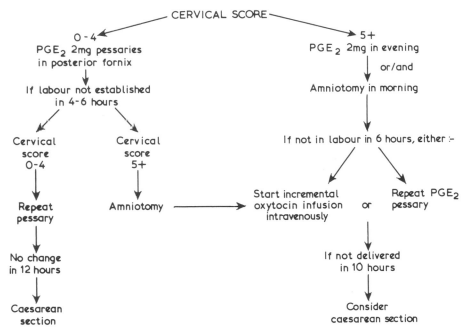

**Fig. 49/5** Induction of labour flow chart

unfavourable (i.e. it is firm or the cervical score is 0–4), the use of prostaglandin $E_2$ vaginal pessaries is preferred to an oxytocin infusion. If the cervix is favourable, low amniotomy, preceded (if desired) the evening before induction with the insertion of a vaginal pessary ($PGE_2$ 2mg in Witespol) is the method of choice. Following either of these methods, either at once or if labour is not established within 6 hours, a further prostaglandin vaginal pessary may be inserted, or a dilute oxytocin infusion started (Fig. **49/5**).

# Chapter 50

# Forceps

In the 400 years since the invention of a secret instrument designed to deliver the fetal head from the birth canal, the obstetric forceps has developed considerably. Two hundred years ago a curve was added to the blades to enable them to be introduced more readily into the curved birth canal, and at about the same time a double-slotted lock to join the two blades was invented by Smellie. One hundred years ago a device which enabled the surgeon to apply traction in the axis of the pelvis was added.

Today the obstetric forceps is a precision-tooled, correctly constructed instrument of great power. But with the increase in precision, and in power, there is an increased need for the obstetrician to know the uses and limitations of the instrument, and to realize that skill, and not strength, is the key to a successful forceps delivery. There are today no dangerous obstetric forceps; unfortunately there are still dangerous obstetricians who misuse the instrument.

## Description of the obstetric forceps

Of more than 600 variants of the obstetric forceps only three types need be considered. These are: (1) *the long-shanked forceps* (Simpson, Barnes–Neville, Luikart); (2) *the light short-shanked forceps* (Wrigley), and (3) *the Kielland forceps*.

The instrument consists of two blades, named right or left, depending on the side of the pelvis in which they will lie after being applied to the fetal head. The blades are usually fenestrated, for lightness, but in Luikart's forceps they are solid. The blades are curved on the flat to fit the fetal head (the *cephalic curve*), and curved on edge to fit the concavity of the sacrum (the *pelvic curve*) (Fig. **50/1**). The essential difference between Kielland's forceps and other types is that the pelvic curve has been largely eliminated.

Each blade is joined to the *handle* by the *shank*

which is of variable length. The two blades are fitted together by a *lock*, which in most forceps consists of opposing *shoulders* with a flange, but in the Kielland's forceps is sliding.

### THE LONG-SHANKED FORCEPS

As its name indicates the shank is long, and in addition the forceps has an attachment for an axis traction device, as in the Barnes–Neville instrument. The axis traction device was originally introduced so that when the head was arrested at the pelvic brim, traction could be made in the axis of the birth canal. Today high forceps is condemned, but the axis traction device is often used for the delivery of the head from the high mid-pelvis. It is not strictly necessary, as the same effect can be obtained by using Pajot's manoeuvre (Fig. **50/2**). If it is employed the surgeon must resist the temptation to pull on the device with all his strength, his feet braced against the foot of the bed. This is not skilful obstetrics, it is brute force and ignorance!

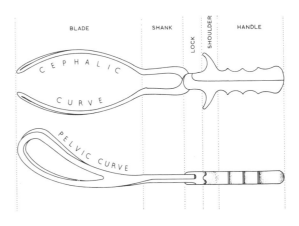

**Fig. 50/1** Simpson's obstetric forceps

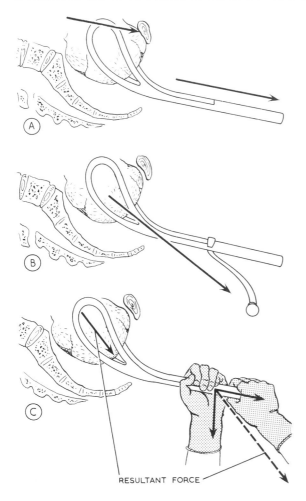

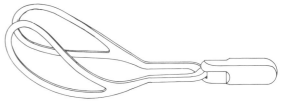

**Fig. 50/3** Wrigley's forceps (scale × half that of Figs **50/1** and **50/4**)

near the vulval outlet, the light Wrigley forceps is a better instrument and can often be applied painlessly, with the minimum of anaesthesia (Fig. **50/3**).

### THE KIELLAND FORCEPS

Originally introduced to deliver the unengaged head, Kielland's forceps is today used exclusively to deliver the baby whose head is arrested in the transverse or posterior diameter of the mid-pelvis (the deep transverse arrest and persistent occipito-posterior positions of the vertex). Since the forceps has no marked pelvic curve the blades can be applied to the sides of the fetal head as it lies, and the forceps and head can then be rotated so that the sagittal suture lies in the favourable antero-posterior diameter of the pelvis (Fig. **50/4**).

**The action of obstetric forceps**

The forceps has two actions, it is a *tractor* and a *compressor*. The Kielland forceps has an additional action as a *rotator*.

### TRACTION

The amount of traction which can be applied by the modern forceps is considerable, so good is the

RESULTANT FORCE

**Fig. 50/2** The mechanics of forceps delivery. (A) Mid-forceps; much of the pull is against the posterior surface of the symphysis. (B) Mid-forceps; with axis traction the force is resolved and the pull is in the axis of the birth canal. (C) Pajot's manoeuvre. The effect of axis traction is obtained with less potential damage

The advantage of the long-shanked forceps is that it permits delivery from the mid-pelvis, provided the head has rotated and the fetal sagittal suture lies in the antero-posterior diameter of the pelvis. It is also the instrument to use for the delivery of the after-coming head of a breech presentation.

### THE LIGHT SHORT-SHANKED FORCEPS

Although the heavier forceps just described can be used satisfactorily to deliver the fetal head which is

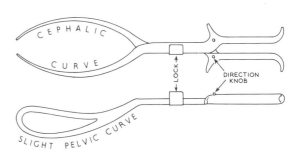

**Fig. 50/4** Kielland's forceps

design. It is for this reason that the instrument can become a dangerous weapon in the hands of the aggressive and inexperienced surgeon. The average pull required to deliver a baby from the mid-pelvis of a primigravida is about 18kg, and of a multigravida 12kg. This amount of pull can be exceeded with the arms alone and the braced weight of the entire body of the surgeon is dangerous and damaging to the fetus.

## COMPRESSION

When forceps blades are properly applied to the sides of the fetal skull, most of the compressive forces are applied to the bony base of the skull. If the handles of the instrument are squeezed during delivery additional compressive forces are applied to the sides of the head, and compression laterally must cause extension in a vertical direction. The danger of this is that the falx cerebri may be torn if too much force is used.

## ROTATION

If the forceps has the normal pelvic curve, rotation of the forceps will cause damage to the vaginal tissues; the absence of a pelvic curve on the Kielland's forceps permits rotation to be used.

**Types and incidence of forceps delivery** (Fig. **50/5**)

## MID-FORCEPS

The forceps is applied to the fetal head, the biparietal diameter of which has passed the pelvic brim but

has not advanced much beyond the ischial spines. The sagittal suture of the fetal head is usually found in the transverse diameter of the pelvis but may be in any diameter.

## LOW FORCEPS

The forceps is applied to the fetal head, the biparietal diameter of which has advanced to, or beyond, the ischial tuberosities, is visible at the vulva, and has wholly rotated so that the sagittal suture lies in the antero-posterior diameter of the pelvic outlet. Low forceps includes outlet forceps, in which the rotated head distends the vulval ring, and would probably deliver spontaneously if an episiotomy were performed.

## INCIDENCE

The incidence of forceps varies from country to country. It is higher in the higher socio-economic groups, and when the patient is attended by a doctor.

In England and Wales in 1985, 10 per cent of all deliveries were effected by forceps (mid-forceps 2 percent; low forceps 8 per cent). In Australia, in 1985, forcep deliveries in teaching hospitals were performed for 20 per cent of all births. In the USA, the forceps rate exceeded 50 per cent. However, it is noteworthy that in all three countries, which have different philosophical attitudes to childbirth, mid-forceps with rotation of the fetal head account for fewer than 3 per cent of all deliveries.

The relatively uniform incidence of mid-forceps deliveries can be contrasted with the wide variation in low forceps deliveries. A low forceps generally is an easy operation; a mid-forceps delivery usually requires as much skill and judgement as a caesarean section and should not be attempted unless the obstetrician has that skill.

**Indications for forceps delivery**

Delivery by forceps is indicated:

1. If the duration of the second stage exceeds $1\frac{1}{2}$ hours (or more than one hour of pushing), or if the fetal head is delayed on the perineum for more than 30 minutes. These cases are generally due to: (a) transverse arrest of the head in the mid-cavity; (b) arrest of the head in a persistent posterior position in the mid-cavity or the lower

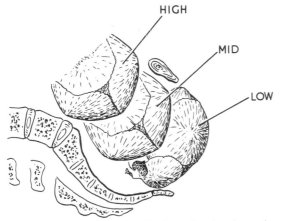

HIGH

MID

LOW

**Fig. 50/5** Types of forceps deliveries – showing the station of the head when the forceps are applied

straight; (c) minor degrees of disproportion; or (d) inadequacy of the uterine powers.

2. If the mother is distressed during the second stage of labour, or has some condition, such as a hypertensive disorder or cardiac disease, which may deteriorate in an energetic second stage. In these cases the use of the forceps to effect delivery is often prophylactic.

3. If the baby shows signs of fetal distress during the second stage.

4. For the delivery of the aftercoming head of a breech presentation.

**Conditions for forceps delivery**

1. The fetal head must be engaged in the maternal pelvis, that is, the greatest diameter of the fetal head must have passed through the pelvic inlet. If the fetal head is engaged there can obviously be no major degree of disproportion.

2. The cervix must be fully dilated. If the baby is dragged through an os which is not fully dilated, the immediate dangers are those of haemorrhage and trauma to the cervix, the vagina and the lower uterine segment; delayed dangers result from damage to the uterine supports predisposing to a uterovaginal prolapse.

3. The membranes should be ruptured before the forceps is applied, and the bladder and bowel should not be distended with urine and faeces respectively.

4. The forceps must only be applied so that the blades lie along the side of the fetal head, just in front of the ears (Fig. **50/6**).

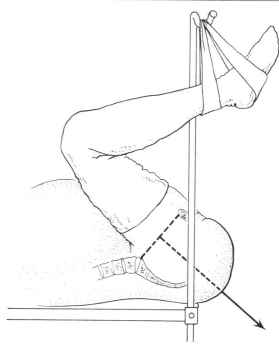

**Fig. 50/7** Position of the patient for mid-forceps delivery

5. A mid-forceps delivery should be considered a 'trial of forceps' and should only be attempted if the obstetrician is able and competent to proceed at once to caesarean section should his attempt fail. In no case should excessive force be used by an aggressive operator unable to admit defeat.

## TECHNIQUE OF FORCEPS DELIVERY

The patient is placed in the lithotomy position, and if a Kielland forceps delivery is to be attempted the buttocks should project over the end of the table, which should be raised (Fig. **50/7**). This enables traction to be made in the pelvic axis irrespective of the station of the head.

### Anaesthesia

If Wrigley's forceps are used, perineal nerve block, supplemented by inhalations of Trilene, or gas and oxygen, is usually adequate, although pudendal nerve block is to be preferred. Pudendal nerve block gives adequate anaesthesia for a mid-forceps application when no rotation is required, but, in general, rotation and extraction by forceps requires general or epidural anaesthesia.

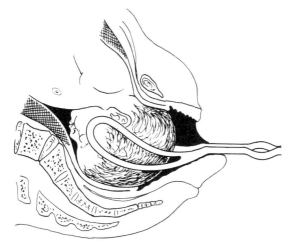

**Fig. 50/6** The ideal application of forceps

## Preliminary procedures

The thighs and vulva are cleansed with antiseptic, and obstetric antiseptic cream is poured over the area and into the vagina. Sterile drapes are applied, and if a mid-forceps is to be attempted a catheter is passed and the bladder emptied. A vaginal examination confirms that all the conditions for forceps delivery have been fulfilled, and re-ascertains the position and station of the fetal head. In many cases much caput will have formed, but a touch picture can be obtained by feeling for the triangular posterior fontanelle. The occipital bone underrides the two parietal bones making this obvious. If this area is obscured by caput, the ear of the fetus must be sought by introducing the whole hand into the vagina. The mastoid process, and its junction with the tragus of the ear, points to the occiput. The perineum is 'ironed out', and if it is proposed to use Kielland's forceps a mediolateral episiotomy is performed. In all other forceps deliveries it is usual to make the episiotomy when the fetal head is distending the perineum.

## Application of forceps with a pelvic curve

This is shown in the illustrations, and the steps explain a procedure which can only be learnt properly by observation of actual deliveries, by practice on the 'phantom' and by applying forceps under expert guidance. This type of forceps should only be applied when the occiput is anterior or within 30° of the anterior position. The blades should only be applied so that they are ideally positioned relative to the child's head.

### STEP 1. APPLICATION

The assembled forceps is held in front of the patient with the pelvic curve uppermost. The left blade is selected, and is held lightly between the thumb and first two fingers of the left hand, the right blade being temporarily laid aside. Two or three fingers of the right hand are introduced into the vagina (in the case of a mid-forceps the whole hand may be introduced) to lie between the fetal head and the posterolateral vaginal wall. The left blade is held over the pubis and is introduced delicately between the fetal head and the operator's fingers (Fig. **50/8A**). The blade is introduced directly between the lateral vaginal wall and the fetal skull and is steered, aided by the fingers, to lie alongside the left side of the child's

head. The whole movement is smooth and gentle, and the blade passes from the vertical to the horizontal in an arc, the handle being lowered as the blade disappears inside the vulva, and comes to lie pressed on the perineum (Fig. **50/8B**). The right blade is introduced in a similar manner, two fingers (or more) of the left hand being introduced into the vagina, and the blade being held in the right hand (Fig. **50/8C**). The depth to which each blade is initially introduced is determined by the station of the head: the higher the head the greater the depth to which it must be introduced.

### STEP 2. ADJUSTMENT

The handles are pressed gently downwards and as the blades adjust to the sides of the fetal skull, the lock is closed. If the lock does not close easily the blades have not been applied properly and if, after a little gentle manoeuvring they still will not close, the forceps should be withdrawn and reintroduced. The lock should not be forced to close. The handles should be fairly close to each other; if they are widely separated, the blades should be re-applied, as it is likely that the position of the head has been misinterpreted.

Only when the blades have been correctly positioned may the axis traction device be applied, and when the securing screw is tightened the handles should never be forcibly approximated.

### STEP 3. EXTRACTION

After locking the blades a gentle pull is made to confirm that they are fitting properly. The handles of the forceps are held with the right hand being placed over the shoulder, the index and middle fingers lying in the space at the lower end of the shank, and the thumbs pressing the under-surface of the handles (Fig. **50/8D**). Only in difficult mid-forceps deliveries are both hands required, or does the axis-traction device need to be used. Traction mimics a uterine contraction, and if contractions are present, as is usual, is applied in time with them. The pull is initially gradual, reaches a peak, is held for a moment and then gradually is relaxed. Between contractions the pressure on the handles or the screw of the axis-traction device is relaxed. It should also be remembered that the forceps move in an arc, simulating the movement the head makes (Fig. **50/8E**). Initially traction is downwards and backwards but

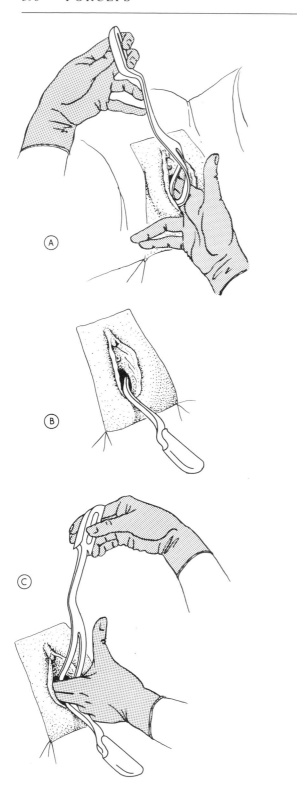

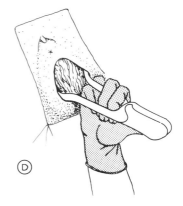

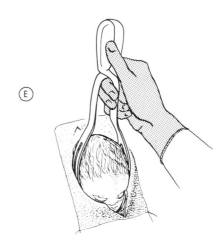

(A)  Introducing the left blade

(B)  The left blade is in position

(C)  The right blade is introduced

(D)  The blades are locked and traction downwards begins

(E)  The head has crowned, traction follows the pelvic curve and is now upwards

**Fig. 50/8**  Low forceps application

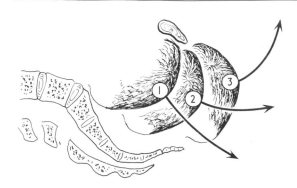

**Fig. 50/9** Diagram of the direction of traction in forceps delivery. In mid-forceps delivery (1) the initial direction of pull is downwards, in low forceps (2) horizontal and in outlet forceps (3) slightly upwards

as the perineum is broached it is progressively upwards (Fig. **50/9**). If the axis-traction device is used the handles are free and the arrow on the device indicates the direction in which to pull. If the perineum is distended a mid-line or, in the case of a difficult forceps, a mediolateral episiotomy is made. Once the head has been born the forceps is removed and the rest of the delivery is effected by the usual method.

**Application of Kielland's forceps in cases of deep transverse arrest**

STEP 1. SELECTION AND INTRODUCTION OF THE BLADE

The assembled forceps is held in front of the patient, the dot on the shoulder pointing to the occiput of the fetus. The blade which is superior is chosen. Two fingers of the hand on the same side as the fetal face are introduced into the vagina to lie posterolaterally between the head and the vaginal wall. The anterior blade is held delicately in the other hand, so that it is almost vertical, the tip of the blade lying on the palmar surface of the intravaginal fingers. The blade is introduced between the fetal scalp and the fingers until all of it, and about half the shank, are in the vagina (Fig. **50/10A**).

STEP 2. THE WANDERING ANTERIOR BLADE

The blade is now manipulated gently around the forehead of the fetus by a combination of the intra-vaginal fingers and the hand holding the handle. The internal fingers push the blade around the head, whilst the external hand aids the wandering and, by steadying and tilting the handle, keeps the leading edge close to the scalp. Ultimately the blade 'wanders' into position over the malar bone of the fetus and the handle lies pressed hard against, and in line with, the vulval cleft (Fig. **50/10B, C, D**).

STEP 3. THE POSTERIOR BLADE

The right hand is introduced into the hollow of the sacrum between the rectum and the scalp. The blade is introduced into the vagina on the side of the first blade which will permit locking without having to cross the blades. It is guided into position until it lies between the head and the sacral promontory or to one or other side of it. Force should not be used, the handle being raised or lowered slightly until resistance disappears (Fig. **50/10E**).

STEP 4. LOCKING AND ROTATION

The sliding lock permits the blades to lock although they may not be at exactly the same level. Any difference will be corrected by the first pull. Before any traction, or rotation, is made, the correct position of the blades is checked by determining that the fetal sagittal suture lies between, and parallel to, each blade. The forceps is grasped at the traction shoulders, and care is taken not to squeeze the handles as this will compress the head. Gentle rotation through 90° to bring the occiput anteriorly (as shown by the dots on the handle) is made, but if rotation proves difficult, it is abandoned and traction applied, and after one or two pulls rotation is attempted again. In this way the head finds the level at which to rotate most easily. Undue force must not be used, and if traction does not bring the head lower into the pelvis, or rotation does not occur easily, the trial forceps should be abandoned, and the patient delivered by caesarean section.

STEP 5. EXTRACTION

Once rotation has occurred the rest of the delivery is carried out as for the long-shanked forceps which has a pelvic curve. But because of the lack of pelvic curve on the Kielland forceps, and the high station of the fetal head, initially traction is downwards. The obstetrician may find it easier to sit on a very low stool so that he may pull in the right direction.

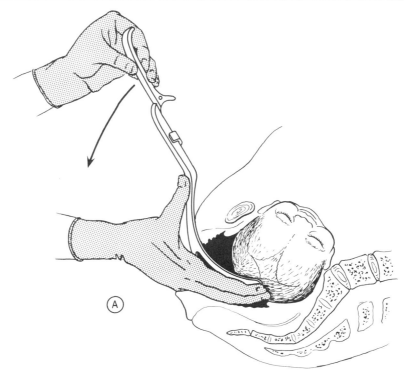

A. The blade is inserted posterolaterally on the same side as the fetal face, between the head and the fingers protecting the vaginal wall

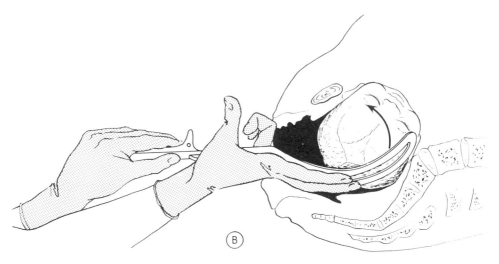

B. The internal fingers, resting behind the blade, guide it anteriorly around the fetus's face. The external hand steadies the handle of the forceps

**Fig. 50/10** Application of Kielland's forceps in cases of deep transverse arrest

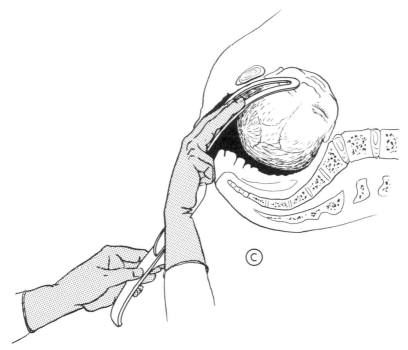

C. The blade 'wanders' around the face and is now almost anterior. The external hand tilts it slightly so that it tends to press more on the head than on the pelvic wall

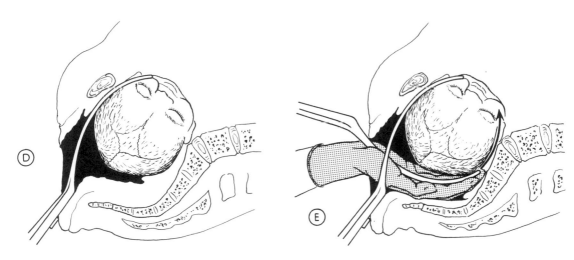

D. The blade is now completely anterior. The handle is elevated to bring the blade to its correct position over the ear and malar bone of the fetus

E. The posterior blade is introduced directly along the curve of the sacrum, the tip being applied closely to the fetal head. To make locking easy, the blade is inserted on the same side as the lock

**Fig. 50/10** Application of Kielland's forceps in cases of deep transverse arrest (cont.)

### Application of Kielland's forceps in cases of persistent occipito-posterior position, arrested in the mid-pelvis

Each blade is introduced between the fetal skull and the lateral vaginal wall, protected by the intravaginal fingers of the obstetrician. The blade is then moved anteriorly by the intravaginal fingers to lie in the ideal position, over the ears and malar eminence of the fetal head. Rotation through 180° is made to bring the occiput into the anterior position, and the remainder of the delivery proceeds normally (Fig. **50/11**).

### Manual rotation and forceps extraction

Until the introduction of Kielland's forceps, delivery of the fetus arrested in the transverse or occipito-posterior position was by manual rotation and forceps extraction, and the method is still popular.

If the occiput lies to the left, the right hand is used; if the occiput is to the right the left hand is used, as it is easier to pronate than to supinate the hand. Before introducing the hand into the vagina the forceps is placed so that it is readily available. The whole hand, well lubricated, is introduced into the vagina and the sinciput grasped, the fingers over one ear, the thumb over the other. It may be necessary to displace the head slightly upwards to do this. The external hand palpates the anterior shoulder and draws it anteriorly, at the same time as the vaginal hand rotates the head (Fig. **50/12**). The vaginal hand rotates the fetal head so that the occiput becomes anterior and, keeping the head in its new position, the left blade of the long-shanked forceps is introduced. After confirming that the occiput is anterior, the right blade is introduced and the blades are locked.

As the whole hand has to be introduced into the vagina, as the head has to be displaced upwards, and as the rotated head is not always stable and easily reverts, it can be appreciated that Kielland's forceps are less traumatic and more successful provided they are skilfully used.

### Forceps in face and brow presentation

The blades are applied as in vertex presentation, if the chin is directly anterior. If the chin is posterior in position, vaginal delivery must not be attempted until it has been rotated into an anterior position. Forceps application to a brow presentation is contraindicated.

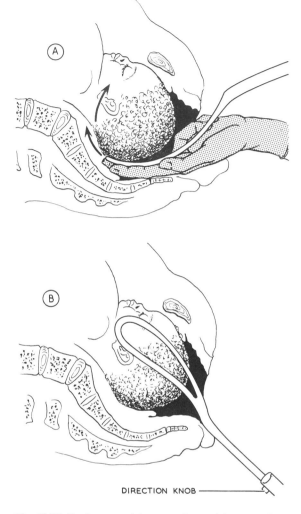

**Fig. 50/11** Persistent occipito-posterior position – application of Kielland's forceps. (A) The correct blade is chosen by holding the assembled forceps in front of the patient, the direction knob pointing to the baby's occiput. The blade is introduced between the head and the posterior vaginal wall and the wandering movement started; (B) to bring it to lie over the ear (redrawn from Parry-Jones, E. *Kielland's Forceps*)

### Forceps delivery of the aftercoming head

The body and arms of the child are held up above the symphysis so that they are not in the way. Since the head is usually in the mid-cavity, the operation is one of mid-forceps delivery, and a long-shanked instrument is used. As a rim of the cervix may still be present, the whole hand is introduced into the

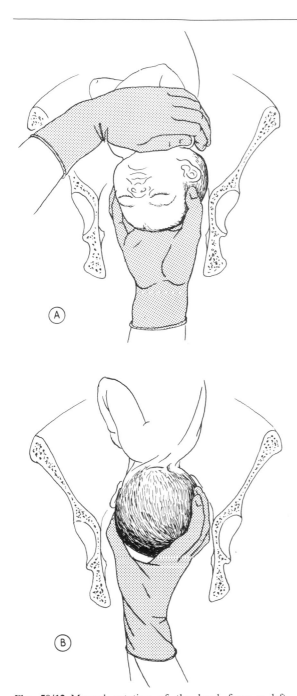

**Fig. 50/12** Manual rotation of the head from a left occipito-posterior position. (A) The left hand is placed on the abdomen and pulls the right shoulder of the baby towards the mother's right side. Simultaneously the right hand, in supination, holds the head by its biparietal diameter and rotates it through 180° to a position of pronation; (B) The occiput becomes anterior at the end of the manoeuvre

vagina to determine this, and the blades guided between the hand and fetal skull to avoid nipping the cervix. Traction is slow and intermittent.

### 'Failed' forceps

The failed forceps case is becoming rarer with the spread of good obstetrical care. It is not to be confused with a controlled trial of forceps conducted in a hospital where a caesarean section can be done if normal force does not produce the delivery of the child. A failed forceps implies that delivery has not occurred despite repeated forceful efforts. Most cases of failed forceps are due to failure to recognize that the cervix is not fully dilated, to an error in determining the exact position of the head and consequently the misapplication of the forceps, or to attempting a high forceps. The danger of failed forceps is trauma to baby and mother, caused by undue, excessive force mistakenly applied. If it is remembered that a mid-forceps delivery requires skill and experience, and if doctors realize that there is no 'loss of face' in seeking help, the high perinatal mortality and maternal morbidity following a failed forceps will be eliminated.

### The dangers of a difficult forceps delivery

A difficult forceps delivery may be accompanied by trauma to the vagina and cervix which may cause haemorrhage and, possibly, infection. Although vaginal lacerations are not uncommon they have no serious import if they are recognized and are sutured immediately after delivery. If a forceps delivery has been difficult, the entire vagina must be inspected in a good light, and lacerations sought and sutured. The main causes of vaginal lacerations are difficult rotation, or the slipping of the blades during traction.

The dangers to the fetus are trauma, compression of the brain or tentorial tearing, fracture of the skull, and facial paresis, due to compression of the nerve as it emerges in front of the mastoid processes. These dangers will be largely avoided if every mid-forceps is treated as a trial forceps.

### Mid-forceps or caesarean section?

Recently, increasing numbers of cases of deep transverse arrest are being delivered by caesarean section, and the skill required to perform a mid-forceps rotation has diminished. The argument for caesarean section is that the neonatal morbidity is decreased; however, when mid-forceps is performed by an experienced obstetrician in a well-equipped hospital, under epidural anaesthesia, and is treated as a trial forceps, the neonatal morbidity is no greater than that following caesarean section and may be less.

## THE VENTOUSE (OR VACUUM EXTRACTOR)

During the 1950s an alternative instrument to forceps was reintroduced by Malstrom. This is the ventouse. The instrument consists of a cup preferably made of silastic and a traction chain. The cup is fixed to the fetal head by creating a vacuum, which draws the scalp into the cavity of the cup and permits considerable traction to be made on the fetus by means of the chain attached to the cup. The baby is pulled into the world by its scalp.

The main mechanical difference is that the compression forces are no longer applied to the bony base of the skull, but diffusely to the entire head, as the scalp presses on the underlying cranial bones. There is no conclusive evidence that less compression force is exerted on the fetal brain than with forceps.

The cup is held in place on the fetal scalp, preferably over the vertex, and the obstetrician ensures that no part of the vaginal wall is included. A vacuum is then created slowly, taking 5 to 10 minutes to obtain 0.8kg per cm². The delivery is accomplished by pulling on the chain intermittently and synchronously with the uterine contractions; but

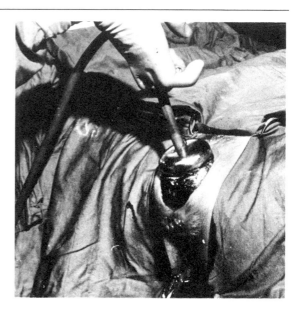

Fig. 50/14 The baby's head is being delivered through the vulva by traction on the ventouse. The position of the cup over the occiput can be seen

if a pull of more than 50kg (110lb) is exerted, the vacuum will be broken. It should not be applied for longer than 30 minutes.

The advantages claimed are that the instrument mimics normal delivery and adds no bulk to the object passing through the birth canal, so that lacerations are uncommon. The disadvantages are that in deliveries from the mid-pelvis the ventouse frequently slips off, and delivery is much slower than with forceps, up to 30 minutes often being required. This taxes mother, baby and obstetrician! Every baby has a large artificial caput (or chignon) which subsides in 12 to 60 hours, and if traction has been prolonged, lacerations at the rim of the caput are common. Between 5 and 20 per cent of babies develop a cephalhaematoma; and 15 per cent of all babies develop neonatal jaundice, twice the rate occurring after forceps delivery.

### The place of the vacuum extractor

The vacuum extractor is as effective as low forceps in delivering the fetal head from the lower pelvis, but takes longer. The discomfort to the patient is not significantly altered, and the perinatal mortality is unchanged. It can be used in place of Kielland's forceps to effect rotation and extraction of the fetal head which is arrested in the transverse or posterior

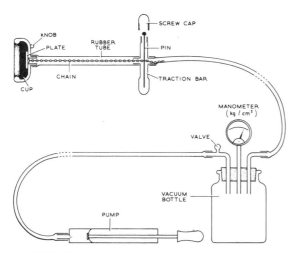

Fig. 50/13 The ventouse or vacuum extractor (after Chalmers)

position. The damage to the vaginal tissues is less with the vacuum extractor, but the failure rate varies between 2 and 20 per cent.

It has been used to secure full dilatation of the cervix and avoid caesarean section in cases where there was cessation in cervical dilatation at 7cm or more, where no obvious disproportion was present and where delivery was urgently required. Intermittent traction usually causes full cervical dilatation within 45 minutes and permits vaginal delivery. It is not yet clear whether this forcible dilatation of the cervix will predispose to cervical incompetence and later uterovaginal prolapse, so this indication must be considered experimental. Finally, the vacuum extractor has been used, with success, to deliver the impacted breech.

# Chapter 51

# Caesarean Section

Caesarean section means the removal of the child from the intact uterus by abdominal operation. In recent years the indications for the operation, and its incidence, have increased considerably (Table 51/1). In Britain, the caesarean section rate in 1980 averaged 8 per cent (with a range in different hospitals of 4 to 22 per cent). In Australia, the proportion of women delivered by caesarean section is higher, averaging 12 per cent (range 5 to 25 per cent) and in the USA, the mean caesarean section rate exceeds 20 per cent (range 8 to 35 per cent). The increased incidence of caesarean section is due in part to fashion, as the operation is now safe for mother and infant and as increasing numbers of malpractice suits are being made, claiming that a vaginal delivery was the cause of damage to the infant. The main reasons for the increase are obstetric factors. Four indications have been identified: (1) dystocia, (2) breech presentation, (3) fetal distress and (4) previous caesarean section. How valid are these indications is difficult to determine as, paradoxically, the caesarean section rate amongst private patients is three times that of the rate amongst public patients, where a higher incidence of complications might be expected. The objective of the higher caesarean section rate is to reduce perinatal mortality and morbidity. However, when a comparison is made between the practice of a Dublin hospital, whose caesarean section rate has remained at 5 per cent, with that of a Boston hospital, whose rate has increased from 5 per cent in 1968 to 20 per cent in 1978, the perinatal mortality rate fell equally in both institutions over the same period of time.

## INDICATIONS

The indication for caesarean section is when, in the opinion of the obstetrician, the risk of leaving the fetus in the uterus, or of fetal damage occurring during labour exceeds that of delivering the baby by operation. In the past two decades the indications have increased, as have the caesarean section rates. Most of the indications have been discussed in earlier chapters, but for convenience they are summarized in Table 51/2 where page references are also given. Two sets of indications which have not been discussed elsewhere need to be mentioned. They are (1) the management of previous unsuccessful pregnancy (poor obstetric history), and (2) the older primigravida.

*Unsuccessful pregnancy* A few women give a history of unsuccessful pregnancies. The woman may have had several abortions, or the baby may have died in utero in the third or early fourth quarter of pregnancy for no apparent reason. Because of the concern of the parents and their obstetrician to obtain a live baby, caesarean section may be decided upon as the best method of delivery. In other cases there may have been intra-uterine growth retardation, and this may be present in the index pregnancy. Provided that a major congenital abnormality is not present, caesarean section may 'rescue' the baby from a hostile intra-uterine environment.

*The older primigravida:* Women who become pregnant for the first time when aged 30 or more are

|  | 1971 | 1976 | 1983 |
|---|---|---|---|
| Australia | 4 | 9 | 15 |
| Denmark | 6 | 8 | 13 |
| England and Wales | 5 | 6 | 10 |
| New Zealand | 4 | 5 | 10 |
| Norway | 2 | 4 | 9 |
| USA | 6 | 12 | 20 |

**Table 51/1** Caesarean section rates per 100 deliveries

1. Failure of labour to progress (dystocia)
   abnormal uterine action (p. 346)
   cephalopelvic disproportion (p. 329)

2. Malpresentations or malpositions
   breech (p. 296)
   face and brow (p. 311)
   transverse lie (p. 312)
   occipito-posterior (p. 310)
   prolapse of umbilical cord (p. 320)
   multiple pregnancy (p. 317)

3. Antepartum haemorrhage
   abruptio placentae (p. 204)
   placenta praevia (p. 201)

4. Hypertensive disease in pregnancy (p. 213)

5. Diabetes mellitus (p. 245)

6. Fetal conditions
   fetal distress (p. 285)
   isoimmunization (p. 258)
   very low birth weight (p. 467)

7. Older primigravidae (p. 405)

8. Failed induction of labour (p. 388)

9. Repeat caesarean section (p. 409)

**Table 51/2** Indications for caesarean section

designated 'older primigravidae'. (In the past they were called 'elderly' primigravidae!) Although most of these women can deliver vaginally, in the absence of antenatal or intrapartum complications, some obstetricians feel that elective caesarean section is preferable. This choice is reinforced if the woman has had a long period of involuntary infertility (> 3 years).

## TYPES OF OPERATION

The incision into the uterus may be vertical through the muscles of the upper, or fundal, portion of the uterus – the classical section – or transversely through the lower uterine segment. Other approaches have been described but are no longer necessary, apart from caesarean hysterectomy which may be required because of placenta accreta, multiple myomata, uterine rupture, or uncontrollable haemorrhage. Today, 95 per cent of caesarean sections are lower uterine segment sections, 4 per cent are classical sections, and less than 1 per cent are caesarean hysterectomies.

**Advantages of the lower segment section**

The lower uterine segment operation is to be preferred as: (1) the risk of rupture of the scar in a subsequent pregnancy is one-tenth that of the classical scar; (2) the healing of the scar is better because the lower segment is at rest during the puerperium; (3) infection is reduced as the wound is extraperitoneal; (4) there are fewer postoperative complications. The disadvantage is that the operation requires more skill and experience, the bladder may be damaged, and haemostasis at the angles of the wound is more difficult to effect.

**Indications for the classical operation**

The classical operation is to be preferred in the following circumstances: (1) when the lower segment is abnormally vascular; (2) when the lower segment cannot be identified because of adhesions to the anterior abdominal wall; (3) when the fetus presents as a transverse lie, particularly with an impacted shoulder; (4) when a constriction ring is present.

## OPERATIVE TECHNIQUE

The patient is prepared by shaving and cleansing the skin with Phisohex. The blood haemoglobin and group are determined and blood is obtained. If the haemoglobin level is less than 11g, a blood transfusion should be started by the anaesthetist. Isotope studies have shown that the mean blood loss in caesarean section is in excess of 1000ml. Because of this, cross-matched blood should always be available.

The type of anaesthetic depends on the experience and skills of the anaesthetist; a general inhalation anaesthetic or an epidural anaesthetic is usually chosen. Rarely, the operation may be performed under local infiltration anaesthesia.

**Lower uterine segment caesarean section**

The technique is show diagrammatically in Fig. **51/1** and only a summary of the steps is given here.

1. The incision is usually transverse, suprapubic (the Pfannenstiel incision) but in some cases a subumbilical mid-line incision may be preferred. On opening the peritoneum the bowel is kept out of the

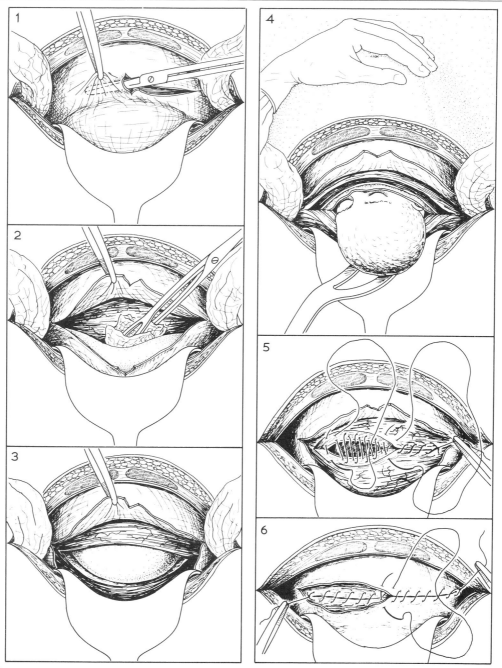

**Fig. 51/1** Lower segment caesarean section

(1) and (2) The loose peritoneum covering the lower uterine segment is divided and pushed down

(3) The exposed muscle of the lower segment is incised so that the membranes bulge into the wound. The incision may be extended with a knife, or the muscle fibres separated with the fingers

(4) The membranes are ruptured and the head delivered using a forceps blade as an inclined plane, counter pressure being exerted on the fundus

(5) The placenta has been expelled and the wound sutured in layers. Great care must be taken at the angles

(6) The peritoneum is sutured

operative field by two moist packs, which are pushed into the lateral part of the uterovesical space on each side, and between the uterine fundus and the anterior abdominal wall superiorly. Any rotation of the uterus is corrected at this time.

2. The loose peritoneum covering the lower uterine segment is lifted, incised and pushed down. This displaces the bladder downwards, and exposes the lower uterine segment (**1 and 2**).

3. The myometrium is incised as far down in the lower uterine segment as possible. The membranes bulge into the incision, which is then extended with the fingers, knife or scissors (**3**).

4. The amniotic membranes are ruptured and the liquor sucked out. The infant's face is rotated so that it appears in the wound and the head is slowly delivered from the uterus using a blade of Wrigley's forceps, or a hand, as an inclined plane, counterpressure being made on the fundus (**4**). An injection of ergometrine 0.25mg is given intravenously with the birth of the head. This expels the placenta.

5. If venous sinuses in the uterine incision bleed they are grasped by Green–Armitage forceps, and the angles of the incision are secured by Allis forceps.

6. The inner half of the muscle is sutured with 0 or 1/0 polyglycolic suture used in a continuous manner. The suture excludes the decidual layer, and approximates the muscle without undue tension. The outer half of the muscle, including the serosal layer, is then sutured (**5**).

7. The peritoneal flap is sutured, again without undue tension, using a 2/0 suture (**6**).

8. The peritoneal cavity is sucked clear of blood and liquor and the packs removed. If desired, an appendicectomy may now be performed.

9. The abdominal wall is repaired in the usual way.

### Classical section

1. The technique is identical to that for the lower segment operation until the packs are inserted. Before these are inserted it is confirmed that the uterus has not rotated by observing the position of the round muscles.

2. A vertical incision is made through the thick muscle layer of the upper uterine segment in the mid-line.

3. The bulging membranes are incised and the fetus extracted by grasping a leg. Ergometrine 0.25mg is given intravenously to expel the placenta.

4. The uterine wound is sutured in three layers using continuous polyglycolic suture. The inner layer takes the inner third of the muscle, excluding the decidua, and firm tension is obtained. The middle layer takes the middle third of the muscle in the same manner. The outer layer penetrates the serosal coat and takes in the outer third of the muscle in the same manner. The sutures of each layer partly interdigitate so that no dead spaces remain. A few additional sutures may be required in the serosal coat to obtain haemostasis.

5. The remainder of the operation is identical with that described for the lower segment operation.

### Caesarean hysterectomy

The technique of this operation differs in no way from the technique of hysterectomy described in books of gynaecological surgery. Three points should be emphasized. First, the ovaries must be preserved, and the ovarian pedicle should be divided as near to the uterus as possible so that the ovarian blood supply is not impaired. The ovarian pedicle should be covered with peritoneum in its normal position, and not attached to the vaginal vault before covering. Secondly, total hysterectomy is the operation of choice and can usually be performed easily because of the mobility of the uterus. Thirdly, it must be ensured that the dilated ureters are not included in the uterine pedicle.

### Tubal ligation

Tubal ligation should be offered to the patient, with her husband's knowledge and agreement, after a second caesarean section, and should be recommended after a third operation. The operation is described elsewhere, and may be performed at the time of the caesarean section, although it is preferable to wait for 2 months so that the decision is made by the patient deliberately and without stress.

## POSTOPERATIVE CARE

In the first 24 hours pain must be controlled and an adequate fluid intake ensured. The former is dealt with by giving adequate doses of pethidine (100 to 150mg) or morphine (15mg) as often as necessary, the latter by continuing intravenous fluids if an infusion has been set up during operation, or by giving oral fluids in small amounts at frequent intervals.

After 12 hours the patient is encouraged to move about in bed, and sits beside the bed whilst it is made. Deep breathing is taught at this time, and practised for 5 minutes each hour. A light diet can be taken. If abdominal distension is marked a rectal tube is passed, or a bisacodyl suppository is given rectally, about 36 hours after operation.

After 48 hours ambulation increases and is encouraged. Antibiotics and anticoagulants are only used if indicated.

## THE COMPLICATIONS OF OPERATION

The immediate complications are haemorrhage from the placental site, or the wound; gut distension and ileus; infection; pulmonary collapse and thromboembolism. These complications are uncommon today. The remote complications are abdominal hernia, intestinal obstruction due to adhesions, and 'vague abdominal pain'.

In countries where fertility can be voluntarily controlled, only 20 per cent of patients who have been delivered by caesarean section subsequently decide to attempt a further pregnancy. The fear of pregnancy must be taken into account when caesarean section is done as an 'easy way out' or for a trivial reason.

## MORBIDITY AND MORTALITY AFTER CAESAREAN SECTION

In cases of elective caesarean section, and when the patient is not admitted exsanguinated, infected or after prolonged labour, the maternal mortality is less than 0.5 per 1000 sections compared with 0.1 per 1000 following vaginal delivery. If the operation is required because of obstructed prolonged labour, or in the presence of infection, the rate is eight times as high. In such cases the alternative methods of treatment are attended by an even higher maternal mortality so the operation is justified.

The maternal mortality will be reduced if the operation is performed in a properly equipped hospital, with adequate blood transfusion facilities, with trained assistants available and, most important, by an experienced obstetrician.

The maternal morbidity varies between 3 and 12 per cent depending on the reason for the caesarean section. It is higher if the operation is performed following prolonged spontaneous rupture of the membranes or if labour has lasted for more than 18 hours. Endometritis accounts for two-thirds of the infections, urinary tract infection and wound infection for the remainder. This finding raises the question about the value of prophylactic antibiotics. The consensus in Britain (but not in the USA) is that prophylactic antibiotics should be given only if the patient is believed to be at a high risk of infection. In this case a short course of ampicillin (3 i.v. doses) or a first generation cephalosporin is chosen, the first injection being given just after the cord has been clamped, to avoid consequences to the baby. An alternative is to give a single dose of piperacillin (4g i.v.) after cord clamping.

The fetal mortality is largely dependent upon the nature of the condition for which the operation was done. When it is 'elective' and the fetus mature, the fetal loss should not exceed that following vaginal delivery.

## DELIVERY AFTER CAESAREAN SECTION

The majority of obstetricians in Commonwealth countries are prepared to allow a patient, who was previously delivered by caesarean section, to undergo a trial of labour in expectation of delivery per vaginam, when no recurrent indication, such as pelvic contraction or tumour, is present. By contrast, in the USA the dictum 'once a caesarean, always a caesarean' holds, with certain exceptions. In 1984 the President of the American College of Obstetricians and Gynecologists stated: 'Once a cesarean always a cesarean is an outmoded dictum. Mortality fears for mother and infant resulting from uterine rupture in a trial of labour are not borne out by existing data.' In spite of this opinion, the argument for repeating the operation persists. Some obstetricians believe that the operation damages the integrity of the uterus which may rupture during the stress of a subsequent labour. Statistics show that 3 per cent of classical scars rupture in late pregnancy or in labour, but the comparable figure for rupture following the lower segment section is only 0.25 per cent. In fact, in properly selected patients, the risk of a maternal death following rupture of a scar is one-fortieth that of the risk to a mother following an elective caesarean section. The risk of perinatal death following a trial of labour, in a woman with a uterine scar, is one-fifth of that following an elective caesarean section.

Against the risk of ruptured uterus must be put

the risk to the patient of repeatedly incising the abdominal cavity. The consequences of multiple laparotomies are rarely analysed, as frequently the patient who develops symptoms seeks attention from a doctor other than the one who did the operation. Although the postoperative mortality of elective caesarean section today is less than 0.1 per cent, immediate postoperative sequelae occur. All patients have pain, some require blood transfusion, some develop bowel distension and require catheterization, pyrexia is not infrequent and wound infection occurs in about 1.5 per cent of patients. Later complications of intestinal obstruction or of divarication of the recti abdominis muscles and abdominal herniation are sufficiently frequent to merit consideration.

For these reasons the dictum 'once a caesarean always a caesarean' cannot be sustained, and should be replaced by 'once a caesarean always confinement in a well-equipped and well-staffed hospital'. Naturally, every case must be considered individually. So that an exact knowledge of the duration of pregnancy may be obtained, the patient should attend the doctor betwen the 6th and 10th week of her next pregnancy. Attendance should be at regular intervals from this time on, and the patient should avoid all heavy work in the last month of pregnancy or, if social conditions are unfavourable, be admitted to hospital for rest. During labour all food is withheld, blood is made available, and the maternal pulse and fetal well-being monitored by cardiotocography. Oxytocin may be used to induce or augment labour, provided it is given via an infusion pump. Delivery is conducted by a doctor who palpates (per vaginam) the lower uterine segment immediately after the birth of the placenta. If it is done at this time, no anaesthetic is required and the procedure is painless. Should the lower uterine segment be found to be ruptured, repair can be performed immediately.

A survey of the world literature in 1984 (excluding the USA), showed that of 4729 women previously delivered by caesarean section, 32 per cent were delivered by elective section, 23 per cent by section after a trial of labour and 45 per cent delivered vaginally after a trial of labour. Twenty-one (0.7 per cent) of the scars ruptured during labour.

## ELECTIVE CAESAREAN SECTION

In spite of the ability of many women to deliver vaginally with safety after caesarean section, many obstetricians (and some patients) elect for a planned caesarean section for the next birth. If this approach is chosen, the timing of the delivery is important, to avoid the preterm birth of the baby. This means that the gestational age must be known with accuracy. The criteria pertaining to gestational age are: (1) a reliable menstrual history; (2) early bimanual examination, preferably between 8 and 12 weeks gestation; and (3) appropriate uterine growth. If any doubt exists about the gestational age, an ultrasonic examination should be made at about the assumed 20th gestational week. If this examination corroborates the clinical examination, a date for the elective caesarean section may be decided upon. However, if any doubt persists in the last quarter of pregnancy, an amniocentesis should be made to determine the L/S ratio before the time of the caesarean section is determined, so that the respiratory distress syndrome may be avoided.

*Chapter 52*

# Other Obstetric Operations

## VERSION

The changing, by manipulation, of the presentation of the baby has great antiquity, having been recorded by Hippocrates, and undoubtedly practised long before his time. If the head is brought to lie over the pelvic brim, the version is cephalic; if the buttocks are brought down it is podalic. Three methods are available to achieve version, first by purely external manipulation (*external version*), secondly by purely internal manipulation (*internal version*) and, thirdly, by combined external and partially internal manipulation (*bipolar version*).

### EXTERNAL VERSION

The manipulation is usually performed if the baby still presents as a breech at the 35th week of pregnancy, when an external cephalic version is attempted; or in late pregnancy if the fetal lie is transverse or oblique, when an external cephalic or podalic version is used, depending on the circumstances.

Before attempting the version, some obstetricians give a tocolytic agent, such as terbutaline sulphate (0.25mg i.v. over 60 seconds). The attempted version is made gently. During the attempt and following it, the patient's blood pressure and pulse are recorded every 5 minutes and the fetal heart rate either continuously or every 2 minutes for 30 minutes. The attempt is given up if the mother complains of pain, if the fetal heart rate drops below 90 beats per minute, or if version does not take place within 10 minutes. If an irregularity of the fetal heart beat occurs, the attempt is stopped, being repeated if the irregularity rapidly subsides. If it persists the attempt should be abandoned.

After version the fetal heart rate occasionally becomes slow and the rhythm irregular, returning to normal within 10 minutes. If the abnormality persists, the baby should be pushed back into the breech position, or, in some cases, a caesarean section performed.

### External cephalic version

For the manipulation to succeed it is essential that the patient should be as relaxed as possible, and her bladder and bowels should be empty. Nervous patients may be given pethidine 100mg intramuscularly half an hour before the manipulation. If the first attempt at cephalic version fails, a second attempt may be made following the use of a tocolytic drug to relax the uterus (see p. 272). Following version the fetal heart is monitored for 1 hour. Some obstetricians attempt external cephalic version under general anaesthesia, if version fails without anaesthesia. Since many babies turn spontaneously after failed version, version under anaesthesia should be delayed for at least 1 week.

The steps of external cephalic version are as follows (Fig. **52/1**).

#### MOBILIZATION OF THE BREECH

The patient is put in a slight Trendelenburg position. The abdominal skin is dusted with talcum powder, and the operator dips his hands into the pelvis, raising the breech and mobilizing it. He then directs it towards one or other iliac fossa.

#### THE VERSION

The breech is pushed out of the iliac fossa with one

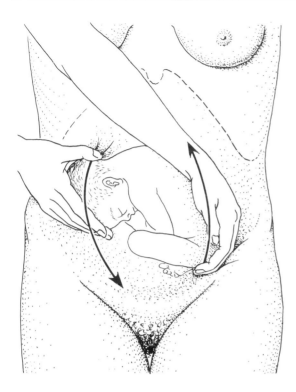

**Fig. 52/1** External version – the obstetrician has lifted the buttocks out of the pelvis, his right thumb controls the baby's head and the direction in which the child is moved encourages flexion

hand, and simultaneously the other hand pushes the head towards the opposite iliac fossa, so that the baby turns 'head over heels'. If the 'forward' version fails, as may occur when the legs are extended, 'backward' version is attempted. The movements during the version should be smooth, the pressure gentle, and made in a circular direction so that the fetus forms a C shape as it turns in a forward somersault.

### Difficulties of version

The commonest difficulty is a tense abdominal wall, especially when the breech has extended legs. In some cases the breech is deeply engaged in the pelvis, or the head is tucked under the costal margin. Version in these cases may be difficult, even if the breech is disimpacted by pushing it up per vaginam. Version should not be persisted with if the breech does not disengage easily.

### Dangers of version

These are infrequent and include placental separation, premature rupture of the membranes, twisting of the cord around one of the fetal limbs and the onset of premature labour. Even with anaesthesia, and greater force, the incidence is no more than 2 per cent. If anaesthesia is avoided the complications are rare.

### Contraindications to version

These include antepartum haemorrhage, multiple pregnancy, maternal hypertension, intra-uterine growth retardation, an anterior placed placenta or a fetal abnormality. Version should not be attempted in cases where caesarean section is to be performed for other reasons, such as in an older infertile primigravida or when the patient has had a previous caesarean section.

### Success of version

Cephalic version without anaesthesia at the 35th to 37th week is successful in breech presentation in 70 per cent of primigravidae and 80 per cent of multigravidae. In those cases where it is unsuccessful the baby usually presents as a breech with extended legs. In transverse and oblique lie, which is usually found in multigravidae, version is 90 per cent successful.

## INTERNAL PODALIC VERSION

Today, with the safety of caesarean section, the use of internal podalic version is limited and is usually restricted to the delivery of a second twin which is lying in the transverse position, or, rarely, to deal with cases of transverse lie in the patient whose cervix is fully dilated and whose membranes are still intact.

The patient is deeply anaesthetized and placed in the lithotomy position. The obstetrician, with full asepsis, his hand liberally anointed with obstetric cream, passes it, the fingers forming a cone, into the uterine cavity. Although either hand will do, manipulation is easier if he uses the right hand when the baby's head is on the mother's left side, and his left hand when the baby's head is on the mother's right side. Inside the uterus the hand passes up along the breech until the limbs are felt, and the heel identified, as this distinguishes that the limb is indeed a leg.

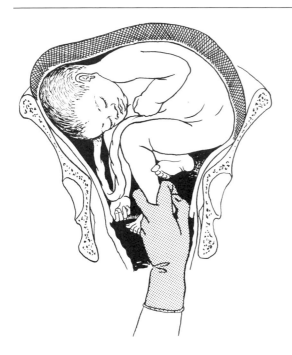

Fig. 52/2 Internal podalic version

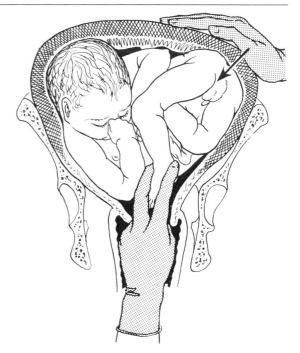

Fig. 52/3 Bipolar version

The foot is grasped, the index and middle finger encircling the ankle, and it is drawn down through the dilated cervix (Fig. **52/2**). The operation must be performed gently and slowly, and no hurried movement made, as the danger of uterine rupture is always present. Internal podalic version should never be used to deliver a big baby from the impacted shoulder presentation.

## BIPOLAR VERSION

The need for this manipulation is very limited, and it is only rarely employed in cases of shoulder pre-sentation in which the membranes are unruptured, or have ruptured recently, and the cervix is only 3 to 5cm dilated, so that the whole hand cannot be introduced into the uterus. Even in these cases caesarean section is to be preferred, as the fetal loss after bipolar version is high.

Under anaesthesia two fingers are introduced through the cervix, and the shoulder is pushed out of the pelvis, whilst the hand on the abdomen pushes the fetal buttocks towards the pelvis (Fig. **52/3**). When the feet are reached, one is grasped by the ankle between the two fingers, it is extracted through the cervix and into the vagina, and secured by a tape to which a weight is attached.

# DESTRUCTIVE OPERATIONS ON THE FETUS

With advances in obstetric care, destructive operations on the living, and indeed the dead fetus are becoming rare. However, in certain circumstances, there is still a place for the operations, particularly in the developing countries of the world, where obstetric care (and the acceptance by patients of such care) may be deficient.

The main operations are: (1) decapitation; (2) craniotomy; (3) evisceration; (4) cleidotomy.

## DECAPITATION

The operation consists of severing the fetal head from the trunk, followed by extraction, per vaginam,

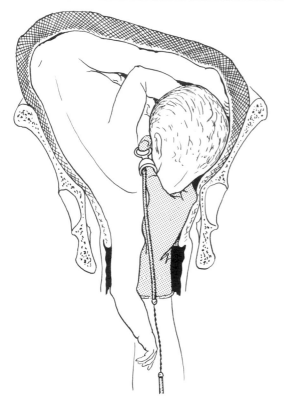

**Fig. 52/4** Decapitation using the Blond–Heidler wire and thimble

of the trunk and finally of the head. The main indication is in cases of impacted shoulder presentation when the child is dead and the cervix fully dilated, and the uterus not in imminent danger of rupture.

The operation is performed with Blond–Heidler thimble and decapitating wire.

### Technique

Traction is put on the arm to bring the neck lower in the pelvis. The wire is then attached to the slot in the thimble and the thimble placed on the thumb. The whole hand is introduced into the vagina, and the neck encircled with the thumb, anteriorly, and the fingers posteriorly (Fig. **52/4**). The index or middle finger feels for the ring, and having found it pulls the thimble and attached wire from the thumb and round the fetal neck. The wire is drawn out of the vagina and attached to the handles, and the neck severed by a to-and-fro movement.

## CRANIOTOMY

The place of craniotomy in operative obstetrics is limited, and if obstetric care has been adequate it should rarely be required. By perforating the fetal head and allowing the brain to escape the volume of the skull is reduced, and the cranial bones collapse, permitting delivery. Obviously there is no place for the operation on the living, normally formed fetus, but in certain cases of hydrocephaly or of disproportion due to an unfavourable position of the child, such as brow or mentoposterior position, in which death of the fetus has occurred, the operation may permit a vaginal delivery. In a few cases a breech delivery will be effected as far as the head, which cannot be delivered and the baby dies. In these cases delivery after craniotomy is less damaging to the mother than forcible delivery of the uncollapsed head.

Craniotomy is usually effected by Simpson's perforator (Fig. **52/5**). This instrument has two cutting blades and these are attached to shanks which are hinged and continue into the handles. The hinge is so arranged that approximation of the handles causes separation of the blades.

### Technique

After anaesthetizing the patient and cleansing the vagina, the perforator, with the blade closed, is introduced to meet the fetal skull under the protection of the obstetrician's fingers. The head of the child is steadied from above by an assistant, and the blades bore a hole into the fetal skull by pressure and a side-to-side movement. The perforator should be maintained at right angles to the skull during this manipulation, and success is increased if the blades and points are sharp. The blades are pushed into the skull as far as the shoulders, and then the handles are closed, which separates the blades and makes a large tear in the skull. The perforator is then turned through 90° and the closing of the handles is repeated. The instrument is now pushed deeply into the brain and the brain tissue broken up. With the collapse of the head the baby can be delivered by

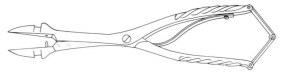

**Fig. 52/5** Simpson's perforator

forceps or the more complicated three-bladed cephalotribe may be used.

If the head is aftercoming, the legs are drawn downwards and backwards and the perforator is introduced into the skull in the region of the posterior occipital bone.

## EVISCERATION

Removal of the thoracic and abdominal contents may be necessary if the baby is a monster, and the enlarged abdomen prevents delivery. The baby is steadied and the abdominal cavity entered with the perforator which is then opened and closed in different directions.

## CLEIDOTOMY

Division of the clavicles reduces the bulk of the shoulder girdle and may be required when large shoulders prevent delivery of the child, which has died during the attempt. The clavicles are divided by a long, strong, straight scissors introduced along the ventral aspect of the child under the protection of the obstetrician's fingers.

## Chapter 53

# Oxytocics

The introduction of safe oxytocic agents has altered considerably the pattern of obstetric practice. The three common oxytocic agents available are prostaglandins, oxytocin and ergometrine. Each causes the uterus to contract, but their actions are different.

## PROSTAGLANDINS

In the 1930s it was discovered that human seminal fluid had a smooth muscle stimulating activity. In the belief that there was a single pharmacological substance present and that it derived from the prostate gland, the compound was named prostaglandin. An expansion of experimental work in the 1960s revealed that human semen contained, not one, but several chemically related smooth muscle stimulatory compounds, and that prostaglandins were present in most, or perhaps all, mammalian tissues.

Two of the prostaglandins $PGE_2$ and $PGE_{2\alpha}$ have special properties in relation to the female genital tract. First, they alter the structure of the connective tissues of the cervix leading to its 'ripening' and effacement. Second, they stimulate or augment uterine contractions. In other words, they are oxytocics. The use of prostaglandins as abortifacients and as post-coital contraceptive agents is now established and the drugs are used for the induction of labour. As the drugs cause smooth muscle contraction, undesirable side-effects of nausea, vomiting and diarrhoea occur, especially when prostaglandins are used orally or intravenously. In early pregnancy these side-effects can be overcome to some extent if prostaglandins are introduced into the amniotic sac or between the amnion and the uterine wall, or if tablets of prostaglandin are placed high in the vagina. Currently two prostaglandins, prostaglandin $E_2$ and prostaglandin $F_{2\alpha}$ are preferred. However, the time during which $PGE_2$ and $PGF_{2\alpha}$ are effective is relatively short, as the molecule is rapidly inactivated by enzymes. This defect has been overcome with the introduction of methyl derivatives of the parent drug.

Prostaglandins have been used as post-conception, post-implantation, anti-fertility agents in women who have an unprotected coitus at ovulation time and have failed to menstruate. In one reported series a single $25\mu g$ dose of intravaginal 15-methyl $PGE_2$ was effective in provoking menstruation in 60 per cent of women, and this rose to over 80 per cent after two doses. However other workers have had less success.

As an abortifacient, prostaglandins have been used with success in the second quarter of pregnancy, particularly intra-amniotically or by the extra-ovular route.

Prostaglandins are being used increasingly to ripen the cervix and to induce labour, particularly when the cervix is 'unfavourable'. Prostaglandins may be administered as vaginal pessaries, or by the intra-cervical or extra-amniotic routes. Experience has shown that vaginal pessaries of prostaglandin effectively induce labour and lead to delivery within 12 hours in $> 50$ per cent of women. The matter is discussed further in Chapter 49.

## OXYTOCIN

Natural oxytocin is produced by cells of the hypothalamus and carried by the neurone axons to the posterior pituitary gland where it is stored. It is released into the bloodstream as required and carried, loosely bound to serum protein, to the uterus where it exercises its biological effect. Synthetic oxytocin is transported in the same way. The action of oxytocin on the uterus is to lower the potential of the cell membrane and to allow the spread of contractions throughout the organ. The action is countered in two ways: oxytocin is destroyed in the bloodstream by oxytocinase, and probably opposed in the uterus by placental progesterone which 'blocks' the action of oxytocin. Various stimuli, such as emotions, cervical stimulation and suckling, cause the release of natural oxytocin from the posterior pituitary gland and increasing amounts are released as pregnancy advances.

Originally extract of posterior pituitary (Pituitrin) was used as a uterine stimulant and, although effective in early pregnancy, its action in late pregnancy was unpredictable, and fatalities followed its intravenous use. Research identified two factions in the extract, one which was mainly uterine-stimulatory (Pitocin), and the other which was mainly a vasopressor and antidiuretic (vasopressin). In 1939 a pure oxytocin, Syntocinon, was made synthetically. This is devoid of any vasopressor activity and is identical in uterine-stimulatory activity with natural oxytocin.

The action of oxytocin on the pregnant, or puerperal, uterus depends upon the time of administration, the dose and the route of administration. The more advanced the pregnancy the greater is the effect. Intramuscular injections in late pregnancy cause uterine contractions which, if the dose is not regulated, can become dangerously strong and lead to tetanic uterine spasm or uterine rupture. The puerperal uterus reacts to an intravenous injection by developing marked spasm within 30 seconds of the injection. The spasm lasts about 8 minutes and is followed by marked contractions for a further 30 minutes when the effect ceases. Intramuscular injection delays the onset of activity to about $2\frac{1}{2}$ minutes, but the type of activity and duration of effect is the same.

Because of the variability of response in pregnancy oxytocin must never be given intramuscularly before the birth of the baby, and even intravenously the drug must be used with care. The following principles apply:

1. Before the birth of the child oxytocin (Syntocinon or Pitocin) should only be given by controlled intravenous infusion in physiological amounts.
2. In the third stage it may safely be given intramuscularly in doses of 5 to 10 units or by dilute intravenous infusion, or directly into the uterine muscle.

# THE USE OF OXYTOCIC DRUGS IN OBSTETRICS

## Abortion

To prevent further bleeding in cases of incomplete or complete abortion, or as a prophylactic measure in therapeutic abortion, ergometrine 0.5mg intramuscularly or 0.25mg intravenously is the drug of choice, but Pituitrin in doses of 5 to 10 units may be used, although the duration of its effect is less. Prostaglandins have been used with considerable success in the induction of therapeutic abortion between the 10th and 19th weeks and in the termination of pregnancy in cases of intra-uterine death of the fetus.

## Induction or stimulation of labour

Since ergometrine produces severe uterine spasm, its use is precluded for the induction or stimulation of labour, and prostaglandins and oxytocin are the drugs of choice for these purposes. Because of the variability of response, oxytocin should never be used intramuscularly, but only given by controlled dilute intravenous infusion.

### INDUCTION OF LABOUR

Although some authorities use an oxytocin infusion to soften the firm cervix, the drug is most effective when administered after amniotomy. If the cervix is firm, the use of prostaglandins is to be preferred (see p. 386).

The oxytocic infusion is made up by adding 15 units of Syntocinon to a litre of normal saline, although a lower dose may be used. The infusion is given via an infusion pump. In calculating the dose of oxytocin given, mU per minute should be recorded, not drops per minute. The relationship between the two is shown in Table 49/4 on p. 387. The infusion is run initially to provide between 2 and 5mU per minute. It is increased by 5mU/min every 20 minutes until contractions lasting 60 seconds and recurring at 3–5-minute intervals are obtained. The patient and the infusion must be monitored by a trained nurse–midwife. No more than 1500ml of fluid is given at any session, and the infusion should be removed after 10 hours to allow the patient to sleep. It may be repeated the following day.

Rates of less than 30mU/minute are usually sufficient, but in certain conditions such as older primigravidity, marked uterine hypotonus or premature induction of labour, higher rates may be required.

## AUGMENTATION OF LABOUR

In cases where there is prolongation of the quiet phase of labour, or the cervix fails to dilate at a rate of 1cm/hour in the active phase, augmentation of labour may be appropriate, using an intravenous infusion of Syntocinon. The reason for the delay must be evaluated and cephalopelvic disproportion excluded before the intravenous infusion is set up. When possible the Syntocinon infusion should be given using an infusion pump. The regimen used is that described in the section on induction of labour (p. 387). The dose should not exceed 10mU/min, as higher concentrations are generally ineffective and possibly harmful.

### Postpartum haemorrhage

The use of oxytocics in the prevention and treatment of postpartum haemorrhage has been one of the great advances in obstetrics. The most efficient oxytocic for this purpose is ergometrine 0.25mg

given intravenously. Oxytocin 5 units given intramuscularly acts in 2½ minutes but unfortunately the effect wears off within 30 minutes and bleeding can occur from the relaxed uterus (Fig. **53/1**). A mixture of oxytocin 5 units with ergometrine 0.5mg (Syntometrine) combines the rapidity of action of intramuscular oxytocin with the duration of action of intramuscular ergometrine. This drug, given intramuscularly as the head of the baby is born, has reduced the incidence of postpartum haemorrhage from 13 per cent to 1 per cent.

For the treatment of established postpartum haemorrhage, intravenous ergometrine 0.25mg is the treatment of choice, but some centres use 10 units of oxytocin added to 500ml of 5 per cent glucose. Ergometrine given intravenously may lead to an increase in the patient's blood pressure. The degree of hypertension appears to be dose related. For this reason a dose of 0.25mg intravenously should, in general, not be exceeded, and intravenous ergo- metrine should be avoided in women with hypertension during late pregnancy or labour.

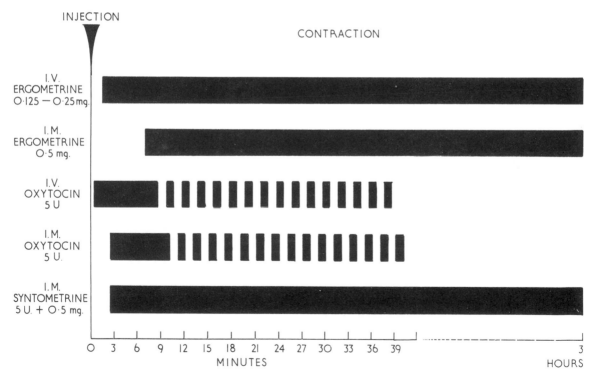

**Fig. 53/1** The diagram is made from direct tocographic measurements of the duration and character of uterine contraction following the injection of various oxytocics given in the third stage of labour. The continuous block shows sustained contraction; the intermittent blocks show intermittent contraction (redrawn from Embry, M. P. *Triangle* 1964, **6**, 199, published by Sandoz)

## ERGOMETRINE

The stimulating effect of extract of ergot on the postpartum uterus was first noted in 1808, but as with many drugs its original controlled use was succeeded by indiscriminate uncontrolled misuse, which resulted in the death of patients and condemnation of the drug. In 1935 the effective alkaloid was extracted from the many which formed ergot, and was called ergometrine. It can be given safely intravenously or intramuscularly, and its effect is to cause an intensive and lasting uterine spasm. Intravenous injection of 0.125 or 0.25mg will cause uterine tetany in 90 seconds, the spasm lasting for 30 minutes, whilst intramuscular injection of 0.5mg is not effective for 7 minutes, but the spasm lasts for up to 3 hours.

The tetanic contraction of the uterus precludes the use of ergometrine as a uterine stimulant whilst the fetus is still in utero, but ergometrine is the drug of choice for the treatment of bleeding after incomplete or complete abortion, and in postpartum haemorrhage.

# Part Six

# EPIDEMIOLOGY OF OBSTETRICS

*Life is an incurable disease.*
    Abraham Cowley (17th century)

## Chapter 54

# The Epidemiology of Obstetrics

The quality of the obstetric care offered to women in a country, or a region, can be measured to some extent by studying the maternal and perinatal mortality rates. In most developed countries the former is studied on a State or Regional basis by properly appointed Maternal Mortality Committees whose function is to analyse the factors causing each death, and to recommend measures to prevent further deaths. Unfortunately, in most of the developing countries the available vital statistics are highly inaccurate, and analysis of maternal deaths can only be made on the basis of experience in individual hospitals. This does not necessarily reflect the conditions in the area. Despite these limitations, the study of maternal mortality trends is of great importance to all doctors who practise obstetrics.

In the developed countries, the maternal mortality has fallen considerably in the past 30 years so that maternal deaths are relatively rare, and attention is now being paid to the perinatal mortality rate, as a sensitive index of the quality of the health services and of the obstetric care offered by a country.

## MATERNAL MORTALITY

The definition of maternal mortality varies slightly between different nations, but most report the rate calculated per 10 000 live births or per 100 000 'maternities', which includes both live and stillbirths. The latter term is used by the Department of Health and Social Security in Britain in their 'Reports on Confidential Enquiries into Maternal Deaths in England and Wales'. In an attempt to resolve the confusion and permit international comparisons, the International Federation of Gynaecologists and Obstetricians has defined a maternal death as 'the death of any woman dying of any cause whilst pregnant or within 42 days of the termination of pregnancy, irrespective of the duration and the site of the pregnancy; from any cause related to or aggravated by the pregnancy or its management but not from accidental or incidental causes.'

Direct causes of maternal death include such conditions as abortion, ectopic gestation, pregnancy-induced hypertension, eclampsia, antepartum and postpartum haemorrhage, and puerperal sepsis. In-direct causes include conditions which, although present before pregnancy, are aggravated by pregnancy: examples are cardiac disease, anaemia, thyroid disease, diabetes and certain malignancies. Non-obstetric causes include car accidents, malaria, typhoid fever and some other infectious diseases.

In Britain, maternal mortality is defined as 'the death of a woman within one year of pregnancy and childbirth'. The deaths are further classified under two headings: maternal deaths and associated deaths.

In Britain and Australia, to take examples of developed countries where statistics are very accurate, the maternal death rate has been falling since 1934 when it was 52 and 60 per 10 000 live births respectively, rates similar to that which had existed for the previous 20 years (Fig. **54/1**). The most striking fall, initially, was of the deaths caused by sepsis, and this was due to the discovery of the sulphonamides and penicillin; but other factors have played a part. In Britain, the wartime food policy provided extra

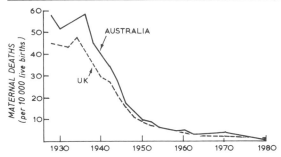

**Fig. 54/1** The secular trend of maternal mortality in Australia and the United Kingdom

rations for pregnant women if they attended for antenatal care, and this led to the increasing use and availability of antenatal clinics where abnormalities of pregnancy were detected early. Simultaneously with this, the blood transfusion services made blood readily available and the spectre of death from haemorrhage receded. In medical schools greater emphasis was laid on adequate obstetric training in the undergraduate period and the Royal College of Obstetricians and Gynaecologists played its part by recommending postgraduate experience for all those doctors who intended to care for pregnant women, and in suggesting improvements in the design of maternity units. In the post-war years the rapidity of the decline in the mortality rate has decreased, but statistics from several developed countries show that the rate is still falling slowly (Table **54/1**).

| Country | *Year* 1939 | 1965 | 1970 | 1985 |
|---|---|---|---|---|
| Australia | 410 | 30 | 19 | 9 |
| United Kingdom | 320 | 25 | 22 | 6 |
| United States | 410 | 33 | 22 | 9 |

**Table 54/1** The decline in the maternal mortality rate (direct causes) in three developed nations since 1939 (rate per 100 000 confinements)

## FACTORS ASSOCIATED WITH MATERNAL MORTALITY

### Parity

The effect of increasing parity upon maternal mortality is considerable. In Britain, the pregnancies in which the rate is below average are the second, third and fourth, the first being slightly above average. The slightly higher risk in first pregnancies is due to

the increased number of extra-marital pregnancies occurring in that group. From the fifth pregnancy onwards the risk rises considerably, the rate for that pregnancy being double the average, and by the tenth pregnancy it is treble the average.

### Age

The United Kingdom studies indicate that the risk of death in pregnancy and childbirth is higher than the mean if the woman is under the age of 20, irrespective of her parity. Obstetrically the safest age to give birth is 20 to 29, and after that age the mortality rate increases.

### Age and parity

In Britain, the last three confidential reports include an age–parity analysis. It was found that the risk of maternal death increased with age, independent of parity. The analysis showed that the safest age for a mother to have her first baby was between 20 and 25, whereas a primigravida aged 40 years or more was at the greatest risk. At all ages the maternal death rate was considerably increased amongst women having their fourth, or subsequent child. Part of the reduction in maternal mortality in England and Wales since 1966, compared with the earlier 20-year period, is due to the fact that fewer women over the age of 30, and fewer women of para 4 or more now give birth. In 1964 to 66, 27.5 per cent of all births were to women aged 30 or more: by 1976–78, the proportion had fallen to 23 per cent. In 1964–66, women, para 4 or more, gave birth to 15.6 per cent of all births, by 1976–78, the percentage had fallen to 7.1 per cent.

The importance of these demographic changes in fertility and fecundity, in reducing maternal mortality is considerable, and has been made possible by the adoption of family planning methods by many couples.

### Social class

In the United Kingdom the maternal mortality rate increases as the social class of the husband falls. The effect of social class cannot be considered in isolation, as women of the lower social classes are likely to have been the least privileged in nutrition, housing, education and social amenities from birth. In Malaysia a similar association was noted, the rate amongst wives of professional and managerial groups, upper echelon clerks and skilled workers being one-sixth that of the wives of unskilled workers. In the USA similar differences are noted when the rates amongst 'Blacks' are compared with the rate amongst 'Whites' (Fig. **54/2**).

## Antenatal care

The most significant immediate factor affecting maternal mortality rates is the availability of antenatal care, and its acceptance by the community. Unfortunately, those very groups which have the highest mortality rate (unmarried primigravidae, high multigravidae and those of the lower socio-economic groups) are the women who least often avail themselves of the facility. This is reflected by a tenfold increase in the mortality rate in Malaysia amongst those who did not attend antenatal clinics, as can be seen in Table **54/2**.

|  | Numbers | Deaths | Rate |
|---|---|---|---|
| Antenatal care | 59 449 | 77 | 1.3 |
| No antenatal care | 13 835 | 206 | 14.9 |
|  | 73 284 | 283 | 3.8 |

**Table 54/2** Effect of antenatal care on the maternal mortality rate (Kuala Lumpur, 1953–62)

## THE CAUSES OF MATERNAL DEATH

The Confidential Enquiries into Maternal Deaths in England and Wales, which have been published every three years since 1952, discuss the deaths

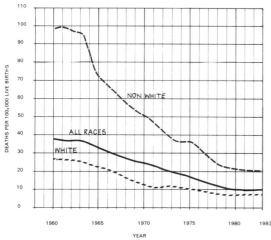

**Fig. 54/2** Maternal mortality rates, by race – United States, 1960 to 1983

analysed by 'main cause of death', when several factors were present. The Maternal Mortality Committee of the National Medical and Research Council in Australia adopts an identical procedure.

In Table **54/3** the direct and indirect causes of maternal death occurring in England and Wales are shown and the steady decline in deaths over the period can be seen. Several matters which appear in the 'Report on Confidential Enquiries into Maternal Deaths in England and Wales' require comment. In 1979–81, 87 women died following but not necessarily due to caesarean section, a death rate of 0.5 per 1000 caesarean sections. In 67 of these deaths, the caesarean section was performed as an emergency and in 20 it was elective. Of these deaths, 59 were classified as direct maternal deaths and they accounted for one-third of all direct deaths; 29 of these women died from causes attributable to anaesthesia, 8 following inhalation of stomach contents; 5 of the 8 developed aspiration pneumonitis (Mendelson's syndrome); 14 women died following an abortion; 5 of the deaths followed a legal abortion (4 from pulmonary embolism and 1 from sepsis); 6 deaths followed a spontaneous abortion and in 3 it was unclear whether the abortion was induced or spontaneous. These 3 women died from sepsis.

In the British Confidential Reports an analysis is made of factors involved in the maternal deaths, and whether these were avoidable or not. In the 1976–78 series avoidable factors were present in 60 per cent of all deaths. The British Confidential Report calculates that the responsibility for permitting the avoidable factor to occur was that of the consultant hospital staff in 55 per cent, other hospital staff (including midwives) in 6 per cent; the general practitioner in 13 per cent, health administrators in 3 per cent and the patient in 23 per cent.

Each chapter of the British Confidential Report ends with a summary of measures which might be taken by doctors, nurse-midwives, or administrators to reduce the number of maternal deaths. Similar analysis of maternal deaths in Australia and New York State also show that a high proportion of avoidable factors are present (Table **54/4**).

In all the countries mentioned the maternal death rate has fallen in the past 27 years. In Figure **54/3**, the decline for the four main causes of maternal death in England and Wales since 1952 is shown.

The reduction in maternal deaths is due to several causes. First, as noted earlier, to a change in demographic patterns of fecundity. Second, to better antenatal, intrapartum and postpartum care. Third,

|  | *1952–54* | *1970–72* | *1979–81* |
|---|---|---|---|
| *DIRECT CAUSES* | | | |
| Hypertensive disease in pregnancy | 246 | 47 | 36 |
| Pulmonary embolism | 138 | 52 | 23 |
| Anaesthesia | * | 37 | 22 |
| Ectopic gestation | 59 | 34 | 20 |
| Amniotic fluid embolism | * | 16 | 18 |
| Haemorrhage | 220 | 27 | 14 |
| Abortion | 244 | 71 | 14 |
| Sepsis, excluding abortion | 68 | 30 | 8 |
| Ruptured uterus | * | 13 | 4 |
| Other direct causes | 219 | 13 | 17 |
|  | 1094 | 340 | 176 |
| *INDIRECT CAUSES* | | | |
| Cardiac disease | * | 39 | 16 |
| Blood diseases | * | 21 | 3 |
| Cerebral haemorrhage/thrombosis | * | 31 | 32 |
| Neoplastic disease | * | 31 | 8 |
| Other | * | 126 | 64 |
|  | | 251 | 123 |
| *DEATH RATE* (per million pregnancies) | | | |
| Direct causes | * | 124 | 72 |
| Indirect causes | * | 109 | 50 |

* information not available

**Table 54/3** The direct and indirect causes of maternal death, England and Wales, 1952–81

| *Cause* | *Percentage of deaths* | *Proportion avoidable* |
|---|---|---|
| Hypertensive disease of pregnancy | 10–25 | 50 |
| Pulmonary embolism | 5–20 | 30 |
| Abortion | 5–15 | 25 |
| Ectopic gestation | 5–15 | 20 |
| Haemorrhage | 5–15 | 50 |
| Sepsis | 5–15 | 30 |
| Cardio-respiratory (including anaesthetic) | 5–15 | 30 |

**Table 54/4** Most common causes of maternal deaths (Australia, England and Wales, New York State)

the ready availability of blood for transfusion. Fourth, to the decline in the virulence of commonly encountered bacteria.

## THE REDUCTION OF MATERNAL MORTALITY

Since the death rate is so much higher in the underdeveloped countries, and in the affluent societies amongst the submerged 20 per cent of the people, the following suggestions for reducing maternal deaths apply, in the main, to these two groups.

1. The provision of conveniently sited antenatal clinics and the education of women to use the facilities provided. Whilst the State, the obstetrician and the family doctor are providing antenatal care, it is up to the community leaders, the press and all educated people to show the poorer and less

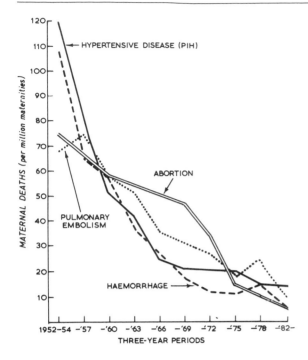

**Fig. 54/3** Main causes of maternal death directly due to pregnancy or childbirth (England and Wales, 1952–82) per 1 000 000 maternities

educated sections of the population that care during the 40 weeks of pregnancy is as important as care during the 12 hours of labour.

2. The provision of facilities for family planning and fertility control, so that the hazard of frequent, repeated childbearing is minimized.

3. The provision of properly designed, adequately equipped obstetric hospitals, which would receive from the peripheral hospitals (or maternity homes), and family doctors, all patients who would more suitably be delivered in units where specialist care is available. These include all women pregnant for the fourth or subsequent time; all primigravidae over the age of 30; all patients with a multiple pregnancy; patients who have had an abnormality in a previous pregnancy or labour, or who develop an abnormality in the present pregnancy; and all women whose labour has lasted more than 18 hours, for whatever cause. The hospitals should have sufficient antenatal beds to admit all patients requiring treatment; in the developed countries an antenatal: postnatal bed ratio of 1 to 8, and in the developing countries a ratio of 1 to 4, is required. The hospitals should also be designed to ensure that the operating theatre is adjacent to the delivery suite and the blood bank and pathological laboratory accessible to both.

4. The provision of facilities for all family doctors who intend to care for pregnant women, to spend 6 months to 1 year after graduation in a selected, properly equipped and adequately staffed obstetric hospital, where continued education is possible. It is also recommended that all family doctors practising obstetrics return every 3 to 5 years for a 2- to 4-week organized course of instruction in the subject.

5. The provision in the central obstetric hospital of medical staff in sufficient numbers to permit teaching and research to be conducted as well as routine clinical care of patients. The specialist obstetricians and gynaecologists in the hospital should have undergone a course of training of not less than 3 years in their specialty.

6. The provision of permanent senior trained nursing staff in the larger obstetric hospitals and, in the developing countries, the intensive training of sufficient midwives to work in the hospitals, the towns, the villages and the rural areas, so that one midwife is available to every 1000 of the population.

The death of a mother in pregnancy or childbirth is the greatest tragedy which can befall a family and the reduction of the maternal mortality is one of the most important indications of the efficiency of the medical care provided in any country. When the rate drops, as it has done in the developed countries, more and more attention is being directed to the perinatal mortality rate.

# PERINATAL MORTALITY

The ability of the infant to survive the first week of life depends largely upon three factors. First, it depends on the physiological reserves with which it is born, and this in turn depends on the health of the mother in pregnancy, and on the quality of the antenatal care which she receives. Secondly, it depends on the care with which labour is conducted, and this, in turn, is related to the quality of training and the skill of the medical attendants. Thirdly, it depends on the quality of care available to the newborn baby and this in turn relates to the availability of intensive neonatal care units.

The factors which may lead to the death of a fetus in utero, with the delivery of a stillbirth, and those which cause neonatal death, in some cases are identical. This has led to the introduction of a new and more precise method of determining the quality of the obstetric services of a country or region. This is the perinatal mortality rate.

**International definitions (WHO, 1979)**

*Live birth* is the complete expulsion or extraction from its mother of a product of conception, irrespective of the duration of the pregnancy, which after such separation, breathes or shows any evidence of life, such as beating of the heart, pulsation of the umbilical cord, or definite movement of the voluntary muscles: whether or not the umbilical cord has been cut or the placenta is attached, each product of such a birth is considered live born.

*Fetal death* is death prior to the complete expulsion or extraction from its mother of a product of conception, irrespective of the duration of pregnancy; the death is indicated by the fact that after such separation the fetus does not breathe or show other evidence of life, such as beating of the heart, pulsation of the umbilical cord, or definite movement of voluntary muscles.

*Early fetal deaths* equate to abortions, and *intermediate fetal deaths* are those occurring between the 22nd and 27th completed gestational weeks, the fetus weighing 500 to 999g (also called stillbirth).

*Late fetal death* is fetal death at 28 completed weeks of gestation and over. The fetus usually weighs 1000g or more (also called stillbirth).

In 1975, the following definitions recommended by the World Health Organization, were accepted by the International Federation of Gynaecologists and Obstetricians (FIGO):

*Neonatal deaths* are deaths of live born infants occurring before 28 completed days of life. Neonatal deaths can be divided into two groups: *early neonatal deaths* and *late neonatal deaths*.

*Early neonatal, or postnatal* death is the death of a live born baby in the first seven completed days (168 hours) of life.

*Late neonatal death* is the death of a live born infant after seven completed days but before 28 completed days of life.

Two definitions of perinatal mortality are therefore possible: (1) the extended perinatal mortality rate; and (2) the basic, or standard, perinatal mortality rate.

The *extended perinatal mortality* is the sum of all fetal deaths (excluding pregnancies terminating before the 20th week of pregnancy in which the conceptus weighed less than 501g) and all neonatal deaths per 1000 births.

The *standard perinatal mortality* is the sum of late fetal deaths and early neonatal deaths, or, put in another way, is the number of stillbirths and first-week deaths of babies weighing 1000g or more at birth per 1000 births.

From these data mortality rates can be inferred and should be used for purposes of international comparison.

*Standard perinatal mortality rate:* The ratio of stillborn infants plus early neonatal deaths of infants weighing 1000g and over × 1000, *divided* by the total births of infants stillborn and live born weighing 1000g and over.

*Stillbirth rate:* Stillborn infants weighing 1000g and over × 1000 *divided* by the total births of infants (stillborn and live born) weighing 1000g and over.

*Early neonatal death rate:* Early neonatal deaths of infants weighing 1000g or more at birth × 1000, *divided* by live born infants weighing 1000g and over.

In the few developing nations which are able to collect data about perinatal mortality, the basic perinatal mortality rate is usually between 35 and 55 per 1000 births. In the developed nations the rate is usually below 20 per 1000 births. Until recently the rate has been dropping, but in the last decade the decline has slowed. There is evidence from many nations that more infants could be saved by the better application of existing knowledge and the better organization of existing medical services. There is a lower limit to which the perinatal mortality ratio can be reduced. This lies between 5 and 10 per 1000 live births.

Only a few nations have adopted the extended perinatal mortality ratio, notably Australia and certain Canadian provinces.

**Social factors affecting the perinatal mortality rate**

Most studies of the effect of social factors take data

CLINICAL ANTECEDENTS

NECROPSY FINDINGS AND PERCENT OF TOTAL DEATHS

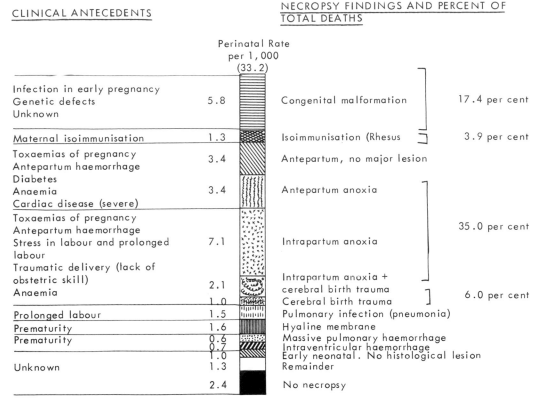

Perinatal Rate
per 1,000
(33.2)

| Clinical antecedents | Rate | Necropsy finding | Per cent |
|---|---|---|---|
| Infection in early pregnancy<br>Genetic defects<br>Unknown | 5.8 | Congenital malformation | 17.4 per cent |
| Maternal isoimmunisation | 1.3 | Isoimmunisation (Rhesus | 3.9 per cent |
| Toxaemias of pregnancy<br>Antepartum haemorrhage | 3.4 | Antepartum, no major lesion | |
| Diabetes<br>Anaemia<br>Cardiac disease (severe) | 3.4 | Antepartum anoxia | |
| Toxaemias of pregnancy<br>Antepartum haemorrhage<br>Stress in labour and prolonged labour | 7.1 | Intrapartum anoxia | 35.0 per cent |
| Traumatic delivery (lack of obstetric skill)<br>Anaemia | 2.1<br>1.0 | Intrapartum anoxia +<br>cerebral birth trauma<br>Cerebral birth trauma | 6.0 per cent |
| Prolonged labour | 1.5 | Pulmonary infection (pneumonia) | |
| Prematurity | 1.6 | Hyaline membrane | |
| Prematurity | 0.6<br>0.7 | Massive pulmonary haemorrhage<br>Intraventricular haemorrhage | |
| | 1.0 | Early neonatal. No histological lesion | |
| Unknown | 1.3 | Remainder | |
| | 2.4 | No necropsy | |

**Fig. 54/4** Primary necropsy findings and clinical correlations in British Perinatal Mortality Survey, 1958 (information obtained from Butler and Bonham (1963). *Perinatal Mortality*, Churchill Livingstone, Edinburgh)

from a single hospital, or from a small region, but two studies in the United Kingdom, one in 1958, and the second in 1970, investigated all singleton births occurring in 1 week and all singleton stillbirths and neonatal deaths occurring over a 3-month period. Information from this study is extremely valuable.

SOCIAL CLASS

In the British Perinatal Mortality Surveys it was confirmed that the social class exerted a profound effect on perinatal mortality, which was 3.5 times as high in the lowest social classes compared with the highest (class I, 7.5 per 1000, Classes IV and V, 26.8 per 1000). Similar findings of the effect of social class have been obtained from Australia and the USA. However, in Britain and Australia the higher perinatal mortality rate (and higher incidence of low birth-weight babies) are due more to life-style factors (e.g. cigarette-smoking and alcohol consumption) then to socio-economic class *per se*.

AGE

An increasing perinatal mortality with maternal age (after 30 years) was noted in Britain, Malaysia and in New South Wales, and this was apparent even amongst patients who had attended antenatal clinics. The rate was also higher under the age of 20 in Britain although this effect was not so marked in Australia.

PARITY

In Britain the risk to the first baby is greater than that to the second, third and probably fourth, which are at average risk. From the fifth baby the risk rises steadily. In New South Wales the risk increased with rising parity, but no significant increase occurred in women delivering their first, second or third baby.

**Effect of antenatal care**

Patients in Britain who did not avail themselves of

antenatal care had five to ten times the average perinatal mortality. Similar findings have been obtained in studies in the USA and Malaysia.

### Medical conditions

Unfavourable social conditions, particularly the absence, or inadequacy, of antenatal care, will influence considerably the incidence and management of disorders occurring in pregnancy and consequently the perinatal mortality rate. Examples are the damaging effect of untreated anaemia, unrecognized cardiac or renal disease, and undetected PIH. Similarly, mismanagement of antepartum haemorrhage will increase the perinatal mortality rate.

### Management of labour

In the British survey no less than 31 per cent of the perinatal loss was due to intrapartum anoxia alone, or associated with birth trauma. In some cases the intrapartum anoxia was a sequel to antepartum anoxia and the fetus entered labour in a precarious condition; in others mismanagement of labour, or the misuse of forceps, aggravated the anoxia and led to the birth of a dead baby, or a damaged baby which died in the first week of life.

### Correlation between social and medical factors

Although a woman of the higher socio-economic groups is usually older when she has her first baby than her sister in the lower groups, she starts pregnancy with better nutritional reserves and is likely to have been well fed since birth. As well as this, she is able to afford a higher standard of obstetric care in the antenatal period and during labour.

A woman of the lower socio-economic groups, on the other hand, is likely to have her first baby when she is under the age of 20 and to have a greater number of pregnancies. Her nutritional state from childhood is likely to have been less adequate, particularly with regard to protein intake, and consequently abnormalities of pelvic shape are more common. In pregnancy she may not receive such skilled attention, and is not so likely to receive antenatal care; pregnancy-induced hypertension and antepartum haemorrhage are more likely to be dangerous. In labour, the attention she receives may not be of such a high standard. That these factors operate can be deduced from a study made in Malaysia. Only primigravidae who had attended the ante-

natal clinics at least twice were included in the survey, and age and social status were analysed. Amongst the higher social classes the incidence of hypertensive disease in pregnancy was half that of patients in the lower socio-economic groups, whilst the reverse was found in operative deliveries (caesarean section and mid-forceps; low forceps are excluded since in many cases the reason was one of convenience only). The rate of operative deliveries in the higher group was three times that of the lower group, but the perinatal mortality rate was 16.7 per 1000 in the higher group, compared with 21.4 per 1000 in the lower group. The differences were particularly marked amongst primigravidae aged 30 or more. Comparable findings have been reported from the USA.

### 'Illegitimacy'

If the mother is unmarried, the perinatal mortality rate of her infant is said to be raised. Studies in the USA have shown this to be so, but in an investigation at The Women's Hospital (Crown Street) Sydney, the perinatal mortality of 'illegitimate'

|  | NSW 1979 | Scotland 1977–81 |
|---|---|---|
| *Environmental* | | |
| Unexplained, low birth-weight | 25.1 | 33.4 |
| Antepartum haemorrhage | 10.4 | 12.1 |
| Congenital anomaly | 20.6 | 24.1 |
| Maternal disorder | 5.5 | 4.1 |
| | | |
| *Obstetric* | | |
| Uexplained, normal birthweight | 19.1 | 7.2 |
| Pregnancy-induced hypertension | 7.2 | 8.4 |
| Mechanical/trauma | 4.7 | 3.6 |
| Iso-immunization | 1.8 | 1.3 |
| Infection/miscellaneous | 5.6 | 2.2 |
| | $n = 866$ | $n = 3781$ |
| Standard perinatal mortality rate | 11.03 | 14.0 |
| Births in period | 78 502 | 270 581 |

**Table 54/5** Comparison of the clinico-pathological classification of perinatal deaths in New South Wales and Scotland, proportional percentages

| Cause of death | High risk mothers |
|---|---|
| 1. Unexplained, low birth-weight (25 to 30 per cent of all) | Low socio-economic status<br>Reduced height<br>In all social classes, highest in women under 20 and over 35<br>Para 4 or more<br>Cigarette smoking |
| 2. Antepartum haemorrhage (10 to 15 per cent of all) | Para 4 or more<br>Low socio-economic status |
| 3. Fetal malformations (20 to 30 per cent of all)<br>    (a) CNS | Increase with diminishing socio-economic status<br>Primiparity<br>Increased rate in primiparae under the age of 20 |
|     (b) Other | Increase with increasing parity and age |
| 4. Maternal disease (3 to 7 per cent of all) | Increase with increasing maternal age: no effect from parity |
| 5. Pregnancy-induced hypertension (6 to 10 per cent of all) | Primiparae<br>Women over 30<br>History of toxaemia in a previous pregnancy |
| 6. Mechanical/trauma (5 to 10 per cent of all) | Primiparity, especially if aged 30 or more<br>Short stature<br>Para 4 or more (inadequate obstetric care) |
| 7. Unexplained, normal birth-weight (10 to 20 per cent of all) | Primiparae, especially aged 30 or more<br>Para 4 or more<br>Post term (i.e. 42 weeks' gestation) especially in older primigravidae |
| 8. Iso-immunization (1 per cent of all) | Increasing parity |
| 9. Infections (1 to 4 per cent of all) | None discerned apart from? increasing age |

**Table 54/6** Standard perinatal mortality by clinico-pathological classification showing mothers likely to have the highest risk. (Information from *Perinatal Problems*, Chapter 12, by Sir Dugald Baird and A. M. Thompson; *Perinatal Mortality Committee Reports*, the Women's Hospital, Crown Street, Sydney)

infants was not raised, provided the mother had availed herself of antenatal care.

### The analysis of perinatal mortality

Most death certificates reporting perinatal mortality only list the immediate causes of death and do not permit a multiple cause analysis so that problems can be identified and solutions introduced to reduce the perinatal death rate.

Until such times as multiple cause analysis is available, the clinico-pathological classification of perinatal mortality suggested by Professor Sir Dugald Baird has much merit. This classification is based on why the baby died rather than the pathological cause

found for its death. For example, autopsy might show that a 2400g baby died in late pregnancy from anoxia, but what is important is to determine why the anoxia occurred.

The clinico-pathological classification of perinatal mortality is shown in Tables **54/5** and **54/6**.

### The reduction of perinatal mortality

First, since the perinatal mortality rate is higher in the most deprived groups, the provision of adequate nutrition from childhood (and this implies that the mothers receive instruction and are educated in the best use of foodstuffs), and the limitation in the number of children each couple chooses to have would reduce the rate. Second, as these patients attend antenatal clinics less frequently and may be supervised in labour by less skilled attendants, there is need for an improvement in the obstetric services available to all the population, and a concerted propaganda effort is required to induce women to avail themselves of the facilities.

Methods of reducing perinatal mortality are similar to methods of reducing maternal mortality with the important addition that well-staffed, well-equipped neonatal care departments are essential. However, such units are only economically viable if they serve a hospital at which more than 3500 babies are delivered each year. This argues for the referral of problem obstetric patients to larger hospitals for confinement.

## SOCIAL FACTORS IN OBSTETRICS

The optimum age at which to be pregnant, as far as maternal and fetal morbidity and mortality is concerned, is between the age of 18 and 30. Women under the age of 18, particularly if primigravida, are at increased risk. Statistically such women account for about 2 to 5 per cent of all pregnancies. They are more likely to give birth to low birth-weight babies, and consequently the pregnancy is associated with a higher perinatal mortality. A pregnant adolescent women is also more likely to develop pregnancy induced hypertension, at least as reported in some studies. Analysis of the data shows that in most instances the increased perinatal risk is due to (1) lack of antenatal care, (2) an inadequate diet, (3) the use of social and addictive drugs and (4) low socio-economic status. If an adolescent primigravida receives and accepts regular antenatal care from early pregnancy, the problems are no greater than amongst older primigravid women: the problems are social rather than biological.

The second group at higher risk are primigravid women aged 35 or older, the so-called 'older primigravidae'. These women have an increased risk of developing hypertensive disease and diabetes in pregnancy; of having a caesarean section or a vaginal operative delivery performed; of giving birth to a preterm baby and of having a baby with a congenital defect.

# Part Seven

# THE INFANT

## Chapter 55

# Neonatal Physiology and Care of the Newborn

In utero the fetus relies upon the placenta to carry out its respiratory function, and its nutritional and excretory exchanges. It therefore has no need to use its lungs, little need for liver function and its energies are mainly concerned in pumping sufficient blood to the placenta, so that the exchanges needed for survival and growth can take place. But with birth, and the separation of the placenta from its bed, the newborn infant is dependent for life upon its own efforts. It must initiate and maintain its own tissue oxygenation, and must alter its circulatory system so that blood is pumped to the lungs instead of the placenta. It must obtain its own food and excrete the waste products of its metabolism. It must maintain its own fluid and electrolyte balance. It must maintain its own body temperature. It must manufacture its own immunoglobulins and mobilize its own defence mechanisms to counter any infection.

The degree to which it succeeds in these complex functions has a broad relationship to maturity, and the shorter the period of gestation the more the chances of survival diminish. Nonetheless many immature infants do survive, and the reason for the loss of many others remains elusive. The primitive nervous responses governing the respiratory and circulatory system mature relatively early. The lungs are capable of exchanging gases sufficient to support life by about the 25th week of gestation, but in other respects, for example the softness of the chest cage and the full quota of surface-active agent in the alveoli, respiratory function is less well developed. The balance is delicate and in the commonly unfavourable circumstances surrounding the birth of premature infants, the interrelated functions of the respiratory and circulatory systems may fail to become established before a damaging cycle of events begins.

Another consideration is the efficiency of placental function while the child was in utero. If this has been inadequate, and the fetus consequently compelled to live in large part from its own resources for some time before birth, even a mature infant may be poorly equipped with energy reserves to withstand the stresses of delivery.

## THE FETAL CIRCULATION IN UTERO

The blood circulation in utero has to maintain adequate tissue oxygenation with erythrocytes which are relatively poorly saturated with oxygen. This is done by maintaining a good flow to the tissues, of which the more rapid fetal heart rate is possibly a reflection, and by certain advantages of fetal blood. These are, first, that the oxygen-carrying capacity of fetal blood is slightly more than that of adult blood, and secondly, that because blood on the fetal side of the placenta is very slightly more acidotic than on the maternal side, transfer of oxygen is favoured. Fetal haemoglobin (HbF) is chemically different from adult, but this is no longer thought to be the explanation for the greater oxygen-carrying capacity of fetal blood. The explanation seems to be that HbF is less affected by the reducing capacity of red cell glycerophosphate than is HbA. This means that red cells containing HbF are more readily able to take up oxygen transferred across the placental membrane.

The fetal circulation can best be described by starting at the umbilical arteries (Fig. **55/1**). Blood leaves the fetus through the umbilical arteries which, in vivo, are large vessels and carry more than half the ventricular output away from the fetus for the purpose of perfusing the placenta. A rapid reduction in blood pressure occurs in the villi and the slowly moving blood takes up oxygen which has been transported across the placental trophoblastic cells

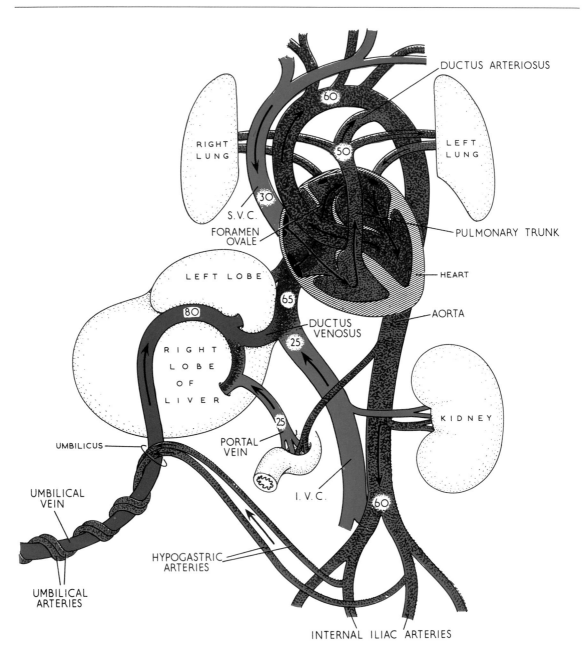

**Fig. 55/1** Normal circulation in the fetus in utero. IVC = inferior vena cava; SVC = superior vena cava. The figures give the approximate oxygen saturation of the blood at given points in the circulatory system

separating the maternal and fetal circulations. The umbilical vein, containing oxygenated blood (80 per cent saturated), goes to the liver where it gives off branches to supply the left lobe and receives the venous blood from the portal vein. The greater por-tion of the oxygenated blood, mixed with some portal venous blood, then bypasses the liver through the ductus venosus to enter the inferior vena cava, and the right atrium of the heart. Here further admix-ture occurs with blood returning from the head and

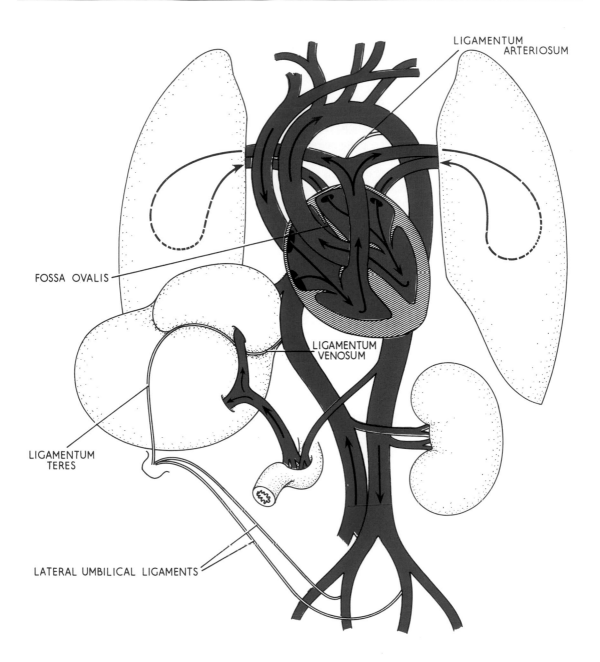

**Fig. 55/2** Normal circulation in the newborn

neck via the superior vena cava. Seventy-five per cent of this mixed blood is deflected through the foramen ovale into the left atrium; 25 per cent enters the right ventricle and is pumped into the pulmonary artery and ductus arteriosus which bypasses the lungs to reach the arch of the aorta. The blood in the left atrium, mixed with the small amount returning from the pulmonary veins, passes into the left ventricle and is pumped, in ventricular systole, into the aorta.

## CIRCULATORY CHANGES AT BIRTH

Within a few moments of birth several events happen almost simultaneously. The large volume of blood returning to the fetus ceases with ligation of the umbilical cord, and hence venous pressure falls in the vena cava. This causes the ductus venosus to close since no blood is available to keep it distended. As well as this the pressure in the right atrium falls. The lungs expand with the first breath and pulmonary vascular resistance falls abruptly with a simultaneous large increase in blood flow through the lungs to enter the left atrium, and the pressure rises within it. Thus venous pressure falls on the right side of the heart and rises on the left, with consequent closure of the flap-like valve of the foramen ovale. Pulmonary arterial pressure falls because of the reduced resistance, systematic arterial pressure rises slightly, and consequently the fetal direction of flow through the ductus arteriosus is reversed and now becomes left-to-right. The ductus contracts over the next few hours by muscular action in response to rising oxygen tension, and blood flow ceases, but a small left-to-right shunt may persist for a few days in some infants. More work is required of each ventricle because, after birth, they work in series and not in parallel, as in utero.

## CIRCULATION IN THE NEONATE

With the closure of the ductus venosus, the foramen ovale and the ductus arteriosus, the adult pattern of circulation is established (Fig. **55/2**). The heart enlarges slightly and this temporary cardiac enlargement is often associated with systolic murmurs which are functional, usually last for a few hours or days, and may be confused with the murmurs due to congenital heart disease. Since metabolic needs are high, the heart continues to beat rapidly and the rate only falls to below 100 beats a minute by the 3rd day of life. As the heart rate drops the cardiac enlargement disappears. With normal oxygen saturation the need for the additional oxygen-carrying qualities of fetal erythrocytes ceases, and they are replaced, as they die, by adult type erythrocytes.

## LUNG DEVELOPMENT IN UTERO

The lung develops by the growth of the bronchial tree into the surrounding mesenchyme. As it grows it branches constantly, and by the 16th week of fetal life a complex branched tubular structure surrounded by

mesenchyme has developed. The tubules are lined by columnar or cuboidal epithelium. At this stage the lung is said to be in the 'glandular' stage of development.

At about the 20th week a rather sudden change takes place. The cuboidal epithelial cells become flattened and their cytoplasm becomes extended at the periphery so that the tubules are lined with a flatter epithelium. Simultaneously a complex capillary network develops beneath the epithelial basement membrane, and secretion of fluid occurs to fill the lung passages, including the trachea. The terminal tubules now dilate and have the appearance of primitive alveoli.

Between the 20th and 24th weeks a further change occurs. Within the cytoplasm of the epithelial cells, inclusion bodies appear, and a surface-active material is secreted into the alveoli. This surfactant is a complex of protein and lipids (mainly dipalmitrol lecithin). It has the important function of forming a film at the interface between the alveolar lining membrane and the oxygen in the alveolus itself. This effectively reduces the alveolar surface tension and improves lung distensibility.

In utero, this is of no importance, but it is of vital concern in the initiation of respiration, as it facilitates the expansion of the lung at birth, making breathing easier, and subsequently has a role of great importance in allowing the air-containing lung to maintain its normal volume.

In normal circumstances substantial amounts of lipid-containing fluid are constantly secreted by the fetal lungs and pass into the nasopharynx. Most of this is swallowed by the fetus and reabsorbed in the intestines. Some is expelled into the amniotic fluid. This has now become important clinically, since measurement of the lipid content of amniotic fluid is an index of fetal lung maturity.

## INITIATION OF BREATHING

The birth of the fetal head occurs simultaneously with a strong contraction and retraction of the uterus which separates the placenta and leads to increasing fetal asphyxia, i.e. decline in blood oxygenation and increase in carbon dioxide content. Asphyxia is an exceedingly powerful stimulus to the respiratory centre acting reflexly on the centre by stimulating the carotid body chemoreceptors. And yet the normal fetus in the later months of pregnancy exists in an environment which is very hypoxic by normal standards without being so stimulated. This apparent paradox has led to much difficulty in explaining the 'cause' of the first breath. The notion that primitive respiratory movements in the young fetus become inhibited by the developing higher centres, with subsequent release at birth, was popular, but is no longer tenable. Sensory stimuli, both thermal and painful, have a role, but since asphyxiation is also present, their relative importance cannot be decided. The problem is to find an explanation which satisfies both the behaviour of the normal 90 per cent or more of newborn babies, and of the minority who are depressed and fail to breathe, in the light of the fact that both categories experience lesser or greater degrees of hypoxia and $CO_2$ retention. The best evidence at present all points to the mild asphyxiation of normal delivery as the stimulus for the first gasp of the healthy baby. Various factors in combination are responsible for abnormal prolongation of apnoea. They include the degree of previous intra-uterine hypoxia which impairs the capacity of the centre to respond, the state of the heart and circulation supplying it with blood, and the possibility of drug effects. When ventilation begins with lung expansion the depressant chain of events is reversed. With the first gasps, the fluid filling the lung passages is driven into the expanding alveoli, from whence it is rapidly absorbed by the lymphatics and the pulmonary circulation. Within about 15 minutes of birth, the fluid has disappeared and the alveoli are distended by air.

Once breathing has been initiated, the rhythmic respirations are maintained by carotid chemoreceptors which are responsible for the ventilating response to hypoxia.

## SEVERE HYPOXIA IN THE NEONATE

The effect of complete anoxia on fetal animals has been studied by immersing them in nitrogen. Four distinct phases of respiratory effort occur before death supervenes. These are: (1) a short period of hyperventilation; (2) a period of primary apnoea lasting 5 minutes; (3) a period of gasping lasting about 15 minutes; and (4) following the 'last gasp' a period of secondary apnoea lasting until death.

Human infants at birth may be in the phases of primary apnoea or secondary apnoea, depending on the severity of hypoxia during birth. If in the former, the infant will rapidly recover provided the airways are clear. If in secondary apnoea, oxygen given by intermittent positive ventilation is essential. In neither condition are analeptic drugs of any value.

## LIVER FUNCTION IN THE NEONATE

Although adult and neonatal liver cells are identical morphologically, in the first few days of life the neonatal liver cells are deficient in certain important functions. The neonatal liver is able to take up oxygen and glucose as efficiently as the adult liver, and glycogen synthesis is more efficient than that of the adult. However, the liver's detoxicating functions are impaired, and this is due to the enzymatic immaturity of the neonatal liver. Amino-acid degradation is also impaired, and this accounts for potentially dangerous levels of tyrosine and phenylalanine found in some premature infants. Conjugation with glucuronic acid is affected particularly, so that the neonate, especially if premature, has difficulty in conjugating bilirubin, cortisol and certain drugs such as morphine, salicylates and chloramphenicol.

The reduced ability to conjugate bilirubin is the most important consequence of the enzymatic immaturity, as each day millions of erythrocytes die and release bilirubin. As the kidney can only excrete bilirubin in the conjugated form, a 'physiological' jaundice may result. It is mild in most cases and occurs between the 3rd and 6th day of life.

The higher serum bilirubin and clinical jaundice found in some neonates, particularly premature infants, dysmature infants and those born to 'high-risk' mothers, appears to be due to a temporary deficiency of the enzyme glucuronyl transferase, which is needed for the conjugation of free bilirubin. It has been suggested that the activity of this enzyme in the microsomes of the liver cells may be enhanced by giving the mothers of high-risk infants small doses of phenobarbitone or alcohol over the last 2 weeks before childbirth. The procedure is still experimental and more information is required before either regimen can be recommended routinely.

In the first few hours of life the newborn infant uses carbohydrate as a source of energy. This is mobilized from liver stores of glycogen by circulating adrenaline and glucagon, and released by the enzymatic action of phosphorylase and glucose-6-phosphatase. The liver stores of glycogen are mainly laid down in the last 8 weeks of intra-uterine life, and should these be depleted from prematurity or from fetal malnutrition due to placental dysfunction, hypoglycaemia may result.

Quite soon after birth the neonate ceases to mobilize carbohydrate, and converts to the oxidization of non-esterified fatty acids, which are held in stores in the adipose tissues. The local oxidization of fats in brown adipose tissue also enables the neonate to produce heat without the method of shivering.

## NUTRITION OF THE NEONATE

The newborn, whether premature or mature, is able to digest monosaccharides and disaccharides, and protein, with little difficulty. Fats are less readily absorbed, particularly by premature babies, although all infants have fat-splitting enzymes present in the gut. Excretion of water also presents a slight problem in the perinatal period, as the neonate has proportionately 10 per cent more body fluid than the adult. Much of the weight loss noted in most infants in the first few days of life is due to the excretion of this water, and as renal physiological efficiency takes a little time to develop, fluid and electrolyte balance may be disturbed during this time.

## TEMPERATURE CONTROL

At birth, vasoconstriction of the skin vessels occurs to preserve body heat, but temperature maintenance is relatively hard for the neonate because of greater surface area and poor insulation in comparison with the adult. In many infants the body temperature falls by 1.5°C (3°F) or more after delivery (because of rapid loss of heat from a wet skin) rising to normal in a few hours. Because of the instability of temperature control, neonates require to be wrapped properly in cold climates, whilst in hot climates avoidance of too many clothes is necessary.

## RESISTANCE TO INFECTION

The fetus has the ability to form antibodies from about the 20th week of gestation, but rarely does so because the intra-uterine environment is relatively sterile, and maternal immunoglobulin G crosses the placenta to give the fetus a degree of passive immunity. The level of maternal IgG in the fetal circulation increases as the gestation period advances. The passively obtained antibodies protect the neonate to some extent for the first 12 to 24 weeks of life, but also impair the efficiency of its own immune response. However, if exposed to antigens, the neonate, whether premature or mature, responds with equal facility by producing immunoglobulins, but because of the passive maternal IgG in its circulation, its response is less marked than that of the adult, and for a variable period hypogammaglobulinaemia is present. The period lasts longer in a premature infant because it has a lower level of passive IgG at birth, and the resistance of the premature baby to infection is therefore likely to be less efficient.

# CARE OF THE NEWBORN

Once respiration has been established, congenital abnormalities have been sought and the parents have celebrated the birth of their child, it is placed in a warmed cot, wrapped in a clean cloth, and in non-tropical countries kept covered to avoid heat loss. Usually the baby is now weighed and measured. Any blood, meconium or mucus on its skin is removed by gentle swabbing with sterile swabs. The baby is not bathed, but its entire body is swabbed with 3 per cent hexachlorophane emulsion (Phisohex), with chlorhexidine cream (Hibitane, 0.5 per cent) or with water, depending on the hospital's regimen. Once this has been done, the baby is returned to its mother's room for 'rooming-in'.

### Care of the umbilical cord

Twenty-four hours after birth the stump of the umbilical cord is retied and cut close to the umbilicus, and the area is smeared with chlorhexidine cream, but no cord dressing or binder is required.

### Weight

Neonates lose between 5 and 10 per cent of their weight during the first 4 days of life and the loss is largely that of fluid. It occurs during the period of starvation before the maternal milk supply is established. It is well withstood by healthy infants born at term, though a few exhibit 'dehydration fever'. From the 4th day the weight begins to rise, and most infants have regained their birth-weight by the 10th day. From then on a weight gain of 120 to 240g (4 to 8 oz) per week may be expected.

## Stools

In the first 2 days of life the stools are of sticky greenish-black meconium. As the gut becomes invaded by micro-organisms, and as feeding starts, the colour changes to yellow with the occasional passage of green stools. The baby is likely to defaecate during feeding because of the gastrocolic reflex. If it is breast-fed the stool will be soft, yellow in colour and non-offensive in smell. However, the formula-fed baby does not defaecate so regularly as the breast-fed, and the stool, when passed, is of a firmer consistency, dark yellow and occasionally offensive.

## Effects of maternal hormones

Breast activity is not uncommon in male and female infants and in a few the mammary gland becomes enlarged and watery fluids can be expressed. The condition is due to the withdrawal of maternal oestrogen and, by 'feed-back', the release of pro-lactin by the fetal pituitary gland. It is without significance and settles rapidly without treatment.

The withdrawal of maternal oestrogen also leads in a few female infants to a 'genital crisis' when a discharge of sero-sanguinous fluid appears at the infant's vulva. Hymenal tags due to the proliferative effect of oestrogen on the infant's vaginal musosa, may also be found but regress in a few weeks and no treatment is required.

## Dehydration fever (heat exhaustion)

The neonate's temperature control is not efficient in the first few days and if the weather is hot and humid it may lose fluid by respiration, during crying and by sweating. Unless this fluid is replaced, heat exhaustion can occur. The baby develops high pyrexia – 39.8°C (103°F) or more, is clearly dehydrated with a dry mouth, depressed fontanelle and marked weight loss. The condition can be avoided by ensuring that babies in these climatic conditions receive sufficient fluid, and if the baby is 'roomed-in' with the mother, dehydration fever will occur rarely. Should a child develop dehydration fever, treatment is to replace the fluid and salt loss by giving oral feeds of 200ml 1/5 normal saline per kg body-weight per 24 hours.

It is important to differentiate dehydration fever from fever due to infection. Babies with dehydration fever are usually large, vigorous and thirsty. Those with infection are usually small and languid.

Extra feeds of water should be offered to the baby. If it drinks the water rapidly and the fever rapidly subsides, the diagnosis is dehydration fever. But if the fever persists despite extra water, infection should be suspected.

## Jaundice

As was mentioned, most babies develop a transient jaundice which is benign and self-limiting. A few infants develop more severe jaundice (serum bilirubin $> 320\mu mol/l$) which may cause kernicterus. Because of this danger, jaundice should be investigated if: (1) it appears within 24 hours of birth; (2) it persists for longer than 8 days; (3) it appears in a baby who is obviously ill; (4) it extends onto the baby's trunk or thighs; (5) the infant's urine is yellow. Investigations include measurement of serum bilirubin, haemoglobin, haematocrit and reticulocyte count. In persistent jaundice $T_3$ and TSH levels should also be measured and the possibility of 'breast-milk' jaundice investigated. In an ill baby, if the jaundice is extensive or if the urine is yellow, urine culture and tests for galactosaemia should be made. Treatment depends on the cause but in most cases phototherapy is also used. In severe cases, exchange transfusion may be needed.

## Feeding

The establishment of lactation in the mother and feeding the neonate have been discussed in Chapter 16.

## Chapter 56

# Examination of the Newborn: Congenital Defects

Once respirations have been established the child should be examined briefly, but systematically, to detect the more obvious congenital malformations. A method is shown in Table **56/1**, Figs **56/1** to **56/8**, and the procedures described in the captions. It should be noted that congenital heart disorders can be very difficult to diagnose as many murmurs are functional, and if any doubt exists the final assessment should not be made until 6 to 8 weeks after birth.

---

Examine baby one hour after a feed when he is likely to be calm, quiet and with open eyes. Get mother to undress the baby.

 1. Observe posture movements, check for skin abnormalities
 2. Palpate neck for goitre or sternomastoid tumour
 3. Look at eyes, see if he will follow side to side movements of examiner's face
 4. Measure occipito-frontal circumference, feel skull and fontanelles
 5. Get baby to open his mouth; examine for cleft palate
 6. Palpate abdomen
 7. Examine external genitalia, feel for femoral pulses
 8. Check Moro and traction manoeuvres:
    *Moro*: When picked up, the baby extends and abducts arms and fingers and opens eyes; he then flexes and abducts arms
    *Traction*: When lifted by grasping hands, the baby flexes his arms and keeps his head in the plane of his trunk
 9. Pick up baby in prone position: check muscle tone, examine spine (scoliosis), anus
10. Examine hips (p. 446)

**Table 56/1** Examination of newborn baby

## CONGENITAL DEFECTS

The chance of a mother giving birth to a baby with a congenital developmental defect varies from country to country, but appears to average about 20 to 30 per 1000 births. One half of these defective infants will be stillborn. The incidence of congenital defects is increased amongst women who are of the lower socio-economic groups and those of higher parity, although the reason for this difference is obscure.

There is no single cause which accounts for all congenital defects. In some cases the cause is genetic; in others it is due to an unfavourable intra-uterine environment consequent on maternal disease or inadequate maternal nutrition; in still others the defect may be due to the maternal ingestion of a drug. In over 65 per cent of cases no identifiable cause is detected. The period of maximum teratogenicity is from day 7 to day 63 after fertilization. This equates to 3 weeks to 11 weeks after the first day of the last menstrual period in a woman with a normal menstrual cycle. During this phase organogenesis is initiated and largely completed, and the type of malformation is directly related to the precise time the agent operates during morphogenesis.

Chromosomal anomalies occur in about 4 per 1000 births. The most common autosomal abnormalities are 18-trisomy and 21-trisomy, which manifest as Down's syndrome, and has an incidence of about 2 per 1000 births, being most frequent amongst women over the age of 40. The most common sex chromosome abnormalities are 47-XXY (Klinefelter's syndrome) and 47-XYY which are found in 2.0 and 1.5 per 1000 newborn male infants; and 47-XXX which is found in about 1.0 per 1000 newborn female infants.

Viruses and bacterial agents are causes of congenital abnormalities in certain undefined circumstances.

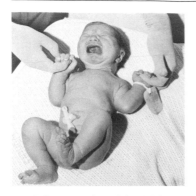

**Fig. 56/1** Inspection of the child as to general appearance and for obvious congenital abnormalities

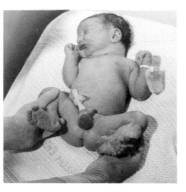

**Fig. 56/2** Congenital dislocation of the hips is sought by testing gross abduction and external rotation of the thigh and by observing for protrusion of the femoral heads

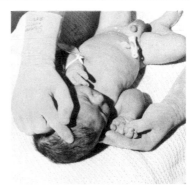

**Fig. 56/3** The fontanelles are palpated to evaluate the intracranial tension

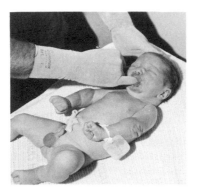

**Fig. 56/4** The mouth is examined to detect cleft palate

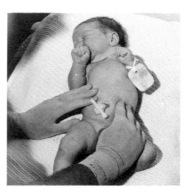

**Fig. 56/5** Gentle abdominal palpation determines the size of liver and spleen

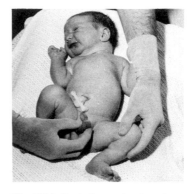

**Fig. 56/6** Genital examination determines the sex of the child and, if male, the position of the testes, which may lie in the scrotum or the inguinal canals. Occasionally they are still intra-abdominal

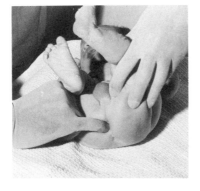

**Fig. 56/7** Rectal examination is made to exclude anal malformations, and a finger or catheter is inserted if the baby has not passed meconium

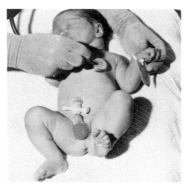

**Fig. 56/8** The chest is auscultated

| Major defects | Per 1000 births |
|---|---|
| Chromosomal (esp. Down's syndrome) | 2–4 |
| CNS defects  (a) Open neural tube defects | 1–3 |
| 1. anencephaly   0.5–1.5 | |
| 2. spina bifida    0.5–1.5 | |
| (b) Hydrocephaly | 1–2 |
| CVS defects. Heart and great vessels | 2–5 |
| Gastro-intestinal defects: | |
| (a) Hare lip, cleft palate | 1–2 |
| (b) Alimentary tract | |
| (esp. pyloric stenosis) | 1–3 |
| Urogenital defects | 0.5–1 |
| Skeletal defects: | 1–3 |
| Talipes | 1–3 |
| Congenital dislocated hip | 2–6 |
| Polydactyly, etc | 0.5–1 |
| Multiple defects | 0.5–1 |
| | |
| MAJOR  DEFECTS:        TOTAL | 13–27 |
| MINOR  DEFECTS (skin blemishes, etc) | 2–15 |

**Table 56/2** Congenital defects, per 1000 births

The most common viruses affecting the developing fetus are rubella (see Chapter 31), cytomegalovirus and toxoplasmosis, although other viruses have been implicated. Cytomegalovirus and toxoplasmosis cause subclinical infections in the adult, and the diagnosis is only possible retrospectively by detecting raised specific antibody titres in the maternal blood after the birth of a malformed fetus or a brain-damaged fetus (in the case of cytomegalovirus infection).

Ingestion of certain drugs in the first quarter of pregnancy may be a rare cause of congenital defects in the infant. However, maternal viral infection and drug ingestion account for less than 2 per cent of all defective neonates. As mentioned, more than one factor may be operative. The environmental factor appears to make a major contribution, whilst the genetic factor is minor and multifactorial (i.e. occurring at many gene loci). It must also be remembered that babies showing congenital malformations are the survivors of a very much larger group which were malformed and eliminated, as abortions, usually before the 14th week of gestation.

The data presented in Table **56/2** are derived from Australian national statistics and from teaching hospital reports from several countries. However, in a total population the frequency of malformations detected at birth would be increased by at least one-third if all the children were followed up for a few years. These two factors may cancel each other out.

In most countries the commonest malformations are anencephaly, hydrocephaly, talipes and cleft palate. The higher incidence of congenital heart lesions in the developed communities may be due to better diagnostic facilities and may not indicate an absolute increase.

## DRUGS AS A CAUSE OF CONGENITAL MALFORMATIONS

The disastrous consequences of the administration of the sedative thalidomide to pregnant women has emphasized the danger of indiscriminate, frequently unnecessary administration of drugs by unthinking doctors. Drugs are of immense value when properly used, they are dangerous when abused. Pregnant women should only be given pharmaceuticals when the need really exists, and then only those drugs proved by extensive testing should be prescribed. New drugs are only of value when they are demonstrably superior to tried ones, and no trial should be made on the pregnant woman.

In Table **56/3** the present knowledge of drugs which may affect the fetus adversely is given. With the exception of cortisone there are proven substitutes for all these drugs and the evidence that cortisone produces cleft palate is not conclusive. Recently, several observers have noted that babies born to epileptic mothers taking anticonvulsant drugs in the first 12 weeks of pregnancy have almost twice as many congenital defects as a control group. The evidence is only suggestive, and the risk small, so that women who require anticonvulsants should continue to take them in early pregnancy, as the anoxia associated with epileptic seizure may be an even more important factor in producing developmental defects. As anticonvulsants lead to subnormal folic acid levels, supplements of folic acid should be prescribed to epileptic women who are pregnant.

Excessive consumption of alcohol, particularly if the mother is undernourished or uses illegal drugs may cause the *fetal alcohol syndrome*. The syndrome includes pre- and post-natal growth retardation, facial abnormalities, organ damage and central nervous dysfunction, especially mental retardation.

| Drug | | Period of pregnancy when contra-indicated | Fetal effect |
|---|---|---|---|
| Alcohol | Alcohol in excess (2 glasses a day are not implicated) | Throughout | Abnormal facies, mental retardation, congenital heart defects |
| Antibacterials | Tetracyclines | From 30 weeks | Yellowing of deciduous teeth |
| | Aminoglycosides | Throughout | Ototoxic after long-term use of streptomycin |
| Anticoagulants | Coumarin group/warfarin | From 30 weeks | Fetal anticoagulation; possible haemorrhage and death in utero |
| Anticonvulsants | Barbiturates with primidone or phenytoin | From 35 weeks | Possible vitamin K deficiency with haemorrhage in neonate |
| | Lithium | First half | |
| Anti-epileptics | Phenytoin + primidone | Throughout | × 3 rate of cleft palate |
| Barbiturates | | In labour | Cross placenta rapidly, can lead to severe depression at birth |
| Benzodiazepines | | In labour, unless indication such as eclampsia | Slowly metabolized and eliminated by fetus and neonate – apnoea, depression for several days |
| Cytotoxic drugs | | Throughout (especially first half) unless essential for maternal survival | Cause fetal death or growth retardation |
| Antihypertensives | Hexamethonium | Late pregnancy | Paralytic ileus |
| | Reserpine | Late pregnancy | Nasal congestion |
| | Thiazides | Last quarter | |
| Antithyroid drugs | Iodine$^{131}$ | Second half | Fetal goitre |
| | Thiouracils | Second half | Fetal goitre |
| Steroids | 19 norsteroids | First 10 weeks | Masculinization of some females |
| | Synthetic oestrogens | First 10 weeks | Possible vaginal adenosis when child adolescent |
| | Corticosteroids (systemic) | Throughout unless essential | Possible growth retardation ?Cleft palate |
| Viruses | | Throughout, but especially in first half | *Live* viral vaccines may infect fetus. *Killed* viruses *not* contra-indicated |

**Table 56/3** Drugs which may affect the fetus

## COMMON CONGENITAL MALFORMATIONS

Only those abnormalities of concern to the obstetrician are mentioned, and then briefly, in this chapter, and further detailed description can be obtained from paediatric textbooks.

*Chromosomal abnormalities* occur in about 4 per 1000 births. The most common autosomal defect is 21-trisomy (Down's syndrome) which accounts for one-third of all chromosomal abnormalities.

### DOWN'S SYNDROME

Previously called 'mongols' from the appearance of their slanting eyes with epicanthic folds, infants with Down's syndrome also have short hands with small fingers, and feet with abnormal skin creases (Fig. **56/9**). The head is short and there are fat pads in the cheeks and on the back of the neck. The upper jaw is smaller than the lower and the mouth small, the nose flat and broad. The ears are squarish, the skin dry and the body hypotonic. Mental defect is general,

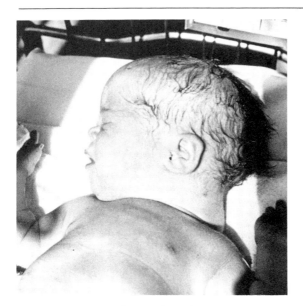

**Fig. 56/9** Down's syndrome

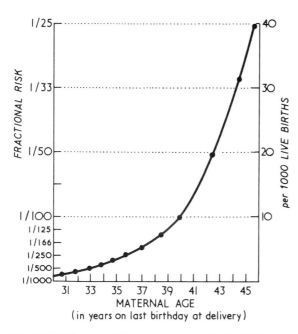

**Fig. 56/10** The rate of Down's syndrome in live births in relation to maternal age (from Cuckle H. S. et al, *Brit Med J*, 1987; **94**, 387–402)

ranging from idiocy to retardation. The condition is due to a non-disjunction of chromosomes 21 during gametogenesis, so that chromosomal studies show 21-trisomy and a total count of 47. The overall incidence is about 1 per 1000 births, but maternal age has a considerable influence (Fig. **56/10**). The incidence amongst mothers aged 30 or less is 1 per 1000 births, but rises to over 20 per 1000 births in women over the age of 45. Two forms of Down's syndrome can be distinguished after chromosomal studies. The common one, 21-trisomy, has been described and the mother has no greater risk than any other mother of having a subsequent child affected with Down's syndrome. The second form, accounting for 2 to 5 per cent of patients with Down's syndrome, is due to a translocation of the extra 21-chromosome which joins with the head of chromosome 15, so that the total count is 46. In this form there is a 30 per cent chance of the disease occurring again. It is recommended that chromosomal studies are made on the amniotic fluid of all pregnant women over the age of 35 and on all women who have had an affected baby. The karyotype of the father of the child should also be studied in cases of 21-trisomy, as in a quarter of cases he may have provided the extra chromosome.

More recently it has been suggested that a higher detection rate would be obtained, irrespective of the mother's age, if alphafetoprotein (AFP) unconjugated oestriol and hCG were also measured. A low AFP, a low unconjugated oestriol and a raised level of hCG, compared with the expected levels for the period of gestation, indicate the need for an amniocentesis to detect or exclude Down's syndrome. An additional marker is a thick nuchal skin fold detected by ultrasound.

Down's syndrome may be confirmed in pregnancy in two ways. The first is by chorionic villus sampling performed about the 8th gestational week. The second is culture of fetal cells obtained by amniocentesis at about the 15th gestational week. These procedures have been discussed on pp. 56–7.

SEX-LINKED GENETIC DISORDERS

Chorionic villus sampling has made the diagnosis of sex-linked genetic disorders more rapid, and their management easier.

**Central nervous system anomalies**

NEURAL TUBE DEFECTS

Anencephaly is the most common major central nervous system malformation, and although many an-

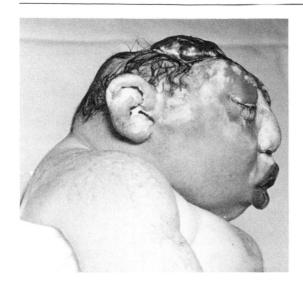

**Fig. 56/11** Anencephaly

encephalic infants are born alive they all die within 5 days (Fig. **56/11**). The babies may cry feebly at birth, and should be removed from the delivery room before the mother hears the cry. *Hydrocephaly* may be detected before birth or may be only noticed after delivery, particularly when difficulty has been experienced in delivering the head. The malforma-tion is recognized by the large head and bulging fontanelle (Fig. **56/12**). If the distended ventricles have not caused too much brain destruction, a shunt from the lateral ventricle to a neck vein can be inserted, but on the whole the prognosis is poor. *Spina bifida* occurs in 0.7 to 1.5 per 1000 live births and is often found in association with myelomen-ingocele, and with hydrocephalus (Fig. **56/13**). Opera-tion should only be attempted in the absence of gross hydrocephaly, if the limbs have adequate muscle power, and in the absence of gross kyphosis or major associated congenital defects.

The risk of delivering a baby with a neural tube defect varies between countries. In Britain the risk is between 3 and 5 per cent; in Australia and the USA it is between 1 and 2 per cent. For babies born alive the risk in all three countries is about half the figures quoted. Over 90 per cent of the babies are born to women who previously have not had an affected child.

Because of this, it has been suggested that for social and economic considerations all women who wish the service should be screened to determine if the fetus has an NTD

In the case of women who previously have had a baby with a neural tube defect, amniotic alphafeto-protein should be routinely estimated at about 15 weeks gestation. A raised level of alphafetoprotein should be followed by discussion with the couple

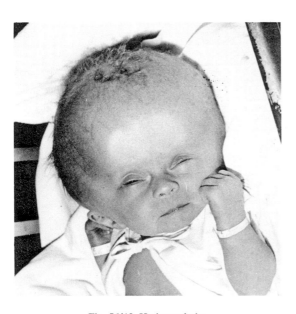

**Fig. 56/12** Hydrocephaly

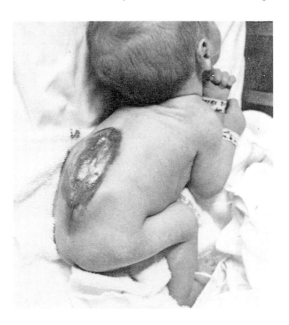

**Fig. 56/13** Spina bifida

and, if they wish, the offer to terminate the pregnancy.

## Cerebral palsy

Cerebral palsy is a descriptive term for a collection of non-progressive neuromotor disorders which are not the result of cerebral malformation. The condition affects between 1.5 and 3.5 per cent of all liveborn children. In most cases the cause of cerebral palsy is unknown, although low birth-weight infants have a greater risk of developing it. If the infant weighs less than 1500g at birth the risk is 25-fold. Birth trauma and hypoxia during labour (judged by a 5-minute Apgar score of 3 or less) are uncommon causes, and in many of these cases the cerebral palsy may have been due to intrinsic fetal defects rather than to events occurring during childbirth.

Clinically cerebral palsy may not be detected in the early neonatal period, although a quarter of the victims have a seizure disorder at this time. The main clinical feature is a lack of motor control, usually presenting as spasticity, or less commonly as involuntary movements or muscle inco-ordination. Any muscle group may be affected, but quadriplegia and diplegia are seen most often. In 15 per cent of affected people, choreo-athetoid, dystonic or ataxic movements predominate. If bulbar involvement occurs, the person will have difficulty in articulating. Over half of all people who have cerebral palsy have normal intelligence.

The stress on the parents and on siblings is considerable, but much can be done to help them.

## Bones and joints

The commonest disorders are *talipes calcaneus* and *talipes equinovarus*. The latter requires early treatment by manipulation and a Denis Browne splint. *Congenital dislocation of the hip* (*CDH*) is defined as a dislocation of the hip joint in which the head of the femur is (or may be) partially or completely displaced from the acetabulum. Between 1.5 and 2.5 of neonates show evidence of hip instability at birth. In most cases the instability resolves spontaneously in a few weeks, but in 10 to 20 per cent of infants with hip instability, congenital dislocation or subluxation persists. Babies are at greater risk of CDH if there is a family history of the disorder, if the baby presented as a breech to term, if there was oligohydramnios or fetal growth retardation.

All neonates should be examined for hip instability within 24 hours of birth. The method is as follows. To examine the left hip, the doctor steadies the infant's pelvis between the thumb of the left hand on the symphysis pubis and the fingers behind the sacrum. The examiner grasps the child's left thigh in the right hand (Fig. **56/14**) and attempts to move the femoral head gently forwards and then backwards out of the acetabulum. If the head of the femur is felt to move, with or without an audible

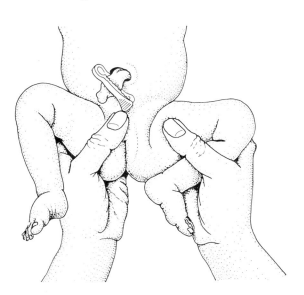

**Fig. 56/14** Detection of congenital dislocation of the hip

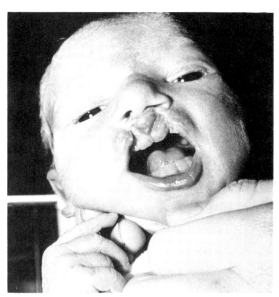

**Fig. 56/15** Hare lip and cleft palate

'clunk', dislocation, or dislocability is diagnosed. If there is any doubt after the examination, real time ultrasound is used to detect a displaced hip. In about 10 per cent of cases the baby's hips produce a soft 'click' rather than a 'clunk', and there is no evidence of abnormal movement of the femoral head. These babies must be examined again before discharge from hospital. If one month later the click has changed into a clunk, and abnormal movement between the femoral head and the acetabulum is found, treatment is needed.

### Alimentary system

*Hare-lip* and *cleft palate* are obvious, as is *absent* or *imperforate anus*. Cleft palate causes some feeding difficulties but most children can be fed using a spoon (Fig. **56/15**). *Atresia of the oesophagus* should be suspected in cases of hydramnios, and a catheter (size 9) should be passed through the mouth. If it meets obstruction about 8 to 10cm from the mouth the defect is likely. The defect should also be suspected in an infant who dribbles considerable volumes of mucus within a few hours of birth. Diagnosis is desirable before the start of feeding, as the passage of milk to the lungs by the associated fistula prejudices the chances of recovery. Atresia of the oesophagus can be confirmed by radiology. Treatment is surgical, and in good hands 70 per cent of affected infants survive. *Duodenal stenosis* or *atresia* should be suspected if persistent bile-stained vomiting occurs, and the higher the obstruction the earlier is the vomiting; but an occasional vomit, light yellow in colour, is common in healthy newborn infants. *Pyloric stenosis*, which is more common in males, is suggested by projectile vomiting in the second or third week of life, and confirmed by feeling the pyloric tumour when the baby is relaxed, during a feed.

### Genito-urinary tract

*Agenesis of the kidneys* is rare and fatal, and can be suspected if the child fails to pass urine and has low-set ears and marked furrows under the eyes. *Circumcision* is never required for medical reasons but in some countries is performed routinely and ritually for irrational reasons. The mothers are said to demand it, the doctors profit by it, and only occasionally does a baby die from the operation (although varying degrees of meatal ulceration are common).

The foreskin of the newborn is normally adherent to the glans and apparent phimosis is observed. It never causes micturition difficulties and the adherent foreskin can be retracted when the infant is 12 months old or more.

In 2 per cent of mature newborn males and in 20 per cent of preterm males, one or both testes will have failed to descend into the scrotum. By one year of age about 0.7 per cent of males will have undescended testes (cryptorchidism). Some of these infants will be found to have retractile testes rather than undescended testes. The treatment of true undescended testes is surgical orchidopexy at the age of 18 months.

### Cardiovascular system

*Gross cardiac defects* are usually demonstrated by cyanosis especially on crying, and by marked cardiac thrills and murmurs, but some severe anomalies produce no murmurs, and many infants with normal hearts have soft systolic murmurs. Care should be taken before diagnosing congenital heart disorders in the newborn, and provided the child is making good progress, the mother should not necessarily be told about a murmur until a reassessment is made at the first postnatal visit.

### The skin

Gross defects such as *ectopia vesicae* and *exomphalos* are obvious. The former has a poor prognosis, but the latter can be corrected surgically provided the defect is not too large. Pending surgical treatment the exomphalos should be covered with a moist sterile saline dressing. Small *superficial angiomata* are found on the nape of the neck, the brow or the upper eyelids in the majority of neonates. All disappear in infancy and no treatment is required. Large *smooth or raised angiomata* ('port wine stains' and 'strawberry marks') are distressing to the mother, and often grow in the first few months, and then decrease in size. The parents should take the child to a surgeon interested in the problem.

The *'Mongolian blue spot'* – these are patches of slate-blue discoloration commonly found over the sacrum or lower lumbar spine, although they may be situated elsewhere. As can be understood from the name they are usually found on children of Asian parents but have been seen in children of parents of Mediterranean stock. No treatment is required.

| Lesion | Operative procedure | Optimal age |
|---|---|---|
| Hare-lip | Cheiloplasty | 6 to 12 weeks |
| Cleft palate | Palatoplasty | 14 to 18 months |
| Dermoid cyst | Excision | Any age, preferably after 6 months |
| Lop ears | Plastic correction | 5 to 6 years |
| Supernumerary ear tags | Excision | Any age |
| Pre-auricular sinus | Excision | After 1 year |
| Branchial cyst and sinus | Excision | After 1 year |
| Thyroglossal cyst and sinus | Excision | After 1 year |
| Cystic hygroma | Excision | Usually as soon as noticed |
| Umbilical hernia | Umbilical herniorrhaphy | After 1 year if required |
| Inguinal hernia | Inguinal herniorrhaphy | Any age |
| Hydrocele | Excision | After 1 year |
| Undescended testicle | Orchidopexy | True ectopic testes 8 to 10 years, otherwise wait till nearer puberty |
| Hypospadias | Meatotomy | 1 to 2 years |
|  | Correction of chordee | 3 to 4 years |
|  | Construction of urethra | 5 to 8 years |
| Exstrophy of bladder | Bilateral uretero-sigmoidostomy | 2 to 4 years |
|  | Excision of bladder | 4 to 5 years |
| Webbed fingers | Plastic repair | 3 to 5 years |
| Supernumerary digits | Excision | Varies; often before 2 years |
| Patent ductus | Division | 3 to 8 years; occasionally sooner |
| Tetralogy of Fallot | Pulmonary-aortic anastomosis | 3 to 10 years |
| Coarctation of aorta | Excision and aortic anastomosis | After 9 years |

**Table 56/4** Optimal ages for elective surgical procedures (Ferguson, C. (1953) *Can Med Assoc. J*, **69**, 381)

## Metabolic diseases

### PHENYLKETONURIA (PKU)

A few infants have a congenital enzyme defect which permits the accumulation of phenylalanine, derived from protein-containing foodstuffs. Accumulation in the body of phenylalanine over a period leads to irreversible mental retardation which can be prevented if susceptible infants are identified and treated from infancy with diets low in phenylalanine content. The 'Guthrie' test detects these infants. A drop of blood is placed on a special filter paper which is sent to the laboratory. The presence of phenylketones is determined by placing the blood spot on a bacteriological plate inoculated with *B. subtilis*. This bacterium requires phenylalanine for growth and the degree of growth correlates with the quantity of the phenylalanine present. About 1 baby of 10 000 born alive is affected.

### CONGENITAL HYPOTHYROIDISM

This disease, which affects 1 baby of every 6000 born alive, can also be detected by measuring the $T_4$ level in blood spots, with supplemental TSH measurements if $T_4$ is low.

### CYSTIC FIBROSIS

This disease, affecting 1 baby in every 2000 can be identified by examining a drop of blood (taken on the 5th day of life and dried on filter paper) for immunoreactive trypsin.

### CONGENITAL ADRENAL HYPERPLASIA (CAH) (incidence 1 in 10 000 neonates)

In cases of CAH due to 21-hydroxylase deficiency, the levels of 17-OH progesterone are raised. A micro-scale filter paper method for measuring 17α-hydroxy-progesterone is now available and can be made on the same filter paper used for screening for PKU and hypothyroidism.

### GALACTOSAEMIA

A Guthrie blood sample (blood spot) is subjected to an assay which detects the presence of galactose deficiency, so that babies with galactosaemia can be given lactose-free milk.

AMINO ACID DISORDERS

Cystinuria, maple syrup disease and other rare disorders can be identified if a urine sample, collected when the baby is six weeks old, is examined in a special laboratory.

## Age for elective surgical correction of anomalies

The present consensus is shown in Table **56/4**, but in all instances the final decision will be determined by the paediatric surgeon.

## Telling the parents of an abnormal child

About 1 per cent of neonates are born with a congenital defect, deformity or disease which will impair their health, and adversely affect their development. Today perhaps 60 per cent of these abnormal children survive and benefit most if they are brought up as a member of their family rather than being segregated in special institutions. It is necessary however for the parents to be informed about the problems of the handicapped child so that it may be accepted into the family.

It is now accepted that parents have a right to all the available medical knowledge about their children, and should be informed of an abnormality as soon as a reliable diagnosis has been made. The fear that this early information may lead to the rejection of the child by the mother has proved to be false, but the way in which the parents are told is crucial. Parental grief and distress seem to be unequally distributed, and to have different appearances. The mother usually feels grief and guilt – that she has delivered an imperfect child. The father is often angry that this 'disaster' has happened to him, seeks to find a reason in his own or his wife's behaviour, and has considerable anxiety about the social and economic consequences of the birth. Consequently, it is not easy, nor pleasant, to be the informant. The informant must be known to and accepted by the parents, able to communicate easily, able to calm the anxieties of the parents and to convey to them his confidence in their ability to undertake the responsibilities of rearing the handicapped child. The parents, moreover, must be able to refer to one person to know the special needs of the child: this requires counselling over a prolonged period.

## Risk of having a further abnormal child

Because congenital defects are due to the interplay between multifactorial genetic inheritance and an adverse environment, the risk of a woman having another abnormal child is difficult to compute. Yet this question will inevitably be asked by anxious parents 'What is the chance of this happening again with the next pregnancy?' Current opinion is listed in Table **56/5**.

| Disorder | Incidence (*per 100 births*) | Risk (*per cent*) | |
|---|---|---|---|
| | | *Normal parent having a second affected child* | *Affected parent having an affected child* |
| Anencephaly | 0.2 | 2 | } 4 |
| Spina bifida | 0.3 | 4 | |
| Cleft palate | 0.04 | 2 | 7 |
| Cleft lip and palate | 0.1 | 4 | 4 |
| Congenital heart disease | 0.6 | 2 | 2 |

**Table 56/5** Risks of recurrence of some congenital defects

## Chapter 57

# Hypoxia in the Newborn

Cutting the umbilical cord finally cuts the baby off from all maternal supplies of oxygen and from now on it is on its own.

The first 24 hours of life is the most hazardous period of the entire life span, and the ability of the baby to survive the birth period depends upon its viability and its ability to obtain oxygen from the atmosphere, so that its tissues, particularly the heart and brain, are adequately oxygenated. For this there are four essentials:

1. The air passages must be patent, and not occluded by inhalation of amniotic fluid during the birth process, so that inhaled oxygen can reach the alveoli.
2. Adequate respiratory exchange must take place in the alveoli. For this to occur expansion of the alveoli must be obtained by spontaneous respiratory efforts, or if this fails to occur, by the resuscitatory efforts of the medical attendants.
3. The circulation must be effective so that oxygen can reach the vital organs.
4. The respiratory centre must not be depressed by excessive sedative drugs.

The old term asphyxia neonatorum, meaning *without pulse*, failed to emphasize that the defect was in oxygenation and further made two classes, asphyxia livida and pallida, which are not particularly helpful in determining treatment. Apart from this mention the terms will not be used in this book and *hypoxia* will be used in their place.

## CAUSES OF HYPOXIA IN THE NEWBORN

### Intra-uterine conditions

Any condition which reduces the oxygen available to the fetus will predispose to hypoxia. As has been shown in Chapter 55, the baby in utero normally lives in an oxygen environment much reduced below the saturation found after birth. The fetus is able to survive in this atmosphere by having additional red cells available, and because fetal blood is better able to attract oxygen and to disassociate the gas in the tissues. Furthermore it is kept at a constant temperature and is relatively inert, so that the reduced oxygen saturation is adequate for the metabolic processes of the brain. In emergency conditions the fetus is able to survive anoxia for about 20 to 30 minutes (a much longer period than the neonate) by obtaining energy from anaerobic breakdown of its large stores of glycogen.

But after birth its total bodily requirements of oxygen increase rapidly, and if this additional oxygen is not supplied quickly, permanent damage to the brain may result. If the respiratory centre has been depressed by intra-uterine hypoxia it may not respond immediately to the normal atmospheric level of oxygen, and high concentrations of gas may be required. Consequently a first step must be to anticipate intra-uterine conditions causing hypoxia. These may be maternal, fetal, or iatrogenic.

Amongst the *maternal conditions* are severe pregnancy-induced hypertension and eclampsia, antepartum haemorrhage, particularly if due to abruptio placentae, severe heart disease, and prolonged pregnancy; whilst cord compression is the main *fetal cause*. The injudicious and excessive use of narcotics, especially morphine analogues, or intramuscular oxytocin which may cause uterine hypertonus, are *iatrogenic causes*. Normal birth always reduces fetal oxygenation, and prolonged labour, particularly a prolonged second stage, a traumatic forceps operation, a difficult breech delivery, or 'holding back the head' pending the arrival of the doctor, can cause gross hypoxia. These episodes may lead to intra-uterine death, but if the baby is born alive, its respiratory centre will be depressed and neonatal hypoxia evident. Most affected babies which survive have no permanent brain damage, but it is impossible to foretell which baby will be damaged, and consequently the possibility of intra-uterine anoxia should be minimized by a policy of careful management of labour.

If the intra-uterine hypoxia has been severe, the infant may be unable to correct the resulting acidaemia by normal respiratory exchange. Failure to do this has two further detrimental effects on its survival. First, blood at a pH of less than 7.20 is able to carry less oxygen than blood which is less acid, and second, acidaemia may lead to a reflex pulmonary vasoconstriction which further impairs pulmonary gas exchange. This increases the degree of hypoxia as blood is shunted away from the lungs through the ductus arteriosus and the foramen ovale. The majority of these infants are in secondary apnoea and have an Apgar score of 3 or less.

## PREVENTION OF HYPOXIA AT BIRTH

When the fetal head has been born, the nose is sucked clear with a soft rubber mucus extractor and the remainder of the delivery is conducted slowly, taking about 60 seconds. Once the baby is delivered it is laid between the mother's legs, with the head lower than the body and the neck extended. Using the mucus extractor any inhaled amniotic fluid contents is gently sucked from the mouth and pharynx. (Alternatively and traditionally, the baby may be held by the heels and the suction performed, but I can see no merit in this.) When the upper respiratory passages are clear, the baby is laid flat. If it is kept head down, not only is cerebral venous engorgement increased but the weight of the large fetal liver presses on the diaphragm and hinders diaphragmatic movement essential to respiration. The majority of babies will have taken their first breath and cried loudly within 60 seconds of birth. Nothing more is required for these babies and once the cord has been severed the child should be given to the mother to cuddle if this has not been done. A minority of infants will not have cried by within 60 seconds of birth and further investigation and treatment is needed.

## APGAR SCORING SYSTEM

The degree to which the intra-uterine hypoxia has affected fetal vitality may be determined by the Apgar score. This system takes into account the fetal heart rate, respiratory effort, muscle tone, reflex irritability and colour, estimated 60 seconds and at 5 minutes after birth, and scored. The two most important signs are heart rate and respiratory effort. A score of 7 to 10 indicates no depression; of 4 to 6 some depression, and of less than 4 severe depression (Table **57/1**).

### Management of the infant according to the Apgar score

1. APGAR SCORE 7 TO 10 – NO DEPRESSION

Apart from observation and confirmation that the mouth and pharynx is clear, no further active treatment is needed.

| *Sign* | *0* | *1* | *2* |
|---|---|---|---|
| Colour | Blue; pale | Body pink; extremities blue | Completely pink |
| Respiratory effort | Absent | Weak cry; hypoventilation | Good; strong cry |
| Muscle tone | Limp | Some flexion of extremities | Active motion; extremities well flexed |
| Reflex irritability (response to stimulation of sole of foot) | No response | Grimace | Cry |
| Heart rate | Absent | Slow (below 100) | Fast (over 100) |

**Table 57/1** Apgar scoring method for evaluating the infant (from Apgar and associates)

## 2. APGAR 4 TO 6 – MILD OR MODERATE DEPRESSION

The baby has cyanosed extremities, the reflexes are present, muscle tone is good, the heart rate rapid, regular and strong, but respiratory efforts have not been made.

1. The pharynx should be sucked out once again.

2. The baby should be placed in a slight Trendelenburg position with the head hyperextended to ensure a patent airway.

3. As the child may be sedated from the effects of pethidine (or other sedation) given to the mother in late labour, it should be aroused by gentle slaps on the feet, or if this fails, by the injection of naloxone 0.02mg into the umbilical vein.

4. Oxygen should be blown gently across the face or given by a baby face mask. Recovery will be shown by the onset of respiration; at first in irregular gasps, or gulps, sometimes at long intervals, which gradually become shorter, and are followed by episodes of rapid irregular respirations. The colour of the child becomes pink, and finally normal respiration is established and the baby cries.

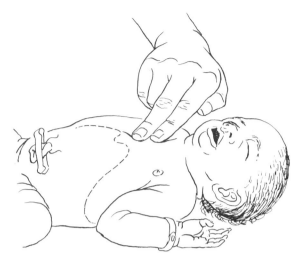

**Fig. 57/1** Closed cardiac massage. Intermittent pressure is applied over the middle-third of the sternum (which is pressed down about half an inch) with two fingers. The heart is compressed between the rib cage and the vertebral column and blood is expelled into the great vessel. For clarity the endotracheal tube has been omitted in the drawing (from Moya, James, Burnard and Hanks. *Anaesthesiology* 1961, **22**, 644)

## 3. APGAR 0 TO 3 – SEVERE DEPRESSION

These babies are markedly depressed and respirations are usually absent or inadequate, muscle tone poor, the heart slow and of poor force, the colour blue or greyish-white. Unless these infants receive rapid, effective treatment they will die or be damaged.

The measures outlined for moderate depression are first instituted, but if not successful within 2 minutes the following further measures are taken:

1. Continuous monitoring of the fetal heart by an assistant.

2. Laryngoscopy of the posterior pharynx and trachea using an infant laryngoscope, and suction, under vision, of all mucus.

3. The passage of a small endotracheal tube (Forreger size 12F) under vision, and suction of the deep trachea.

4. Intermittent positive pressure ventilation with oxygen through the endotracheal tube until spontaneous respirations start, and are maintained, and the fetal heart rate exceeds 100.

5. If the heart beat is not heard or if the rate does not increase above 60 after a few lung expansions with intratracheal ventilation, firm regular external cardiac massage is practised intermittently (5 or 6 chest compressions followed by 2 ventilations and repeated) until the rate increases considerably (Fig. **57/1**).

6. Should the infant fail to become pink, or fail to gasp after becoming pink following intermittent positive pressure ventilation over a period of 1 minute, or if the heart rate does not increase after external cardiac massage, an injection of 2ml of 25 per cent dextrose and 5mmol bicarbonate per estimated kg body-weight, should be given into the umbilical vein, to correct the acidaemia which is present and increasing in severity.

7. Continuous observation of the child and treatment of cyanotic attacks for the first 24 hours after delivery is essential.

Recently there has been criticism of Apgar scoring and suggestions made that it be abandoned. However no suggestions (apart from those in the next section) for its replacement have been made. Probably the best discriminants to detect an asphyxiated baby are its failure to establish regular respirations by two minutes after birth, and a heart beat of less than 80 per minute persisting for more than two minutes after birth.

**Umbilical artery blood pH**

The sensitivity and specificity of the Apgar score is not high. Because of this it is recommended that if the birth has been difficult, a sample of blood from the umbilical artery should be taken and its pH measured. A pH $\leqslant 7.10$ indicates severe neonatal acidaemia, which requires urgent action to resuscitate the baby by giving oxygen and bicarbonate.

## SEVERE PROLONGED HYPOXIA

Severe hypoxia may be followed by some degree of permanent neurological handicap in about 10 per cent of babies. If a hypoxic baby is apathetic in the first days of life and this is followed by excitability and extensor muscle hypertonia, neurological handicap is likely to persist.

The infant may develop convulsions in the neonatal period and later be diagnosed as having cerebral palsy, although hypoxia during childbirth is an uncommon cause of this condition. Cerebral palsy is discussed on p. 446.

## THE RESPIRATORY DISTRESS SYNDROME (HYALINE MEMBRANE DISEASE)

The respiratory distress syndrome, or hyaline membrane disease, affects 0.5 to 1.0 per cent of all neonates, and the lower the birth-weight of the baby the higher is its incidence. The disease is rare amongst babies of 37 weeks or more gestation who weigh 2500g or more at birth, but affects 10 per cent of low birth-weight babies. It is particularly dangerous in babies weighing less than 1500g at birth, when up to 50 per cent of infants may be affected.

Pregnancy has frequently been complicated so that premature labour began spontaneously or was induced. The mother may have had PIH or antepartum haemorrhage, and delivery by forceps or caesarean section may have been required. Such conditions are usual when a baby weighing 2500g or more at birth develops the disease.

Hyaline membrane disease is due to a relative lack of surfactant in the alveoli. As mentioned in Chapter 55, surfactant, which is a lipoprotein composed mainly of lecithin, begins to be secreted by the fetal lung from about the 20th to 25th week of pregnancy. The amount secreted increases with increasing gesta-

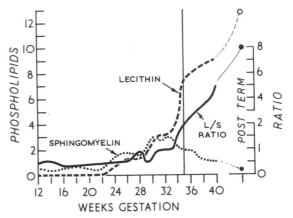

Fig. 57/2 Changes in the concentrations of lecithin and sphingomyelin in amniotic fluid during pregnancy. The figure also shows the alteration in the L/S ratio after the 36th week

tional age, and the substance passes into the amniotic fluid.

Lecithin is not the only lipoprotein detectable in amniotic fluid. Sphingomyelin also appears in the fluid. However, the concentration of sphingomyelin does not increase greatly throughout pregnancy, whilst that of surface-active lecithin increases quite dramatically from about the 32nd to 34th gestation weeks (Fig. **57/2**). The ratio between lecithin and sphingomyelin concentrations (the L/S ratio) in amniotic fluid thus gives an indication of maturation of the fetal lung, and an L/S ratio of 2 or more suggests that hyaline membrane disease is unlikely to occur.

The exact function of surfactant has not yet been clearly elucidated. It is known that surfactant determines the stability of the lung after birth, ensuring a normal residual volume of air and the capacity for gas exchange. In the absence of surfactant, the alveoli become airless at the end of each breath, and their ability to re-expand against the forces of surface tension requires great effort. In this way lung compliance is reduced. This has further undesirable consequences. The relative hypoxaemia due to lack of oxygen intake causes pulmonary vasoconstriction and the bypassing of the lung as the ductus arteriosus and foramen ovale are kept open. In effect the circulation returns towards the fetal pattern. In turn, this reduces the pulmonary capillary blood flow and less surfactant is secreted, so that a vicious circle is set up. The hypoxaemia stimulates increased physical activity as the infant strives to obtain extra oxygen, but increasing respiratory and metabolic acidosis results.

These physiopathological considerations account for the symptoms and signs of hyaline membrane disease.

### Clinical aspects

At birth, respiration in the low birth-weight infant may have been established with difficulty and low Apgar scores are usual. Within a few hours of birth the neonate shows an increased respiratory rate, with nasal flaring, expiratory grunting, and sternal or intercostal retraction. The legs and hands may be oedematous, and cyanosis in ambient air is usual. The characteristic picture by the age of 4 to 6 hours is that of an infant who lies limply with hips flexed and abducted, making few spontaneous movements (though he may react strongly if irritated) in the presence of intense dyspnoea (rate 60 to 100), a noisy expiratory grunt and paradoxical indrawing of chest and upper abdomen with each inspiration. This state of affairs may last 24 to 48 hours, the baby becoming increasingly inert and showing the pallor of supervening circulatory failure. The lungs are collapsed and congested at autopsy and the terminal air passages lined with hyaline material.

The diagnosis is confirmed by radiology when a recticulogranular, ground glass or 'snowstorm' pattern is seen.

In between 70 and 90 per cent of infants the disease is only moderately severe, but in the remaining 10 to 30 per cent the child is critically ill. The management of the two groups differs in degree, but in both an acute phase and a recovery phase can be noted.

### Treatment

In the acute phase, which lasts until it is reasonably certain that the baby will survive, treatment is active. The neonate is placed in a warm (thermo-neutral) environment to reduce oxygen requirements, and oxygen is provided. The temperature in the incubator is adjusted to 35°C, radiant heat loss is prevented, and the humidity is maintained at more than 60 per cent. Adequate oxygen is essential so that normal oxygenation of the arterial blood is obtained. The accepted level is an oxygen saturation of at least 95 per cent, and a tension of 60–80mmHg. If this is achieved the vicious circle outlined may be broken. Unfortunately there is no adequate bedside guide. Obviously, it is necessary to avoid cyanosis since the blood is then only 70 to 80 per cent saturated, and

tension in the region of 40mmHg. But knowledge that hyperoxygenation may damage the premature retina imposes limitations to its use. In the first place the concentration supplied should always be measured with an oxygen analyser. Secondly, the provision of high concentrations (above 40 per cent) which may be essential at times, should be reviewed every few hours.

Damage to the retina shows histologically as retrolental fibroplasia and is a leading cause of childhood blindness. High $O_2$ concentrations apparently lead to vaso-occlusion and the resulting tissue ischaemia causes a fibroplastic reaction. Recently the use of oral tocopherol (vitamin E) in a daily dose of 100mg/kg body-weight has been shown to reduce the incidence of retrolental fibroplasia amongst small preterm infants ($\leqslant 1500$g) significantly.

It will be obvious that optimal conditions for the survival of an affected infant require that it be managed in a neonatal unit provided with full facilities for biochemical and physical methods of investigation and care.

Optimal care involves frequent monitoring of arterial blood gases, continuous transcutaneous $pO_2$ and the provision of oxygen based on the biochemical findings. The measurements made include arterial blood pH, $pO_2$, $pCO_2$ and $HCO_3$.

A notable advance in the management of hyaline membrane disease has been the introduction of continuous positive airways pressure (CPAP). This technique should be used if the condition of the infant deteriorates despite therapy or if the arterial oxygen tension remains below 40mmHg.

CPAP can be provided by a variety of techniques, all of which require skilled supervision. The principle is to compel the baby to expire against pressure and thus hold the alveoli more open. This manoeuvre often dramatically improves fetal oxygenation, which in turn necessitates frequent arterial blood gas monitoring and readjustment of oxygen supplies. It is not always successful. If CPAP is shown to be failing, recourse has to be made to assisting ventilation with a machine.

Because of the dangers of metabolic acidosis, the blood pH is monitored and corrected using alkali. Once the metabolic acidosis is corrected, pulmonary capillary resistance is reduced, permitting a greater blood flow, and myocardial contractility is increased.

Adequate feeding is needed as the baby is rapidly using his stores of energy and losing much fluid in the form of water vapour from his lungs. To maintain fluid and energy requirements, the infant is fed intravenously using a glucose electrolyte solution. A total of 65 to 150ml per kg body-weight per 24 hours is given. The alternative is to give expressed breast milk via a nasogastric tube at a rate of 1 to 2ml per hour.

The decision whether to feed orally or intravenously is often difficult, and emphasizes the importance of treating affected infants in specialized neonatal intensive care units.

The development of hypoglycaemia is avoided by early feeding but the blood glucose levels must be monitored 4-hourly (using Dextrostix) to ensure that normal levels are maintained.

Although an essential part of treatment is to avoid disturbing the infant, some disturbance is inevitable. The prophylactic use of antibiotics remains controversial, as does the choice of antibiotic to be given. Experts continue to disagree, and students would be advised to follow local custom in the matter.

Between 72 and 98 hours after birth most surviving infants will enter the recovery phase. In this period the oxygen is reduced gradually, checking the infant's $pO_2$ before reducing the percentage concentration.

The mortality of hyaline membrane disease varies from 15 to 50 per cent and the smaller the infant, the higher the mortality. The best results are obtained in neonatal intensive care units, where expert staff is on duty and where facilities are available on a 24-hour basis for estimation of blood gases, blood pH and blood glucose, and where mechanical ventilators are available.

A method of prevention of hyaline membrane disease has been suggested. It is based on the observation that steroids given to immature fetal lambs induce the production of surfactant. Hyaline membrane disease may largely be prevented if a woman with intact membranes, who is threatening to go into labour prematurely, is given betamethasone (Celestone Chronodose) 24mg, intramuscularly repeated after 24 hours, and the onset of labour is delayed for 24 hours. If the membranes have ruptured for more than 24 hours this therapy is unnecessary, as the baby will have been 'stressed' and will be producing surfactant. It is also unnecessary if the amniotic L/S ratio is greater than 2.

A protein-free 'artificial' surfactant has been developed. The substance called 'artificial lung expand-ing compound' (ALEC) given into the pharynx of very low birth-weight babies has reduced the neonatal mortality from hyaline membrane disease by 50 per cent in a controlled trial.

**Other causes for dyspnoea in the newborn**

Several other conditions may cause dyspnoea in the newborn, and although they occur in premature infants their practical importance is mainly in babies born at term. The aspiration syndrome is the most important to recognize because it is fairly common and may lead to death if not promptly treated. All require radiography and other special measures for diagnosis.

1. *Aspiration syndrome.* Aspiration of liquor and meconium in the course of an unduly asphyxial birth results in obstruction of air passages with collapse of parts of the lung and over-inflation of others. The baby may become very dyspnoeic within an hour or two of delivery. As in the baby with hyaline membrane disease, there is considerable right-to-left shunting of blood and cyanosis is pronounced. Oxygen is the necessary form of treatment, and may be given freely in high concentrations since there is no danger to the mature retina. Antibiotics should also be administered in appropriate doses.

2. *Pneumothorax.* This arises as a result of rupture of a bulla following a ball-valve mechanism of obstruction in small airways typically due to meconium aspirated into the lungs. A small pneumothorax is not uncommonly found when babies are routinely x-rayed. It resolves spontaneously. A large tension pneumothorax may cause urgent dyspnoea and requires surgical relief.

3. *Congenital abnormalities*, e.g. diaphragmatic hernia, pulmonary hypoplasia, congenital lobar emphysema, and acute heart failure in some forms of congenital heart disease.

4. *Intra-uterine pneumonia.* In some cases of premature rupture of the membranes the amniotic fluid becomes infected, and if inhaled by the fetus may cause intra-uterine pneumonia. Considering the frequency of premature rupture, pneumonia from this cause is remarkably uncommon. The most helpful alerting sign is maternal fever indicating that infection has taken place, but the prophylactic use of antibiotics unfortunately offers no protection to the baby. The baby should be assessed carefully after delivery with a view to prompt antibiotic treatment should there be evidence that he has become infected.

## Chapter 58

# Birth Injuries

With increasingly good obstetric care the incidence of fatal birth injuries has been reduced in recent years.

The main forms of birth injury are cranial, or intracranial, and both are more likely to occur in breech delivery, amongst premature infants and when cephalopelvic disproportion requiring forceps delivery is present. There can be little credit to the obstetrician who persists with a difficult forceps delivery and succeeds in delivering a live, but damaged, baby which subsequently dies.

The majority of birth injuries can be avoided by treating all mid-forceps deliveries as trial forceps, by assessing carefully the size of the baby presenting as a breech and by avoiding excessive prolongation of labour. Despite all precautions, however, some babies will be injured at birth.

## CRANIAL INJURY

During labour, when the head is being pushed deeply into the pelvis, the venous return from the scalp veins is impeded, and extravasation of fluid may occur causing a *caput succedaneum*. The incidence of this condition is 2 per 1000 births. No treatment is required and re-absorption of the fluid is rapid. Occasionally, either due to continued pressure on the head or, more often, to trauma from forceps, and particularly the ventouse, the periosteum is dragged from the underlying bone with subperiosteal haemorrhage and the formation of a *cephalhaematoma* (Fig. **58/1**). The condition arises in 2 per cent of births, most commonly one or other parietal bone being involved, and since the periosteum is bound to the edge of the bone, the spread of the haematoma is limited to the area occupied by the bone. The swelling is fluctuant, and may increase in size over the first 2 days of life. The edges then become hard, as a rim of calcification occurs beneath the raised periosteum. The haema-

toma stays much the same size for 2 to 3 weeks, and then is slowly absorbed. Unless the haematoma is very large treatment should be expectant, and the alternative, aspiration, is rarely practised.

### Fracture of the skull

Occasionally, a *linear fracture* of the skull is found in the parietal bone beneath a cephalhaematoma.

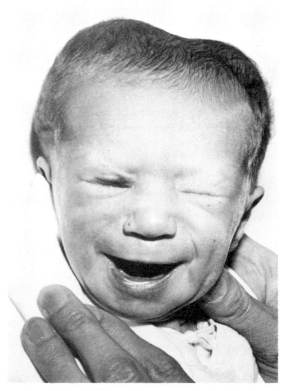

**Fig. 58/1** Bilateral cephalhaematomata. As shown the subperiosteal haemorrhage is limited to the area of the bone by the periosteum

No treatment is required. *Depressed fractures*, or depression of a portion of the cranial bones, may occur following marked cephalopelvic disproportion, particularly due to a flat pelvis, but are rare. No active treatment is required unless there is evidence of intracranial bleeding.

## INTRACRANIAL HAEMORRHAGE

This is of two kinds, *subdural* and *intraventricular*; the former was once fairly common but is nowadays rare unless the obstetrical policy outlined above has been contravened. Then, excessive moulding, or twisting strain from misuse of forceps, may lead to rupture of the large venous sinuses in the falx or the tentorium, with massive bleeding into the subdural space which may break through into the subarachnoid. The infant, if born alive, is deeply shocked and shows little response to resuscitative efforts. A lesser, and potentially remediable lesion, is when the rupture is confined to smaller venous tributaries traversing the subdural space, leading to an acute subdural haematoma. Once again, since delivery usually involves considerable asphyxiation, the infant is depressed at birth. The lesion develops rather slowly, and declares itself by signs of increasing irritability, a tense bulging fontanelle, and often

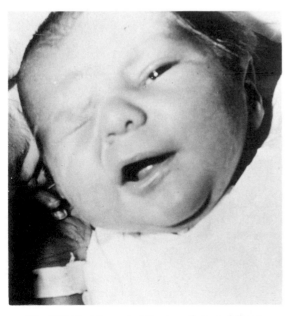

**Fig. 58/2** Facial paresis following a forceps delivery

a convulsion, some 24 to 72 hours after birth. A surgeon should be consulted. Withdrawal of blood through a 20-gauge needle inserted to a depth of 3 to 4mm at the lateral corner of the fontanelle (subdural tap) confirms the diagnosis.

### Intraventricular haemorrhage

This is still fairly common. It begins in small veins beneath the ependyma which become congested, and perhaps also altered in permeability, during prolonged or recurrent episodes of hypoxia, and then these rupture into the ventricles; rupture into the brain substance may also occur. Bleeding of this type is most often found in premature infants and is related to the steadily worsening hypoxia of such babies. Intraventricular haemorrhage is not due to maternal obstetrical complications, the duration of labour, or to the method of delivery. Most IVH occurs within the first 72 hours of life and may be suspected if the infant's condition suddenly deteriorates. The condition may be diagnosed by a CAT scan or by serial ultrasound examinations.

### Excessive irritability or cerebral irritation

This is not uncommon amongst larger infants who have suffered considerable hypoxia during delivery. Such babies pass through an initial stage of depression for a few hours, when tone is excessively lax and the Moro reflex depressed, to one of excessive activity and tremulousness, with a high-pitched cry, and sometimes convulsions. The fontanelle may bulge somewhat as an indication of the oedematous brain beneath. Such babies occasionally suffer an intraventricular haemorrhage too, and the fontanelle then is tense. Treatment of intraventricular bleeding in these circumstances is by repeated lumbar punctures, and survival is possible.

Treatment of the irritability resulting from hypoxia is by suitable sedation.

## INJURIES TO NERVES

This form of injury is relatively uncommon and accounts for less than 6 per cent of all birth injuries. The common form is a unilateral *facial palsy* due to pressure from the tip of the forceps blade on the facial nerve as it emerges from the skull. It should be stated, however, that at least as many cases of facial palsy occur amongst babies delivered vaginally without the use of forceps. The paralysis is of the lower motor neurone type with paresis or paralysis of the facial muscles and inability to close the eye on the affected side (Fig. **58/2**). Apart from attention to the eye to avoid corneal damage, no treatment is required as recovery occurs within 2 to 3 weeks.

*Brachial plexus palsy* can occur in cases of breech delivery when there is difficulty in delivering the aftercoming head, or in shoulder dystocia. Fortunately the frequency is low, and with good obstetric care should not exceed 0.5 per 1000 births. In most cases the nerve sheath is torn, the nerve maintaining its integrity, but becoming compressed by haemorrhage and oedema. *Erb's paralysis* is due to compression of the fibres of the fifth and sixth cervical nerves in the brachial plexus. The arm hangs limply at the side with the elbow extended, the forearm pronated and the wrist flexed (Fig. **58/3**). It does not respond to the Moro reflex. Treatment consists of putting the arm into abduction with flexion of the elbow and extension of the wrist. This can best be achieved by tying the arm to the head of the cot or by the use of a light aeroplane splint. This should be combined with repeated passive movements until power returns to the limb. Recovery of function is good but in about 30 per cent of infants minor sensory or motor defects persist for about a year. In the rare *Klumpke's paralysis*, the seventh and eighth cervical nerves are damaged and the infant presents with wrist drop and paralysis of muscles of the hand. The prognosis is worse than for Erb's paralysis.

### Bone injury

Fracture of the clavicle or the humerus may occur in difficult breech delivery, particularly if the arms are extended, whilst fracture of the femur may occur during attempts to bring down extended legs. The fractures are invariably of the 'greenstick' variety, and union is excellent provided splinting is adequate.

### Muscle injury

Occasionally, following a difficult delivery a haematoma of the sternomastoid muscle may occur. It is difficult to detect but should be sought in all babies whose birth has been difficult as, unless treated, it can lead to permanent muscle shortening and torticollis. Treatment is by passive stretching of the muscle several times daily.

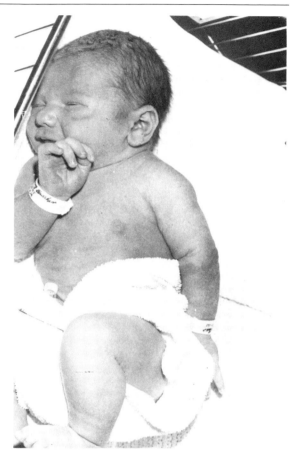

**Fig. 58/3** Erb's palsy

## NEONATAL CONVULSIONS

About 1 per cent of newborn babies will develop convulsions which are of two clinical types – tonic, characterized by extension of the trunk and lower limbs, often associated with apnoea and cyanosis, and clonic, which may be generalized, multifocal or focal. In the generalized form, the convulsions occur at a rate of one to three a minute; whilst focal jerking of a limb cannot be stopped by flexing it.

Convulsions may be due to brain damage or to metabolic disturbance, and it is important to differentiate the two. Convulsions due to brain damage occur, typically, in the first 3 days of life. The baby has usually had a 1-minute Apgar score of 4 or less, and has required resuscitation using intermittent positive pressure. It sucks poorly and needs tube feeding. It is generally lethargic, with a low level of motor activity, and poor muscle tone. Frequently there are few spontaneous eye movements and an absent Moro reflex. Prognosis is poor; 10 to 20 per cent of the infants die, and 10 to 20 per cent are moderately or severely handicapped.

Convulsions due to metabolic disturbance show none of the signs mentioned in the previous paragraph. The fits are clonic in over 95 per cent of cases, and usually occur after the 3rd day of life. The prognosis is much better, death and mental retardation being relatively uncommon.

*Chapter 59*

# Neonatal Infections

Infection in the neonatal period may have begun during late pregnancy, during labour and delivery or, more commonly, begun in the postnatal period.

In pregnancy, fetal infections occur by the transfer of viruses, parasites or, rarely, bacteria from the mother's blood via the placenta. Such infections have been considered in Chapter 31, and may persist into the neonatal period. Intrapartum infections may develop, particularly if labour is prolonged or if the amniotic membranes have been ruptured for more than 24 hours, but are not as common as would appear from some reports. After early rupture of the membranes, the infection reaches the amniotic cavity and the fetus, from the upper vagina. The pathogen is usually a Gram-negative bacillus, particularly *E. coli* or *B. proteus*. Although fulminating fetal infection is unusual in these cases, the early warning sign of maternal fever in labour should lead to the clinical evaluation of the situation and the administration of appropriate antibiotics. In the USA, infection of the amnion is reported as a significant cause of fetal disability, but the diagnosis is frequently equivocal, and the fetus is only occasionally infected. During its passage through the birth canal in labour, the fetus may acquire an infection from the vaginal fungus, *Candida albicans*.

The most usual type of infection of the newborn baby is that acquired after birth. Postnatal infections are introduced to the infant from the mother, the doctors and nurses, or by contaminated dust, laundry articles or feeding utensils. The bacteria responsible are most often staphylococci; but occasionally streptococcal, *E. coli* or pneumococcal infections occur. In most hospitals staphylococci are endemic, and within 3 days of birth colonies are growing in the nose of 50 per cent of the neonates. The umbilical area is usually colonized first, followed by the groins, the neck and the nose. *E. coli* are usually transferred from the mother to her baby, but may also be introduced from contaminated incubators when care is not meticulous.

The incidence of neonatal infection can be reduced considerably (1) if 'rooming-in' is practised; (2) if control of infection in all staff is made by routine nasal swabs, and by the treatment of those with positive swabs; (3) by avoiding bathing the baby at birth, and by smearing its entire body, which has previously been cleaned, with Phisohex or Hibitane cream, once or twice during the period it is in hospital.

**Staphylococcal infections**

These infections are the most common encountered and usually present as skin pustules, peri-umbilical infection, paronychia or blepharoconjunctivitis. Undetected staphylococcal infection may spread in the bloodstream and produce osteomyelitis, meningitis or arthritis, but these are rare and are not seen until the infant is 3 or 4 weeks old.

**Candida albicans**

This is relatively common and presents as a monilial infection of the infant's mouth. The fungus almost certainly derives from the mother's vagina. On opening the child's mouth small white patches are seen, which, if removed, leave a reddened base. Examination of a smear, stained with methylene blue, will demonstrate the branched fungi. Treatment is by painting the mouth twice daily with 1 per cent aqueous gentian violet.

**Gonococcal infection**

Gonococcal conjunctivitis is acquired by the baby during the birth process. It is now uncommon in the developed countries. Within a few days of birth, a purulent conjunctivitis occurs. The diagnosis is made by examining the pus microscopically and by culture. Treatment is to give systemic benzylpenicillin (25 000U/kg body-weight) twice daily for 3 days. Prophylactic eye drops are no longer recommended.

### Chlamydia infection

Most babies acquiring *Chlamydia trachomatis* infection during birth develop conjunctivitis (60 per cent); and a few (10 per cent) develop pneumonia. Conjunctivitis occurs 1 to 3 weeks after birth; whilst pneumonia often occurs later (8 to 12 weeks after birth). Treatment is to give systemic erythromycin 25mg/kg body-weight twice daily for 10 days.

### Gram-negative organisms

Salmonella, and some specifically pathogenic strains of *E. coli*, are dangerous causes of gastro-enteritis in neonates, should the bacteria be introduced into a nursery. Low birth-weight infants are at especial risk, since they have to be kept in hospital for long periods. The severity of the epidemic can only be reduced if all babies who develop watery diarrhoea are promptly isolated and are properly investigated. Such investigations include enquiring if the mother or any of the medical attendants has gastro-intestinal symptoms. It should be understood that loose stools (especially in babies fed on 'formula' milks), or even frank diarrhoea, may have a dietetic origin, but the preventive measures should be initiated.

*E. coli* is also a cause of renal infection in infants, which may be difficult to diagnose. The only signs may be a low fever, prolonged jaundice or failure to thrive. Diagnosis is made in such cases by examining a specimen of urine obtained by suprapubic puncture for organisms and leucocytes. The infection may arise in infants with congenital anomaly of the urinary tract, or it may be the result of a subacute bloodstream infection acquired during birth.

## MANAGEMENT OF NEONATAL INFECTION

### a. Preventive

The prevention of infection has already been mentioned and may be summarized as follows:

1. Appointment of an infection officer whose duty it is to investigate all cases of maternal or infant infections, to seek infection in the staff and to keep the staff constantly aware of the problem.
2. Careful nursing technique.
3. 'Rooming-in' of babies, and provision of isolation nurseries or areas for 'infected' babies.

### b. Curative

Any baby showing signs of infection should be isolated until adequate treatment has controlled the disease. One of the many antibiotics available should be given as soon as possible in adequate doses. The most suitable drugs at present available are shown in Table 59/1. Gonococcal or staphylococcal conjunctivitis should be treated by local instillation of the antibiotic as well as systemic administration. Changes in bacterial sensitivity are rapid, and new drugs become available at intervals, so that different drugs may be more appropriate in different areas and at different times. For these reasons, the reader should consult with local neonatologists before making a final decision about which drug to use.

| Infection | Drug | Route | Dose in 24 hours |
|---|---|---|---|
| Staphylococci | Methicillin | Parenteral | 100 to 200mg/kg, 4 to 6 doses |
| Streptococci | Penicillin G 'crystalline' | IM or IV | 100 000 U/kg (in 2 doses) |
| *E. coli* | Kanamycin | IM | 10 to 30mg/kg (in 2 doses) |
| | Amoxycillin | Orally or IM | 150mg/kg (in 4 doses) |
| *Candida* | Nystatin | Oral | 600 000U (in 6 doses) |
| Gonorrhoea | Penicillin G | Parenteral | 50 000 units/kg/day in 2 doses for 7 days |
| | Tetracycline | Locally to eye | Eye ointment |
| *Pseudomonas* | Carbenicillin | Parenteral | 200mg/kg (4 doses) |
| | Gentamicin | Parenteral | 5mg/kg/day (2 doses) |

**Table 59/1** Treatment of neonatal infections

# Chapter 60

# The Low Birth-Weight Baby

The birth-weight of any infant depends on a complex relationship between its genetically inherited growth potential, and the effectiveness of the support to its growth provided by the uteroplacental environment, the latter being the more important of the two.

The genetically inherited growth potential is unalterable for the individual fetus, but the uteroplacental environment (mainly the uterine blood flow) is modified by a variety of factors, some affecting all fetuses, others affecting only certain fetuses. An example of inherited growth potential is that after the 34th to 36th week of gestation, male fetuses tend to be 50 to 150g heavier than female fetuses; and the infants of multigravid mothers tend to be 100 to 120g heavier than those of primigravidae. Examples of the altered uteroplacental environment are the effects of intra-uterine growth retardation due to multiple pregnancy (see Chapter 40), to fetal malformation and maternal disease (see Chapter 36).

The relationship between fetal growth potential and maternal growth support has been considered in detail by Gruenwald. So long as the growth support exceeds the growth potential, growth will continue. But when the maternal growth support is inadequate, fetal growth potential is severely limited. This means that given the same fetal growth potential, variations in growth support will produce deviations from the straight line of fetal growth potential (Fig. **60/1**). These deviations usually arise after the 30th week of gestation, and are most marked after the 35th week.

Charts have been constructed to show fetal growth as related to gestational age (Fig. **60/2**). Fetal growth retardation has been arbitrarily delineated if the weight of the infant is more than 2 standard deviations below the mean for the given gestational age. Because of the inability of some women to remember with accuracy the date of the last menstrual period, a low birth-weight baby in the developed countries is arbitrarily defined as any infant weighing less than 2500g at birth. In the developing countries, where the mean birth-weight at all gestational stages in the second half of pregnancy is lower, this figure would be unrealistic, and lower birth-weights are arbitrarily accepted (Table **60/1**). These weights have been determined by a scrutiny of birth records of normal births, by studying the perinatal mortality rates and the neonatal death rates of babies of various birth-weights. In Malaysia a birth-weight of less than 2000g defined a low birth-weight baby, and in the Philippines 2250g has proved a reasonable measure of low birth-weight. Studies in which these reduced weights have been adopted have shown that the incidence of prematurity (as redefined) is close to the 4 to 7 per cent encountered in Western countries, but the mortality rates for each weight group are less. Thus a Malaysian baby weighing 1800g has the

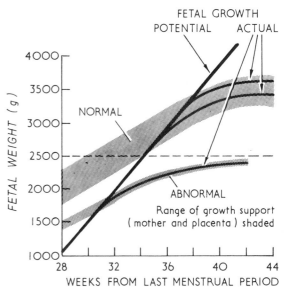

**Fig. 60/1** Fetal growth potential and maternal growth support (source: *Perinatal Problems*)

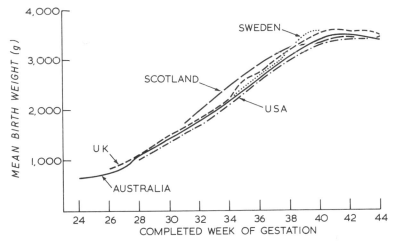

**Fig. 60/2** The mean birth-weight at various gestational ages in several developed nations. Note that the mean birth-weight at the end of the 35th gestational week is approximately 2500g

| Race | Country | Socio-economic Group | |
|---|---|---|---|
| | | High (g) | Low (g) |
| European | Australia, New Zealand | 3400 | 3200 |
| | USA (Caucasian) | 3400 | 3200 |
| | UK | 3400 | 3100 |
| Malay | Malaysia | 2905 | 2750 |
| | Indonesia | 3020 | 2815 |
| Chinese | Hong Kong | 3100 | 2900 |
| | Malaysia | 3090 | 2885 |
| Indian | Madras | 2985 | 2750 |
| | Malaysia | 2915 | 2645 |
| African | Nigeria | 3200 | 2850 |
| | Congo | 3000 | 2850 |
| | South Africa | 3050 | |

**Table 60/1** Mean birth-weights in different countries

same chance of survival as a European baby weighing 2200g. The variations in birth-weight in different racial groups are largely due to socio-economic influences, but some genetic influence also operates.

Low birth-weight babies comprise two populations: (1) preterm babies and (2) small-for-dates babies.

*Preterm babies,* previously called premature babies, are babies whose weight is correct for the gestational period but who are born when the pregnancy is less than 37 weeks advanced. Usually their birth-weight is less than 2500g.

*Small-for-dates babies* are babies whose weight is less than expected for the gestational age. They are also termed intra-uterine growth retarded babies, or dysmature babies. Small-for-dates babies are usually wasted with little subcutaneous fat, and are probably at greater risk of dying in the neonatal period than preterm babies. Combinations of the two forms also occur and in some cases it is hard to classify a particular baby. In such a case, the management is that of a 'small-for-dates' baby.

The Perinatal Mortality Survey in Britain studied the correlation between birth-weight and period of gestation for the first time in a national sample, and scrutiny of Table **60/2** shows that the mortality is more closely related to birth-weight than to period of gestation, but that the combination of curtailment of pregnancy and low birth-weight carries a greater risk of fetal mortality.

| Weight (g) | Gestation (in weeks) | Percentage of all births | Perinatal mortality (per 1000) | Live birth per cent survival |
|---|---|---|---|---|
| < 500 | All | | 990 | 1 |
| 501–750 | All | 0.5 | 750 | 25 |
| 751–1000 | All | | 500 | 50 |
| 1001–1500 | All | 0.8 | 250 | 75 |
| 1501–2000 | less than 37 | 1.0 | 200 | 80 |
| | more than 37 | | 150 | 85 |
| 2001–2500 | less than 37 | 5.0 | 100 | 90 |
| | more than 37 | | 50 | 95 |
| 2501–3000 | All | 18.0 | | |
| 3001–3500 | All | 39.0 | 30 | 97 |
| 3501–4000 | All | 27.7 | | |
| > 4000 | All | 8.0 | 50 | 95 |

**Table 60/2** Perinatal mortality related to weight and period of gestation (UK, Australia 1975–85)

Low birth-weight infants, therefore, include both premature and 'small-for-dates' (or dysmature) babies, and comprise between 4 and 8 per cent of all births (two-thirds preterm; one-third small-for-dates or dysmature). The rate is influenced by many factors such as maternal age and parity, the socio-economic status, health and physique of the parents, and the incidence of pregnancy-induced hypertension, chronic nephritis and fetal malformations in the population.

The higher proportion of babies weighing < 2500g in the developing nations (range 12 to 30 per cent) compared with the developed nations (range 3 to 9 per cent) is largely due to the increased proportion of small-for-dates babies in the former, presumably due to chronic intra-uterine malnutrition. There are six times as many small-for-dates babies in the developing nations, compared with the developed nations and only twice as many preterm babies.

## AETIOLOGICAL FACTORS (Table 60/3)

### Socio-economic conditions

Studies in several communities show that even in the developed countries of the world, the prevalence of low birth-weight babies is related to socio-economic conditions. To some extent the higher prevalence is due to the more frequent onset of preterm labour, and to some extent to the birth of dysmature babies amongst women in lower socio-economic groups. The proportional incidence of the two groups may vary considerably when different populations are investigated. Nor is it clear to what extent

| Social | Maternal age < 17 > 35 |
|---|---|
| | Socio-economic class IV and V |
| | Pre-pregnancy weight < 50kg > 75kg |
| | Excessive alcohol consumption |
| Obstetric | Previous preterm labour |
| | Previous low birth-weight baby |
| Present pregnancy | Hypertensive disease in pregnancy |
| | Renal disease |
| Fetal | Congenital defect (malformation) |
| | Intra-uterine infection |

**Table 60/3** Risk factors in incidence of low birth-weight babies

the higher prevalence in the lower socio-economic groups is due to poor maternal nutrition in childhood, the less ready acceptance of antenatal care, and the greater the likelihood of heavy work in late pregnancy.

In the study made in Aberdeen, Baird found that if the mother was the daughter of a professional or business man, and married to a man of similar status, the risk of her baby being preterm was half that of a woman whose father and husband were in a semi- or an unskilled job. Baird also found that the superior health, nourishment and physique of the woman in social classes I and II were advantages at all stages of gestation: a baby born to an affluent woman was heavier than that born to a woman in social classes III and IV, and this latter factor did more to produce the lower 'prematurity' rate (if defined by weight alone) than the diminished risk of premature onset of labour. Substantially similar findings have been reported from England by Fedrick and from Malaysia by Llewellyn-Jones.

A further social factor which has recently been observed to influence birth-weight is smoking. Heavy smokers tend to have smaller babies. It is not clear whether this is a direct effect, or whether the woman who smokes heavily is less well nourished than the non-smoker.

### Maternal conditions

#### PREMATURE LABOUR – UNEXPLAINED

This group accounts for about one-third of preterm births which lead to the delivery of a low birth-weight baby. It includes premature labour and spontaneous rupture of the membranes. Cervical incompetence is often alleged to be a cause, but the evidence is tenuous that it is, except rarely.

#### DISORDERS OF PREGNANCY

In some communities teenage pregnancy (especially amongst primigravidae aged 17 or less) is associated with low birth-weight of the baby. Other associations are with a previous history of low birth-weight, and with threatened abortion in the current pregnancy.

Pregnancy-induced hypertension (PIH) and antepartum haemorrhage may cause the onset of premature labour, or labour may have to be induced prematurely to 'rescue' the fetus from a hostile intra-uterine environment.

Twins (and triplets) account for between 12 and 18 per cent of all low birth-weight infants, and a proportion of the infants are dysmature. For example, it is not unusual to deliver a pair of twins, one of which weighs 3000g and is normal, the other weighing only 1500g and being clinically dysmature. In most instances the smaller twin has been malnourished in utero, its fellow having obtained the main share of nutrients transferred. Since PIH is four times as common in multiple as in singleton pregnancy, additional factors conducive to low birth-weight also operate.

#### MATERNAL DISEASE

It has been mentioned that although the babies of diabetic mothers are born preterm and are functionally immature, their birth-weight is often greater than normal for the period of gestation. The reverse of this is found in severe anaemia, both iron-deficient and megaloblastic. In these conditions, pregnancy does not necessarily terminate prematurely, but the incidence of low birth-weight babies is three times that found amongst non-anaemic mothers. Severe essential hypertension (especially if protein is found in the urine) and chronic nephritis are often associated with the birth of a dysmature infant. Pyelonephritis and symptomless bacteriuria are possible causes of low birth-weight infants, but the association is not constant. Viral infections, especially rubella, occurring in pregnancy may also produce retarded fetal growth, due to the effects of the virus on the developing fetal organs, and lead to the birth of a dysmature infant.

#### FETAL AND PLACENTAL DISEASE

A malformed fetus is both of low birth-weight and liable to be born preterm, but this is an infrequent cause of low birth-weight. More common, but less understood, is the factor of placental dysfunction, which may be associated with hypertensive disorders (in 60 per cent of cases), pyelonephritis during pregnancy (in 5 per cent), or have no known cause (in 35 per cent). The babies are smaller than expected at each period of gestation, and even at term may weigh less than 2500g. Except for the higher incidence of maternal disease (mainly anaemia) as a factor in the developing countries, the proportion of the various factors considered responsible is similar in developed and developing lands (Table **60/4**).

### The reduction of low birth-weight

The association of low birth-weight babies and the mother's socio-economic status suggests a nutritional factor. However, controlled trials of supplementary feeding during pregnancy failed to show any benefit in reducing the numbers of low birth-weight babies born. If poor nutrition is a factor, it must operate long before the childbearing years of the woman. Nor have any other methods of prevention – more frequent antenatal visits, cervical circlage, hospital

|  | Percentage |
|---|---|
| Premature labour, unexplained | 35–45 |
| Pregnancy induced hypertension | 10–20 |
| Multiple pregnancy—uncomplicated | 5–15 |
| Antepartum haemorrhage | 5–10 |
| Congenital malformations | 2–5 |
| Maternal disease; intra-uterine infections | 2–5 |

**Table 60/4** Aetiological factors in low birth-weight

admission, education, reduced the rate of spontaneous preterm delivery.

During pregnancy, smoking, drugs and the excessive consumption of alcohol should be avoided. About one-quarter of women whose first infant was of low birth-weight due to dysmaturity have a second baby which is also small for gestational age (SGA). This finding suggests that some 'intrinsic' factor exists and would explain the failure of nutritional supplements, the avoidance of drugs and good prenatal care to eliminate low birth-weight babies.

## CLINICAL ASPECTS

### Preterm (premature) babies

Apart from low birth-weight, the preterm baby is frail with a relatively large head and hands. Its skin is thin and pale, and blood vessels are easily seen. Adipose tissue is deficient, and its features are angular, occasionally the face looking old and wizened. Its abdomen is protuberant (Fig. **60/3**). There is also strong evidence that motor nerve conduction velocity

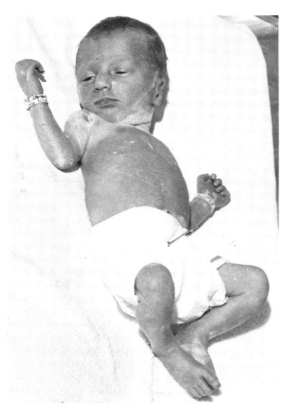

**Fig. 60/3** The preterm baby

is correlated with gestational age rather than birthweight. This means that the more preterm the infant, the less efficient are its motor functions, including respiration and feeding. For these reasons its cry is feeble and whining, and expansion of its lungs is poor, with episodes of apnoea, so that during handling or feeding, cyanotic episodes are common. The temperature control is poor, and its body temperature often below normal. Since maternal immunoglobulins are only transferred in any quantity in late pregnancy, the preterm baby may be immunodeficient, so that infection is readily acquired and may give few signs. Enzyme systems, particularly those involving bilirubin conjugation, are defective so that physiological jaundice may be intense and prolonged. Sucking and swallowing are less efficient, and mucus may accumulate in the mouth. Fat absorption from the gut is poor. Capillary fragility is increased and hypoprothrombinaemia may be present. Haemorrhagic manifestations, particularly cerebral intraventricular haemorrhage, may occur; most of these are hypoxic in origin. The iron stores are likely to be depleted, as most of the iron is transferred to the fetus in the last 8 weeks of pregnancy. The lungs are less able to expand and to ventilate properly because of a relative lack of surfactant. This has been discussed in Chapter 57. Renal function is immature with the result its excretory capacity is limited, as is its capacity to re-absorb bicarbonate. This predisposes the baby to metabolic acidosis. As well, the kidney of a preterm baby is less well able to handle sodium, so that hypernatraemia or hyponatraemia may occur.

These various defects are most marked in the smaller preterm babies (less than 1500g). The greatest hazards to survival are poor pulmonary ventilation; the development of the respiratory distress syndrome; and intraventricular haemorrhage.

At any given birth-weight, the true premature baby has a higher mortality than the gestationally more advanced dysmature baby.

### 'Small-for-dates' (dysmature) babies

In most 'small-for-dates' infants the size of the spleen, the liver, the adrenals and the thymus are reduced, with a reduction both in the numbers and size of the individual cells. By contrast the heart and the brain are disproportionately large so that the 'small-for-dates' baby has a relatively large head. The main metabolic defect of the 'small-for-dates' infant is lipid malnutrition. The infant has inadequate stores of both brown and white fat. It is not clear if this is due to inadequate transfer of carbohydrate and fatty acids through a dysfunctional placenta, or if there is insufficient fetal insulin secreted and thus insufficient intracellular glucose deposition, both of which are necessary for triglyceride synthesis and storage. There may also be inadequate production, or activation, of the enzymes involved in triglyceride deposition. For these reasons the body fat (both brown and white) is reduced, and glycogen stores in the liver and cardiac muscle are less than in a preterm baby of similar birth-weight. As the dysmature infant has a relatively large amount of actively metabolizing tissue, the oxygen consumption per unit weight is increased. This makes the transitional period between birth and the establishment of feeding especially hazardous. In this period hypoglycaemia, metabolic acidosis and hypothermia are fairly common. Clinically, hypoglycaemia is the most important metabolic defect. It is entirely preventable if blood glucose levels are monitored, and if early feeding is practised. Pulmonary alveolar haemorrhage is an additional hazard.

Clinically the 'small-for-dates' infant is not always easy to distinguish from the preterm infant. In general, its appearance is of a small, thin, skinny, dry, wrinkled infant which has the features of a more mature baby despite its small size. As noted, its head is relatively large. Its skin is often meconium-stained at delivery, and there is a complexity of skin creases on the soles of the feet. The 'small-for-dates' infant tends to be far more alert, lively and restless than the preterm infant, and has mature reflex responses.

METHOD OF BIRTH

Recently controversy has arisen about the most appropriate method of delivering a preterm baby, especially if its birth-weight is estimated as being less than 1500g. Many obstetric units routinely perform caesarean section arguing that the trauma to the soft fetal head and intraventricular haemorrhage may occur during vaginal delivery. However, prospective studies show that caesarean section is no safer for the baby, unless a breech presentation, severe PIH, antepartum haemorrhage or fetal distress is a complicating factor.

## COMPLICATIONS IN LOW BIRTH-WEIGHT BABIES

The following complications occur amongst low birth-weight babies, and are more common in premature babies.

1. *Failure of the lungs to expand* (atelectasis) and the respiratory distress syndrome (see Chapter 57).

2. *Inhalation of feeds.* Despite careful handling, inhalation of regurgitated stomach contents occurs more commonly than might be expected. Any low birth-weight infant who has difficulty with breathing should be suspected of having inhaled food or vomit, and the pharynx should be aspirated carefully.

3. *Cyanotic attacks.* These are common in infants below 1500g birth-weight and may be due to inadequate ventilation of the lungs or to cerebral damage.

4. *Development of infection.* The great majority of babies over 1500g birth-weight who survive the first 48 to 72 hours of life will remain alive unless infection supervenes. Still smaller babies who begin life vigorously may gradually deteriorate in the absence of infection because their lungs are not fully competent.

5. *Jaundice.* Since early feeding was introduced, the incidence of marked jaundice in preterm babies has fallen considerably. However, serum bilirubin levels in excess of $250\mu mol/litre$ (15mg/dl) cause concern because of potential kernicterus.

As jaundice may be a sign of infection, the child should be examined carefully to exclude or treat this before giving specific therapy. The usual method of treating jaundice is to perform an exchange transfusion. This is a rapid and effective way of diminishing the hyperbilirubinaemia. Recently, a secondary method has been recommended. This may be used in milder cases, if exchange transfusion is technically difficult (as, for example, in infants with umbilical infection) or if the bilirubin levels begin to rise again after exchange transfusion. The method is to use phototherapy either by brightly illuminating nurseries, or by using 'blue light'. Light emits streams of protons which oxidize bilirubin in skin capillaries to the harmless biliverdin and other water-soluble substances. Phototherapy with white light (using about 500 foot-candles) is safer than 'blue light', but both may cause retinal damage unless the eyes are covered, and dehydration, due to insensible water loss may occur. Phototherapy seems of value in the hyperbilirubinaemia of prematurity and in mild haemolytic disease.

6. *Hypoglycaemia.* This condition affects about 4 in every 1000 babies born, but increases to 15 per 100 small-for-dates babies. It may affect the infants of diabetic mothers, and babies who have erythroblastosis, but is more common in small-for-dates

babies than others. It is due to a lack of fetal reserve of glycogen. A dysmature baby is also less able to convert glycogen into glucose. Hypoglycaemia may cause apathy, listlessness, irritability and convulsions. Some babies have bradycardia and are cyanosed. The symptom complex is not diagnostic, as infection may also cause some of the signs. The diagnosis is made by measuring blood glucose levels (by Dextrostix). If the level is less than 30ml/dl (1.67mmol/l) in a term infant, or less than 20mg/dl (1.11mmol/l) in a preterm infant hypoglycaemia is probable. Hypoglycaemia is confirmed by a biochemical estimation of blood glucose levels and treatment given. In 'at risk' babies, the blood glucose levels should be monitored every 2 hours in the first 12 hours of life and 4 hourly until feeding has been established.

The incidence of hypoglycaemia can be reduced by preventing heat loss, and by establishing early feeding to obtain an adequate calorie intake. Treatment is to give glucose by intravenous infusion at a rate of 6 to 9mg/kg/minute.

7. *Hypocalcaemia.* Low blood calcium levels may occur in low birth-weight babies, usually in the first 24 hours of life. If a plasma calcium level of 8mg/dl or less is found, intravenous calcium gluconate (200mg/kg) is given.

8. *Intracranial haemorrhage.* Periventricular haemorrhage (intraventricular and parenchymal haemorrhage) is relatively common among babies weighing 1500g or less. Between 20 and 30 per cent of these babies have the condition. It is diagnosed by real-time ultrasonography (echo-encephalography) or CAT scan.

The incidence is not affected by the route or mode of delivery, the state of the membranes (intact or ruptured), or the duration of labour. If the 1-minute Apgar score is 6 or less, if the fetus has been acidotic, hypercapnic, or develops hyaline membrane disease, periventricular haemorrhage is more likely to occur.

The incidence of periventricular haemorrhage is reduced significantly if ethamsylate in a dose of 12.5mg/kg body-weight is given 6-hourly for the first 4 days of life.

## MANAGEMENT OF THE LOW BIRTH-WEIGHT INFANT

The objectives of management are: (1) to provide an environment as close to that found in utero as possible; (2) to prevent the development of infection; and (3) to provide adequate nourishment by carefully

controlled feeding, so that the infant may grow and mature. The most successful results in management occur in units where low birth-weight babies are attended by devoted nurses and doctors who have continuous experience of their problems. Special equipment is helpful but the most important factor in the survival of low birth-weight babies is the constant observation and intelligent action by skilled attendants.

At birth the low birth-weight baby is received into a warmed bassinette or a Humidicrib, and laid on one side. Phytomenadione (vitamin K) 1 mg is given intramuscularly and oxygen provided until the infant can be taken to a 'premature' baby unit.

### Control of the environment

The neonatal intensive care nursery should be kept at a temperature of no less than 24°C (75°F), and the humidity at no less than 65 per cent. In temperate countries the babies are nursed in incubators which provide a controlled temperature of 26 to 32°C (80 to 90°F), and allow a controlled supply of oxygen to be provided at a humidity of 65 to 75 per cent. In tropical countries where temperature and humidity are high, incubators are not necessary, provided oxygen can be supplied to the baby at proper concentrations. Simple head boxes will achieve this end, but devices to measure the oxygen concentration are essential if the dangers of oxygen in the treatment of low birth-weight babies are to be avoided. Too much oxygen supplied for too long at too high a concentration led in recent years to the development of retrolental fibroplasia and blindness in a proportion of surviving prematures. With proper control this iatrogenic disease will not occur.

### Control of infection

The most important single factor is a high standard of nursing by sufficient trained nurses. One nurse can only adequately care for two or three infants. Visitors, apart from the baby's parents, should be excluded from the section of the nursery treating babies weighing 1500g or less, as they are particularly prone to infection. It is important for 'bonding' between parents and baby that the parents should have access. However, they should be visited by the neonatologist before they go to the nursery, as they may be considerably disturbed to see a scrawny baby, with respiratory difficulties, lying naked inside an incubator, connected by various tubes and wires to machines. An explanation of the reason for the apparatus will prevent parental anxiety. The involvement of the mother, particularly in the care of her baby, is important and the provision of fresh breast milk is now believed desirable. The cots may either be placed in cubicles or in an open area, provided that 1.8 to 2.7 m² is available for each cot. Infection may enter through the upper respiratory tract, the umbilical area and through abrasions on the skin. Over-enthusiastic washing will reduce normal resistance. The low birth-weight baby should be cleaned at birth, to remove blood and mucus, but thereafter it should not be bathed until it weighs 1750g. Only the diaper area needs attention. Chlorhexidine powder applied to the perineum, umbilical area, groins and axillae will reduce the incidence of staphylococcal invasion.

Babies known or suspected to be infected should be attended in a special part of the unit by nurses who do not come into contact with other babies, if this is possible.

### Feeding

Feeding is started between 6 and 24 hours of birth, depending upon the vigour of the baby. Modern practice is to start feeding for all babies, and particularly for 'small-for-dates' babies as early as possible. After a short initial period, when saline or water is given, expressed breast milk or half-cream spray-dried milk is given 3-hourly. There is evidence that fresh breast milk is the most suitable food, particularly if the baby weighs less than 1500g, as it provides anti-infective agents which reduce the risk of necrotizing enterocolitis considerably.

The baby is fed by gavage or spoon, as appropriate, and as soon as it is strong enough is put to the breast if possible, or given its feeds by bottle. The amount of formula milk is calculated from the formula that a preterm baby requires about 225ml per kg per day. Breast-fed babies are suckled often.

Total parenteral feeding should be used only in special circumstances, when oral feeding is contraindicated, as it offers no greater survival, is extremely expensive and has potential dangers to the baby. The dysmature baby is especially susceptible to hypoglycaemia. But it is commonly thirsty and feeds well from the early hours. Feeds, preferably milk, should therefore be given very early to avoid the risk of hypoglycaemia and its possible conse-

quence, brain damage. As well, the infant's blood sugar levels should be monitored and if the level falls below 1.11mmol/litre (20mg/dl) additional glucose should be given.

### Supplements

Vitamin $K_1$ (phytomenadione) 1mg should be given at birth and vitamin C 25mg is recommended on the first day.

Within the first two weeks, regular vitamin supplements should be given with feeds. Recommended daily doses are 1000 units of vitamin D and 5000 units of vitamin A, 50mg of ascorbic acid, 1mg of thiamine, 1mg of riboflavin and 6mg of niacin. A number of preparations are marketed in slightly different combinations. It is at present uncertain to what extent the low birth-weight baby's vitamin requirement exceed those of the ordinary baby, and also whether more effort should be taken to secure a good intake of the B-group of vitamins.

### Drugs

The routine administration of antibiotics with the object of improving the survival rate of low birth-weight infants has proved disappointing, and all authorities now advise against this. Similarly the administration of gammaglobulin is not recommended. The low birth-weight baby is slow in producing gammaglobulin because of the passively transferred IgG, and by the 3rd month when the supply received from across the placenta has been degraded, the gammaglobulin levels in his serum tend to be depressed. Although the level can be raised by intramuscular injection of immunoglobulin, which would theoretically improve his resistance to infection at this stage, such administration will still further depress his own production of antibodies. As it is known that in response to infection the preterm infant can gain immunocompetence at the same rate as the full term infant, the use of allogenic immunoglobulin is contraindicated.

## PROGNOSIS

Although babies of low birth-weight (whether dysmature or preterm) form < 10 per cent of births, these babies contribute 70 per cent of first-week deaths, and the smaller the baby at birth, the less is its chance of survival. Of those babies dying, more than 70 per cent do so within the first 48 hours of birth, and if the baby can survive these critical two days, it has a reasonably good chance of living. Because of their greater gestational maturity, dysmature infants have a better prognosis for survival than preterm babies of the same birth-weight.

With the development of intensive neonatal care units, fewer low birth-weight babies die, and those that survive are likely to be healthy.

Today, about 25 per cent of babies weighing 501 to 750g will live, as will 50 per cent of babies weighing 751 to 1000g. Babies weighing from 1001 to 1500g at birth today have a 75 per cent chance of living.

With the improvements of neonatal care such as early feeding, early treatment of hypoglycaemia, hyperkalaemia, hypothermia, regular measurement of blood gases, controlled oxygen and CPAP, the number of babies who show severe physical or mental defects has diminished.

Babies weighing more than 1500g at birth who survive the neonatal period, as most do, have a low incidence of residual physical or mental handicaps. Babies whose birth-weight is 1500g or less, have a greater chance of survival than in the past, but are a vulnerable group for disabilities. The post-neonatal death rate is 7 times that of the general population, as is the likelihood of the sudden infant death syndrome. Between 5 and 10 per cent of these very low birth-weight babies will have major physical handicaps (mostly cerebral palsy, sensorineural deafness or blindness), and about another 5 to 15 per cent will have minor physical handicaps. About the same proportion will be found to have marked mental developmental delay when assessed at age 3 to 4. Over 70 per cent of babies weighing 1000g or less will be stillborn or will die, usually in the first 48 hours of life. One in three of the survivors will have a severe physical or mental handicap, and the lower the birth-weight, the greater is the chance of handicap.

Assessment of very low birth-weight babies at 1 and 3 years gives a strong indication of later difficulties. It has also been noted that children whose parents are poor are more likely to have poorer mental ability.

# Bibliography

I have intentionally kept this bibliography short for two reasons. First, few students use a bibliography and second, the availability of electronic search systems makes a long bibliography unnecessary. However, if a reader has a specific question about a statement made in this book, I shall try to answer it with the appropriate reference.

## GENERAL REFERENCES

BEARD RW, NATHANIELSZ PW. *Fetal Physiology and Medicine*, 2nd ed. Decker, London, 1984.

DANFORTH DN. *Textbook of Obstetrics and Gynaecology*, 5th ed. Harper and Row, New York, 1986.

DE SWIET M (ed). *Medical Disorders in Pregnancy*, 2nd ed., Blackwell, Oxford, 1989.

ENKIN M, CHALMERS I (jt eds). *Effectiveness and Satisfaction in Antenatal Care*. Heinemann, London, 1982.

KLAUS M, FANAROFF A. *Care of the High Risk Neonate*, 2nd ed. WB Saunders, Philadelphia, 1979.

MACDONALD RR. *Scientific Basis of Obstetrics and Gynaecology*, 3rd ed., Churchill-Livingstone, Edinburgh, 1985.

PRITCHARD JA, MACDONALD PC (jt eds & contribs). *Williams Obstetrics*, 17th ed. Appleton Century Crofts, New York, 1985.

SCHAFFER A, AVERY MA. *Diseases of the Newborn*, 5th ed. WB Saunders, Philadelphia, 1983.

SHEARMAN RP (ed). *Reproductive Endocrinology*. Churchill Livingstone, Edinburgh, 1985.

WETHERALL DJ, LEDINGHAM JGG, WARRELL DA. *The Oxford Textbook of Medicine*, 2nd ed., OUP, Oxford, 1987. (2 vols).

WHITEFIELD CR. *Dewhurst's Integrated Obstetrics and Gynaecology for Postgraduates*, 4th ed. Blackwell Scientific Publications Limited, Oxford, 1985.

## CHAPTER REFERENCES

### Chapter 1

EDWARDS RG et al. The growth of human pre-implantation embryos in vitro. *Amer J Obst Gynecol*, 1981; **141**, 408–13.

MARX J. The mating game. *Science*, 1978; **200**, 1256–9.

MOORE KL. *The Developing Human*. WB Saunders, Philadelphia, 1973.

### Chapter 2

BOYD JD, HAMILTON WJ. *The Human Placenta*. Heffer, Cambridge, 1970.

GLEIGHER N, DEPPE G, COHEN LJ. Common aspects of immunological tolerance in pregnancy. *Obst Gynecol*, 1979; **54**, 339–42.

WHO. Maturation of fetal body systems. *Tech Rep*, **540**, Geneva, 1974.

### Chapter 3

BARNES AC (ed). *Intra-Uterine Development*. Lea and Febiger, Philadelphia, 1965.

DAWES GS. *Fetal and Neonatal Physiology*. Year Book Publishers, Chicago, 1973.

FUCHS F, KLOPPER A. (eds). *Endocrinology of Pregnancy*. 2nd ed. Harper and Row, New York, 1980.

PECILE A, FINZI C. *The Feto-Placental Unit*. Excerpta Medica, Amsterdam, 1969.

WAISMAN HA, KERR G. *Fetal Growth and Development*. McGraw-Hill, New York, 1970.

### Chapter 4

GILLESPIE EC. *Amer J Obst Gynecol*, 1950; **59**, 949.

HEALY D. The clinical significance of endometrial prolactin. *Aust NZ J Obst Gynaecol*, 1984; **24**, 111–15.

HYTTEN FE, CHAMBERLAIN G. *Clinical Physiology in Obstetrics.* Blackwell Scientific Publications, Oxford, 1980.

SHORT RV (ed). Reproduction. *Brit Med Bull,* 1979; **35**, 97–208.

## Chapter 5

CALVERT JP et al. Antenatal screening by measurement of the symphysis-fundal weight. *Brit Med J,* 1982; **285**, 846–9.

## Chapter 6

DAVIDSON S, PASSMORE R, BROCKS JF. *Human Nutrition and Dietetics,* 7th ed. Churchill Livingstone, Edinburgh, 1979.

EDITORIAL. Diagnostic ultrasound in pregnancy. *Lancet,* 1984; **1**, 201–2.

ELKIN M, CHALMERS I. *Effectiveness and Satisfaction in Antenatal Care.* Heinemann, London, 1982.

MacGILLIVRAY I. *Pre-eclampsia, the Hypertensive Disease of Pregnancy.* WB Saunders, London, 1983.

NATIONAL ACADEMY OF SCIENCES. *Maternal Nutrition and the Course of Pregnancy.* Washington, 1970.

### TOBACCO AND ALCOHOL

See Lumley J, Astbury J in Elkin and Chalmers (above)

### SEXUALITY

KLEBANOFF MA et al. Coitus during pregnancy. *Lancet,* 1984; **2**, 914–17.

PERKINS PR. *Obst Gynecol,* 1982; **59**, 189–98.

### ULTRASOUND

WARSOFF SL, PEARCE JM, CAMPBELL S. The present place of routine ultrasound screening. *Clin. Obst Gynaecol,* 1983; **10**, 445–57.

## Chapter 9

CALDEYRO-BARCIA O. *Modern Trends in Obstetrics and Gynaecology.* Librairie Beauchemin, Montreal, 1959.

DUMOULIN JG, FOULKES JEB. Ketonuria during labour. *Brit J Obst Gynaecol,* 1984; **91**, 96–8.

HUSZAR G, ROBERTS JM. Biochemistry and pharmacology of the myometrium and labour. *Amer J Obst Gynecol,* 1982; **142**, 225–35.

LIGGINS GC et al. Control of parturition in man. *Biol Reprod,* 1977; **16**, 39–47.

REYNOLDS RM. *Physiology of the Uterus,* 2nd ed. Hafner, New York, 1965.

## Chapter 10

BERGSJO L et al. Duration of spontaneous labour. *Acta Obst Gynecol Scand,* 1979; **58**, 129–36.

## Chapter 12

PEISNER DB, ROSEN MG. Transition from latent to active labour. *Obstet Gynecol,* 1986; **68**, 448–50.

## Chapter 13

DUMOULIN JG, FOULKES JEB. Ketonuria in labour. *Brit J Obst Gynaecol,* 1984; **91**, 970–98.

O'DRISCOLL K et al. The active management of labour. *Brit Med J,* 1973; **3**, 135. and *Obst Gynecol,* 1984; **63**, 435.

PHILPOTT RH, CASTLE WM. *J Obstet Gynaecol Brit Cwlth,* 1972; **79**, 592.

SAWYERS RS. Fetal monitoring during labour. *Brit Med J,* 1983; **287**, 1649–50.

STUDD J. *Brit Med J,* 1973; **4**, 451.

### MATERNAL–INFANT BONDING

ANISFELD E et al. *Pediatrics,* 1983; **72**, 569–72.

KLAUS M, KENNELL J. *Parent-Infant Bonding.* CV Mosby, St Louis, 1982.

LAMB NE. *J Paediatrics,* 1982; **101**, 555–7.

## Chapter 15

BOURNE S, LEWIS E. Delayed psychological effects of perinatal death. *Brit Med J,* 1984; **289**, 147–8.

OUNSTED C et al. Fourth goal of perinatal medicine. *Brit Med J,* 1982; **284**, 879.

## Chapter 16

APPLEBAUM RM. The modern management of successful breast feeding. *Pediatric Clin of N Amer,* 1970; **17**, 203.

LLEWELLYN-JONES D. *Breast Feeding*. Faber and Faber, London, 1983.

McNEILLY AS. Physiology of lactation. *J Biosoc Sci*, 1977; Suppl. **4**, 5–21. and *Brit Med Bull*, 1979; **35**, 151.

WALKER S et al. *Lancet*, 1975; **2**, 542.

WHO. Physiology of lactation. *Tech Rep Series* No. 305, Geneva, 1965.

YUEN BH et al. Human prolactin: secretion, regulation and pathophysiology. *Obstet Gynaecol Surv*, 1973; **28**, 527.

## Chapter 17

LLEWELLYN-JONES D. *Human Reproduction and Society* (Chapters 10–14). Faber, London, 1974. (Now out of print, available in reference libraries.)

## Chapter 18

CRAWFORD JS. *Principles and Practice of Obstetric Anaesthesia*, 4th ed. Blackwell Scientific Publications Limited, Oxford, 1978.

FOLDES FF, CRAWFORD JS. *Acta Anaesth Scand*, Suppl. 1959; **11**, 15.

MORGAN B et al. Effectiveness of pain relief in labour, *Brit Med J*, 1982; **285**, 684–90.

SHNIDER S, MOYA F. *The Anesthesiologist, Mother and Newborn*. Williams and Wilkins, Baltimore, 1974.

## Chapter 19

ALLEN, EP. *Brit J Radiol*, 1947; **20**, 45, 108, 164, 205.

CALDWELL WE, MOLOY HC. *Amer J Obst Gynecol*, 1933; **26**, 479.

MOIR JC. *J Obstet Gynaecol Brit Emp*, 1949; **56**, 189.

THOMS H. *Pelvimetry*. Hoeber Inc, New York, 1956.

## Chapter 20

ELKIN M, CHALMERS I. Symptomatic treatment in pregnancy. In Elkin M and Chalmers I, *Effectiveness and Satisfaction in Antenatal Care*. Heinemann Medical Books, 1982.

## Chapter 22

SIMPSON JL et al. Low fetal loss after ultrasound proved viability in early pregnancy. *J Amer Med Assoc,* 1988; **258**, 2555–8.

## Chapter 24

ABRUPTIO PLACENTAE

HIBBARD BM. *Clin Obstet Gynaecol*, 1966; **9**, 93.

KINCAID-SMITH P, LAVER MC, FAIRLEY KF. *Med J Aust*, 1970; **1**, 145.

LLEWELLYN-JONES D. *Aust NZ J Obstet Gynaecol*, 1963; **3**, 97.

## Chapters 25, 26

BONNAR J (ed). *Pregnancy Hypertension*. MTP Press, Lancaster, 1980.

MACGILLIVRAY I, *Pre-eclampsia, the Hypertensive Disease of Pregnancy*, W. B. Saunders, London, 1983.

RUBIN PC et al. Beta-blockers in pregnancy. *New Engl J Med*, 1981; **315**, 232–5.

RUBIN PC et al. Atenolol in treatment of pregnancy associated hypertension. *Lancet*, 1983; **1**, 431–4.

## Chapter 27

EISENBACH G, BOYD J. *Kidney and Pregnancy*. Karger, Basel, 1981.

KASS EH, BRUMFELT W. *Infections of the Urinary Tract*. Chicago University Press, 1978.

KATZ AJ et al. *Kidney International*, 1980; **18**, 192.

## Chapter 28

ALGER LS et al. Thalassaemia and pregnancy. *Amer J Obst Gynecol*, 1979; **134**, 662.

HENDRICKSE JP, WATSON-WILLIAMS EJ. Haemoglobinopathies. *Amer J Obstet Gynecol*, 1966; **94**, 739.

LLEWELLYN-JONES D. Iron deficiency and megaloblastic anaemia. *Aust NZ J Obstet Gynaecol*, 1963; **5**, 191.

TUCK SH et al. Sickle-cell haemoglobinopathy. *Brit J Obst Gynaecol*, 1983; **90**, 112–17.

WHO. Nutritional anaemias. *Tech Rep Series*, No. 503. Geneva, 1972.

## Chapter 29

ELKAYAM U, GLEICHER N. Cardiac problems in pregnancy. *J Amer Med Assoc*, 1984; **251**, 2838–9.

## Chapter 30

EDITORIAL. Diabetes in pregnancy. *Lancet*, 1985, **1**, 961–2.

EDITORIAL. Glucose testing in pregnancy – the who and how of testing. *Lancet*, 1988; **2**, 1173–4.

PEDERSEN J. *The Pregnant Diabetic*. Munksgaard, Copenhagen, 1967.

PLEHWE WE. Management of pregnant diabetics. *Curr Therapeut*, 1984; **8**, 53–66.

SYMPOSIUM. Gestational diabetes. *Diabetic Care*, 1980; **3**, 399–501.

WHO. Diabetes mellitus. *Tech Rep Series*, No. 648, Geneva, 1980.

### Chapter 31

EDITORIAL. Hepatitis B. *Lancet*, 1984; **1**, 939–40.

GIBBS RS. The management of genital herpes infection in pregnancy. *Obstet Gynecol*, 1988; **71**, 779–84.

KILBRICK S. Herpes virus infection at term. *J Amer Med Assoc*, 1980; **243**, 157.

LLEWELLYN-JONES D. *Herpes, AIDS and Other Sexually Transmitted Diseases*. Faber and Faber, London, 1985.

MENSER MA. Prevention of congenital rubella. *Med J Aust*, 1984; **140**, 636–7.

WATERSON AP. Virus infections during pregnancy. *Brit Med J*, 1979; **2**, 564.

### Chapter 32

PEDDLE LJ. The antenatal management of the Rh sensitized woman. *Clin Perinatol*, 1984; **11**, 251–66.

TOVEY LAD et al. Antenatal anti D immunoglobulin trial. *Lancet*, 1983; **2**, 244–7.

WHITFIELD CR. Future challenges in the management of rhesus disease, in *Progress in Obstetrics and Gynaecology*, Vol. 2 (ed J Studd). Churchill Livingstone, Edinburgh, 1982: pp. 48–59.

### Chapter 35

ELDER MG (ed). *Preterm Labour*. Butterworths, London, 1981.

ELDER MG et al. Low dose aspirin in pregnancy. *Lancet*, 1988; **1**, 410.

KING JF et al. Betamimetics in preterm labour – an overview of randomized controlled trials. *Brit J Obst Gynaecol*, 1988; **95**, 211–22.

LIPSHUTZ J. *Seminars in Pediatrics*, 1981; **5**, 252–63.

### Chapter 36

ANTA D, THACKER SB. Costs and benefits of electronic fetal monitoring. *Obst Gynacol Surv*, 1979; **34**, 627.

LEVENO KJ et al. A prospective comparison of selective and universal electronic fetal monitoring. *New Engl J Med*, 1986; **315**, 615–22.

NELDAM S. Fetal movements as indication of fetal well-being. *Lancet*, 1980; **1**, 1222–5.

PARSONS RJ et al. Fetal monitoring in labour, in *Progress in Obstetrics and Gynaecology*, Vol. 1 (ed. J Studd). Churchill Livingstone, Edinburgh, 1981.

PEARSON JF, WEAVER JB. Fetal activity and fetal well-being. *Brit Med J*, 1976; **1**, 1305–7.

PRENTICE A, LIND T. Fetal heart monitoring in labour. *Lancet*, 1987; **2**, 1375–7.

### Chapter 38

EDITORIAL. Delivery of small breech babies. *Lancet*, 1983; **1**, 336–7.

EDITORIAL. External cephalic version. *Lancet*, 1984; **2**, 385.

HYTTEN FE. Breech presentation: is it a bad omen? *Brit J Obst Gynaecol*, 1982; **89**, 879–80.

### Chapter 40

CHERVENAK FA et al. Is routine caesarean section necessary for vertex-breech and vertex-transverse twin gestations? *Amer J Obst Gynecol*, 1984; **148**, 1–5.

GRANT A et al. In Elkin M and Chalmers I, *Effectiveness and Satisfaction in Antenatal Care*. London, Heinemann, 1982; pp 203–6.

RHYDSTROM H et al. Routine hospital care does not improve prognosis in twin gestation. *Acta Obstet Gynaecol Scand*, 1987; **66**, 361–4.

### Chapter 44

FRIEDMAN EA. *Labour – Clinical Evaluation and Management*. Appleton Century Crofts, New York, 1967.

### Chapter 46

LUCAS WE. Postpartum haemorrhage. *Clin Obst Gynecol*, 1980; **23**, 637.

**Chapter 47**

WOINARSKI JE, WRIGHT JT. Morbidity of episiotomy. *J Obst Gynaecol*, 1982; **3**, 66–70.

**Chapter 48**

CLARKE-PEARSON DL et al. Postoperative venous thrombo-emboli. *Amer J Obst Gynecol*, 1984; **48**, 1047–54.

DEAN C, KENDELL RE. The symptomatology of puerperal illness. *Brit J Psych*, 1981; **139**, 128–33.

**Chapter 49**

CAMERON IT, BAIRD D. Early pregnancy termination. *Brit J Obst Gynaecol*, 1988; **95**, 271–6.

EMBREY MP. Prostaglandins in human reproduction. *Brit Med J*, 1981; **283**, 1563–6.

**Chapter 50**

DRIFE JO. Kielland's or caesar? *Brit Med J*, 1983; **287**, 309–10.

PARRY-JONES E. *Kielland's Forceps*. Butterworths, London, 1952.

QUILLIGAN E (ed) Caesarean section. *Clin Obst Gynecol*, 1985; **28**, 689–782.

RADCLIFFE W. *The Secret Instrument*. Heinemann Medical Books, London, 1947.

**Chapter 51**

LAVIN BT et al. Vaginal delivery in patients with a previous caesarean section. *Obstet Gynecol*, 1982; **59**, 135–42.

O'DRISCOLL K, FOLEY M. Correlation of decrease in perinatal mortality and increase in caesarean section rates. *Obstet Gynecol*, 1983; **61**, 1–5.

**Chapter 54**

DEPARTMENT OF HEALTH AND SOCIAL SECURITY. *Reports on Confidential Enquiries into Maternal Death*. HMSO, London.

WHO. Recommendations for statistical tables related to the perinatal period. *Acta Obst Gynaecol Scand*, 1977; **56**, 247–53.

**Chapter 55**

DAWES GS. *Fetal and Neonatal Physiology*. Year Book Publishers, Chicago, 1973.

OLSHAN AF et al. Caesarean section and neonatal mortality in very low birth weight infants. *Obstet Gynecol*, 1984; **67**, 267–71.

**Chapter 56**

PANETH N. Birth and origins of cerebral palsy. *New Engl J Med*, 1986; **315**, 124–6.

SCRIMGEOUR JG, COCKBURN F. Congenital abnormalities. *Lancet*, 1979; **2**, 1349–52.

STANDING MEDICAL ADVISORY COMMITTEE. Screening for the detection of congenital dislocation of the hip. *Arch Dis Child*, 1986; **61**, 921–6.

**Chapter 57**

KLAUS MS, FANAROFF A. *Care of the High Risk Neonate*, 2nd ed. WB Saunders, Philadelphia, 1979.

**Chapter 60**

KLAUS MS, FANAROFF A. *Care of the High Risk Neonate*, 2nd ed. WB Saunders, Philadelphia, 1979.

# Glossary

This glossary, which precedes the index, is included so that students may have a readily available reference to the definition of certain frequently encountered terms.

### Abortion

The process of expulsion of a fetus which weighs less than 500g.

### Abortus

An expelled embryo or fetus weighing less than 500g.

### Embryo

The product of conception (conceptus) from fertilization until the 50th day, by which time all major structures have formed.

### Fetus

The product of conception from the 50th day (end of 7th week) until birth at whatever period of gestation that this may be.

### Immature infant

An infant weight from 500 to 999g at birth. Also called a *'previable' infant*. It has a poor chance of survival.

### Miscarriage

Spontaneous abortion.

### Pregnancy-induced hypertension (PIH)

The preferred term for pre-eclampsia or pre-eclamptic toxaemia.

### Preterm (premature) infant

An infant weighing between 1000 and 2499g. The upper limit is lowered in certain developing countries to 1999g.

### Vernix caseosa

The greasy, cheese-like deposit found in patches on the skin of the newborn infant. It is derived from desquamated epithelial cells and sebaceous gland secretions.

---

### Gravida

A pregnant woman.

### High multigravida

A patient who is pregnant for the 5th or subsequent time.

### Multigravida

A patient who has previously been pregnant. She may have aborted or have delivered a viable baby.

### Multipara

A patient who has delivered two or more children.

### Primigravida

A patient pregnant for the first time.

**Primipara**

A patient who has delivered one viable child.

**Note:** The terms gravida and para are erroneously used interchangeably. A patient may be gravida 3 (having been pregnant twice previously), but para 0 (as the two previous pregnancies ended in abortion). During her first pregnancy, a patient is gravida 1 but para 0. She only becomes para 1 (or primiparous) after delivering her first child. In view of this confusion, it is best to use the term gravida, and in detailing the previous obstetric history, to write a chronological list of details of each pregnancy. In the USA a shorthand notation of 4 digits is used: as 3-0-1-3. The first figure refers to the number of mature infants delivered; the second to the number of premature infants; the third to the number of abortions; and the fourth to the number of infants surviving.

# Index

cardiotocography, *contd.*
  oxytocin test 279
cardiovascular system, changes in
      pregnancy 37–8
cellulitis, pelvic 372
cephalhaematoma 456
cephalopelvic disproportion *see*
      disproportion,
      cephalopelvic
cerebral palsy 446
cervix:
  carcinoma 264
  cautery of 146
  changes:
    labour, in 80
    pregnancy, during 37, 80
    puerperium, in 131, 146
  circlage 271
  conization 264
  cytology 264
  dilatation, estimation of 121
  dystocia 342
  effacement 82, 84
  'erosion' 146
  eversion 146, 177
  incompetent 188
  induction of labour 384, 385,
      389
  infection, puerperal (cervicitis)
      372
  laceration 362
  mucus 4
    plug 82
  oedema 178
  postpartum 131
  'ripening' 82
  'score' 390
child abuse 136
childbirth:
  actively managed 119
  conventional 119
  prepared, participatory 117
chignon 402
chorioadenoma destruens *see*
      trophoblastic disease
choriocarcinoma *see* trophoblastic
      disease
chorion:
  biopsy 56
  development 11
  frondosum 11
  infection of 273
  laeve 11
  villus sampling 56
chromosomes:
  anomalies in abortion 181
  fetal malformations, in 443
  sex-linked disorders 444
  translocation 444
  trisomy 444

chronic hypertension *see* essential
      hypertension
circulation, maternal, changes in
      pregnancy 37–9
circumcision 447
cleft palate 447
cleidotomy 414
clubfoot 446
coagulation defects 191, 203, 209,
      214
coelom, extraembryonic 8
colostrum 137
compound presentation 314
congenital malformations 440–449
  adrenal hyperplasia 448
  aminoacid disorders 449
  anencephaly 326, 444
  antenatal detection of 56, 66–7,
      454
  anus, imperforate 447
  cardiac defects 447
  chromosomal, due to 443
  cleft palate 447
  congenital hypothyroidism 448
  cystic fibrosis 448
  diabetes mellitus 246
  diagnosis:
    by amniocentesis 57
    by chorionic villus sampling 56
    by ultrasound 59
  Down's syndrome 443–4
  drugs 442–3
  duodenal stenosis 447
  ectopia vesicae 447
  exomphalos 447
  galactosaemia, 448
  hare-lip 447
  heart disease, congenital 447
  hip, congenital dislocation 446
  hydrocephaly 324, 445
  incidence 442
  iniencephaly 324
  kidneys, agenesis 447
  meningocele 445
  metabolism, inborn errors 448
  mongolism *see* Down's syndrome
  neural tube defects 444–5
  prevention by vitamins 58
  oesophageal atresia 447
  phenylketonuria 448
  pyloric stenosis 447
  recurrence of 449
  rubella and 249
  screening, prenatal 56–9
  spina bifida 445
  talipes calcaneus and equinovarus
      446
constipation 173
constriction ring 349
consumption coagulopathy 203

contraception:
  barrier methods 149
  breastfeeding 143
  hormonal 147
    oral 147–8
    injection 148
  intra-uterine device 149
  periodic abstinence 149
  permanent methods 149
  progestogen 148
contractions *see* uterus,
      contractions
Coombs' test 259
cord *see* umbilical cord
corona radiata 3
corpus luteum 3
cotyledon, fetal 12
Couvelaire uterus 202
cramps, leg 173
craniotomy 413
Credé's expression of placenta 353
crowning 108
curtailed pregnancy 269
cystitis 223
cystocele *see* prolapse
cystic fibrosis 448
cytomegalovirus infection 250
cytotrophoblast, formation 11

deafness, rubella 249
decapitation 412
decidua 7
dehydration fever 439
delivery:
  date expected 61
  fetus:
    head of 108
    shoulders of 108
dental care 70
depression 135
destructive operations on fetus:
  cleidotomy 414
  craniotomy 413
  decapitation 412
  evisceration 414
diabetes mellitus 240
  carbohydrate metabolism 240
  classification 241
  congenital malformations 243
  diagnosis 241
  management 243–6
  newborn, management 246
diet:
  daily allowance 54
  in diabetes 244
  in pregnancy 54
disproportion, cephalopelvic 329–38
disseminated intravascular
      coagulation 203, 209
Döderlein bacillus 179

# THE DEFEAT OF COLLECTIVE SECURITY, 1932–33

*I regard neutrality as the greatest gift that
God has put in the hands of the American
people.*

EDWIN BORCHARD, March 28, 1933

On the evening of September 18, 1931, Japan announced that a group of Chinese soldiers had exploded a bomb on the South Manchurian Railway a few miles north of Mukden. The Japanese army quickly began to occupy the line of the railway and then gradually spread out into the remainder of Manchuria. Though at first foreign observers believed this was only another in a series of minor skirmishes between Japan and China in Manchuria, the Mukden incident soon developed into the most serious international crisis since World War I, challenging the fragile structure of collective security embodied in the League of Nations and the Kellogg-Briand Pact.[1]

For the United States, the abstract question of American neutrality toward aggression became a real and pressing issue. President Herbert Hoover, deeply concerned about the depression which had steadily worsened since 1929, quickly made his decision —facing catastrophe at home, the nation must avoid any risk of entanglement in foreign war. But Secretary of State Stimson, a

[1] Robert H. Ferrell, *American Diplomacy in the Great Depression* (New Haven, 1957), pp. 122–24.

23

dedicated advocate of collective security, was equally determined to use American influence and prestige to curb Japan's aggression in Manchuria. Throughout the remainder of the Hoover administration, these two leaders disagreed on the role the United States should play in the Far Eastern crisis, and though they finally compromised on the principle of non-recognition, this moralistic formula only disguised their fundamental divergence on American policy toward aggression overseas.[2]

## I

In the fall of 1931, before the extent of the Manchurian crisis became known, the United States followed a very cautious policy. Stimson, believing that moderate elements in the Japanese government could restrain the army, refrained from sending strong protests to Japan. In October, the United States did begin to cooperate with the League, dispatching Prentiss Gilbert, an American consular officer at Geneva, and later Charles G. Dawes, the ambassador to Britain, to attend meetings of the League Council. Stimson realized that economic sanctions would be the only effective action the League could undertake against Japan, and in late October he suggested to Hoover that the United States should cooperate with the League by refusing to interfere with any economic measures directed against a violator of the Kellogg pact. Though Hoover firmly denounced military and economic sanctions as "roads to war," on November 19 Stimson informed Dawes that while the United States could not participate in any embargo of Japan, "we would not probably in any way interfere through our fleet with any embargo by anybody else."[3] This suggestion of a limited surrender of traditional neutral rights evidently had little

[2] Richard Current, Secretary Stimson: A Study in Statecraft (New Brunswick, N.J., 1954), p. 113.

[3] Henry L. Stimson and McGeorge Bundy, On Active Service in Peace and War (New York, 1947), p. 233; Current, Secretary Stimson, pp. 80–81; Papers Relating to the Foreign Relations of the United States: 1931 (Washington, 1946), III, 496. Hereafter cited as "FR."